Essentials of
HAEMATOLOGY

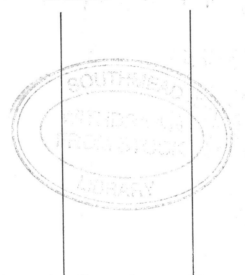

Essentials of
HAEMATOLOGY

SECOND EDITION

Shirish M Kawthalkar MD (Pathology)
Associate Professor
Department of Pathology
Government Medical College
Nagpur, Maharashtra, India

JAYPEE BROTHERS MEDICAL PUBLISHERS (P) LTD

New Delhi • Panama City • London • Dhaka • Kathmandu

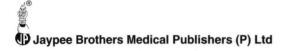

Jaypee Brothers Medical Publishers (P) Ltd

Headquarters

Jaypee Brothers Medical Publishers (P) Ltd
4838/24, Ansari Road, Daryaganj
New Delhi 110 002, India
Phone: +91-11-43574357
Fax: +91-11-43574314
Email: jaypee@jaypeebrothers.com

Overseas Offices

J.P. Medical Ltd
83 Victoria Street, London
SW1H 0HW (UK)
Phone: +44-2031708910
Fax: +02-03-0086180
Email: info@jpmedpub.com

Jaypee-Highlights Medical Publishers Inc.
City of Knowledge, Bld. 237, Clayton
Panama City, Panama
Phone: +507-301-0496
Fax: +507-301-0499
Email: cservice@jphmedical.com

Jaypee Brothers Medical Publishers (P) Ltd
17/1-B Babar Road, Block-B, Shaymali
Mohammadpur, Dhaka-1207
Bangladesh
Mobile: +08801912003485
Email: jaypeedhaka@gmail.com

Jaypee Brothers Medical Publishers (P) Ltd
Shorakhute, Kathmandu
Nepal
Phone: +00977-9841528578
Email: jaypee.nepal@gmail.com

Website: www.jaypeebrothers.com
Website: www.jaypeedigital.com

Inquiries for bulk sales may be solicited at: jaypee@jaypeebrothers.com

This book has been published in good faith that the contents provided by the author contained herein are original, and is intended for educational purposes only. While every effort is made to ensure accuracy of information, the publisher and the author specifically disclaim any damage, liability, or loss incurred, directly or indirectly, from the use or application of any of the contents of this work. If not specifically stated, all figures and tables are courtesy of the author. Where appropriate, the readers should consult with a specialist or contact the manufacturer of the drug or device.

Essentials of Haematology

First Edition: 2006
Second Edition: 2013

ISBN 978-93-5090-184-7

Printed at Sanat Printers, Kundli.

Preface to the Second Edition

The second edition of *Essentials of Haematology* has become necessary because of continuous, fast-paced expansion of knowledge in laboratory techniques, immunology, molecular biology, and genetics that has directly affected the speciality of haematology. The task of preparing second edition was difficult as it was also important to maintain the concise and illustrated format of the book. I have tried to retain the basic intention of the book, i.e. to present haematology and blood transfusion in a concise and simplified manner which is mainly aimed at undergraduate students (MBBS) and residents of pathology and medicine. As stated in the preface of the earlier edition, the publication is not intended to be an all-inclusive textbook but rather a simplified and up-to-date introduction to haematology. I have not incorporated any new chapters but rather incorporated new and essential information in almost all chapters which is of significance and relevance in pathogenesis, diagnosis, and management of blood disorders.

In this edition, almost all the figures and illustrations have been maintained as in previous edition and many have been added and where required suitable modifications have been made in the text. Depiction of many figures is diagrammatic for easier understanding as actual images are somewhat difficult to understand at basic level of learning, especially figures of blood cells, genetics, and flow cytometry. I take full responsibility for any errors of omission and commission that may have occurred. All suggestions and constructive criticism are most welcome.

After many years of working and teaching in the field of haematology, I feel that there often appears to be a misconception among students that blood tests are all that is required for a haematological disease to be diagnosed. Understanding haematology requires knowledge of physiology, insight into pathogenesis and essential pathological processes, laboratory tests (with their limitations and strengths), and clinical medicine. For diagnosis of a haematological disease, integration of clinical examination findings and haematological tests is necessary and final evaluation and judgement has to come from co-ordination between the pathologist and the clinician. *Essentials of Haematology* is an effort to make understanding of haematology easier so that it will facilitate learning by students and help them solve haematological problems in their clinical practice.

I am thankful to Dr RM Powar, Dean, Government Medical College and Hospital, Nagpur and Dr DT Kumbhalkar, Professor and Head, Department of Pathology, Government Medical College, Nagpur, Maharashtra, India for their encouragement and valuable guidance.

I am eternally indebted to my parents for their constant encouragement, guidance, and blessings. It is not possible to express in words my feelings for the unwavering and inspirational support and patience of my wife Dr Anjali, a gynaecologist and of my children Ameya and Ashish.

I am indebted to Shri Jitendar P Vij (Group Chairman), Mr Ankit Vij (Managing Director) and Mr Tarun Duneja (Director-Publishing) of M/s Jaypee Brothers Medical Publishers (P) Ltd, New Delhi, India and his expert staff for excellent presentation of this book.

Shirish M Kawthalkar

Preface to the First Edition

This book is an attempt to present haematology and blood transfusion in a concise and simplified manner and is primarily intended for undergraduate students (second and final year MBBS and BDS). At the same time, it will also be useful for postgraduate students of pathology, medicine, paediatrics, and obstetrics and gynaecology. One comes across a haematological problem frequently in all branches of medicine. Haematology and blood transfusion are closely related, and blood bank forms an integral and life-saving support system of a multidisciplinary hospital. A concise textbook of haematology and blood transfusion is needed for undergraduates who have to take on major subjects during their MBBS years. The coverage of haematology in available books is either too extensive or too short for their requirements. I have tried to strike a balance based on my experience in teaching and in diagnostic haematology.

This book was published in 1998 as *Essentials of Haematology and Blood Transfusion*. Changes are constantly occurring in haematology especially in molecular diagnostics, classification, and treatment of malignant disorders. I have tried to update each chapter to ensure that current knowledge and practices are reflected. Laboratory investigations play a major role in proper diagnosis and management of blood diseases. Therefore, laboratory aspects have been given relatively more coverage. As the scope of this book is limited, it has not been possible to give treatment of blood disorders in detail, especially dosages and drug schedules.

During preparation of this book help has been taken from various well-known textbooks and numerous journals that have been duly acknowledged at the end of each chapter. Figures of blood and bone marrow cells have been presented in a manner that highlights the important morphological details and helps in better understanding. Undoubtedly, there will be errors of omission and commission for which I take the full responsibility. Suggestions and constructive criticism are most welcome.

I am indebted to my parents for their constant support, value-based guidance, and blessings that I have received throughout my life. The friendship, love, care, and support of my wife Anjali, herself a gynaecologist, can never be adequately acknowledged and my children Ameya and Ashish, have made everything in life meaningful, worthwhile, and enjoyable.

I am thankful to Dr (Mrs) VS Dani, Dean, Government Medical College, Nagpur and Dr SK Bobhate, Professor and Head, Department of Pathology, Government Medical College, Nagpur, Maharashtra, India for their valuable guidance. I express my appreciation and gratitude to M/s Jaypee Brothers Medical Publishers (P) Ltd, New Delhi, India for their sensible and valuable advice during publication of this book and also for bringing out the book in an excellent, easy-to-read format.

Shirish M Kawthalkar

Contents

SECTION 3: DISORDERS OF WHITE BLOOD CELLS

SECTION 4: DISORDERS OF HAEMOSTASIS

SECTION 5: BLOOD TRANSFUSION

CHAPTER

1

Overview of Physiology of Blood

❑ NORMAL HAEMATOPOIESIS

The physiologic process of formation of blood cells is known as haematopoiesis. It proceeds through different stages starting from early embryonic life—mesoblastic stage (yolk sac), hepatic stage, and myeloid (bone marrow) stage. During embryonic and early foetal life, haematopoiesis occurs in the yolk sac (only erythoblasts) and the liver (all blood cells). Blood cell precursors first appear in yolk sac during third week of embryonic development. Definitive haematopoiesis, however, first begins in the mesoderm of intraembryonic aorta/gonad/mesonephros (AGM) region after several weeks. Some blood cell formation also occurs in the spleen (all blood cells), lymph nodes and thymus (mostly lymphocytes). Bone marrow starts producing blood cells around 3rd to 4th month and by birth becomes the exclusive site of blood cell formation (Fig. 1.1). In younger age, whole of the skeletal marrow participates in blood cell production. By late childhood, haematopoiesis becomes restricted to the flat bones such as sternum, ribs, iliac bones and vertebrae and proximal ends of long bones. At other skeletal sites haematopoietic areas are replaced by fat cells. However, when there is increased demand for blood cell production, conversion of yellow fatty inactive marrow to red active marrow can occur. In extremely severe case s (e.g. severe chronic anaemia), resumption of haematopoietic activity in organs other than bone marrow such as liver and spleen (extramedullary haematopoiesis) can occur.

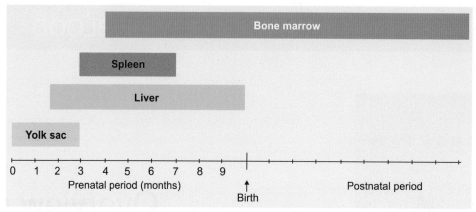

Figure 1.1: Stages of haematopoiesis

Hierarchy of Haematopoiesis

The scheme of haematopoiesis is shown in Figure 1.2. All blood cells are derived from pleuripotent haematopoietic stem cells, which are present in small numbers in the bone marrow. The haematopoietic stem cell is the most primitive cell in the bone marrow. It has the ability of proliferation, self-renewal, and differentiation along several lineages. The capacity of self-renewal permits life-long continuation of the process. The myeloid and lymphoid stem cells originate from the pleuripotent haematopoietic stem cell. From myeloid and lymphoid stem cells progressively more committed progenitors arise having progressively restricted potential to generate different types of blood cells. Ultimately progenitor cells committed to produce only a single type of cell are derived. These single-lineage progenitors further differentiate to produce morphologically identifiable blood cells (Fig. 1.3). Red cells, granulocytes, monocytes, and platelets are derived from myeloid stem cell while B and T lymphocytes are formed from lymphoid stem cell through intermediate stages.

The factors, which influence the commitment of stem cells and progenitor cells to different lineages, are unknown; the bone marrow microenvironment and responsiveness of progenitors to haematopoietic growth factors appear to play a role.

Haematopoietic Growth Factors (HGFs)

HGFs are a group of proteins that (i) regulate proliferation, differentiation, and maturation of haematopoietic progenitor cells, (ii) influence the commitment of progenitors to specific lineages, and (iii) affect the function and survival of mature blood cells. HGFs are produced by different types of cells, which include T lymphocytes, macrophages, fibroblasts, endothelial cells, and renal interstitial cells (Fig. 1.4 and Table 1.1).

HGFs may bind to specific cell receptors on the surface of the cells to directly induce their proliferation and differentiation or may stimulate the production of other cytokines that then act on the target cells. Two types of HGFs may be distinguished — multilineage

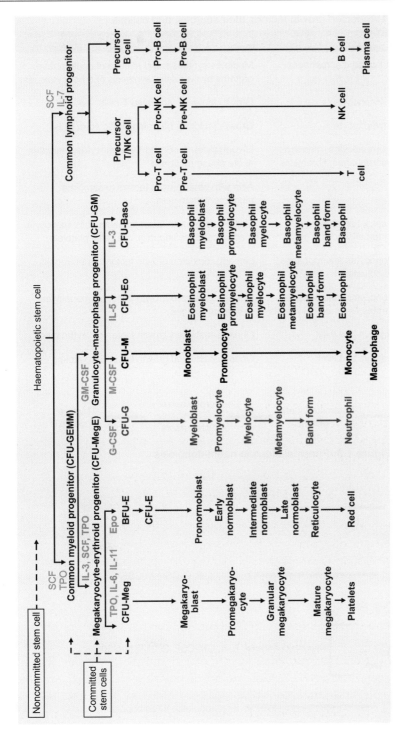

Figure 1.2: Normal haematopoiesis

Abbreviations: SCF: Stem cell factor; TPO: Thrombopoietin; IL: Interleukin; EPO: Erythropoietin; G-CSF: Granulocyte colony stimulating factor; GM-CSF: Granulocyte-macrophage colony stimulating factor; M-CSF: Macrophage colony stimulating factor; CFU-GEMM: Colony-forming unit-Granulocyte Erythroid Megakaryocyte Macrophage; CFU-GM: Colony forming unit-Granulocyte Macrophage; CFU-MegE: Colony forming unit-Megakaryocyte Erythroid; BFU-E: Burst forming unit-Erythroid; CFU-E: Colony forming unit-Erythroid; CFU-G: Colony forming unit-Granulocyte; CFU-M: Colony forming unit-Macrophage; CFU-Eo: Colony forming unit-Eosinophil; CFU-Baso: Colony forming unit-Basophil; NK: Natural killer.

Table 1.1: Selected growth factors, their sources, and actions

Growth factor	Source	Action
1. Interleukin-1 (IL-1)	Activated macrophages	Mediates synthesis and release of acute phase proteins by liver cells; synthesis of other cytokines
2. Interleukin-2 (IL-2)	T lymphocyte	Growth factor for activated T cells
3. Interleukin-3 (IL-3)	T lymphocyte	Growth factor for haematopoietic stem cells
4. Interleukin-6 (IL-6)	T lymphocytes, monocytes/ macrophages, fibroblasts	Growth factor for B and T lymphocytes; mediates acute phase response
5. C-kit ligand (stem cell factor)		Acts with other growth factors to stimulate pluripotent stem cells
6. GM-CSF	T cells, fibroblasts, endothelial cells	Multilineage growth factor for neutrophils, monocyte/ macrophage, eosinophils, red cells, platelets
7. G-CSF	Monocytes/macrophages, fibroblasts	Lineage-restricted growth factor for neutrophils
8. M-CSF	Monocytes/macrophages, fibroblasts, endothelial cells	Lineage-restricted growth factor for monocytes and macrophages
9. Erythropoietin	Kidneys and liver	Lineage-restricted growth factor for erythrocytes
10. Thrombopoietin	Kidneys and liver	Lineage-restricted growth factor for platelets

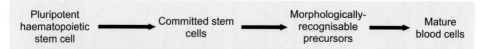

Figure 1.3: Principal steps in haematopoiesis

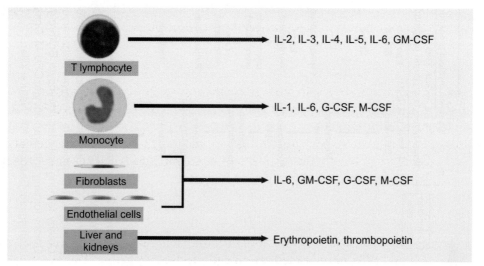

Figure 1.4: Selected HGFs and their sources

HGFs that have action on more than one cell line and lineage-restricted HGFs that act on one specific cell line. Examples of multilineage HGFs are GM-CSF (granulocyte macrophage colony stimulating factor) and IL-3 (interleukin-3) while lineage-restricted HGFs are erythropoietin, G-CSF (granulocyte colony stimulating factor), and M-CSF (macrophage colony stimulating factor). For proliferation and differentiation of myeloid progenitors, either GM-GSF or IL-3 and a lineage-specific cytokine (erythropoietin, G-CSF, or M-CSF) are required.

Many of the HGFs have been produced by the recombinant DNA technology and are undergoing clinical trials in various disorders. Recently, recombinant GM-CSF, G-CSF and erythropoietin have been approved for clinical use in certain conditions in USA.

GM-CSF

1. GM-CSF stimulates proliferation, differentiation, and maturation of lineages committed to neutrophil and monocyte/macrophage cell lines (CFU-GEMM and CFU-GM) and also enhances the functional activity of mature neutrophils and monocytes.
2. Recombinant GM-CSF is used to enhance the myeloid recovery following autologous bone marrow transplantation in non-myeloid malignancies. It is also being used to increase stem cell harvest from peripheral blood in peripheral blood stem cell transplantation. It is being tried in chemotherapy-induced myelosuppression and in myelodysplastic syndrome with neutropaenia.

G-CSF

1. G-CSF stimulates myeloid progenitor cells (CFU-G) to form mature neutrophils.
2. Recombinant G-CSF is used to reduce duration and severity of neutropaenia in non-myeloid malignancies that are being treated with myelosuppressive chemotherapy and in autologous bone marrow transplantation.

Erythropoietin

1. Erythropoietin is a glycoprotein produced in the kidneys (90%) and in the liver (10%). It stimulates progenitor cells committed to erythroid lineage (CFU-E and BFU-E) to proliferate and differentiate.
2. It is indicated in patients with anaemia of chronic renal failure who are on dialysis. It is also being tried in zidovudine-treated human immunodeficiency virus-positive patients having anaemia, and in anaemia of cancer.

The Haematopoietic Microenvironment

The existence of haematopoietic microenvironment is suggested by the fact that formation of blood cells is restricted specifically to bone marrow. The exact nature of the microenvironment is poorly understood; however it appears to be composed

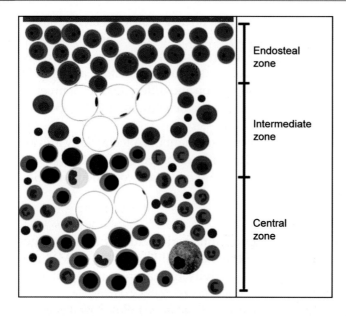

Endosteal zone

Intermediate zone

Central zone

Figure 1.5: Bone marrow organisation. Bone marrow is located in the intertrabecular space beneath the cortex. Organisation of various cells in the normal bone marrow is characteristic. (1) Endosteal zone: myeloid precursors (myeloblasts, promyelocytes); (2) Intermediate zone: myelocytes, erythroid islands; (3) Central zone: metamyelocytes, bands, segmented neutrophils, erythroid islands, and megakaryocytes

of endothelial cells, fibroblasts, adipocytes, macrophages, and extracellular matrix. Bone marrow microenvironment provides supporting stroma and growth factors for haematopoiesis. Stem cells and progenitors are bound to the stromal cells or to adhesion molecules within the matrix. Release of mature blood cells from the marrow is regulated by the microenvironment.

Organisation of bone marrow: Organisation of normal bone marrow is shown in Figure 1.5.

❑ RED BLOOD CELLS

Stages of Erythropoiesis

Within the bone marrow, erythroid cells are arranged in the form of islands (Fig. 1.6). The earliest morphologically identifiable erythroid cell in the bone marrow is the **proerythroblast** (pronormoblast), a large (15–20 μm) cell with a fine, uniform chromatin pattern, one or more nucleoli, and dark blue cytoplasm.

The next cell in the maturation process is the **basophilic (early) normoblast**. This cell is smaller in size (12–16 μm) and has a coarser nuclear chromatin with barely visible nucleoli. The cytoplasm is deeply basophilic.

The more differentiated erythroid cell is the **polychromatic (intermediate) normoblast** (size 12–15 μm). The nuclear size is smaller and the chromatin becomes clumped. Polychromasia of cytoplasm results from admixture of blue ribonucleic acid and pink haemoglobin. This is the last erythroid precursor capable of mitotic division.

The orthochromatic (late) normoblast is 8 to 12 μm in size. The nucleus is small, dense and pyknotic and commonly eccentrically-located. The cytoplasm stains mostly pink due to haemoglobinisation. It is called as orthochromatic because cytoplasmic staining is largely similar to that of erythrocytes. The nucleus is ultimately expelled from the orthochromatic normoblast with the formation of a reticulocyte. The reticulocyte still has remnants of ribosomal RNA in the form of a cytoplasmic reticulum. After 1 to 2 days in the bone marrow and 1 to 2 days in peripheral blood reticulocytes lose RNA and become mature pink-staining erythrocytes (Figs 1.7 and 1.8).

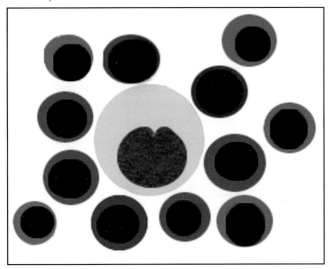

Figure 1.6: Erythroid island: Within the bone marrow, erythroid progenitors are found in the form of 'islands' (erythroid colonies). An erythroid island is composed of erythroblasts surrounding a central macrophage. The more immature precursors are present close to the macrophage and maturing forms are towards the periphery. The macrophage has dendritic processes which extend between erythroid progenitors, support them, and supply iron for haemoglobin synthesis

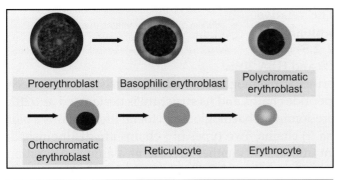

Figure 1.7: Stages in the formation of a mature red cell. With each stage, cell size and nuclear size become smaller, chromatin clumping increases, and ultimately nucleus is extruded. Colour of cytoplasm gradually changes from basophilic to orange-red

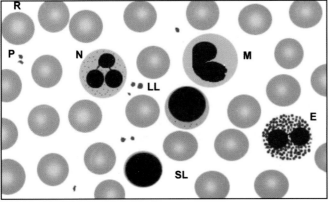

Figure 1.8: Normal peripheral blood smear showing normocytic normochromic—red cells (R), neutrophil (N), eosinophil (E), monocyte (M), small lymphocyte (SL), large lymphocyte (LL), and platelets (P)

About four mitotic divisions and continued differentiation lead to the production of 16 mature erythrocytes from each pronormoblast.

Structure and Function of Erythrocytes

Mature erythrocyte is a round biconcave disc about 7 to 8 μm in diameter. Basic structural properties of various red cell components (haemoglobin, enzymes, and membrane) are outlined below.

Haemoglobin

Haemoglobin is responsible for transport of oxygen from lungs to the tissues and of carbon dioxide from tissues to the lungs. Haemoglobin (MW 64,500 daltons) is composed of haem (consisting of iron and protoporphyrin) and globin. The globin portion of the molecule consists of four (or two pairs of) polypeptide chains. One haem group is bound to each polypeptide chain.

Variants of haemoglobin: Haemoglobin is not homogeneous and normally different variants exist such as A, A2, F, Gower I, Gower II, and Portland (Box 1.1). The last three are present only during embryonic life. Others are present in varying proportions during foetal and adult life. **The relative proportions of different haemoglobins are: Adults—HbA 97%, HbA2 2.5%, and HbF 0.5%; Newborns—HbF 80% and HbA 20%.**

Box 1.1   Normal haemoglobin variants
• Hb Gower I: $\zeta 2 \varepsilon 2$
• Hb Gower II: $\alpha 2 \varepsilon 2$
• Hb Portland: $\zeta 2 \gamma 2$
The above three haemoglobins are embryonic haemoglobins
• HbF: $\alpha 2 \gamma 2$: Predominates in foetal life
• HbA: $\alpha 2 \beta 2$: Predominates in adult life
• HbA2: $\alpha 2 \delta 2$

Haemoglobin A (HbA), the principle haemoglobin of adults, consists of a pair each of alpha (α) and of beta (β) polypeptide chains and its structure is designated as $\alpha 2\beta 2$. Foetal haemoglobin (HbF), the predominant haemoglobin in foetal life, contains a pair of alpha (α) and a pair of gamma (γ) chains. Two types of γ chains are distinguished, Gγ and Aγ, which have different amino acids (either glycine or alanine) at position 136. Thus, HbF is heterogeneous and contains $\alpha 2 \gamma 2$ 136Gly and $\alpha 2 \gamma 2$ 136Ala. During embryonic life, there are three haemoglobins: Gower I ($\zeta 2 \varepsilon 2$), Gower II ($\alpha 2 \varepsilon 2$) and Portland ($\zeta 2 \gamma 2$). With foetal development, synthesis of zeta (ζ) and epsilon (ε) chains is replaced by that of α and γ chains, respectively. After birth, production of γ chains switches to that of β and delta (δ) chains.

Structure of globin genes: Normal haemoglobin is a tetramer composed of a pair of α-like and a pair of β-like polypeptide chains. Each chain is linked to one molecule of haem. The α-like polypeptide chains (ζ and α) and β-like polypeptide chains (ε, γ, β, and δ) are encoded by α- and β-globin gene clusters on chromosomes 16 and 11, respectively. The order of genes in α-globin gene cluster from 5′ to 3′ end is ζ-ψζ-ψα2-ψα1-α2-α1. The order of genes in β-globin gene cluster from 5′ to 3′ end is ε-Gγ-Aγ-ψβ-δ-β (Fig. 1.9). The

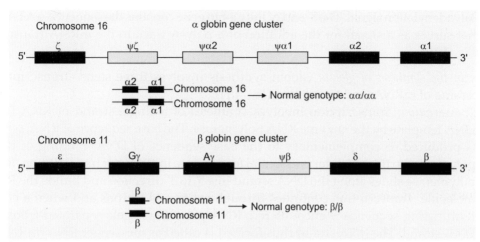

Figure 1.9: α and β globin gene clusters. Open boxes represent pseudogenes while filled boxes represent active genes. Normal genotype is shown below each gene cluster

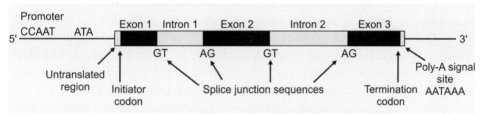

Figure 1.10: A schematic diagram of β globin gene

ψζ, ψα2, ψα1, and ψβ are pseudogenes. A pseudogene (ψ) contains sequences similar to a functional gene but is rendered inactive due to mutation during evolutionary process.

In humans, autosomal chromosomes occur in pairs. As each member of chromosome 16 has two α gene loci (a locus refers to specific physical position of a gene on chromosome), there are total four α genes. However, there is only one β globin gene locus on chromosome 11, and therefore β genes are two in number.

Genes are the base sequences, which are present along the DNA strands and are necessary for the formation of a protein. The different functional areas of a globin gene are:

1. Exons and introns: The regions of DNA strand which encode amino acids in the protein product are known as exons while non-coding regions which interrupt the coding sequences are known as introns or intervening sequences. Each globin gene contains three exons and two introns.

2. Splice junction sequences: These are sequences at the junction of exons and introns and are required for precise splicing (or removal) of introns during the formation of mRNA.

3. Promoter: The promoter region is present towards 5′ end of the gene and contains sequences to which the RNA polymerase binds; it is necessary for correct initiation of transcription. Two promoter sequences are TATA and CCAAT.

4. Polyadenylation signal: The 3′ end of the globin gene contains the sequence AATAAA that serves as a signal for the addition of a poly-A track to the mRNA transcript (Fig. 1.10).

Steps in the synthesis of globin: Globin synthesis involves three steps—transcription, processing of mRNA, and translation (Fig. 1.11).

   i. *Transcription:* Transcription involves synthesis of a single strand of RNA from DNA template by the enzyme RNA polymerase. The base sequence of RNA, which is produced, is complementary to the base sequence of DNA. Binding of RNA polymerase to the promoter is essential for accurate initiation of transcription. RNA polymerase slides along the DNA strand in a 5′ to 3′ direction and builds the RNA molecule. Transcription continues through exons and introns and when a chain terminating sequence is encountered, RNA polymerase gets separated from the DNA strand. The RNA strand thus formed is called as messenger RNA (mRNA).

   ii. *Processing of mRNA:* In the next stage, mRNA molecule is processed by addition of a cap structure and a poly-A tail and by removal of introns. A cap structure (modified nucleotides) is added at the 5′ end of mRNA; though the exact role is unknown, capping appears to be necessary for initiation of translation. At the 3′ end a poly-A tail consisting of about 150 adenylic acid residues is added. AAUAAA sequence at the 3′ end signals the addition of poly-A tail about 20 bases downstream from the polyadenylation site. Polyadenylation is required for stability of the transcript and its transport to the cytoplasm. Excision of

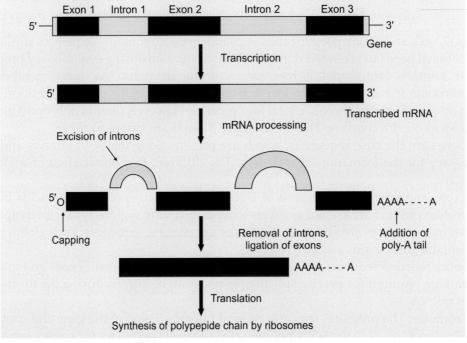

Figure 1.11: Globin chain synthesis

introns and joining together of exons in the mRNA transcript are essential before mRNA is transported from the nucleus to the cytoplasm. Accurate splicing is guided by the presence of GT dinucleotide at the exon-intron boundary (5′ end of intron) and AG dinucleotide at the intron-exon boundary (3′ end of intron). Intron 1 is excised before intron 2. During splicing, excision at 5′ exon-intron boundary occurs initially with the formation of 'lariat' structures; subsequently excision at the 3′ intron-exon boundary occurs followed by joining of exons.

iii. *Translation:* This process, which occurs on ribosomes, consists of synthesis of a polypeptide chain according to the directions provided by the mRNA template. There are three kinds of RNA which take part in the synthesis of polypeptides— messenger RNA (mRNA), transfer RNA (tRNA) and ribosomal RNA (rRNA). The mRNA, transcribed from the DNA template, carries the genetic code from the nucleus to the cytoplasm and determines the sequence of amino acids in the formation of a polypeptide. The tRNA transports specific amino acids from the cytoplasm to the specific locations (codons) along the mRNA strand; each tRNA binds and transports a specific amino acid. The rRNA, along with certain structural proteins, constitutes the ribosome which serves as a site for protein synthesis.

The different steps of protein synthesis (translation) are activation, initiation, elongation, and termination. In activation, an amino acid combines with its specific tRNA molecule in the cytoplasm; such tRNA is called as activated or charged tRNA. Translation always begins at a codon that specifies methionine (AUG, the initiator codon). The process of translation is initiated when a methionine-bearing specific tRNA binds with initiator codon in mRNA. Elongation of polypeptide chain occurs when successive amino acids are added after methionine according to the pattern provided by the genetic code. During this process, movement of ribosomes occurs along the mRNA strand and ribosome slides to the next codon when an amino acid specified by preceding codon is added to the growing polypeptide chain. Amino acids are attached to each other by peptide bonds. Termination of translation occurs when a chain-terminating (or a stop) codon is encountered (UAA, UAG, or UGA). This is followed by release of the completed polypeptide chain from the ribosomes.

The primary polypeptide chain is then organised into a secondary and a tertiary structure from interactions in its amino acids. One molecule of haem is attached to each polypeptide chain. Two different pairs of polypeptide chains with their attached haem moieties associate with each other to form a tetrameric haemoglobin molecule.

Changes in globin gene expression during development (Globin 'switching'): Hb Gower I, Hb Gower II, and Hb Portland are the predominant haemoglobins during embryonic life (upto 12 weeks). HbF (α2γ2) is the major haemoglobin of foetal life; it starts gradually declining after 36 weeks of gestation and constitutes less than 1% of haemoglobin in adults. Beta (β) chain synthesis starts around 10th week of gestation and is significantly augmented around the time of birth. HbA (α2β2) gradually becomes the predominant haemoglobin by 3 to 4 months of age. Delta (δ) globin gene is expressed late in the third trimester but HbA2 (α2δ2) remains at a low level (about 2.5%) in adults.

The developmental changes in the expression of the globin genes can be correlated with the time of appearance of clinical features in haemoglobinopathies. Thus, α-thalassaemia manifests at birth while clinical features of β-thalassaemia appear a few months after birth.

Biosynthesis of haem: Haem is a complex of protoporphyrin and iron. Biosynthesis of haem requires mitochondrial (as well as cytosolic) enzymes and therefore only erythroid precursors but not mature red cells can synthesize haem.

Structure and function of haemoglobin: Haemoglobin is a tetramer composed of four polypeptide chains (α1, α2, β1, and β2) and four haem groups. α chain consists of 141 amino acids while β chain has 146 amino acids. Each polypeptide chain is arranged in a helical conformation. There are eight helical segments designated A to H. Iron of haem is covalently bound to histidine at the eighth position of the F helical segment. Charged or polar residues are arranged on the outer surface while the uncharged or nonpolar residues are arranged towards the inner part of the molecule. Haem is suspended in a 'pocket' formed by the folding of the polypeptide chain and residues in contact with haem are nonpolar. The four polypeptide chains make contact at α1β1 and α1β2 interfaces. The former is a stabilizing contact while the latter is the functional contact across which movement of chains occurs during oxygenation and deoxygenation.

The function of haemoglobin is transport of oxygen from the lungs to the tissues. As partial pressure of oxygen increases, haemoglobin shows progressively increasing affinity for oxygen. When first oxygen binds to the haem group, it successively increases the oxygen affinity of the remaining three haem groups. When the percent saturation of haemoglobin with oxygen is plotted against the partial pressure of oxygen, a sigmoid-shaped oxygen dissociation curve is obtained. Small changes in oxygen tension allow significant amount of oxygen to be released or bound.

Factors affecting oxygen affinity of haemoglobin are pH, temperature, intraerythrocyte level of 2,3-diphosphoglycerate (2,3-DPG) and presence of haemoglobin variants. The Bohr effect refers to the alteration in oxygen affinity due to alteration in pH. Low pH (e.g. in tissues) reduces the oxygen affinity while higher pH (e.g. in lungs) increases the oxygen affinity of haemoglobin. High temperature reduces the oxygen affinity while low temperature increases the oxygen affinity. 2,3-DPG binds to deoxy-haemoglobin with considerably more affinity than to oxyhaemoglobin and stabilizes the deoxyhaemoglobin state. Low levels of 2,3-DPG in red cells in stored blood in blood bank are associated with reduced release of oxygen after blood transfusion. Haemoglobin variants with high oxygen affinity are methaemoglobin, Hb Bart's, and Hb H.

Red Cell Enzymes

The mature red cell requires energy to preserve the integrity of the cell membrane, for active transport of cations, for nucleotide salvage, and for synthesis of glutathione. This is mostly provided by glycolysis (Embden-Meyerhof pathway). In this metabolic pathway, glucose is converted to pyruvate and lactate through a series of enzymatic reactions with generation of ATP (Fig. 1.12). In the middle of the glycolytic pathway, a Rapoport-Luebering shunt exists in red cells for the synthesis of 2,3-DPG. The net yield of ATP from glycolysis is dependent upon the amount of glucose utilised by this shunt. 2,3-DPG is an important determinant of the oxygen affinity of haemoglobin. Apart from ATP and 2,3-DPG, another important product of glycolysis is NADH that is required for reduction of methaemoglobin to oxyhaemoglobin.

The aerobic hexose monophosphate shunt (pentose phosphate shunt) is another metabolic pathway in red cells. The two dehydrogenase enzymes, glucose-6-phosphate

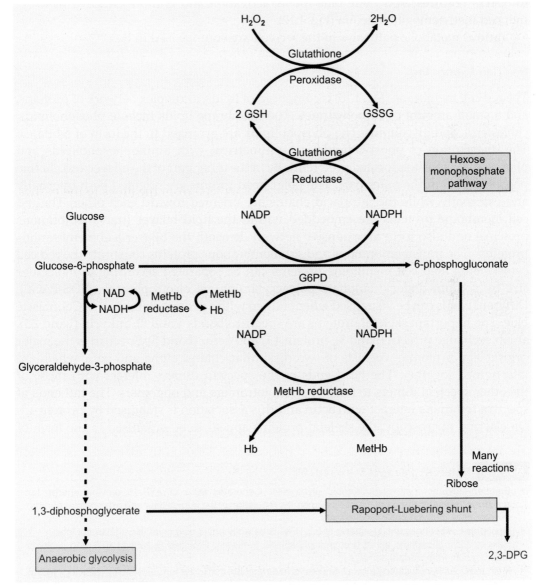

Figure 1.12: Metabolic pathways in red cell. For simplicity, only some of the steps are shown

dehydrogenase (G6PD) and 6-phosphogluconate dehydrogenase (6-PGD), cyclically generate NADPH from NADP. These two enzymes also convert glucose-6-phosphate to pentose, which is returned to the main glycolytic pathway. NADPH and the enzyme glutathione reductase are required for the regeneration of reduced glutathione (GSH) from oxidised glutathione (GSSG). GSH along with glutathione peroxidase detoxifies hydrogen peroxide and protects haemoglobin from oxidant damage.

Most of the methaemoglobin produced in the normal cell is reduced to haemoglobin by NAD-linked methaemoglobin reductase. Methaemoglobin reductase that is linked to NADP requires methylene blue for its activation and is more effective in drug-induced methaemoglobinaemia (Fig. 1.12).

Various metabolic pathways in the red cell are summarised in Box 1.2.

Red Cell Membrane

The red cell membrane (Fig. 1.13) is composed of lipids, a complex network of proteins, and a small amount of carbohydrates. The membrane lipids include phospholipids, cholesterol, and glycolipids. The phospholipids are arranged in the form of a bilayer. The distribution of phospholipids is asymmetrical with aminophospholipids and phosphatidyl inositols located preferentially in the inner part of the bilayer and choline phospholipids in the outer part. The polar head groups are oriented both internally and externally while the fatty acid chains are oriented toward each other. The red cell membrane proteins are embedded within the lipid bilayer (transmembranous proteins) and also form an extensive network beneath the bilayer (submembranous proteins). The transmembranous and submembranous proteins constitute the red cell cytoskeleton. Red cell membrane proteins can be separated according to molecular size by sodium dodecyl sulphate polyacrylamide gel electrophoresis (SDS-PAGE). Different bands can be visualised when stained with a protein stain such as Coomassie blue. The important skeletal proteins are spectrin (bands 1 and 2), ankyrin (band 2.1), anion exchange protein (band 3), protein 4.1, and actin (band 5). Spectrin is the major cytoskeletal protein; it consists of two dissimilar chains, alpha and beta, which are intertwined together. The head ends of the spectrin dimers interact with those of the other spectrin dimers to form spectrin tetramers and oligomers. The tail ends of spectrin tetramers interact with actin and this association is stabilised by protein 4.1. On electron microscopy, the skeletal proteins appear to be organised in the form of

---

Box 1.2   Metabolic pathways in the red cell

- Embden-Meyerhof pathway(Anaerobic glycolysis): Generates 90% of ATP to provide energy for reactions like maintenance of membrane integrity, regulation of the intracellular and extracellular pumps, maintenance of hemoglobin function, etc.
- Rapoport-Luebering shunt: Synthesis of 2,3-DPG, a determinant of oxygen affinity of haemoglobin
- Hexose monophosphate shunt (Pentose phosphate pathway): Provides 5–10% of ATP and protects haemoglobin from oxidant damage
- Methaemoglobin reductase pathway: Maintains haemoglobin iron in the ferrous state by reducing NAD to NADH and prevents accumulation of methaemoglobin in red cell.

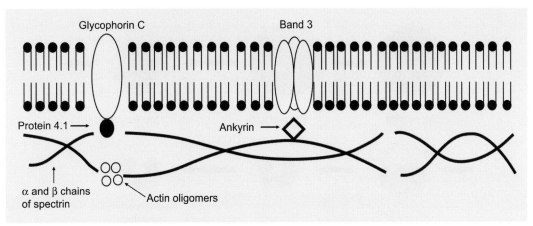

Figure 1.13: Schematic illustration of red cell membrane

a hexagonal lattice; the arms of the hexagon are formed by spectrin and corners by actin, protein 4.1, and adducin. The anchorage of the cytoskeleton to the overlying lipid bilayer is achieved by two associations: band 3-ankyrin-spectrin association and glycophorin C-protein 4.1 association. Band 3 is the anion exchange channel through which the exchange of HCO_3^- and Cl^- occurs.

The membrane provides mechanical strength and flexibility to the red cell to withstand the shearing forces in circulation. The cell membrane also serves to maintain the red cell volume by the cation pump. The cation pump, operated by the membrane enzyme ATPase, regulates the intracellular concentration of Na^+ and K^+. The membrane ATPase also drives the calcium pump, which keeps the intracellular Ca^{++} at a very low level. The red cells exchange HCO_3^- (formed from tissue CO_2) in the lungs with Cl^- through the anion exchange channel (band 3) in the membrane.

Red cell destruction: The life span of normal erythrocytes is about 120 days. The senile red cells are recognized by macrophages of reticuloendothelial system and are destroyed mainly in the spleen. Globin is converted to amino acids, which are stored to be recycled again. Degradation of haem liberates iron and porphyrin. Iron is stored as ferritin in macrophages or is released in circulation where it is taken up by transferrin and transported to erythroid precursors in bone marrow. The porphyrin is converted to bilirubin.

❑ WHITE BLOOD CELLS

Neutrophils

Stages of Granulopoiesis

The maturation sequence in granulopoiesis is—myeloblast, promyelocyte, myelocyte, metamyelocyte, band cell, and segmented granulocyte (Fig. 1.14). This process occurs within the marrow.

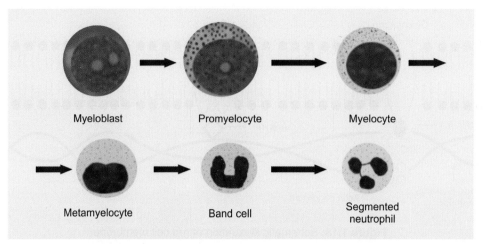

Figure 1.14: Stages in the formation of mature neutrophils

Myeloblast: Myeloblast is the earliest recognizable cell in the granulocytic maturation process. It is about 15 to 20 µm in diameter, with a large round to oval nucleus, and small amount of basophilic cytoplasm. The nucleus contains 2 to 5 nucleoli and nuclear chromatin is fine and reticular.

Promyelocyte: The next stage in the maturation is promyelocyte which is slightly larger in size than myeloblast. Primary or azurophil granules appear at the promyelocyte stage. The nucleus contains nucleoli as in myeloblast stage, but nuclear chromatin shows slight condensation.

Myelocyte: Myelocyte stage is characterised by the appearance of secondary or specific granules (neutrophilic, eosinophilic, or basophilic). Myelocyte is a smaller cell with round to oval eccentrically placed nucleus, more condensation of chromatin than in promyelocyte stage, and absence of nucleoli. Cytoplasm is relatively greater in amount than in promyelocyte stage and contains both primary and secondary granules. Myelocyte is the last cell capable of mitotic division.

Metamyelocyte: In the metamyelocyte stage, the nucleus becomes indented and kidneyshaped, and the nuclear chromatin becomes moderately coarse. Cytoplasm contains both primary and secondary granules.

Band stage (stab form): This is characterised by band-like shape of the nucleus with constant diameter throughout and condensed nuclear chromatin.

Segmented neutrophil (polymorphonuclear neutrophil): With Leishman's stain, nucleus appears deep purple with 2 to 5 lobes which are joined by thin filamentous strands. Nuclear chromatin pattern is coarse. The cytoplasm stains light pink and has small, specific granules (Fig. 1.15).

Primary and secondary granules: The neutrophil granules are of two types: primary or azurophilic granules and secondary or specific granules. Azurophil granules

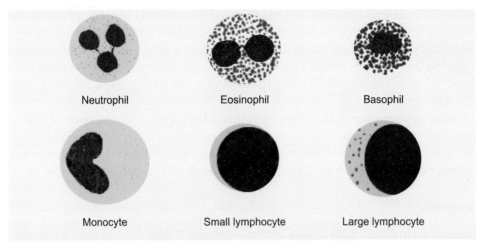

Figure 1.15: Mature white blood cells

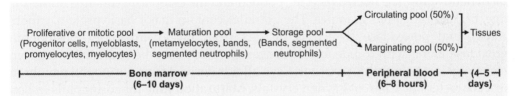

Figure 1.16: Neutrophil kinetics. After release from the marrow, neutrophils in peripheral blood can be divided into two compartments: circulating pool (measured by leucocyte count) and marginating pool (neutrophils adhering to endothelium via adhesion molecules; this portion is not measured by leucocyte count)

contain myeloperoxidase, lysozyme, acid phosphatase, elastases, collagenases, and acid hydrolases. Specific granules contain lysozyme, lactoferrin, alkaline phosphatases, vitamin B_{12}-binding protein and other substances.

Function of neutrophils: After their formation, neutrophils remain in marrow for 5 more days as a reserve pool. Neutrophils have a life span of only 1 to 2 days in circulation. Neutrophil compartments and kinetics is shown in Figure 1.16.

In response to infection and inflammation, neutrophils come to lie closer to endothelium (margination) and adhere to endothelial surface (sticking). This is followed by escape of neutrophils from blood vessels to extravascular tissue (emigration). The escape of neutrophils is guided by chemotactic factors present in the inflammatory zone. Chemotactic factors for neutrophils include bacterial factors, complement components such as C3a and C5a, breakdown products of neutrophils, fibrin fragments, and leukotriene B4. Phagocytosis follows which involves three steps—antigen recognition, engulfment, and killing of organism. Neutrophils have receptors for Fc portion of immunoglobulins and for complement. Many organisms are identified by neutrophils after they are coated with opsonins (IgG1, IgG3, and C3b). Cytoplasm of the neutrophil extends in the form of pseudopods around the microorganism, and the organism is eventually completely enclosed within the membrane-bound vacuole (phagosome). Lysosomal granules fuse with phagosome and discharge their contents into the phagolysosome. The last step in phagocytosis is killing of micro-organism, which may be either oxygen-dependent or oxygen-independent. Oxygen-dependent mechanism involves conversion of oxygen to hydrogen peroxide by oxidase in phagolysosome; myeloperoxidase in the presence of halide ion (e.g. Cl^-) converts hydrogen peroxide to $HOCl$· that has a strong bactericidal activity.

Another oxygen-dependent bactericidal mechanism is independent of myeloperoxidase and involves formation of superoxide radicals. Oxygen independent bactericidal mechanism occurs in lysosomal granules and is mediated by substances such as lysozyme, major basic protein, bactericidal permeability increasing protein, etc.

Eosinophils

Eosinophil forms via same stages as the neutrophil and the specific granules first become evident at the myelocyte stage. The size of the eosinophil is slightly greater than that of neutrophil. The nucleus is often bilobed and the cytoplasm contains numerous, large, bright orange-red granules. The granules contain major basic protein, cationic protein, and peroxidase (which is distinct from myeloperoxidase). Eosinophilic peroxidase along with iodide and hydrogen peroxide may be responsible for some defense against helminthic parasites. Crystalloids derived from eosinophil membrane form characteristic Charcot-Leyden crystals. Maturation time for eosinophils in bone marrow is 2 to 6 days and half-life in blood is less than 8 hours. In tissues, they reside in skin, lungs, and GIT.

Basophils

Basophils are small, round to oval cells which contain very large, coarse, deep purple granules. The nucleus has condensed chromatin and is covered by granules.

Mast cells in connective tissue or bone marrow differ morphologically from basophils in following respects: mast cells (10–15 μm) are larger than basophils (5–7 μm); mast cells have a single round to oval eccentrically placed nucleus while nucleus of the basophils is multilobed; and the cytoplasmic granules in mast cells are more uniform. Tissue mast cells are of mesenchymal origin.

Basophil granules contain histamine, chondroitin sulfate, heparin, proteases, and peroxidase. Basophils bear surface membrane receptors for IgE. Upon reaction of antigen with membrane-bound IgE, histamine and other granular contents are released which play a role in immediate hypersensitivity reaction. Basophils are also involved in some cutaneous basophil hypersensitivity reactions.

Monocytes

The initial cell in development is monoblast, which is indistinguishable from myeloblast. The next cell is promonocyte which has an oval or clefted nucleus with fine chromatin pattern and 2 to 5 nucleoli. The monocyte is a large cell (15–20 μm),

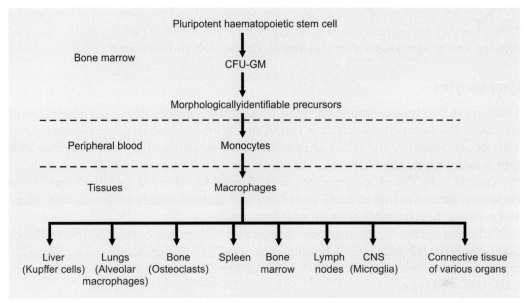

Figure 1.17: The mononuclear phagocyte system

with irregular shape, oval or clefted (often kidney-shaped) nucleus and fine, delicate chromatin. Cytoplasm is abundant, blue-grey with ground glass appearance and often contains fine azurophil granules and vacuoles.

Monocytes circulate in blood for about 1 day and then enter and settle in tissues where they are called as macrophages or histiocytes. In some organs, macrophages have distinctive morphologic and functional characteristics (Fig. 1.17).

Macrophage phagocytosis is slower as compared to neutrophils. Macrophages have receptors for Fc portion of IgG and C3b and cause phagocytosis of organisms that are coated with these substances. Macrophages also recognise and phagocytose some target substances by their surface characteristics.

Macrophages may be activated by certain stimuli such as lymphokines (interferon γ secreted by T lymphocytes), direct contact with micro-organism, phagocytized material and complement components. Activated macrophages are larger and have enhanced metabolic and phagocytic activity.

Activated macrophages secrete a variety of biologically active substances:
1. Cytokines—interleukin-1, tumour necrosis factor α, interferons α and β;
2. Growth factors—fibroblast growth factors, haematopoietic growth factors (GM-CSF and G-CSF), angiogenesis factor, transforming growth factor β;
3. Complement proteins;
4. Coagulation factors, e.g. thromboplastin;
5. Oxygen-derived free radicals—hydrogen peroxide, superoxide, hydroxyl radical;
6. Prostaglandins and leukotrienes which are chemical mediators in inflammation;
7. Enzymes—elastases, collagenases, lysozyme, plasminogen activator, lipases;
8. Fibronectin;
9. Transferrin, transcobalamin II, apolipoprotein E.

The major functions of macrophages are processing and presentation of antigens to T lymphocytes during immune response, killing of intracellular pathogens, tumoricidal activity, and phagocytosis of organisms and of injured and senescent cells.

Lymphocytes

These are of two types—small and large. Most of the lymphocytes in peripheral blood are small (7–10 µm). The nucleus is round or slightly clefted with coarse chromatin and occupies most of the cell. The cytoplasm is basophilic, slight and is visible as a thin border around the nucleus.

Around 10 to 15% of lymphocytes in peripheral blood are large (10–15 µm). Their nucleus is similar to that of small lymphocytes but their cytoplasm is relatively more and contains few azurophilic (dark red) granules.

On immunophenotyping, there are two major types of lymphocytes in peripheral blood: B lymphocytes (10–20%) and T lymphocytes (60–70%). Differences between B and T lymphocytes are presented in Table 1.2. About 10 to 15% of lymphocytes are of natural killer (NK) cell type.

B Lymphocytes

B lymphocytes arise from the lymphoid stem cells in the bone marrow. Initial development occurs in primary lymphoid organ (bone marrow) from where B cells migrate to the secondary lymphoid organs (lymph nodes and spleen) where further differentiation occurs on antigenic stimulation. On activation by antigen, B cells undergo differentiation and proliferation to form plasma cells and memory cells. Plasma cells secrete immunoglobulins while memory cells have a lifespan of many years and upon restimulation with the same antigen undergo proliferation and differentiation. Plasma cell is a round to oval cell with eccentrically placed nucleus and deeply basophilic cytoplasm. Nuclear chromatin is dense and arranged in a radiating or cartwheel pattern. The function of B lymphocytes is production of antibodies after differentiation to plasma cells. Antibodies can cause destruction of target cells/organisms either directly or by opsonisation.

Table 1.2: Comparison of B and T lymphocytes

Parameter	B lymphocytes	T lymphocytes
1. Origin	Lymphoid stem cell in bone marrow	Lymphoid stem cell in bone marrow, maturation in thymus
2. Surface antigens	CD19, CD20, CD22	CD2, CD5, CD6, CD4/CD8
3. Surface receptor	Surface membrane immunoglobulin (SmIg)	T cell receptor associated with CD3
4. Percentage in peripheral blood	30%	70%
5. Location in lymph node	Follicles, medullary cords	Paracortex, medullary sinuses
6. Function	Humoral immunity (maturation into plasma cell which produce immunoglobulins)	Cell-mediated immunity, graft rejection, delayed hypersensitivity, regulation of B cell function

Immunoglobulin gene rearrangement: There are 5 classes of immunoglobulins: IgM, IgG, IgA, IgD, and IgE. Each immunoglobulin molecule consists of two heavy chains and two light chains. Heavy chain (μ, δ, γ, ε, and α) determines the class of the immunoglobulin molecule. The two light chains are kappa (κ) and lambda (λ). Both heavy and light chains have constant and variable regions. The antigen-specificity of a particular immunoglobulin molecule depends upon amino acid sequence in the variable region (antigen-binding site). To react with a vast array of antigens, the immune system must have the capability to produce a large number of antigen-specific variable regions. The amino acid sequences in constant regions of heavy and light chains remain same for particular class and do not determine antigen specificity.

The heavy chain genes are located on chromosome 14. Light chain genes are located on chromosomes 2 (κ chain) and 22 (λ chain).

An immunoglobulin gene consists of V (Variable) and J (Joining) exons which code for amino acid sequences in variable region, and C (Constant) exon which codes for amino acid sequences in constant region. In heavy chain genes, another exon called D (Diversity) is present which codes for amino acids in variable region (in addition to V and J) (Fig. 1.18). There are several gene segments in V, D, and J regions, and therefore numerous antigen specificities can arise by various combinatorial rearrangements.

The unrearranged heavy and light chain genes are present in all the cells of the body (germ-line configuration); complete rearrangement occurs only in B cells. During development of B cells, rearrangement of heavy chain genes precedes the rearrangement of light chain genes.

Heavy chain gene rearrangement (Fig. 1.18): First, a D gene segment combines with a J segment (to form DJ), followed by combination of DJ with a V gene segment. The VDJ thus formed codes for amino acid sequence in variable region. From the C region, initially Cμ segment (which is located immediately 3' to the VDJ exon) is transcribed so as to form VDJCμ mRNA. This causes expression of μ heavy chains in the cytoplasm of pre-B cells, and after rearrangement of light chain genes expression of IgM on the surface of early B cells. Usually Cδ locus, which lies very close to Cμ locus, is also transcribed so that the cell expresses both IgM and IgD (with identical variable region sequences) on the surface.

Light chain gene rearrangement: During light chain gene rearrangement, initially a VJ exon is formed by fusion of one V and one J segment. The VJ exon is transcribed along with C exon and after splicing forms VJC mRNA.

Second immunoglobulin gene rearrangement can occur in activated B cells in which switching to new C segment of heavy chain gene occurs, i.e. Cμ to Cγ1 or Cα1 or Cε, etc. This causes change in the class of the immunoglobulin molecule, i.e. IgM to IgG1 or IgA or IgE, etc. Switching does not affect VDJ exon so that antigen specificity is not altered.

B cell ontogeny (Fig. 1.19): During B cell development, sequential genotypic and phenotypic changes occur which can be detected by immunological markers and gene rearrangement studies. Important features in B cell ontogeny are outlined below.

  i. There are two stages of B cell development: antigen-independent and antigen-dependent. Antigen-independent development occurs in bone marrow while antigen-dependent development occurs in peripheral lymphoid tissues.

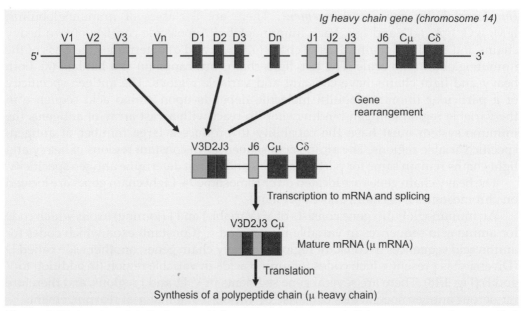

Figure 1.18: Immunoglobulin heavy chain gene rearrangement. DJ rearrangement occurs first followed by VDJ joining (V3D2J3 in this example). V and D regions other than V3 and D2 are deleted. The rearranged gene is transcribed into μRNA and intervening sequences between J3 and Cμ are spliced. The mRNA formed is translated into a μ heavy chain in cytoplasm

ii. Rearrangement of immunoglobulin genes and immunoglobulin expression: Initially there is rearrangement of heavy chain genes which is followed by rearrangement of light chain genes. In pre-B cell, rearrangement of heavy chain gene causes appearance of μ heavy chain in cytoplasm (Cμ). This is followed by rearrangement of light chain genes. Light chains associate with μ heavy chain in cytoplasm and IgM is expressed on the cell surface. Mature B cells express both IgM and IgD. In activated B cells, class switching of heavy chains occurs such as IgM to IgG or IgA or IgE. Plasma cells do not have surface expression of immunoglobulin but synthesize and secrete large amounts of immunoglobulins of one class.

iii. Cell surface antigens: The earliest antigens expressed during B cell development are TdT (within the nucleus) and HLA-DR (on cell surface); these are, however, not specific for B cells. There is a sequential appearance of antigens on developing B cells: CD19, CD10, and CD20. With development and maturation new antigens are expressed while some of the previous ones are lost. Plasma cells express specific antigens such as CD38 (Fig. 1.19).

iv. According to the fundamental theory of lymphoid neoplasms, the neoplastic cells represent cells arrested at various stages of normal lymphocyte development.

T lymphocytes

T lymphocytes originate from the progenitor cells in the bone marrow and undergo maturation in thymus. After their release from thymus, T cells circulate in peripheral

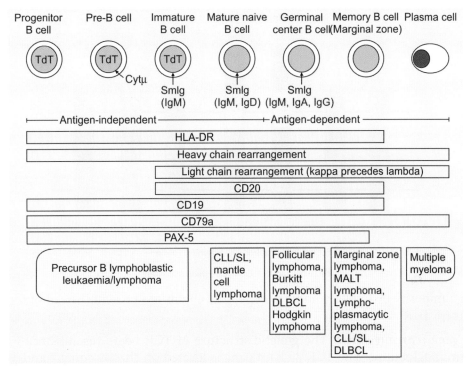

Figure 1.19: Normal stages of B cell development showing sequential expression of various antigens and heavy and light chain gene rearrangement. As shown at the bottom, lymphoid neoplasms represent cells arrested at various stages of normal development
Abbreviations: CLL/SL: Chronic lymphocytic leukaemia/small lymphocytic lymphoma; DLBCL: Diffuse large B cell lymphoma; MALT: Mucosa associated lymphoid tissue.

blood and are transported to secondary lymphoid organs (i.e. paracortex of lymph nodes and periarteriolar lymphoid sheaths in spleen).

There are two major subsets of mature T cells: T helper-inducer cells and T cytotoxic cells. Helper-inducer T cells regulate the functions of B cells and cytotoxic T cells. T helper-inducer cells recognise antigen presented by antigen-presenting cells in association with MHC class II molecules. Cytotoxic T cells recognize antigen in association with MHC class I molecules and play an important role in cell-mediated immunity. T lymphocytes secrete cytokines such as interferon-γ, GM-CSF, tumour necrosis factor, and certain interleukins.

T cell receptor (TCR): The T cell receptor complex consists of seven polypeptide chains. In the majority (95%) of T cells, α and β chains form the antigen-binding site of TCR ($\alpha\beta$ TCR); each of these chains has a variable and a constant region similar to immunoglobulins. α and β chains are linked together by a disulfide bond to form α-β heterodimer. The α-β heterodimer is non-covalently associated with CD3 molecular complex which is composed of five polypeptide chains (Fig. 1.20). The variable regions of α and β chains bind antigen, while CD3 converts this antigenic recognition into intracellular activating signals.

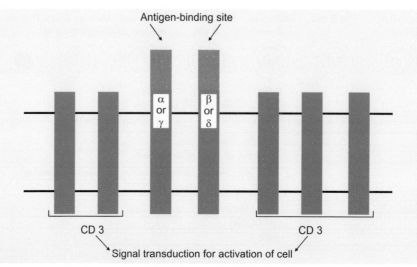

Figure 1.20: T cell receptor complex

In a minority of T cells, γ and δ polypeptide chains are present instead of α and β chains (γδ TCR).

TCR gene rearrangement: The genetic structure of TCR bears resemblance to that of immunoglobulins. The TCR β chain gene is located on chromosome 7 and TCR α chain gene is located on chromosome 14.

Although all somatic cells contain T cell receptor gene in germ-line configuration, rearrangement occurs only in T cells. The TCR β gene consists of variable (V), diversity (D), joining (J), and constant (C) regions. One segment each from V, D, and J regions join together with deletion of intervening sequences. The rearranged gene is transcribed into mRNA. Splicing in transcribed mRNA causes fusion of VDJ to C region to generate TCR β mRNA. Rearrangement of other polypeptide chain occurs similarly. As there are a number of V, D, and J segments which code for amino acid sequences in variable region, it is possible to generate T cell receptors with different antigen specificities by various combinations during rearrangement.

Rearrangement of TCR β gene precedes the rearrangement of TCR α gene.

T cell ontogeny (Fig. 1.21): Progenitor T cells from the bone marrow are transported to thymus where they undergo maturation. During maturation, there is rearrangement of TCR genes, expression of some cell surface proteins, and acquisition of ability to distinguish self-antigen from foreign antigens.

Initially, immature cortical thymocytes express CD7, TdT, and cytoplasmic CD3 (cCD3). Those T cells which subsequently are going to form α and β polypeptides (αβ TCR) first rearrange TCR β gene followed by TCR α gene. Expression of αβ TCR occurs in association with expression of CD3 on surface of cells. Initially, both CD4 and CD8 antigens are acquired; with further maturation cell retains either CD4 or CD8 antigen. CD4+ cells are called as helper-inducer T cells whereas CD8+ cells are called as cytotoxic T cells. The mature T cells are released from thymus, circulate in peripheral blood, and are transported to peripheral lymphoid organs.

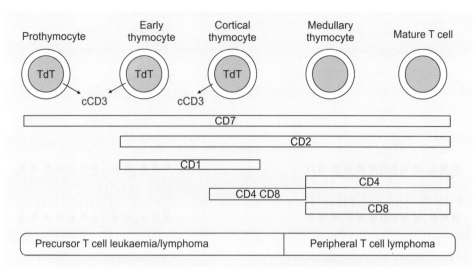

Figure 1.21: Stages of T cell development. Correlation of stages with
T cell neoplasms is shown at the bottom

Natural Killer (NK) Cells

About 10 to 15% of peripheral blood lymphocytes are natural killer cells. These cells do not require previous exposure or sensitisation for their cytotoxic action. They play a significant role in host defense against tumour cells and virally-infected cells. Morphologically, these cells are large granular lymphocytes.

White Cell Antigens

The HLA System

The HLA or human leucocyte antigens are encoded by a cluster of genes on short arm of chromosome 6 called as major histocompatibility complex (MHC). There are numerous allelic genes at each locus which makes the HLA system extremely polymorphic. The antigens are called as HLA because they were first detected on white blood cells, although they are present on several other cells also.

Types of HLA antigens: There are three types of HLA antigens: class I, class II, and class III.

Class I antigens: Genes at HLA-A, HLA-B, and HLA-C positions specify class I antigens. Class I antigens are glycoproteins which are associated noncovalently with $\beta2$ microglobulin. Almost all nucleated cells possess class I antigens (Fig. 1.22).

Class II antigens: HLA-D region (HLA-DR, HLA-DQ, and HLA-DP) encodes class II antigens. These consist of two glycoprotein chains α and β which are bound noncovalently. Class II antigens are present on monocytes, macrophages, B-lymphocytes, and stimulated T lymphocytes (Fig. 1.22).

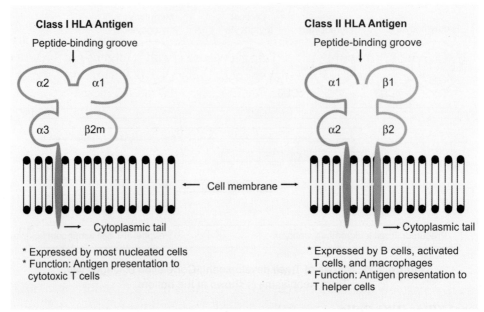

Figure 1.22: Structure of class I and class II HLA antigens

Class III antigens: Genes specifying class III antigens are situated between genes which specify class I and class II antigens. Class III genes encode certain complement components and cytokines (tumour necrosis factor).

The HLA genes are closely linked and are inherited by an individual as a haplotype from each parent. In a given population, certain HLA haplotypes occur much more frequently than expected by chance alone (linkage disequilibrium).

Significance of HLA antigens: (1) They are important as histocompatibility antigens in organ transplantation; (2) HLA antigens play a major role in recognition of foreign antigens and in immunity; (3) In transfusion medicine, HLA antigens are responsible for alloimmunization against platelet antigens and refractoriness to platelet transfusions, febrile transfusion reactions, and graft-verus-host disease; (4) A relationship exists between presence of some HLA antigens and susceptibility to certain diseases; (5) HLA antigen typing can be used for paternity testing.

Tests for detection of HLA antigens:
1. *Lymphocytotoxicity test:* Class I HLA antigens are detected by lymphocytotoxicity test. In this test, lymphocytes are first isolated from peripheral blood by density gradient separation. These lymphocytes are then added to known specific antisera in microwell plates and incubated to allow the antibodies to bind to target antigens. Complement is added to the lymphocyte-antiserum mixture followed by further incubation. If particular antigen is present on lymphocytes, then antigen-antibody reaction occurs which activates and fixes the complement, leading to cell membrane injury and cell death. A vital dye (eosin Y or trypan blue) is then added to differentiate living

from dead cells. Damaged cells take up the dye due to the increased permeability of injured cell membrane while living cells remain unstained.

For detection of class II antigens (HLA-DR and HLA-DQ), lymphocytotoxicity test is carried out on B lymphocytes. This is because class II antigens are present on B lymphocytes and not on unstimulated T cells. Separation of B lymphocytes is usually achieved by magnetic beads, which are coated with monoclonal antibodies against B cells.

2. *Mixed lymphocyte culture (MLC) or mixed lymphocyte reaction (MLR):* This test is used for detection of class II antigens. Lymphocytes from two different individuals are cultured together. Lymphocytes from one individual are inactivated by irradiation or by mitomycin C before the test to suppress their division; these lymphocytes are called stimulator cells. During incubation in culture, lymphocytes from the other individual recognise the foreign class II HLA antigens on stimulator cells and respond by enlarging in size, synthesizing DNA, and proliferating (blastogenic response); these cells are called as responder cells. If HLA class II antigens on responder and stimulator cells are identical, there is no blastogenic response. After 5 to 7 days 3H-thymidine is added to the culture and radioactive material incorporated into the dividing (responder) cells is quantitated. The amount of radioactive thymidine incorporated into the dividing cells is proportional to DNA synthesis.

3. *Primed lymphocyte typing (PLT) test:* This test is used for detection of HLA-DP antigens. It is based on mixed lymphocyte culture. In this method the culture of lymphocytes is extended for 2 weeks during which death of stimulator cells occurs and proliferation of responder cells halts. As these responder cells have been primed (i.e. sensitised), their re-encounter with the cells, which carry the same HLA-DP antigen as the initial stimulator cells, causes their rapid proliferation.

4. *DNA analysis:* Allelic genes at HLA-D loci can be identified by allele-specific oligonucleotide probe analysis. With the advent of polymerase chain reaction technology, which amplifies the desired DNA sequence several times, sensitivity of DNA analysis for HLA typing has greatly increased.

Neutrophil-specific Antigens

Apart from HLA antigens, granulocytes also possess neutrophil-specific antigens. These are NA1, NA2, NB1, NB2, NC1, ND1, NE1, 9a, and HGA-3a, 3b, 3c, 3d and 3e. Neutrophil-specific antigens play an important role in immune neutropaenias and in febrile nonhaemolytic transfusion reactions.

❏ IMMUNE SYSTEM

As white cells play a major role in immunity, it is appropriate to consider antibodies and complement here.

Antibodies

Antibodies are immunoglobulins that react with antigens. They are produced by plasma cells, which in turn are derived from B lymphocytes.

Structure of Immunoglobulins

The immunoglobulin molecule consists of two identical heavy (H) chains and two identical light (L) chains. The H and L chains are linked together by disulfide (s-s) bonds. Five classes of immunoglobulins are recognised based on the type of H chain: IgA (α or alpha H chain), IgD (δ or delta), IgE (ε or epsilon) IgG (γ or gamma), and IgM (μ or mu). Light chains are of two varieties—κ (kappa) and λ (lambda).

A molecule of immunoglobulin consists of light chains of the same type (either κ or λ); both types of light chains are never present together. Kappa and lambda chains are present in 2:1 proportion in immunoglobulins.

Each chain has a constant and a variable region (Fig. 1.23). Amino acid composition in the carboxy terminal region of heavy chain and light chain is the constant region; in the heavy chain it determines the class of the immunoglobulin molecule. The CH2 domain in IgG binds complement while CH3 domain binds to Fc receptor of monocytes. The variable region of the molecule (VL and VH) is the specific antigen-binding site and is in the amino-terminal part of the molecule. The area J of the heavy chains in the constant regions between CH1 and CH2 domains is flexible and is called hinge region; due to this the two antigen-binding sites can move in relation to each other spanning variable distances.

Each immunoglobulin molecule can be digested by a proteolytic enzyme papain just above the disulphide bond joining the two heavy chains into three parts: one Fc and two Fab fragments. The fragment, which contains the carboxy terminal and constant parts of both heavy chains, is called the Fc (fragment crystallizable) fragment. Each Fab (fragment antigen binding) fragment contains amino terminal portion of H chain and complete light chain and has the antigen-combining site (Fig. 1.23).

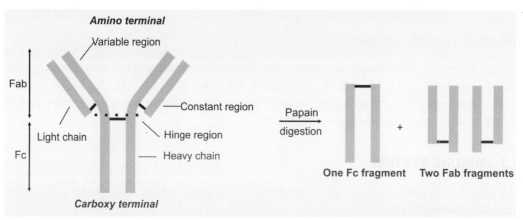

Figure 1.23: Structure of immunoglobulin molecule. Broken line indicates site of papain digestion

Classes of Immunoglobulins

IgG: This is the major immunoglobulin in plasma comprising about 75% of all circulating immunoglobulins. IgG is the monomer of the basic immunoglobulin structure. There are four subclasses of IgG: IgG1, IgG2, IgG3, and IgG4. Relative concentration in serum can be represented as IgG1 >IgG2>IgG3>IgG4. IgG is usually produced during secondary immune response. It is the only immunoglobulin, which is transferred transplacentally to the foetus from the mother. The foetus cannot synthesize IgG and therefore IgG antibodies in the newborn represent those passively gained from the mother. IgG is capable of fixing complement with order of efficacy being IgG3, IgG1 and IgG2. IgG4 cannot bind complement in the classical pathway. Only IgG3 and IgG 1 can bind to Fc receptors on macrophages.

IgM: This has high molecular weight and is also called as macroglobulin due to its large size. IgM molecules have a pentameric structure (i.e. five immunoglobulin units joined together) and also have an additional short polypeptide chain (J or joining chain). It comprises 5–10% of circulating immunoglobulins. IgM is the first antibody produced in response to the antigen (primary response). In contrast to IgG, IgM cannot cross the placenta. The foetus is able to produce IgM after maturation of its immune system. IgM is highly efficient in binding complement. A single molecule of IgM can bind complement while two molecules of IgG (IgG doublets) are necessary for complement-binding. The order of efficiency of complement binding of immunoglobulins is IgM, IgG3, IgG1 and IgG2. There are no receptors on macrophages for IgM.

IgA: There are two subclasses of IgA: IgA1 and IgA2. IgA is present mostly in body secretions such as gastrointestinal and respiratory mucosal secretions, saliva, tears, etc. Secretory IgA is mostly IgA2 and exists as a dimer. Serum IgA, which is mostly IgA1, is a monomer.

IgD and IgE: Both are present in trace amounts in serum and are monomeric.

Most IgD is expressed on the surface of resting B lymphocytes where it serves as an antigen receptor.

Most IgE is bound to basophils or mast cells through heavy chain. When a specific antigen combines with IgE, vasoactive substances are released from these cells and lead to anaphylaxis.

Alloantibodies vs autoantibodies: Alloantibodies are those which are produced by an individual against antigens present in another individual of the same species. Autoantibodies are those, which are produced by an individual against one's own antigens.

Warm vs cold antibodies: Warm antibodies react maximally at 37°C while cold antibodies show maximum activity at 0 to 4°C. Most IgG antibodies are of warm type while most IgM antibodies are of cold type. Characteristic features of different immunoglobulins are presented in Table 1.3.

Table 1.3: Characteristics of immunoglobulins

Parameter	IgM	IgG	IgA	IgE	IgD
1. Approx % of total Ig	5%	80%	15%	Trace	Trace
2. Molecular weight	900,000	150,000	150,000 or 300,000	190,000	180,000
3. Heavy chain	μ	γ	α	ε	δ
4. Structure	Pentamer	Monomer	Dimer (secretions), monomer (serum)	Monomer	Monomer
5. Half-life (days)	5	21	6	2	3
6. Complement activation	Yes	Yes	No	No	No
7. Placental transfer	No	Yes	No	No	No
8. Main function	Primary immune response	Secondary immune response	Mucosal immunity	Anaphylactic reaction	Unknown

Complement

Complement are serum proteins which when activated react in an orderly manner with each other to cause immunologic destruction of target cells (lysis or phagocytosis). There are three pathways of complement activation: classical, alternate and mannose-binding pathway (Fig. 1.24).

Classical Pathway

Classical pathway is usually initiated by reaction of antibody (IgG or IgM) with antigen (e.g. red cells). Binding of only a single IgM pentameric molecule or of IgG doublet to an antigen are necessary for complement activation.

The complements are activated in the following order: Ag-Ab complex—C1 C4 C2 C3 C5 C6 C7 C8 C9. This process occurs on the surface of target cells (e.g. red cells). Binding of antibody to antigen causes exposure of complement-binding site on immunoglobulin. The activated C1 cleaves C4 to form C4a and C4b; C4a is released into the body fluid while C4b attaches to the red cell membrane. Activated C1 also cleaves C2 to form C2a. The C4b2a complex (C3 convertase) is formed. The C4b2a complex attached to cell membrane has enzymatic activity and can cleave several hundred C3 molecules. The C3a is released into plasma while C3b attaches to the cell membrane. C3b however is rapidly degraded into C3dg. C3b is not enzymatically active by itself, but presence of C3b on the cell surface is recognized by specific receptors on the surface of macrophages and this causes phagocytosis of C3b-bearing cells. C3dg cannot adhere to macrophages because macrophages do not have receptors for C3dg. Once C3b is converted to C3dg, then complement cascade is terminated; C3dg coated red cells in circulation are resistant to further complement-mediated cell destruction.

Some C3b joins C4b2a to form C4b2a3b (C5 convertase). C5 convertase cleaves C5 into C5a and C5b. C5a is released in circulation. C5b joins with C6 C7 C8 C9 to form membrane attack complex (MAC), which fixes on cell membranes and causes cell lysis. The MAC creates pores in red cell membrane through which water enters into red cells, cells swell and are lysed.

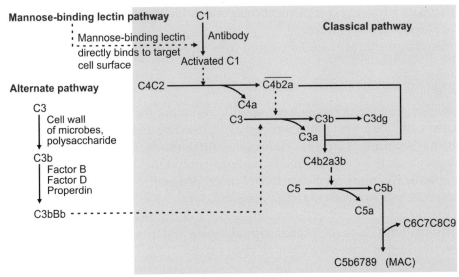

Figure 1.24: The complement pathway. Solid arrow indicates transformation of a complement component. Dashed arrow indicates enzymatic action of complement component that causes cleavage of that component

Alternate Pathway

In alternate pathway, C3 is activated directly with no role of earlier complement components. It does not require antigen-antibody reaction.

C3 can be activated by endotoxins, complex carbohydrates such as are present on some micro-organisms, and aggregates of IgA. A serum protein called properdin, factors B and D, and magnesium ions are needed for activation of alternate pathway.

Normally, C3 is being continuously cleaved at low level, probably by factor B, resulting C3b is rapidly cleared from the plasma. However, when C3b comes in contact with certain substances (e.g. complex carbohydrates on the surface of micro-organisms) then association of C3bB occurs on the surface of micro-organisms in the presence of Mg^{++} ions. Factor B is cleaved by factor D to form C3bBb. Properdin may stabilise C3bBb. C3bBb splits C3 to generate more C3b thus forming an amplification loop.

Alternate pathway plays an important role in initial defense against infection in nonimmune persons.

Mannose-binding lectin pathway: Mannose-binding lectin directly binds to target cell surface; this resembles binding of C1 to immune complexes and directly activates the classical pathway (without the need for immune complex formation).

Regulation of Complement Activity

Following factors act as a control mechanism against prolonged complement action:
  i. Specific inhibitors of activation of some complement components (particularly C1 and C3) are present in plasma.

ii. Enzymatically active complement components have a very short life and are rapidly degraded to inactive forms.

iii. Active fragments are rapidly cleared from circulation.

Various Effects of Complement Activation

1. *Opsonisation:* Macrophages have specific receptors for C3b and thus target cells coated with C3b are recognised and phagocytosed by them (Opsonins are substances which when present on the surface of the antigen such as red cells facilitate immune phagocytosis; these are C3b and Fc portion of immunoglobulin which are recognized by specific receptors on the surface of macrophages).

2. *Target cell lysis by membrane attack complex C5b-9.*

3. *Acute inflammation:* Certain complement components play a role in acute inflammation. C3a and C5a are anaphylatoxins and increase vascular permeability. C5a, in addition, causes neutrophil chemotaxis.

❑ MEGAKARYOPOIESIS

The process of development of megakaryocytes and platelets in bone marrow is known as megakaryopoiesis. It is divided into four stages (Fig. 1.25). Megakaryoblasts (stage I) are the earliest morphologically recognizable precursors; they are 6 to 24 μ in diameter, contain a single, large, oval, kidney-shaped, or lobed nucleus with loose chromatin and multiple nucleoli, and have deeply basophilic agranular cytoplasm. Promegakaryocytes (stage II) are larger than megakaryoblasts (15–30 μ), have lobulated or horseshoe-shaped nucleus, more abundant and less basophilic cytoplasm which may contain azurophil granules. Granular megakaryocytes (stage III) are 40 to 60 μ in diameter, contain a large multilobed nucleus with coarsely granular chromatin, and have abundant mildly basophilic cytoplasm containing numerous azurophil granules. Mature megakaryocytes (stage IV) are of similar size, contain a tightly packed multilobed and pyknotic nucleus, and have acidophilic cytoplasm; granules are arranged as 'platelet fields' (groups of 10–12 azurophil granules). Sometimes neutrophils or other marrow cells are seen traversing through the cytoplasm (emperipolesis); it has no clinical significance.

Mature megakaryocytes extend long and slender cytoplasmic processes (proplatelets) between endothelial cells of sinusoids in bone marrow and platelets are released from fragmentation of these processes. Each meakaryocyte produces 1000 to 5000 platelets, leaving behind a 'bare' nucleus which is removed by macrophages.

A unique feature of thrombocytopoiesis is endomitosis. This refers to nuclear division with cytoplasmic maturation but without cell division. As the cell matures from megakaryoblast to the megakaryocyte, there is gradual increase in cell size, number of nuclear lobes, and red-pink granules and gradual decrease in cytoplasmic basophilia. Megakaryocytes, the most abundant cells of the platelet series in the marrow, are large and contain numerous nuclear lobes with dense nuclear chromatin, and small aggregates of granules in the cytoplasm. The megakaryocytes possess well-developed membrane

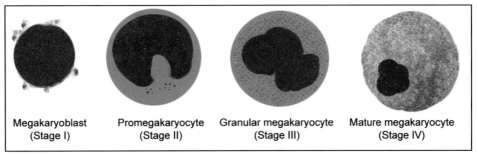

| Megakaryoblast (Stage I) | Promegakaryocyte (Stage II) | Granular megakaryocyte (Stage III) | Mature megakaryocyte (Stage IV) |

Figure 1.25: Megakaryopoiesis

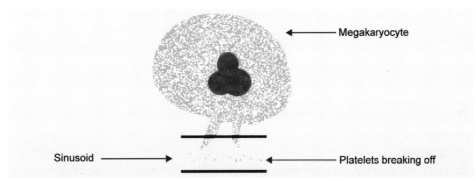

Figure 1.26: Formation and release of platelets from a megakaryocyte

demarcation system. Upon complete maturation, megakaryocytes extend pseudopods through the walls of the marrow sinusoids and individual platelets break-off into the peripheral circulation (Fig. 1.26). There is evidence that some of the megakaryocytes are carried to the lungs where platelets are released. A humoral factor, thrombopoietin, controls the maturation of megakaryocytes.

❏ NORMAL HAEMOSTASIS

Haemostasis is the mechanism by which loss of blood from the vascular system is controlled by a complex interaction of vessel wall, platelets, and plasma proteins. Following vessel injury, haemostasis can be considered as occurring in two stages: primary and secondary. Primary haemostasis is the initial stage during which vascular wall and platelets interact to limit the blood loss from damaged vessel. During secondary haemostasis, a stable fibrin clot is formed from coagulation factors by enzymatic reactions. Although formation of blood clot is necessary to arrest blood loss, ultimately blood clot needs to be dissolved to resume the normal blood flow. The process of dissolution of blood clot is called as fibrinolysis.

The roles of vascular wall, platelets, and plasma proteins in normal haemostasis are briefly outlined below.

Vascular Wall

Endothelial cells synthesise certain substances which have inhibitory influence on haemostasis. These include—thrombomodulin, protein S, heparin-related substances, prostacycline (PGI2), and tissue plasminogen activator (tPA). Binding of thrombomodulin to thrombin causes activation of protein C. Protein C inactivates factors V and VIII: C and is a potent inhibitor of coagulation. Protein S is a cofactor for protein C. Deficiency of protein C or protein S is associated with tendency towards thrombosis. Heparin-like substances on the surface of endothelial cells potentiate the action of antithrombin. Prostacycline, a prostaglandin synthesised by endothelial cells, induces vasodilatation and also inhibits platelet aggregation. Endothelial cells also synthesise tissue plasminogen activator, which converts plasminogen to plasmin, and activates fibrinolytic system.

Certain factors synthesised by endothelial cells promote haemostasis and include tissue factor, von Willebrand factor and platelet activating factor. Tissue factor or thromboplastin activates extrinsic system of coagulation. von Willebrand factor mediates adhesion of platelets to subendothelium. Platelet activating factor induces aggregation of platelets (Fig. 1.27).

Another vascular factor promoting haemostasis is vasoconstriction of small vessels following injury.

Subendothelial collagen promotes platelet adhesion and also activates factor XII (intrinsic pathway).

Platelets

Platelets are derived from cytoplasmic fragmentation of bone marrow cells called megakaryocytes. They measure 2 to 3 μ in diameter. Normal platelet count in peripheral blood is 1.5 to 4 lacs/cmm. Platelets remain viable in circulation for approximately 10 days. About one-third of the total platelets in the body are in the spleen and remainder in peripheral blood. Under light microscope, in peripheral blood smears stained with one of the Romanowsky stains, platelets appear as small, irregular with fine cytoplasmic processes. Cytoplasmic granules are often visible. These granules may

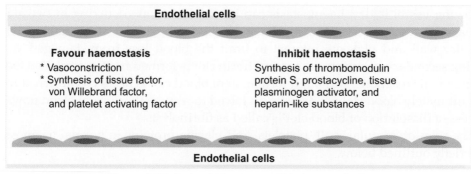

Figure 1.27: Role of blood vessels in haemostasis

be packed in the central portion (granulomere) with peripheral cytoplasm appearing clear (hyalomere).

Ultrastructure of Platelets

Ultrastructurally, following three zones can be distinguished: (1) Peripheral zone: exterior coat (glycocalyx), cell membrane, open canalicular system; (2) Sol-gel zone: microfilaments, circumferential microtubules, dense tubular system; (3) Organelle zone: alpha granules, dense granules, mitochondria, lysosomes (Fig. 1.28).

Peripheral zone: Exterior or surface coat (glycocalyx) overlies the cell membrane. It is made of proteins, glycoproteins, and mucopolysaccharides. Some of the glycoproteins are polysaccharide side chains of the integral membrane proteins while others are adsorbed from the plasma.

The cell membrane is a trilaminar membrane composed of proteins, lipids, and carbohydrates. The chief membrane lipids are phospholipids which are arranged as a bilayer; the polar head groups are oriented both externally (towards plasma) and internally (towards cytoplasm) while the fatty acid chains are oriented toward each other. Phospholipids are distributed asymmetrically in the membrane with phosphatidylinositol concentrated on the inner half of the bilayer and phosphati-dylethanolamine on the outer half. The phospholipids play an important role in prostaglandin synthesis and in platelet procoagulant activity.

An extensive open canalicular system, formed by invagination of the cell membrane, communicates with the exterior. It functions as a route through which platelet contents are secreted outside the cell.

Sol-gel zone: Microtubules provide structural support to the platelets. Microfilaments have contractile function. The dense tubular system, derived from smooth endoplasmic reticulum, is the site of pooling of calcium and formation of prostaglandin and thromboxane.

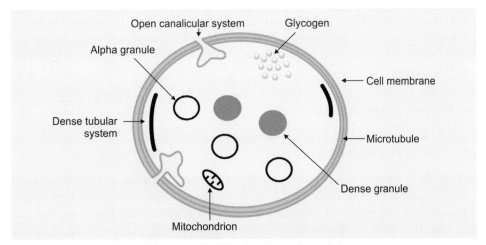

Figure 1.28: Ultrastructure of platelet

Table 1.4: Platelet organelles and their contents

Alpha granules
• Platelet-specific proteins: platelet factor-4, β thromboglobulin, platelet-derived growth factor, thrombospondin
• Coagulation system proteins: fibrinogen, factor V, von Willebrand factor, high molecular weight kininogen
• Fibrinolytic system proteins: α2-antiplasmin, plasminogen, PAI-1
• Others: fibronectin, albumin
Dense granules
• Anions: ADP, ATP, GTP, GDP
• Cations: calcium, serotonin

Organelle zone: Platelet organelles are alpha granules, dense granules, lysosomes and peroxisomes. Contents of platelet organelles are shown in Table 1.4.

Platelet Membrane Glycoproteins

The cell membrane contains integral membrane glycoproteins (Gp), which play an important role in haemostasis. Important platelet membrane glycoproteins and their functions are as follows:

Gp Ib-IX-V: This is a constitutively active receptor that mediates vWF-dependent adhesion of platelets to subendothelial collagen.

Gp IIb/IIIa: On activation, serves to bind fibrinogen and thus mediates aggregation. Also receptor for vWF, fibronectin, and thrombospondin.

Gp Ia-IIa: Constitutively active receptor for collagen and mediates platelet adhesion independent of vWF.

Platelet Antigens

Platelets possess HLA antigens and platelet-specific antigens. HLA class I antigens induce alloimmunisation and cause refractoriness to platelet transfusions when platelets are obtained from random donors. The platelet-specific antigen systems are now known as human platelet antigen (HPA) systems. Platelet specific antigens play an important role in neonatal alloimmune thrombocytopaenic purpura (NATP) and in post transfusion purpura.

Role of Platelets in Haemostasis

Activation of platelets refers to adhesion, aggregation, and release reaction of platelets which occurs after platelet stimulation (i.e. after vascular damage).

Adhesion: This means binding of platelets to nonendothelial surfaces, particularly subendothelium which is uncovered following vascular injury. von Willebrand factor (vWF) mediates adhesion of platelets to subendothelium via GpIb on the surface of platelets (Fig. 1.29). Congenital absence of glycoprotein receptor GpIb (Bernard-

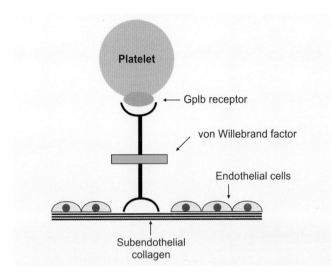

Figure 1.29: Platelet adhesion to subendothelial collagen. Gplb receptor on platelets and von Willebrand factor are necessary for attachment of platelets to subendothelial collagen

Soulier syndrome) or of von Willebrand factor in plasma (von Willebrand's disease) causes defective platelet adhesion and bleeding disorder.

Platelets normally circulate as round to oval disc-like structures. With activation, platelets undergo shape change, i.e. they become more spherical and form pseudopodia.

This shape change is due to reorganisation of microtubules and contraction of actomyosin of microfilaments.

Release reaction (secretion): Immediately after adhesion and shape change, process of release reaction or secretion begins. In this process, contents of platelet organelles are released to the exterior. ADP released from dense granules promotes platelet aggregation. Platelet factor 4 released from alpha granules neutralises the anticoagulant activity of heparin while platelet-derived growth factor stimulates proliferation of vascular smooth muscle cells and skin fibroblasts and plays a role in wound healing.

Activated platelets also synthesise and secrete thromboxane A2 (TxA2) (Fig. 1.30). Platelet agonists such as ADP, epinephrine, and low-dose thrombin bind to their specific receptors on platelet surface, and activate phospholipase enzymes, which release arachidonic acid from membrane phospholipids. Arachidonic acid is converted to cyclic endoperoxides PGG2 and PGH2 by the enzyme cyclo-oxygenase. These are then converted to thromboxane A2 by thromboxane synthetase. Thromboxane A2 has a very short half-life and is degraded into thromboxane B2 which is biologically inactive. TxA2 causes shape change and stimulates release reaction from alpha and dense granules. TxA2 also induces aggregation of other platelets and local vasoconstriction.

Aggregation: This may be defined as binding of platelets to each other. ADP released from platelets or from damaged cells binds to specific receptors on platelet surface. This causes inhibition of adenyl cyclase and reduction in the level of cyclic AMP in platelets. A configurational change in the membrane occurs so that receptors for fibrinogen (GpIIb and IIIa) become exposed on the surface. Binding of fibrinogen

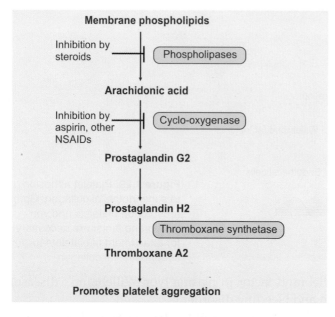

Figure 1.30: Synthesis of thromboxane A2. Modes of action of certain antiplatelet drugs are also shown

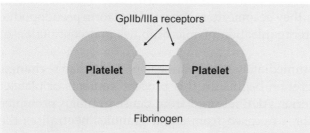

Figure 1.31: Platelet aggregation. This requires binding of fibrinogen molecules to GpIIb/IIIa receptors on platelets

molecules to GPIIb/IIIa receptors on adjacent platelets causes platelet aggregation (Fig. 1.31). The activated platelets release ADP and TxA2 and so a self-sustaining reaction is generated leading to the formation of a platelet plug. Thrombin generated from activation of coagulation system is a potent platelet-aggregating agent and also converts fibrinogen to fibrin. Fibrin and aggregated mass of platelets at the site of injury constitute the haemostatic plug.

Platelet procoagulant activity: When platelets are activated, negatively charged phospholipids (phosphotidylserine and phosphatidylinositol) located in the inner half of the lipid bilayer become exposed on the outer surface. These phospholipids play active role in coagulation by providing surface for interaction of some coagulation factors. Critical coagulation reactions for which activated platelets provide a negatively charged phospholipid (PL) surface are shown in Figure 1.32.

Platelets may play a role in the activation of F XII in the presence of ADP and kallikrein. Platelets also can directly activate F XI independent of F XII. This may explain the absence of bleeding diathesis in persons with F XII deficiency.

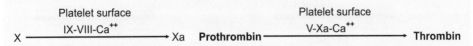

Figure 1.32: Platelet procoagulant activity. Platelets provide surface for some important coagulation reactions

In addition platelets also secrete calcium, FV, fibrinogen, and FXII and contribute to the coagulation system.

Plasma Proteins in Haemostasis

Plasma proteins in haemostasis can be divided into following groups:
1. *Coagulation system:* Factors I, II, III, IV, V, VII, VIII, IX, X, XI, XII, XIII, prekallikrein, high molecular weight kininogen.
2. *Fibrinolytic system:* Plasminogen, plasmin, tPA, α2- antiplasmin, PAI-1, PAI-2.
3. *Inhibitor system:* Protein C, protein S, antithrombin.

Coagulation System

A number of coagulation proteins (factors) participate in coagulation reactions, which ultimately lead to the formation of a fibrin clot. According to the International System of Nomenclature, coagulation factors are designated by Roman numerals (I to XIII). Table 1.5 lists the blood coagulation factors; common names and synonyms are given on the right side. Coagulation proteins can be divided into following categories: (1) Fibrinogen (F I); (2) Serine proteases: (a) Vitamin K-dependent Factors—II, VII, IX, X, (b) Contact factors—XI, XII, high molecular weight kininogen, prekallikrein; (3) Cofactors—V, VIII, tissue factor (F III); and (4) Transglutaminase: F XIII.

The coagulation factors have been assigned Roman numerals according to the order of their discovery. Except calcium and thromboplastin, all the coagulation factors listed in Table 1.5 are glycoproteins. When coagulation factors become activated, they are converted from an inactive zymogen form to a serine protease. However, factors V and VIII, when activated, do not develop enzymatic activity but become modified and are called as cofactors; in their absence the reactions, which they modify, become markedly slow. Activation of fibrinogen denotes cleavage of fibrinopeptides A and B from the molecule with formation of fibrin. Factors II, VII, IX, and X are called as vitamin K-dependent factors. Vitamin K is required for γ-carboxylation of these proteins, which is necessary for calcium binding. Calcium in turn, is necessary for binding of these coagulation factors to phospholipid surface. Attachment of coagulation factors to phospholipid is essential for coagulation reactions to occur. In the absence of vitamin K, carboxylation fails to occur and functionally inactive forms of vitamin K-dependent factors are produced. Factors XII, XI, high molecular weight kininogen, and prekallikrein are called as contact factors; they are involved in the activation of coagulation via intrinsic pathway.

Table 1.5: Blood coagulation factors

Factor	Synonym
I	Fibrinogen
II	Prothrombin
III	Tissue factor, thromboplastin
IV	Calcium
V	Labile factor, proaccelerin
VI	F VI has been determined to be activated form of F V and the term FVI is no longer used
VII	Stable factor
VIII	Antihaemophilic factor or globulin
IX	Christmas factor, Plasma thromboplastin component
X	Stuart-Prower factor
XI	Plasma thromboplastin antecedent
XII	Hageman factor
XIII	Fibrin stabilising factor, Laki-Lorand factor
Fletcher factor	Prekallikrein
Fitzgerald factor	High molecular weight kininogen

The liver is the site of synthesis of most coagulation factors. However, F XIII is derived from megakaryocytes, while vascular endothelial cells and megakaryocytes synthesize von Willebrand factor.

Individual coagulation factors are considered briefly below:

Fibrinogen (Molecular weight (MW) 340,000; 1/2 life 90 hours): The level of fibrinogen in plasma is the greatest among the coagulation proteins and ranges from 200 to 400 mg/dl. Fibrinogen molecule consists of three pairs of polypeptide chains Aα, Bβ, and γ which are held together by disulfide bonds. The complete molecule is represented as Aα2 Bβ2 γ2. Fibrinogen consists of three domains—two outer D domains and a central E domain. Fibrinopeptides A and B are located in the central domain at the N-terminals of Aα and Bβ chains, respectively. Thrombin releases fibrinopeptides A and B from these chains to form fibrin monomers (Fig. 1.38). Fibrinogen is an acute phase reactant and its concentration rises in a variety of non-specific conditions such as inflammation, trauma, and myocardial infarction.

Prothrombin (MW 72,000; 1/2 life 60 hours): Factor II or prothrombin is converted to thrombin by the enzyme complex Xa-V-phospholipid-calcium (called as prothrombinase). Thrombin has multiple functions in haemostasis (Fig. 1.33).
1. Thrombin splits fibrinopeptides A and B from fibrinogen to form fibrin monomers;
2. Thrombin activates F XIII which is necessary for cross-linking of fibrin and stabilisation of the clot.
3. Thrombin activates Factors VIII and V which in turn enhance the activation of F X and prothrombin, respectively.

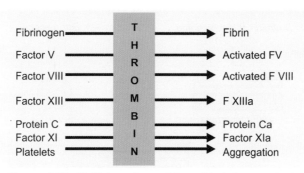

Figure 1.33: Multiple actions of thrombin in haemostasis

4. Thrombin is a powerful platelet agonist.
5. Thrombin activates protein C, a natural anticoagulant.

Thromboplastin: Tissue factor is required for activation of F VII in extrinsic pathway. It is composed of two parts: protein and phospholipid. Tissue factor is distributed in all tissues, but especially high concentrations are present in brain, placenta, and lungs.

Factor V (MW 330,000; 1/2 life 12–36 hours): F V is a heat-labile factor, which is inactivated rapidly at room temperature *in vitro*. F V is activated by thrombin and functions as a cofactor in the conversion of prothrombin to thrombin by the prothrombinase complex. About one-fifth of the FV in blood is stored in platelet alpha granules, which is released when platelets are activated.

Factor VII (MW 48,000; 1/2 life 6 hours): Tissue injury results in the formation of a complex between single chain form of F VII, tissue factor, and calcium which generates small amount of F Xa from F X. Factor Xa then in the reverse reaction cleaves F VII to yield F VIIa (two chain form); the F VIIa- tissue factor-calcium complex has greatly increased activity. This complex can also activate F IX.

Factor VIII (MW of F VIII: C-200,000; 1/2 life of F VIII: C approx 12 hours): The F VIII circulates in plasma as a noncovalently bound complex of two components—F VIII:C and von Willebrand factor. F VIII:C is the low molecular weight portion which has procoagulant activity and its synthesis is X-linked. F VIII mRNA is detected in various tissues; liver however, appears to be the primary source of F VIII. von Willebrand factor is the high molecular weight component which is autosomal in inheritance and synthesised by endothelial cells and megakaryocytes (Fig. 1.34). von Willebrand factor functions as a carrier protein for F VIII:C and also mediates adhesion of platelets to the subendothelium at sites of vessel damage.

The gene that codes for F VIII is located on the long arm of the X chromosome. It is 186 kilobases long and consists of 26 exons. The RNA is approximately 9 kilobases in length. The F VIII protein is composed of various domains, which are arranged as A1-A2-B-A3-C1-C2. A1 and A2 domains constitute the heavy chain of the molecule while A3, C1, and C2 make up the light chain. B is the connecting region (Fig. 1.35).

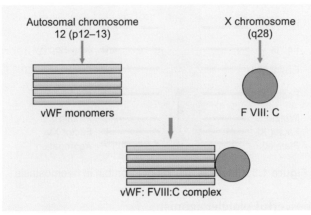

Figure 1.34: Formation of F VIII:vWF complex

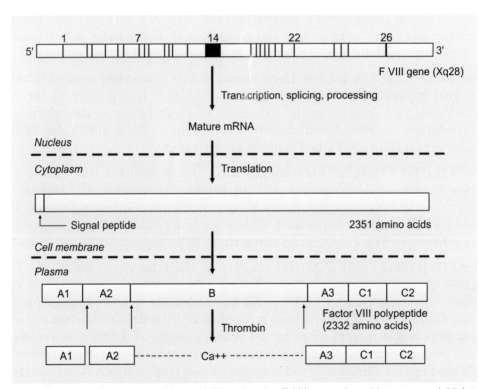

Figure 1.35: Factor VIII gene and factor VIII molecule. F VIII gene has 26 exons and 25 introns. Polypeptide chain encoded by the gene has six regions: A1, A2, B, A3, C1, and C2. Proteolytic action by thrombin (small arrows) produces activated F VIII molecule

Thrombin proteolytically cleaves F VIII molecule at three different positions to form activated F VIII. Activated F VIII functions as a cofactor in the reaction $F X \rightarrow FXa$ and enhances the velocity of this reaction several thousand-fold. Further cleavage by thrombin and activated protein C inactivates VIII.

Various terms and definitions related to F VIII and von Willebrand factor are given below:

- *VIII vWF:* Complex of FVIII procoagulant protein and von Willebrand factor
- *F VIII: C:* F VIII coagulant activity which is measured by clotting assay
- *F VIII: C Ag:* Antigenic expression of F VIII measured by immunologic technique
- *VWF:* A multimeric protein necessary for platelet adhesion
- *VWF:RCo:* Ristocetin cofactor activity, the activity of von Willebrand factor required for ristocetin-induced platelet aggregation
- *VWF Ag:* Antigenic expression of von Willebrand factor measured by immunological technique.

Factor IX (MW 57,000; 1/2 life 24 hours): F IX, a vitamin K-dependent glycoprotein, is activated by F XIa or by F VIIa-tissue factor complex to F IXa, a two-chain molecule. F IX is inherited in a sex-linked manner.

Factor X (MW 58,000; 1/2 life 20–40 hours): F X, a vitamin K-dependent protein, is activated by both intrinsic (i.e. F IXa-VIII-phospholipid-calcium complex) and extrinsic (i.e. tissue factor-VII complex) pathways. It is necessary for the formation of prothrombinase (Xa-V-phospholipid-calcium) in the common pathway.

Factor XI (MW 160,000; 1/2 life 40–80 hours): F XI is activated by F XIIa in the presence of high molecular weight kininogen. Its activity increases upon storage.

Factor XII (MW 80,000; 1/2 life 40–50 hours): F XII is activated when it comes in contact with substances such as collagen, glass, celite, ellagic acid, etc. F XIIa converts F XI to its active form and also prekallikrein to kallikrein. F XII plays a role in contact activation of coagulation system, inflammatory response, complement system, fibrinolysis, and formation of kallikrein and kinin.

Factor XIII (MW 320,000; 1/2 life 3–7 days): In contrast to all other coagulation factors, F XIII is a transglutaminase. Activated F XIII catalyzes the formation of covalent bonds between adjacent molecules of fibrin monomer (cross-linking) which provides stability to the fibrin clot.

Prekallikrein (MW 88,000; 1/2 life 35 hours): Prekallikrein is activated by F XIIa to kallikrein. Kallikrein in turn further activates F XII and thus serves to amplify the initial stimulus. Kallikrein plays a role in chemotaxis and in activation of fibrinolysis. Kallikrein also converts high molecular weight kininogen to bradykinin, a chemical mediator of inflammation.

High molecular weight kininogen (MW 110,000; 1/2 life 6.5 days): This circulates in plasma complexed to pre-kallikrein and F XI. It promotes contact activation.

Mechanism of Blood Coagulation

Scheme of blood coagulation is divided into intrinsic, extrinsic, and common pathways (Fig. 1.36). The intrinsic pathway is initiated by contact activation and consists of

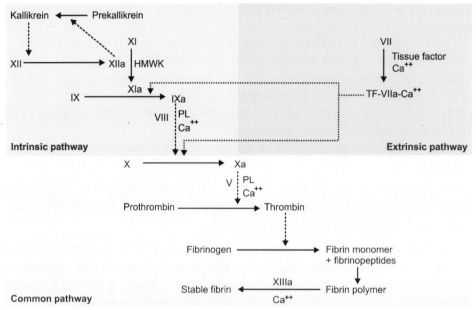

Figure 1.36: Scheme of blood coagulation. Solid arrows indicate transformation. Broken lines indicate action. Abbreviations: HMWK: High molecular weight kininogen; TF: Tissue factor; PL: Phospholipid; Ca^{++}: Calcium

interaction of contact factors (F XII, F XI, prekallikrein, and high molecular weight kininogen), F IX, F VIII, phospholipid, and calcium; these reactions generate a complex which causes activation of F X to F Xa. The extrinsic pathway is initiated by tissue injury with release of tissue thromboplastin which causes activation of F VII; the enzyme which is formed activates F X. Both intrinsic and extrinsic pathways proceed to common pathway which begins with activation of F X, involves interaction of F X, F V, prothrombin, phospholipid, calcium, and F XIII and leads to the formation of fibrin.

Intrinsic pathway: Initiation of intrinsic pathway occurs when plasma comes in contact with a negatively charged surface such as glass, kaolin, celite, or ellagic acid *in vitro*. *In vivo*, this surface is probably provided by subendothelium of a damaged vessel. Following contact with a negatively charged surface, a conformational change in FXII with exposure of enzymatically active site probably occurs and in this way a small amount of F XIIa is formed. F XIIa converts prekallikrein to kallikrein and F XI to FXIa in the presence of high molecular weight kininogen. Kallikrein in turn activates more F XII thus providing autoamplification of the reaction. F XIa cleaves F IX to yield F IXa; this reaction requires the presence of phospholipid and calcium. F IXa complexes with activated F VIII, phospholipid, and calcium and activates F X to F Xa. F VIII is activated by thrombin and also by F Xa. F VIII does not possess enzymatic activity but functions as a cofactor; in its presence the reaction rate is enhanced several thousand times.

Extrinsic pathway: F VII complexes with tissue factor released after tissue injury in the presence of calcium ions and activates F X and F IX. F Xa and thrombin convert the single-chain form of F VII to the two-chain form, which has greatly increased enzymatic activity as compared to the single-chain form. This reciprocal activation of F VII leads to autoamplification of the reaction.

The concept of intrinsic and extrinsic pathways of blood coagulation is applicable to *in vitro* blood clotting. It is uncertain whether intrinsic pathway plays any significant role *in vivo*. This is because of observed absence of haemorrhagic tendencies in patients of F XII, prekallikrein, or HMWK deficiency. Also, in addition to F VII of extrinsic pathway, tissue factor has also been shown to activate F IX to F IXa in intrinsic pathway. *In vivo*, blood clotting seems to be initiated primarily by tissue factor.

Common pathway: Common pathway begins with the activation of F X. F Xa generated by intrinsic or extrinsic pathway complexes with F V, phospholipid and calcium. This is called as prothrombinase complex, which activates prothrombin to thrombin. FV is modified by thrombin or F Xa to form activated F V which functions as a cofactor in the above reaction. Thrombin removes fibrinopeptides A and B from α and β chains of the fibrinogen molecule to form fibrin monomer. Free fibrin monomers spontaneously polymerize by forming end-to-end and side-to-side non-covalent bonds with each other. This is called as fibrin polymer. F XIIIa (generated from F XIII by thrombin), in the presence of calcium, mediates the formation of covalent bonds between adjacent polypeptide chains. This cross-linking of fibrin monomers imparts structural stability to the clot (Fig. 1.38).

Physiologic mechanism of coagulation: Under physiologic conditions *in vivo*, tissue factor (TF) and F VIIa initiate coagulation. F VIIa-TF complex activates F IX to F IXa, which then activates F X to F Xa. F Xa in turn activates prothrombin to thrombin, which converts fibrinogen to fibrin. If stimulus for thrombin formation is strong enough, coagulation is maintained through the activation of F XI by thrombin. Thrombin also activates F VIII, F V, and F XIII (Fig. 1.37).

Fibrinolytic System

Fibrinolysis is the process of dissolution of blood clots which is necessary to maintain the free flow of blood in the vascular system. The major enzyme of the fibrinolytic system is plasmin, which is generated from proteolytic cleavage of plasminogen. Plasmin can cause cleavage of both fibrinogen as well as fibrin. Plasmin digests insoluble or cross-linked fibrin to release fibrin degradation products or FDPs which are then cleared from the circulation by macrophages of the mononuclear phagocytic system.

Plasminogen is converted to plasmin by plasminogen activators. This reaction occurs on the surface of fibrin. The plasminogen activators include—(1) tissue plasminogen activator (tPA): This is synthesized by endothelial cells and is the most important physiological plasminogen activator. tPA most efficiently converts plasminogen to plasmin when plasminogen is bound to the fibrin clot; (2) kallikrein (formed from prekallikrein by the action of F XIIa) converts plasminogen to plasmin (Fig. 1.39).

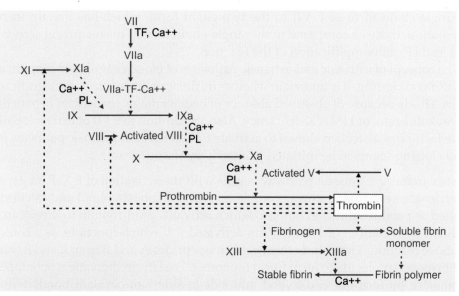

Figure 1.37: Physiologic mechanism of coagulation: Under physiologic conditions *in vivo*, tissue factor (TF) and F VIIa initiate coagulation. F VIIa-TF complex activates F IX to F IXa, which then activates F X to F Xa. F Xa in turn activates prothrombin to thrombin, which converts fibrinogen to fibrin. If stimulus for thrombin formation is strong enough, coagulation is maintained through the activation of F XI by thrombin. Thrombin also activates F VIII, F V, and F XIII and plays a central role in coagulation

Inhibitors of fibrinolysis: These include (1) α2-antiplasmin which combines rapidly with plasmin in circulation to form plasmin-antiplasmin complex; (2) α2-macroglobulin which inhibits plasmin; (3) plasminogen activator inhibitors PAI-1 and PAI-2 released from endothelial cells which neutralize tPA and (4) thrombin-activated fibrinolytic inhibitor (TAFI) which cleaves specific fibrin lysine residues, thus removing binding sites for plasminogen and tPA.

Fibrinogen degradation products: Plasmin initially attacks α chains of the fibrinogen molecule and removes small fragments designated as A, B, and C from the C-terminals of the Aα chains. This is followed by degradation of Bβ chains with removal of first 42 amino acids. This leads to the formation of a large fragment X that still retains fibrinopeptide A. The next cleavage involves all the three chains in an asymmetrical manner with the release of fragment Y and fragment D. Fragment Y is rapidly degraded by plasmin liberating two fragments D and E (Fig. 1.40).

Fibrin degradation products: Degradation of cross-linked fibrin is different from that of fibrinogen. Firstly, the fibrin degradation products are different because of the presence of covalent bonding. Thus, the characteristic fragments are oligomers of X and Y, D-dimer, D2E complex, and Y-D complex. Secondly, fibrin degradation is slower due to the presence of cross-linkages (Fig. 1.41)

Effects of FDPs: Normally, the FDPs are cleared from the circulation by macrophages of the reticuloendothelial system. However, when FDPs increase they have a potent

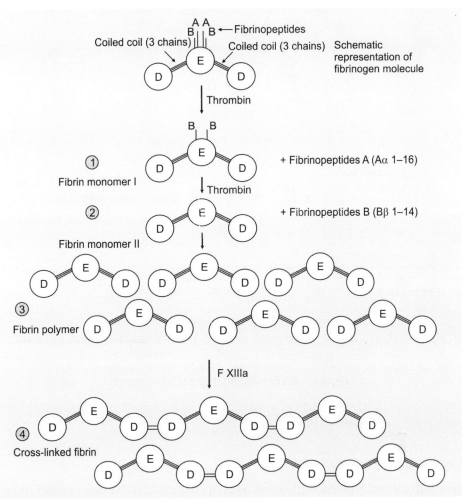

Figure 1.38: Steps in the formation of cross-linked fibrin. 1 and 2: Cleaving of fibrinopeptides from fibrinogen by thrombin to form fibrin monomers. 3: Spontaneous polymerisation of fibrin monomers. 4: Cross-linking of fibrin monomers mediated by F XIIIa. During this stage, covalent bonds form mainly between adjacent γ chains. For simplicity Aα chains are not shown

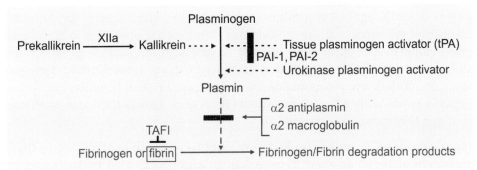

Figure 1.39: The fibrinolytic system

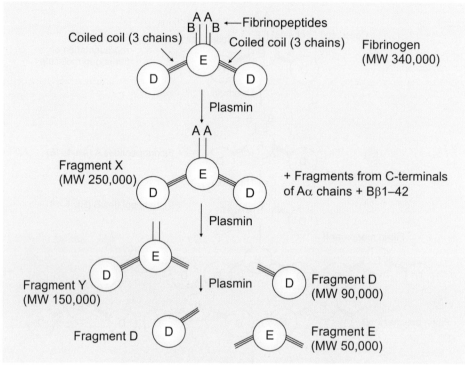

Figure 1.40: Fibrinogen degradation products

anticoagulant action in the form of inhibition of polymerisation of fibrin, antithrombin activity, and impairment of platelet function.

Natural Inhibitors of Coagulation

There are three main physiologic inhibitors of coagulation that are present in normal plasma. These are antithrombin (previously called antithrombin III), protein C and protein S system, and tissue factor pathway inhibitor (Fig. 1.42).

Antithrombin (AT): AT is the most important physiologic inhibitor of coagulation. This is a single chain glycoprotein synthesized by the liver. AT possesses inhibitory activity principally against thrombin and to a lesser extent against factors Xa, XIa, XIIa, and IXa. AT binds with thrombin and other serine proteases to form a stable complex. Heparin-like substances present on the luminal surface of blood vessels promote activity of AT. The importance of AT as a natural anticoagulant derives from the fact that AT deficiency is associated with increased risk of thrombosis.

Heparin binds with AT and potentiates its action. This is the basis of efficacy of heparin as a therapeutic anticoagulant.

Protein C: Protein C is a vitamin K-dependent glycoprotein synthesized in the liver. Protein C circulates in an inert zymogen form and is activated by thrombin in the

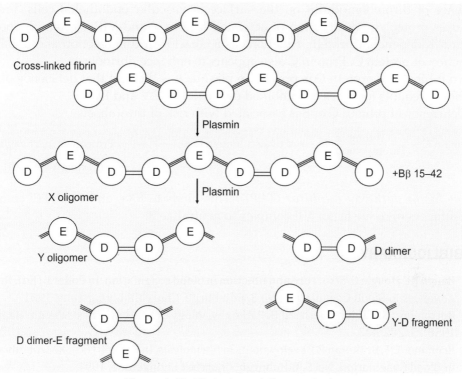

Figure 1.41: Fibrin degradation products

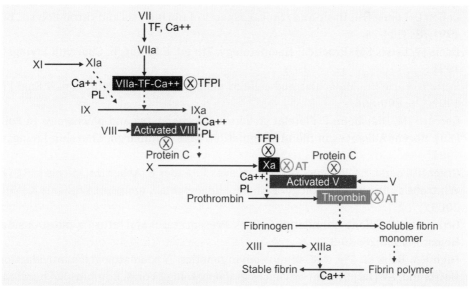

Figure 1.42: Natural inhibitors of coagulation: These include (1) tissue factor pathway inhibitor (TFPI) (binds to F Xa and then to VIIa-TF-Ca++ complex), (2) antithrombin (AT) (inhibits mainly thrombin and F Xa) and (3) protein C pathway (inactivates activated forms of F VIII and F V)

presence of thrombomodulin on the surface of vascular endothelial cells. Protein C causes proteolytic destruction of activated factors V and VIII. Protein S, another vitamin K-dependent protein, functions as a cofactor in this reaction and enhances the action of protein C. Protein C also appears to enhance fibrinolysis.

An inhibitor of protein C is present in plasma; it is thought that deficiency of this inhibitor accounts for cases of combined deficiency of F V and FVIII.

Deficiency of protein C or S is associated with risk of thrombosis.

$$\text{Protein C} \xrightarrow[\text{Thrombomodulin}]{\text{Thrombin}} \text{Activated protein C} \xrightarrow{\text{Protein S}} \text{Proteolytic inactivation of factors V and VIII}$$

Tissue factor pathway inhibitor (TFPI): This binds to FXa, and FXa-TFPI complex then attaches to tissue factor-VII complex to neutralize it.

❏ BIBLIOGRAPHY

1. Baugh RF, Hougie C. Structure and function in blood coagulation. In Poller L (Ed): Recent Advances in Blood Coagulation. No.3. Edinburgh. Churchill Livingstone. 1981.
2. Bottomley SS, Muller-Eberhard U. Pathophysiology of heme synthesis. Semin Hematol. 1988;25: 282-302.
3. Brommer EJP, Brakman P. Developments in fibrinolysis. In Poller L (Ed): Recent Advances in Blood Coagulation. No. 5. Edinburgh. Churchill Livingstone, 1991.
4. Cannistra SA, Griffin JD. Regulation of the production and function of granulocytes and monocytes. Semin Hematol. 1988;25: 173-88.
5. Collen D, Lijnen HR. Basic and clinical aspects of fibrinolysis and thrombolysis. Blood. 1991;78: 3114-24.
6. Dacie JV, Lewis SM. Practical Haematology. 7th ed. Edinburgh. Churchill Livingstone. 1991.
7. Furie B, Furie BC. Molecular and cellular biology of blood coagulation. N Engl J Med. 1992;326: 800-806.
8. Gerrard JM, Didisheim P. Platelet structure, biochemistry and physiology. In Poller L (Ed): Recent Advances in Blood Coagulation. No.3. Edinburgh. Churchill Livingstone. 1981.
9. Greer JP, Foerster J, Rodgers GM, Paraskevas F, Glader B, Arber DA, Means Jr RT (Eds): Wintrobe's clinical hematology. 12th ed. Philadelphia. Lippincott Williams & Wilkins. 2009.
10. Groopman JE. Colony-stimulating factors: Present status and future applications. Semin Hematol. 1988;25: 30-37.
11. High KA, Benz EJ. The ABC of molecular genetics. A haematologist's introduction. In Hoffbrand, AV (Ed): Recent Advances in Haematology Vol. 4. Edinburgh. Churchill Livingstone. 1985.
12. Holmsen H. Platelet metabolism and activation. Semin Hematol. 1985;22: 219-40.

13.   Imboden JB, Jr. T lymphocytes and natural killer cells. In Stites DP, Terr AL, Parslow TG (Eds): Basic and Clinical Immunology. 8th ed. Connecticut. Appleton and Lange. 1994.

14.   Johnston RB. Monocytes and macrophages. N Engl J Med. 1988;318: 747-752.

15.   Kumar V, Abbas AK, Fausto N, Aster JC: Robbins and Cotran Pathologic basis of disease. 8th Ed. Philadelphia. Saunders Elsevier. 2010.

16.   Lenting PJ, van Mourik JA, Mertens K. The life cycle of coagulation factor VIII in view of its structure and function. Blood. 1998;92: 3983-96.

17.   McPherson RA, Pincus MR (Eds): Henry's clinical diagnosis and management by laboratory methods. 21st ed. Philadelphia. Elsevier Saunders. 2007.

18.   Mohandas N, Chasis JA. Red blood cell deformability, membrane material properties and shape: Regulation by transmembrane, skeletal, and cytosolic proteins and lipids. Semin Hematol. 1993;30: 171-92.

19.   Nathan CF. Secretory products of macrophages. J Clin Invest. 1987;79: 319-26.

20.   Ogston D, Bennett B. Blood coagulation mechanism. In Poller L (Ed): Recent Advances in Blood Coaguation. No.5. Edinburgh. Churchill Livingstone. 1991.

21.   Parslow TG. Immunoglobulin genes, B cells, and the humoral immune response. In Stites DP, Terr AL, Parslow TG (Eds): Basic and Clinical Immunology. 8th ed. Connecticut. Appleton and Lange. 1994.

22.   Sixma JJ. The haemostatic plug. In Poller L (Ed): Recent Advances in Blood Coagulation. No. 3. Edinburgh. Churchill Livingstone. 1981.

23.   Spangrude GJ. Biologic and clinical aspects of hematopoietic stem cells. Annu Rev Med. 1994;45: 93-104.

24.   Swerdlow SH, Campo E, Harris NL, Jaffe ES, Pileri SA, Stein H, Thiele J, Vardiman JW (Eds): WHO classification of tumours of haematopoietic and lymphoid tissues. 4th ed. Lyon. International Agency for Research on Cancer. 2008.

25.   Van der Valk P, Herman CJ. Leucocyte functions. Lab Invest. 1987;56: 127-37.

26.   Williams D and Nathan DG. Introduction: The molecular biology of hematopoiesis. Semin Hematol. 1991;28: 114-116.

CHAPTER

2

Approach to Diagnosis of Anaemias

Anaemia is defined as a reduction in the concentration of circulating haemoglobin or oxygen-carrying capacity of blood below the level that is expected for healthy persons of same age and sex in the same environment. Normal haemoglobin (and packed cell volume or PCV) levels are given in Table 2.1. Anaemia exists if haemoglobin or PCV level is below the lower limit of normal for the particular age and sex.

The normal haemoglobin level depends upon age and sex of the individual and the environment. The difference of haemoglobin level between sexes is related to the androgens that have stimulatory effect on erythropoiesis. The lower level of haemoglobin during pregnancy as compared to the nonpregnant state is due to haemodilution caused by expansion of plasma volume. The normal haemoglobin level in newborn period is highest; subsequently haemoglobin level falls and reaches minimum level by 2 months of age. Haemoglobin level reaches adult levels by puberty. Persons living at high altitudes who are exposed to low oxygen tensions have a higher haemoglobin concentration than persons living at sea level.

Table 2.1: Normal levels of haemoglobin and packed cell volume

Age/Sex	Haemoglobin (g/dl)	PCV (%)
Adult males	13–17	40–50
Adult females (nonpregnant)	12–15	38–45
Adult females (pregnant)	11–14	36–42
Children, 6–12 years	11.5–15.5	37–46
Children, 6 months–6 years	11–14	36–42
Infants, 2–6 months	9.5–14	32–42
Newborns	13.6–19.6	44–60

❏ APPROACH TO DIAGNOSIS

Anaemia can result from a variety of causes. Investigations in a case of anaemia should be directed towards answering following questions—(1) Is anaemia present and if so, what is its severity? (2) What is the cause of anaemia? In most cases, presence of anaemia can be established and its cause determined with the help of clinical findings and a few simple investigations.

Establishing the Presence and Severity of Anaemia

The tests used for this purpose are estimation of **haemoglobin concentration and packed cell volume.** The results of these tests are influenced by plasma volume. Increase in plasma volume with red cell count remaining normal causes haemodilution and measurement of haemoglobin or packed cell volume yields a subnormal result; this is known as "spurious" or "pseudo" anaemia and occurs in 3rd trimester of pregnancy (due to rise in plasma volume), splenomegaly (due to pooling of red cells in spleen), congestive cardiac failure (due to fluid retention), and paraproteinaemias (rise in globulins).

Determination of Haemoglobin Concentration

Various methods are available for estimation of haemoglobin (Table 2.2). Out of these, **cyanmethaemoglobin method is the most accurate** and is recommended by the International Committee for Standardization in Haematology. In this method a specified

Table 2.2: Methods for estimation of haemoglobin

Colorimetric methods
Colour comparison is made between the known standard and the test sample, either visually or by photoelectric colorimeter

- *Visual methods*
  - **Tallqvist blotting paper method:** Highly inaccurate and now obsolete
  - **Sahli's acid haematin method:** Inaccurate
  - **WHO haemoglobin colour scale:** Simple, inexpensive, and reliable; especially suitable for those laboratories where photoelectric colorimeter is not available
- *Methods using photoelectric colorimeter*
  - **Cyanmethaemoglobin method:** Most accurate and recommended method
  - **Oxyhaemoglobin method:** Reliable method; however, no stable standard is available
  - **Alkaline haematin method:** Accurate method

Gasometric method
Oxygen-carrying capacity of blood is measured in van Slyke apparatus; not suitable for routine use

Chemical method
Iron content of blood is measured and value of haemoglobin is calculated indirectly; tedious and time-consuming method

Specific gravity method
Simple, rapid and inexpensive method in which a rough estimate of haemoglobin is obtained from specific gravity of blood; used for mass screening like selection of blood donors.

amount of blood is mixed with a solution containing potassium ferricyanide and potassium cyanide (Drabkin's solution); potassium ferricyanide converts haemoglobin to methaemoglobin while methaemoglobin combines with potassium cyanide to form cyanmethaemoglobin. Most forms of haemoglobins present in blood (e.g. oxyhaemoglobin, carboxyhaemoglobin, methaemoglobin, etc.) except sulfhaemoglobin are completely converted to a single compound, cyanmethaemoglobin. After completion of the reaction, absorbance of the solution is measured in a spectrophotometer at 540 nm. To obtain the haemoglobin concentration of the unknown sample, its absorbance is compared with that of the standard cyanmethaemoglobin solution the haemoglobin concentration of which is known. The absorbance can be converted to haemoglobin concentration by using a formula or from previously constructed calibration graph or table.

Anaemia can be graded according to haemoglobin concentration as shown in Box 2.1.

Determination of Packed Cell Volume or PCV (Haematocrit)

PCV is the volume of packed red cells obtained after centrifugation of a sample of anticoagulated venous or capillary blood. It is expressed either as a percentage of volume of whole blood or as a decimal fraction.

Uses of PCV are: (i) Detection of anaemia and polycythaemia; PCV is normally about three times the haemoglobin concentration when the latter is expressed in g/dl (Box 2.2); (ii) Calculation of red cell indices such as mean cell volume (MCV) and mean cell haemoglobin concentration (MCHC); (iii) checking the accuracy of haemoglobin value.

There are two methods for determining PCV—macromethod (Wintrobe method) and micromethod (microhaematocrit method).

Wintrobe method: Anticoagulated whole blood is centrifuged in a Wintrobe tube at 2300 G for 30 minutes to pack the red cells. The level of the column of the red cells is directly read from the tube. Wintrobe tube is 110 mm in length with 3 mm internal bore, is marked at every 1 mm upto 100 and has a capacity for about 1 ml of blood. After centrifugation, three layers can be distinguished—a column of straw-coloured plasma

---

Box 2.1   Grading of anaemia

- Mild: Haemoglobin from lower limit of normal to 10.0 g/dl
- Moderate: 10.0–7.0 g/dl
- Severe: < 7.0 g/dl

Box 2.2   "Rule of 3"

- Red cell count in millions/cmm × 3= Haemoglobin in g/dl
- Haemoglobin in g/dl × 3 = PCV in %

Rule of 3 is used as a mathematical check by clinicians and technologists

Rule of 3 applies mainly to normocytic normochromic specimens

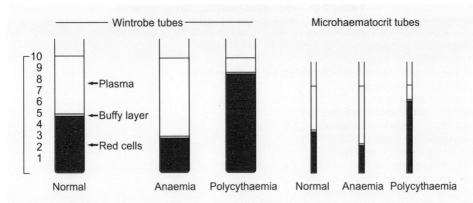

Figure 2.1: Packed cell volume showing comparison of normal, anaemic, and polycythaemic blood samples. Red: Column of red cells; Grey: Buffy coat layer; Yellow: Column of plasma

at the top, a thin greyish-layer of white cells and platelets in the middle ("buffy layer"), and a column of red cells at the bottom (Fig. 2.1). Sometimes additional information can be derived by observing the colour of the plasma (pink in haemolysis, yellow in the presence of jaundice, colourless in iron deficiency anaemia) and the thickness of the buffy layer (thick buffy layer indicates leucocytosis, thrombocytosis, or leukaemia). Smears can also be prepared from the buffy coat layer for demonstration of blast cells and for malaria parasites (if they are few in number in blood).

Microhaematocrit method: This method is simple, rapid, and needs only a small quantity of blood. Micromethod, however, requires microhaematocrit centrifuge (or table top centrifuge with microhaematocrit head) and capillary haematocrit tubes (75 mm long with a 1 mm bore). Two types of capillary haematocrit tubes are available: anticoagulated (coated with heparin so that capillary blood can be directly collected) and plain (without anticoagulant so that anticoagulated blood is needed). The capillary tube is filled about 3/4th with blood, sealed at one end, and centrifuged in a microhaematocrit centrifuge at high speed for 5 minutes. The result is derived by using microhaematocrit tube reading device or an arithmetic graph paper.

Determining the Cause of Anaemia

When the presence of anaemia is established, the next step is to determine the cause of anaemia. Various causes of anaemia are listed in Table 2.3. Main causes of anaemia in India are shown in Box 2.3. Ascertaining the underlying cause of anaemia requires correlation of clinical findings with results of laboratory investigations.

Box 2.3	Important causes of anaemia in India

- Nutritional deficiency: Iron, folate, less commonly vitamin B_{12}
- Infections: Tuberculosis, malaria, kala-azar, HIV infection/AIDS, hookworm
- Inherited anaemias: Thalassaemias, sickle cell disorders, glucose-6-phosphate dehydrogenase deficiency
- Blood loss: Obstetrical problems

Table 2.3: Aetiological classification of anaemia

Anaemias due to impaired red cell production

1. Anaemias due to deficiency of nutrients
   - Iron deficiency anaemia
   - Megaloblastic anaemia due to deficiency of folate or vitamin B_{12}
2. Anaemia of chronic disease
3. Sideroblastic anaemia
4. Aplastic anaemia and related disorders
5. Anaemia of chronic renal disease
6. Anaemia of liver disease
7. Anaemia in endocrine disorders
8. Myelophthisic anaemia (Anaemia due to replacement of marrow by metastatic carcinoma, leukaemia, lymphoma, infections, storage disorders, etc.)
9. Congenital dyserythropoietic anaemia

Anaemias due to excessive red cell destruction (Haemolytic anaemias)	
Abnormality intrinsic to red cells	*Abnormality extrinsic to red cells*

1. **Defects in red cell membrane**
  • Hereditary spherocytosis
  • Hereditary elliptocytosis
	1. **Immune haemolytic anaemias**
	  • Autoimmune
	  • Alloimmune
	  • Drug-induced

2. **Defects in haemoglobin**
  • Quantitative: Thalassaemias
  • Qualitative: Sickle-cell disease; Haemoglobin D, E, or C disease
	2. **Mechanical haemolytic anaemia**
	  • Microangiopathic
	  • Cardiac
	  • March haemoglobinuria

3. **Defects in enzymes**
  • Glucose-6-phosphate dehydrogenase deficiency
  • Pyruvate kinase deficiency
	3. **Direct action of physical, chemical, or infectious agents**

	4. **Hypersplenism**

Anaemias due to excess blood loss

Clinical Evaluation

The symptoms and signs in an anaemic patient may result from anaemia *per se* and the underlying disorder causing anaemia. The **symptoms and signs of anaemia** include easy fatiguability, effort dyspnoea, tachycardia, and pallor. In severe cases, congestive cardiac failure can develop. The associated symptomatology may point towards the probable diagnosis and suggest the direction for laboratory investigation. A **history of chronic blood loss** such as menorrhagia or haemorrhoids suggests iron deficiency as the cause of anaemia. Anaemia manifesting during **pregnancy** is usually nutritional due to deficiency of folate and iron. An intense and abnormal desire to eat strange substances such as starch or earth (pica) is a peculiar feature of iron deficiency. When a **chronic alcoholic** presents with anaemia, aetiological considerations include vitamin B_{12} and folate deficiency, iron deficiency secondary to bleeding, chronic liver disease, and sideroblastic anaemia. History of malabsorption such as in coeliac disease and tropical sprue indicates combined deficiency of folate, vitamin B_{12}, and iron. Drugs can cause various types of anaemias such as hypoplastic anaemia (e.g. cytotoxic

---

Box 2.4   Prevalence of hereditary haemolytic anaemia

- β thalassaemias: Mediterranean countries, Africa, Middle East, India (North India especially in Sindhis, Bhanushalis, Lohanas, Jains), Pakistan, South-East Asia
- α thalassaemias: Southeast Asia
- Sickle cell disorders: Africa, Middle East, Central and Southern India
- Haemoglobin D disease: North India (Punjab)
- Haemoglobin E disease: South-East Asia, East India (Bengal, Assam)
- Hereditary spherocytosis: Northern European descent
- Glucose-6-phosphate dehydrogenase (G6PD) deficiency: Africa, Middle East, India (especially in Parsees)

---

drugs, chloramphenicol, phenylbutazone), megaloblastic anaemia (e.g. methotrexate, trimethoprim, anticonvulsants), iron deficiency anaemia (e.g. aspirin secondary to gastric blood loss), and haemolytic anaemia (e.g. antimalarials, penicillins, methyldopa). A detailed drug history is therefore essential. A history of jaundice or gallstones in the patient and in a close relative may point towards inherited haemolytic anaemia. In some cases, **primary underlying disease** may be responsible for anaemia, e.g. collagen vascular disease, malignancy, chronic infection, acquired immunodeficiency syndrome, cirrhosis of liver, chronic renal disease, or endocrine disorder. Sometimes population studies conducted in the past can provide valuable information regarding the **prevalent form of anaemia in a geographic area or in a particular community**. This applies particularly to sickle cell anaemia, thalassaemia, and G6PD deficiency (Box 2.4).

Laboratory Evaluation

Initial investigations to define the underlying cause of anaemia include examination of peripheral blood smear, reticulocyte count, and red cell indices. Depending on the results of these studies further specialized laboratory procedures may be carried out to arrive at a definitive diagnosis such as bone marrow examination, determination of serum iron and total iron binding capacity, haemoglobin electrophoresis, etc.

Examination of peripheral blood smear: Peripheral blood smear or film provides important information regarding the underlying cause of anaemia. Peripheral blood smear is prepared by spreading a drop of capillary or venous blood across a glass slide and staining it with a Romanowsky stain. A well-made blood film should show three zones—thick area or the 'head', 'body', and the thin portion or the 'tail' of the smear. The smear should be smooth and uniform in appearance with gradual transition from thick to thin portion. It should not cover the entire area of the slide.

The blood film should be examined in an orderly manner under low and high powers and oil immersion lens for red cell morphology, presence of nucleated red cells, approximate number of white blood cells, differential leucocyte count, abnormal white blood cells, parasites, and adequacy of platelets. Valuable information regarding the cause of anaemia can be obtained by observing the red cell morphology (Fig. 2.2 and Box 2.5).

Reticulocyte count: Reticulocytes are young red cells that contain RNA remnants. RNA stains with supravital dyes such as brilliant cresyl blue or new methylene blue

---

Box 2.5   Red cell terminology

- *Normocytic normochromic:* Red cells with normal size and colour (i.e. normal haemoglobin content); 7–8 μ size; pink with small area of central pallor (1/3rd the diameter of red cell)
- *Anisocytosis:* Significant variation in size of red cells
- *Poikilocytosis:* Significant variation in shape of red cells; both aniso- and poikilocytosis are nonspecific features of a variety of anaemias
- *Microcytic hypochromic:* Red cells smaller than normal with increased area of central pallor due to deficiency of haemoglobin
- *Macrocytic:* Red cells larger in size than normal; may be round or oval
- *Sickle cells:* Elongated and narrow cells with one or both ends curved and pointed
- *Spherocytes:* Small and densely staining red cells without central area of pallor
- *Target cells:* Cells with accumulation of haemoglobin in centre and periphery with clear intervening area producing a bull's eye or target-like appearance
- *Schistocytes:* Irregular fragmented cells appearing as helmet-shaped and triangular
- *Burr cells:* Cells with many spiny, small, regularly spaced projections on surface
- *Tear drop red cells:* Cells with a tapering drop-like shape
- *Polychromatic red cells:* Slightly larger red cells with faint blue-grey tint due to presence of ribosomal RNA
- *Basophilic stippling (punctate basophilia):* Presence of fine (megaloblastic anaemia) or coarse (lead poisoning) purple-blue granules (representing ribosomal aggregates) in red cells
- *Howell-Jolly bodies:* Round, purple nuclear remnants in red cells
- *Rouleaux:* Arrangement of red cells like a stack of coins
- *Dimorphic red cells:* Presence of two different populations of red cells, e.g. macrocytic and hypochromic, normocytic and hypochromic, etc. Seen in sideroblastic anaemia, partially treated anaemia, myelodysplasia, and post-blood transfusion

---

with formation of blue precipitates of granules or filaments (Fig. 2.3). After staining, smears are made on a glass slide, reticulocytes are counted among 1,000 red cells, and the result is expressed as a percentage. **Reticulocyte count is performed to assess erythropoietic activity of the bone marrow in a case of anaemia.** In anaemia due to decreased red cell production or ineffective erythropoiesis, reticulocyte count is low. In anaemia with effective red cell production, reticulocyte count is high.

Measures of reticulocytes: Reticulocyte count can be expressed in various ways as follows:

1. *Reticulocyte count:* This is the number of reticulocytes counted amongst 1000 red cells and expressed as a percentage.

$$\text{Reticulocyte count} = \frac{\text{Reticulocytes counted}}{\text{Number of red cells}} \times 100$$

In adults and children, the normal reticulocyte count is 0.5 to 2.5%. In newborns, reticulocyte count is 2 to 5%.

2. *Corrected reticulocyte count:* This is the reticulocyte count corrected for the degree of anaemia.

$$\text{Corrected reticulocyte} = \frac{\text{Reticulocyte count} \times \text{PCV of patient in \%}}{\text{Average PCV for age}}$$

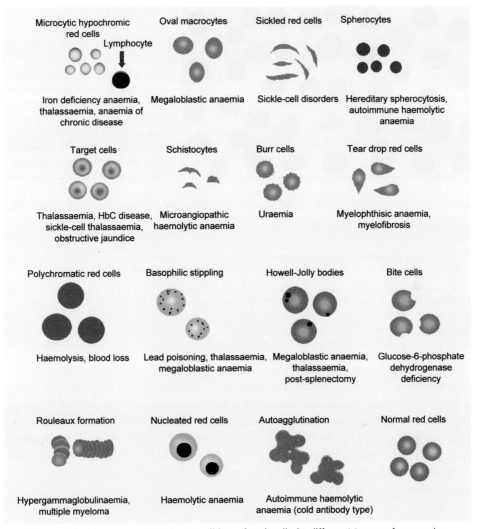

Figure 2.2: Morphological abnormalities of red cells in different types of anaemias. Size of red cells is compared with the nucleus of a small lymphocyte (7 μ).

3. *Absolute reticulocyte count:* This is the number of reticulocytes in 1 cmm of blood.

$$\text{Absolute reticulocyte count} = \frac{\text{Reticulocyte percentage} \times \text{Red cell count}}{\text{in million/cmm}}$$

Normal absolute reticulocyte count is 50,000 to 100,000/cmm.

4. *Reticulocyte production index:* After their formation in bone marrow the reticulocytes normally spend about 2 days in bone marrow and one day in peripheral blood before they become fully mature red cells. However in severe haemolytic anaemia and acute blood loss, reticulocytes are released prematurely in peripheral circulation where they require more time (2 days) for maturation. This results in doubling of reticulocytes in blood. In such cases to avoid the overestimation of daily red

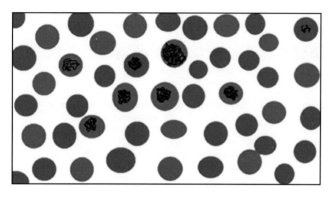

Figure 2.3: Reticulocytes stained with a supravital stain. Following supravital staining, any non-nucleated red cell containing 2 or more granules of blue-stained material is considered as a reticulocyte. The blue-stained material represents ribosomal RNA and is more in immature reticulocytes

cell production and to get idea about actual erythropoietic activity, reticulocyte production index is derived.

$$\text{Reticulocyte production index} = \frac{\text{Corrected reticulocyte count}}{\text{Maturation time in days}}$$

Maturation times in days according to PCV are:
- PCV > 35%: 1
- PCV 25–35%: 1.5
- PCV 15–25%: 2
- PCV 5–15%: 2.5

Reticulocytes should ideally be reported as absolute count or as corrected reticulocyte count for proper assessment of bone marrow response (low or appropriate) to anaemia. For example, a reticulocyte count of 1% in a patient with 42% PCV and a reticulocyte count of 1% in another patient with 20% PCV may both appear to be normal. However, when corrected for PCV, the corrected reticulocyte counts are respectively 0.9% (normal, indicating normal erythropoietic activity) and 0.3% (low, indicating inadequate erythropoietic activity).

Causes of reticulocytosis:
- Acute blood loss
- Haemolytic anaemia
- Response to specific therapy in nutritional anaemias.

Causes of reticulocytopaenia:
- Deficient red cell production
  - Iron deficiency anaemia
  - Anaemia of chronic disease
  - Aplastic anaemia
  - Anaemia due to marrow infiltration (leukaemia, lymphoma, metastatic cancer).
- Ineffective erythropoiesis
  - Megaloblastic anaemia.

Classification of anaemias according to the reticulocyte response is presented in Table 2.4.

Table 2.4: Classification of anaemia according to the reticulocyte response

Reticulocyte response	Reticulocyte production index (Absolute reticulocyte count)	Causes
1. Appropriate for the degree of anaemia	≥ 2% (>100,000/μl)	Hyperproliferative anaemias (blood loss, haemolytic anaemias)
2. Inappropriately low for the degree of anaemia	< 2% (<75,000/μl)	Hypoproliferative anaemias (iron deficiency anaemia, megaloblastic anaemia, anaemia of chronic disease, thalassaemia, endocrine diseases, sideroblastic anaemia, aplastic anaemia, myelodysplasia)

Table 2.5: Morphological classification of anaemias

Macrocytic anaemias (MCV > 100 fl)	Microcytic anaemias (MCV < 80 fl)	Normocytic anaemias (MCV 80–100 fl)
Megaloblastic anaemia	Iron deficiency anaemia	Reticulocyte production normal
Nonmegaloblastic anaemia	Thalassaemias	• Recent blood loss
• Liver disease	Sideroblastic anaemia	• Haemolytic anaemia
• Haemolytic anaemia	Anaemia of chronic disease	Reticulocyte production deficient
• Alcoholism		• Aplastic anaemia
• Myelodysplastic syndrome		• Myelophthisic anaemia
• Hypothyroidism		• Chronic renal failure
		• Anaemia of chronic disease
		• Hypothyroidism

Red cell indices: Red cell indices are helpful in the morphological classification of anaemias (Table 2.5). They are derived from the values of red cell count, haemoglobin (Hb) concentration, and packed cell volume (PCV). Red cell indices obtained by manual methods are often inaccurate. Electronic haematology cell analysers more reliably perform them.

The normal ranges of red cell indices in adults are as follows:

MCV = 80–100 fl

MCH = 27–32 pg

MCHC= 32–36 g/dl

1. **Mean corpuscular volume (MCV):** MCV represents the average volume of a single red cell. It is expressed in femtolitres or fl (1 fl = 10^{-15} litres). MCV is performed manually as follows:

$$\text{Mean cell volume (MCV) in femtolitres} = \frac{\text{Packed cell volume in \%}}{\text{Red cell count in million per cmm}} \times 10$$

Anaemias are classified as normocytic, microcytic, and macrocytic on the basis of MCV. Since MCV measures average cell volume, it may be normal even though there is marked variation in size of red cells (anisocytosis). Some haematology cell analysers measure this degree of variation in size of red cells as red cell distribution width or RDW.

2. **Mean corpuscular haemoglobin (MCH):** This is the average amount of haemoglobin in each red cell. It is expressed in picograms or pg (1 pg = 10^{-12} of a gram) and is derived manually from the following formula:

$$\text{Mean cell haemoglobin (MCH) in picograms (pg)} = \frac{\text{Haemoglobin (g/dl)} \times 10}{\text{Red cell count in million/cmm}}$$

Low MCH is found in microcytic hypochromic anaemia, while high MCH in macrocytic anaemia.

3. **Mean corpuscular haemoglobin concentration (MCHC):** This represents the average concentration of haemoglobin in a given volume of packed red cells. It is expressed in grams/dl and calculated as follows:

$$\text{Mean cell haemoglobin concentration (MCHC) in g/dl} = \frac{\text{Hb (g/dl)}}{\text{PCV (\%)}} \times 100$$

Low MCHC occurs in microcytic hypochromic anaemia. An increase in MCHC occurs in hereditary spherocytosis.

4. **Red cell distribution width (RDW):** RDW is the degree of variation of red cell size and can be determined on some blood cell analysers. This parameter may sometimes be helpful for distinguishing iron deficiency anaemia from β thalassaemia minor (low MCV with high RDW: iron deficiency anaemia; low MCV with normal RDW: β thalassaemia minor).

Apart from morphological categorisation of anaemias, red cell indices are also helpful in differentiating mild iron deficiency anaemia from thalassaemia trait. In microcytic hypochromic anaemia of iron deficiency, MCV, MCH, and MCHC are low. In thalassaemia, MCV and MCH are low but MCHC is normal; target cells and basophilic stippling may also be present on peripheral blood smear. In severe anaemias, peripheral blood smear is sufficiently characteristic and red cell indices do not provide additional information. **The red cell indices are mainly helpful in detecting mild or early red cell abnormalities.**

Sometimes in a non-anaemic individual, increase or decrease of MCV is detected on a routine haemogram on electronic cell counters. This mandates further investigations, as elevation of MCV is an early indicator of deficiency of folate or vitamin B_{12}, myelodysplastic syndrome, and aplastic anaemia. Decreased MCV without anaemia occurs in thalassaemia trait.

Table 2.6: Differential diagnosis of anaemias based on MCV and RDW

MCV	RDW	Causes
1. Low	Normal	Thalassaemia carrier, anaemia of chronic disease
2. Low	High	Iron deficiency anaemia, haemoglobin H disease, sickle-cell-β thalassaemia
3. High	Normal	Myelodysplastic syndrome, aplastic anaemia
4. High	High	Megaloblastic anaemia, immune haemolytic anaemia
5. Normal	Normal	Anaemia of chronic disease, sickle-cell trait, hereditary spherocytosis
6. Normal	High	Early iron deficiency or megaloblastic anaemia, sideroblastic anaemia, myelofibrosis, sickle-cell anaemia

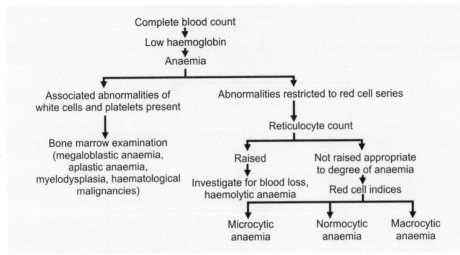

Figure 2.4: A simplified approach for evaluation of anaemia based on complete blood count

Differential diagnosis of anaemias based on MCV and RDW is given in Table 2.6.

Based on findings of complete blood count, a simplified approach for diagnosis of anaemias is presented in Figure 2.4.

Classification of Anaemias into Three Morphological Types

With the help of the information gained from the clinical data and these basic laboratory studies, further investigations can be undertaken to define the underlying cause of anaemia.

Evaluation of Macrocytic Anaemias

In macrocytic anaemia MCV is greater than 100 fl. In most cases, various causes of macrocytic anaemia can be differentiated on the basis of reticulocyte count and examinations of peripheral blood smear and bone marrow (Fig. 2.5).

Two types of macrocytosis can be distinguished on blood smear: round and oval. Their causes are listed in Box 2.6.

> **Box 2.6**   Oval and round macrocytosis
>
> **Oval macrocytosis**
> Megaloblastic anaemia due to deficiency of folate or vitamin B_{12}, Drug therapy (hydroxyurea, zidovudine, chemotherapy), myelodysplasia
>
> **Round macrocytosis**
> Alcoholism, liver disease, hypothyroidism

Typical features of megaloblastic anaemia due to deficiency of vitamin B_{12} or folate are—(1) Peripheral blood smear: macrocytic anaemia, leucopenia, and thrombocytopenia (pancytopenia); marked anisopoikilocytosis (variation in size and shape of red cells); Howell-Jolly bodies; and hypersegmented neutrophils (5 or more lobes in more than 5% neutrophils); (2) Bone marrow examination: Bone marrow examination confirms the diagnosis of megaloblastic anaemia. It shows ineffective erythropoiesis (increase in early erythroid precursors due to premature destruction of more mature erythroid

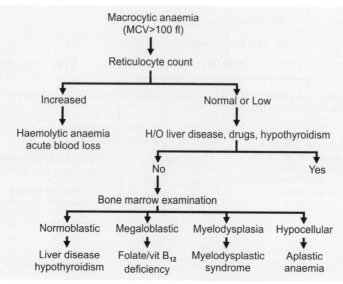

Figure 2.5: Evaluation of macrocytic anaemia

cells resulting in anaemia), megaloblasts with nuclear cytoplasmic asynchrony (nuclear chromatin is open or sieve-like while cytoplasm shows haemoglobinisation), and presence of giant bands and metamyelocytes. The distinction between folate and vitamin B_{12} deficiencies is based on estimation of serum and red cell folate and serum vitamin B_{12}. Therapeutic trial can also be given to distinguish between the two deficiencies (See chapter on megaloblastic anaemias).

Reticulocytosis in haemolytic anaemias is another cause of macrocytosis. As reticulocytes are larger than mature red cells MCV is increased. Chronic extravascular haemolysis is associated with mild icterus, variable splenomegaly, and unconjugated hyperbilirubinaemia. Peripheral smear shows polychromatic cells and normoblasts. Intravascular destruction of red cells is associated with haemoglobinaemia, haemoglobinuria, and haemosiderinuria.

Macrocytosis in liver disease is uniform, round, and is associated with target cells and abnormal liver function tests.

Most patients with myelodysplastic syndrome are elderly and have bi- or pancytopenia. Bone marrow examination reveals dysmyelopoiesis and sometimes abnormal localization of immature precursors.

In alcoholic patients, macrocytosis can occur in the absence of megaloblastic marrow or alcoholic cirrhosis. The mechanism is unknown.

Macrocytosis also occurs in pregnancy, newborns, during cytotoxic chemotherapy and in aplastic anaemia.

Evaluation of Microcytic Hypochromic Anaemia

Causes of microcytic hypochromic anaemia are listed in Table 2.5. The most common cause of microcytic hypochromic anaemia is iron deficiency. In early stages of iron deficiency, the red cell morphology is normal (normocytic and normochromic). With progressive fall in haemoglobin concentration, anaemia becomes microcytic and hypochromic. The degree of reduction in MCV and MCHC is proportional to the severity of anaemia. The biochemical parameters of iron deficiency are low serum iron, increased total iron binding capacity (TIBC), low transferrin saturation (<15%), and low serum ferritin (<12 μg/L). Bone marrow examination shows micronormoblastic erythropoiesis and on prussian blue staining absence of stainable iron.

In β thalassaemia major, severe anaemia develops during first few years of life that requires regular blood transfusion therapy. Hepatosplenomegaly is present. Peripheral blood smear shows marked anisopoikilocytosis, severe microcytosis and hypochromia, frequent target cells, basophilic stippling, and normoblasts. Haemoglobin electrophoresis shows predominance of HbF.

In β thalassaemia minor, anaemia is either absent or mild and peripheral blood smear shows prominent red cell abnormalities such as microcytosis, hypochromia, basophilic stippling, and target cells. Haemoglobin electrophoresis typically shows increase in HbA2 (3.5–7%).

Sideroblastic anaemia exhibits dimorphic population of red blood cells in peripheral blood (normocytic normochromic and microcytic hypochromic) and ringed sideroblasts in bone marrow.

Patient may be evaluated for anaemia of chronic disease if there is a history of chronic inflammation, chronic infection or malignant disease. The anaemia is usually mild to moderate, serum iron and total iron binding capacity are reduced, serum ferritin is elevated, bone marrow morphology is normal and storage iron in marrow is normal or increased. Erythrocyte sedimentation rate is raised and does not correspond with the degree of anaemia.

A scheme for evaluation of microcytic hypochromic anaemia is presented in Figure 2.6.

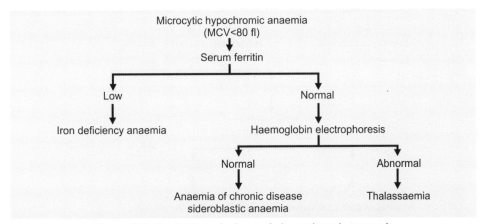

Figure 2.6: Evaluation of microcytic hypochromic anaemia

Evaluation of Normocytic Normochromic Anaemia

Depending upon bone marrow erythropoietic activity, normocytic anaemias are divided into two types (Fig. 2.7 and Table 2.5).

Normocytic anaemias with increased reticulocyte count—Two possible causes are acute blood loss and haemolysis.

1. *Acute posthaemorrhagic anaemia:* Acute blood loss can occur either externally or internally (e.g. haemothorax, fracture of hip). Significant blood loss occurring rapidly over a short period of time causes acute blood loss anaemia.

   After haemorrhage, to compensate for hypovolaemia, there is an increase in plasma volume due to movement of fluid from extravascular sites. This causes haemodilution and fall in haematocrit and haemoglobin levels. Anaemia does not become evident for 1 to 3 days after haemorrhage due to the time needed for restoration of plasma volume. Acute posthaemorrhagic anaemia is normocytic and normochromic. Stimulation of bone marrow by erythropoietin causes erythroid hyperplasia. Reticulocytosis begins about 3 days after the episode and reaches its peak around 9 to 10 days. During this period, nucleated red cells may appear in peripheral blood. Thrombocytosis and neutrophilic leucocytosis with mild shift to left (i.e. increase in immature white blood cells) are common findings. If haemorrhage is internal, destruction of extravasated red cells and catabolism of haem cause increase in serum bilirubin. If internal haemorrhage is not detected, these findings may be misinterpreted as indicative of haemolytic anaemia.

2. *Haemolytic anaemia:* Once the possibility of blood loss is ruled out, haemolytic anaemia is the prime consideration. Haemolytic anaemias are due to increased

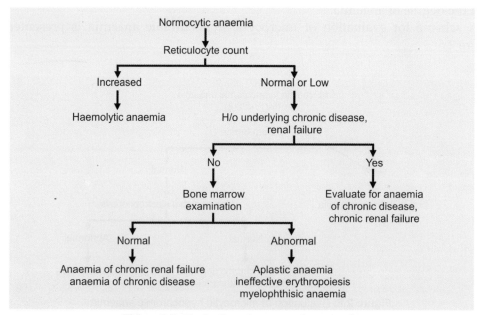

Figure 2.7: Evaluation of normocytic anaemia

rate of red cell destruction. When the red cell destruction is balanced by increased red cell production by the bone marrow, anaemia may not develop (compensated haemolysis). Haemolytic anaemia results when the bone marrow is unable to compensate for the increased rate of red cell destruction.

Tests to establish the presence of haemolysis: Various laboratory tests are used to detect haemolysis.

Red cell destruction can occur either extra- or intravascularly (Figs 2.8 and 2.9, and Table 2.7). **Extravascular destruction of red cells** by macrophages occurs mostly in spleen and liver. This leads to unconjugated hyperbilirubinaemia. Increased level of serum unconjugated bilirubin also occurs in other conditions such as ineffective erythropoiesis, internal haemorrhage, and certain liver disorders. It is, therefore, not a specific marker of haemolysis.

Serum lactate dehydrogenase level rises due to the release of the enzyme from the haemolysed red cells. Raised levels of lactate dehydrogenase are also observed in megaloblastic anaemia, haematologic malignancies, infarction of various organs, and skeletal muscle disorders. Thus increased lactate dehydrogenase alone is not a reliable marker of haemolysis.

Intravascular haemolysis causes release of haemoglobin in circulation. Free haemoglobin combines with haptoglobin in plasma and this complex is then cleared from the circulation by hepatocytes. This causes reduction in the level of plasma haptoglobin. Low plasma haptoglobin levels also occur in extravascular haemolysis,

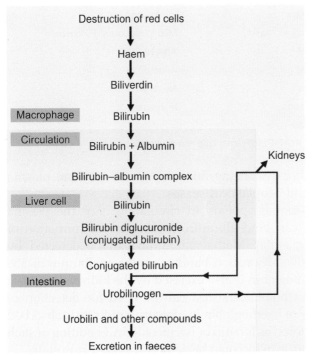

Figure 2.8: Mechanism of extravascular haemolysis in macrophages of reticuloendothelial system with formation of bilirubin

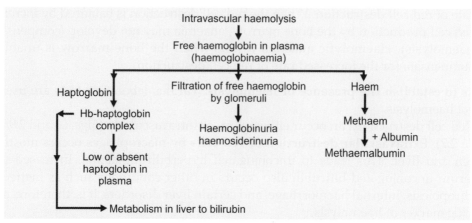

Figure 2.9: Intravascular haemolysis

Table 2.7: Comparison of extravascular and intravascular haemolysis

Parameter	Intravascular haemolysis	Extravascular haemolysis
1. Site of haemolysis	Within circulation	Macrophages of spleen, liver, bone marrow, etc.
2. Causes	Blackwater fever, incompatible blood transfusion, PNH, PCH	Haemoglobinopathies, hereditary haemolytic anaemias, autoimmune haemolytic anaemia
3. Splenomegaly	Absent	Present
4. Reticulocyte count	Increased	Increased
5. Indirect serum bilirubin	Increased	Increased
6. Plasma haemoglobin	Markedly increased	Mild to moderately-increased
7. Haemoglobin in urine	Present	Absent
8. Haemosiderin in urine	Present	Absent
9. Methaemalbumin (Schumm's test)	Positive	Negative
10. Serum haptoglobin	Decreased	Decreased
11. Serum LDH	Increased	Increased

PNH: Paroxysmal nocturnal haemoglobinuria; PCH: Paroxysmal cold haemoglobinuria

megaloblastic anaemia, and liver diseases. Being an acute phase reactant, plasma haptoglobin rises in inflammatory and neoplastic diseases.

Free haemoglobin (haemoglobinaemia) appears in circulation once the plasma haptoglobin disappears. Free haem can bind albumin, leading to the formation of methaemalbumin (methaemalbuminaemia). Methaemalbumin can be detected by Schumm's test (detection of distinctive absorption band of methaemalbumin at 558 nm on spectrophotometry). Free haemoglobin is also excreted by the kidneys resulting in haemoglobinuria. Benzidine or orthotoluidine test can be used for detection of haemoglobin in urine. Some quantity of haemoglobin in glomerular filtrate is absorbed by renal tubular epithelial cells and stored as ferritin or haemosiderin. Shedding of such cells in urine results in haemosiderinuria, which can be demonstrated by iron stain.

Excessive red cell destruction causes compensatory erythroid hyperplasia in the bone marrow. Enhanced erythropoietic activity is associated with reticulocytosis, presence of nucleated red cells, and increased numbers of white cells and platelets in peripheral blood. Young red cells with ribosomal remnants are called as polychromatic cells on Romanowsky stained smears and as reticulocytes when stained supravitally with brilliant cresyl blue or new methylene blue. Polychromatic cells are slightly larger than mature red cells and have a faint blue-grey tint due to the presence of residual RNA. Staining of haemoglobin with acid dyes and staining of RNA with basic dyes produces polychromasia. These signs of accelerated erythropoiesis are also seen in acute blood loss anaemia and recovery phase of nutritional anaemias. Features common to all haemolytic anaemias are presented in Box 2.7.

Box 2.7	Features common to all haemolytic anaemias

- Clinical: pallor, mild jaundice
- Laboratory:
  a. Biochemical: Increased unconjugated serum bilirubin, increased lactate dehydrogenase, decreased or absent serum haptoglobin
  b. Haematological: Increased reticulocyte count, polychromasia on blood smear, erythroid hyperplasia in bone marrow

No single test is specific for haemolysis and therefore a combination of laboratory tests is usually obtained to document the presence of haemolysis.

Tests to determine the cause of haemolysis: Various causes of haemolytic anaemia are listed in Table 2.3. Once the presence of haemolysis is established, further work-up is guided by the clinical information and peripheral smear findings (e.g. sickled forms, spherocytes). Some of the laboratory tests used for demonstrating the cause of haemolysis are–haemoglobin electrophoresis (for abnormal haemoglobins), test for glucose-6-phosphate dehydrogenase deficiency, osmotic fragility test for hereditary spherocytosis, antiglobulin (Coombs') test for immune haemolysis, isopropanol precipitation test for unstable haemoglobins, Ham's test for paroxysmal nocturnal haemoglobinuria, etc. These tests are discussed in respective chapters.

Approach to diagnosis of haemolytic anaemia involves establishing the presence of haemolysis followed by determination of the cause of haemolytic anaemia (Figs 2.10 and 2.11).

Normocytic anaemias with reduced reticulocyte count: This type of anaemia results from hypoproliferation in the bone marrow. Peripheral blood smear shows pancytopaenia with relative predominance of lymphocytes in aplastic anaemia. Leucoerythroblastic picture is a characteristic feature of myelophthisic anaemia.

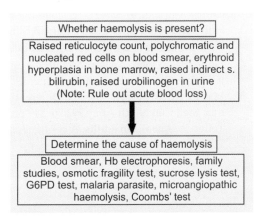

Figure 2.10: Evaluation of haemolytic anaemia

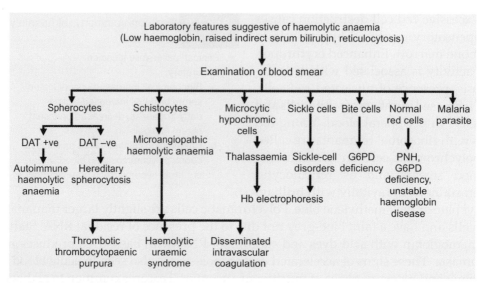

Figure 2.11: A simplified approach to diagnosis of haemolytic anaemias. Abbreviations: DAT: Direct antiglobulin test; G6PD: Glucose-6-phosphate dehydrogenase; PNH: Paroxysmal nocturnal haemoglobinuria; Hb: Haemoglobin

In both these conditions, bone marrow examination is essential for diagnosis. In renal failure, anaemia of chronic disorders, and hypothyroidism, clinical manifestations and ancillary laboratory studies (e.g. renal function tests) are helpful in establishing the diagnosis.

❑ BIBLIOGRAPHY

1. Colon-Otero G, Menke D, Hook CC. A practical approach to the differential diagnosis and evaluation of the adult patient with macrocytic anemia. Med Clin North Am. 1992;76: 581-597.
2. Hermiston ML, Mentzer WC: A practical approach to the evaluation of the anemic child. Pediatr Clin N Am. 2002;49:877-91.
3. Hoffman R, Benz EJ, Shattil SJ, Furie B, Silberstein LE, McGlave P, Heslop H (Eds): Hematology. Basic principles and practice. 5th ed. Philadelphia. Churchill Livingstone Elsevier. 2008.
4. Lindenbaum John. An approach to the anemias. In Wyngaarden JB, Smith LH Jr, and Bennett JC (Eds.): Cecil Textbook of Medicine. 19th ed. Philadelphia. W.B. Saunders Co. 1992.
5. Massey AC. Microcytic anemia: Differential diagnosis and management of iron deficiency anemia. Med Clin North Am. 1992;76: 549-66.
6. Tefferi A. Anemia in adults: A contemporary approach to diagnosis. Mayo Clin Proc. 2003;78: 1274-280.

CHAPTER

3

Anaemias due to Impaired Red Cell Production

IRON DEFICIENCY ANAEMIA

Deficiency of iron is the most common cause of anaemia worldwide. Iron deficiency is a state of low total body iron content. Iron deficiency anaemia develops when body iron stores are depleted, level of circulating iron is reduced, and there is insufficient iron available for erythropoiesis.

❑ NORMAL IRON METABOLISM

Normal iron metabolism is diagrammatically represented in Figure 3.1.

Iron Requirements

Normally in adult males only a small quantity of iron is lost by exfoliation of epithelial cells from gastrointestinal and urinary tracts and skin. This loss is about 1 mg per day, which needs to be matched by absorption of similar quantity of iron from food. Iron requirement is increased during adolescence due to growth. In females, iron need (and vulnerability to iron deficiency) is greater due to menstrual blood loss and increased demand for iron by the foetus during pregnancy.

The **daily iron requirement**, which varies according to the age and sex, is shown in Box 3.1.

Box 3.1	Daily iron requirements

- Infants upto 4 months: 0.5 mg
- Infants 5–12 months and children: 1 mg
- Menstruating women: 3 mg
- Pregnancy: 3–4 mg
- Adult men and postmenopausal women: 1 mg

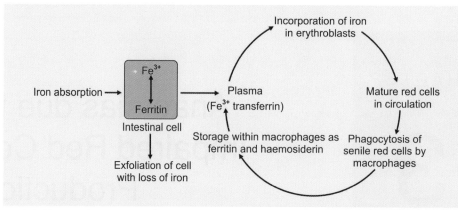

Figure 3.1: Normal iron metabolism. After absorption iron binds with transferrin and is transported to various tissues. In the bone marrow, iron is internalised by erythroblasts to form haem. Some iron is also stored as ferritin and such erythroblasts containing ferritin aggregates are called sideroblasts. Macrophages contain ferritin and haemosiderin derived mostly from catabolism of senescent red cells. Macrophage iron can be mobilised to circulating iron when required. Iron is lost from desquamation of intestinal cells

The normal daily diet (western) of an adult contains about 10 to 20 mg of iron. **To balance the daily iron loss of 1 mg, about 10% of the daily iron intake is absorbed.** Iron absorption is augmented in the presence of iron deficiency and decreased in conditions associated with iron overload. Women absorb more iron as compared to men due to increased iron demand caused by menstrual blood loss and pregnancy.

Body iron compartments: These are shown in Box 3.2.

Box 3.2	Body iron compartments
• Total body iron: 50 mg/kg body weight in males; 40 mg/kg body weight in females
• Haemoglobin iron: 65%
• Storage iron (ferritin, haemosiderin): 30%
• Transport iron (transferring-bound iron): 1%
• Tissue iron (myoglobin, enzymes): 4%

Dietary Sources of Iron

The main sources are meats, eggs, and green leafy vegetables. Milk is a poor source of iron.

Absorption of Iron

Iron absorption mostly occurs in duodenum and upper jejunum. Absorption is in ferrous form.

Meat contains haem iron about one-fourth of which is directly absorbed by intestinal epithelial cells. After cellular uptake haem is broken down and iron is released in the cytoplasm.

Green vegetables contain inorganic iron only 1 to 2% of which is absorbed. The absorption is usually in the ferrous form. In contrast to haem iron absorption of inorganic iron is affected by certain substances in the diet, i.e. tannates, phytates,

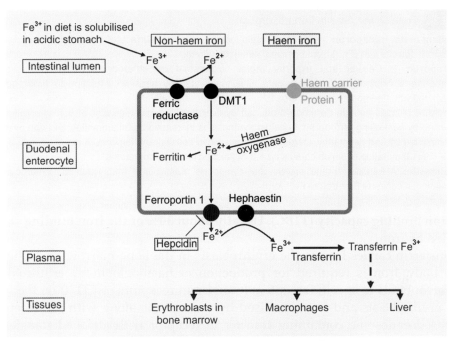

Figure 3.2: Mechanism of iron absorption

phosphates and certain drugs (antacids, proton pump inhibitors, tetracyclines) retard absorption while ascorbate and amino acids facilitate absorption.

Iron absorption mainly occurs in epithelial cells lining the villi close to gastroduodenal junction. Low pH of gastroduodenal contents facilitates dissolution of ingested iron. Ferric iron (Fe^{3+}) is converted to ferrous form (Fe^{2+}) by an enzyme (ferric reductase) located along the brush border of the epithelial cells. Iron is transported from the apical cell surface into the cell by DMT1 (divalent metal transporter 1). Inside the cell iron is either stored as ferritin or is transported to plasma. Iron is released from the cell through ferroportin 1 at the basolateral surface in Fe^{2+} state. Hepcidin regulates expression of ferroportin and is the central regulator of iron metabolism (Fig. 3.2). In plasma, iron is converted back to Fe^{3+} state by an enzyme (hephaestin) located on the basal border of the enterocyte. Fe^{3+} then combines with plasma transferrin and is transported to various body tissues.

Body iron stores and rate of erythropoiesis regulate iron absorption. Iron absorption is stimulated by ineffective erythropoiesis (as occurs in thalassaemia). Summary of proteins involved in iron absorption is presented in Box 3.3.

Transport of Iron

After absorption, iron is transported in plasma by transferrin. Transferrin is a glycoprotein that is produced in the liver. A molecule of transferrin can carry two atoms of iron. **The iron-binding sites of all the circulating transferrin constitute the**

Box 3.3   Proteins involved in iron absorption

- **Divalent metal transporter 1 (DMT1):** Protein located on apical surface of duodenal enterocytes that transports ferrous iron (Fe^{2+}) from intestinal lumen to cytosol
- **Ferroportin 1:** Cellular iron exporter protein expressed on enterocytes (basolateral surface), macrophages, hepatocytes, and placenta; it is inactivated by hepcidin; mutation in *FPN1* gene is associated with haemochromatosis type IV
- **Hepcidin:** A small peptide hormone produced by liver that is a key regulator of iron absorption and recycling by controlling ferroportin; hepcidin synthesis is increased by inflammation and iron overload, and inhibited by iron deficiency, increased erythropoietic activity, and hypoxia. It is encoded by *HAMP* gene (19q13) mutation of which causes type II or juvenile haemochromatosis
- **Hephaestin:** A transmembrane protein that transports dietary iron from duodenal enterocytes to circulation; it converts Fe^{2+} iron to Fe^{3+} form.

---

total iron binding capacity (TIBC). Usually about 30% of the iron binding sites are occupied by iron.

Transferrin carries iron to the erythroblasts in the bone marrow and other cells in the body. Iron is required for production of haemoglobin by erythroid cells. Transferrin binds to specific receptors (transferrin receptors or CD71) on the surface of the erythroblasts and is internalised by endocytosis along with the receptor. A specialised endosome containing transferrin receptor with attached transferrin is formed. A proton pump increases the pH within the endosome that causes release of iron into the cytoplasm. Transferrin devoid of iron (apotransferrin) and transferrin receptor are returned back to the cell surface for further cycles of iron transport and uptake (Fig. 3.3).

Incorporation of Iron in Erythroid Precursors

Once inside the cytoplasm of erythroid precursors, iron is inserted into protoporphyrin to form haem. This reaction occurs in the mitochondria of erythroid precursors and is mediated by the enzyme ferrochelatase. Iron is also stored as ferritin in lysosomes of erythroblasts. Erythroblasts which contain aggregates of ferritin are known as sideroblasts. Sideroblasts constitute about 25 to 30% of nucleated red cells in bone marrow.

Storage of iron

Storage iron is of two types: ferritin and haemosiderin.

Ferritin consists of a protein shell and an iron core. The protein portion is called as apoferritin that is spherical in shape. The central core of apoferritin consists of numerous ferric oxyhydroxide molecules. Ferritin is water-soluble and is readily mobilised for haemoglobin synthesis when required. **A direct relationship exists between amount of circulating ferritin and body iron stores.** Serum ferritin concentration decreases to less than 12 µg/L in iron deficiency anaemia and increases in iron overload disorders.

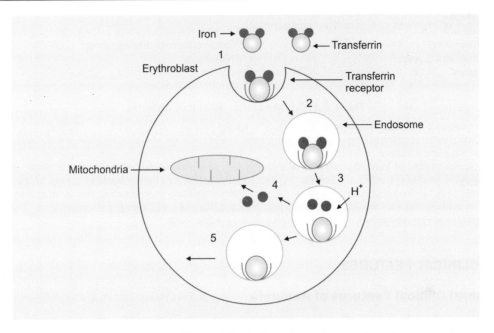

Figure 3.3: Uptake of iron in erythroblasts. (1) Binding of transferrin to transferrin receptor on cell surface. (2) Transferrin-transferrin receptor complex is internalised by endocytosis with formation of endosome. (3) Inside the endosome, pH is raised by proton pump which causes release of iron molecule from transferrin. (4) Iron is released in cytoplasm and reaches mitochondria where it is inserted into protoporphyrin ring to form haem. (5) Apotransferrin (transferrrin devoid of iron) and transferrin receptor are returned back to cell surface for further cycles of iron uptake and delivery

Haemosiderin represents aggregations of ferritin from which most of the protein (apoferritin) portion has been removed. Normally haemosiderin is stored in cells of mononuclear phagocyte system in bone marrow, liver, and spleen. Haemosiderin is water-insoluble and is less easily available for haemoglobin synthesis. Haemosiderin appears as a golden-brown, coarsely granular pigment when stained with haematoxylin and eosin. Prussian blue reaction is used for demonstration of haemosiderin in bone marrow. Lack of stainable iron in the bone marrow is a diagnostic feature of iron deficiency anaemia.

❑ CAUSES OF IRON DEFICIENCY ANAEMIA

Causes of iron deficiency can be broadly classified into four groups: inadequate dietary intake, defective absorption, excessive loss of iron, or increased requirements (Table 3.1).

In **infants and children** (esp. 6–18 months of age), iron deficiency usually results from poor dietary intake. In **adults** iron deficiency occurs usually secondary to chronic blood loss particularly from gastrointestinal tract. In **women of reproductive age group** iron deficiency is usually the result of menstrual disorders and pregnancy (Box 3.4).

| Box 3.4 | High risk of iron deficiency anaemia |

- Pregnancy
- Children < 5 years
- Elderly
- Women of reproductive age group
- Adolescents

Table 3.1: Causes of iron deficiency anaemia

1. **Inadequate dietary intake of iron**
2. **Defective absorption of iron**—Subtotal gastrectomy, coeliac disease, *Helicobacter pylori* gastritis, antacids, proton pump inhibitors
3. **Excessive loss of iron**—Gastrointestinal bleeding (e.g. oesophageal varices, hiatus hernia, peptic ulcer, gastritis, Meckel's diverticulum, Crohn's disease, ulcerative colitis, hookworm infestation, various neoplasms especially carcinoma of colon, marathon runners); uterine bleeding (menorrhagia); urinary tract bleeding (haematuria, haemoglobinuria); respiratory tract bleeding (haemoptysis); bleeding disorders
4. **Increased requirements for iron**—Pregnancy, infancy, adolescents

❑ CLINICAL FEATURES

General Clinical Features of Anaemia

Patients may present with non-specific symptoms and signs of anaemia such as weakness, easy fatiguability, breathlessness on exertion, tachycardia, and systolic heart murmur.

Clinical Features Related to Iron Deficiency

One of the characteristic symptoms of iron deficiency anaemia is **pica**. It refers to an abnormal and intense desire to eat strange substances such as clay, paint, cardboard, coal, etc. Atrophic glossitis, angular stomatitis, and nail changes are other manifestations. The fingernails become brittle, lusterless, and flat; in advanced cases their shape changes from normal convex to concave (koilonychia). These changes are due to loss of enzymes that contain iron.

The association of iron deficiency anaemia, dysphagia, and glossitis is known as Plummer-Vinson (or Patterson-Kelly) syndrome. This syndrome is rare, but is associated with increased risk of post-cricoid carcinoma.

Clinical Features due to Underlying Cause of Iron Deficiency

There may be bleeding from gastrointestinal tract, menorrhagia, poor diet in small children and adolescents, alteration of bowel habits (in adults with colon cancer), etc.

❑ LABORATORY FEATURES

Sequence of events in iron deficiency is presented first followed by various laboratory investigations.

There are **three stages in the development of iron deficiency anaemia** (Box 3.5 and Fig. 3.5)—depletion of iron stores, reduction in circulating iron with iron-deficient erythropoiesis, and development of iron deficiency anaemia. (1) The first event in

Box 3.5	Stages in the development of iron deficiency anaemia
	Depletion of iron stores → Decrease in transport iron with reduced availability of iron for erythropoiesis → Normocytic normochromic anaemia → Microcytic anaemia → Microcytic hypochromic anaemia

iron deficiency is exhaustion of iron stores and reduction in serum ferritin concentration (<12 µg/L). There is absence of stainable iron in the bone marrow. (2) After depletion of iron stores, the circulating iron level falls and the level of transferrin devoid of iron increases. This manifests as decreased serum iron and transferrin saturation and increased TIBC. This leads to insufficient availability of iron for erythropoiesis. Free erythrocyte protoporphyrin (FEP) increases as combination of protoporphyrin with iron cannot occur. (3) If the state of iron deficiency persists then anaemia develops. To start with anaemia is normocytic and normochromic. This is followed by appearance of microcytic red cells. The last stage of iron deficiency is microcytic hypochromic anaemia with MCV less than 80 fl and MCHC less than 30 g%.

Peripheral Blood Examination

Initially anamia is normocytic and normochromic. Later the red cells show **microcytosis and hypochromia**. The red cells often show variation in size and shape along with elongated cells and **pencil cells**. The white cell count may be normal or mildly decreased. Platelets are often increased, especially in the presence of blood loss (Fig. 3.4).

Red Cell Indices

Although red cell indices may be derived manually after obtaining values of haemoglobin level, red cell count and packed cell volume, they are best measured by electronic cell counters. There is reduction of MCV and MCH with degree of

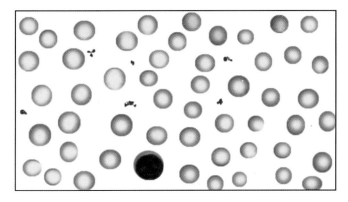

Figure 3.4: Peripheral blood smear in iron deficiency anaemia. Compare the size of red cells with the nucleus of a small lymphocyte

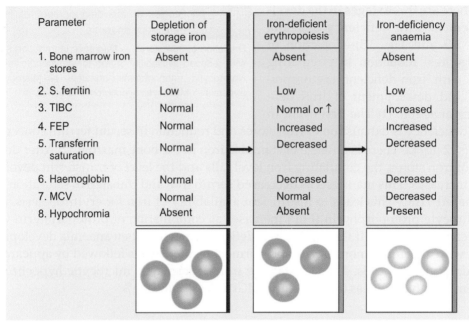

Parameter	Depletion of storage iron	Iron-deficient erythropoiesis	Iron-deficiency anaemia
1. Bone marrow iron stores	Absent	Absent	Absent
2. S. ferritin	Low	Low	Low
3. TIBC	Normal	Normal or ↑	Increased
4. FEP	Normal	Increased	Increased
5. Transferrin saturation	Normal	Decreased	Decreased
6. Haemoglobin	Normal	Decreased	Decreased
7. MCV	Normal	Normal	Decreased
8. Hypochromia	Absent	Absent	Present

Figure 3.5: Stages in the development of iron deficiency anaemia. Microcytic hypochromic anaemia is the late stage of iron deficiency

reduction being proportional to the severity of anaemia. Red cell distribution width is increased in iron deficiency anaemia, while in thalassaemia minor it is often normal. Combination of low MCV and high RDW is one of the best screening tests for iron deficiency anaemia.

Bone Marrow Examination

In iron deficiency anaemia, erythropoiesis is micronormoblastic. The micronormoblasts are smaller than normal with reduced amount of cytoplasm that is vacuolated and has ragged cell borders. Haemoglobinisation of cytoplasm is defective. Granulocytic and megakaryocytic lines are normal. **Absence of stainable iron in the bone marrow on Perl's Prussian blue reaction is a specific and a reliable test for diagnosis of iron deficiency anaemia (Fig. 3.6).**

Serum Ferritin

There is a **direct correlation between amount of storage iron and serum ferritin level** and therefore estimation of serum ferritin is commonly employed for diagnosis of iron deficiency and iron overload. One µg/L of plasma ferritin represents about 8 to 10 mg of storage iron. Normal level of serum ferritin varies between 15 and 300 µg/L. Values below 12 µg/L strongly indicate lack of storage iron. Usefulness of this assay, however, is limited by the non-specific increase in concentration in inflammation, neoplastic disorders, and liver disease. (Serum ferritin is an acute phase reactant). If iron deficiency

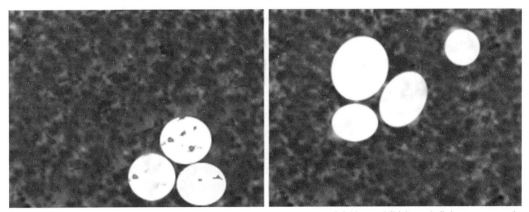

Figure 3.6: Prussian blue stain on bone marrow aspiration smear (a) Normal (b) Iron deficiency anaemia

anaemia is associated with these conditions (as is the case in most hospitalized patients), then its diagnosis may require (i) therapeutic trial of iron, (ii) assay of serum transferrin receptor, or (iii) demonstration of lack of stainable iron in the bone marrow (Box 3.6).

Serum Iron, TIBC, and Percent Transferrin Saturation

Alteration in these measurements occurs after depletion of storage iron and are thus normal in early stage.

The normal serum iron level is 50 to 150 µg/dl with values in women being slightly lower. In addition to iron deficiency anaemia, serum iron levels are also low in chronic inflammation and malignancies. In iron deficiency anaemia, Serum iron is usually < 50 µg/dl. This test is affected by many variables and values should be interpreted along with other tests.

TIBC (normal range 300–400 µg/dl), which reflects amount of transferrin in circulation, is increased in iron deficiency anaemia (> 400 µg/dl) and reduced in chronic infections.

Transferrin saturation is the ratio of serum iron to total iron binding capacity expressed as a percentage and indicates proportion of transferrin to which iron is bound. The average normal value is 30% (normal range is 20–55%). In iron deficiency anaemia, transferrin saturation is less than 15%.

$$\% \text{ transferrin saturation} = \frac{\text{Serum iron} \times 100}{\text{TIBC}}$$

Box 3.6	Serum ferritin

- Most sensitive and specific test for diagnosis of iron deficiency anaemia. Serum ferritin decreases even before the appearance of anaemia
- Serum ferritin correlates with body iron stores (1 µg/L serum ferritin ≈10 mg storage iron)
- Serum ferritin < 12 µg/L is highly specific for diagnosis of iron deficiency anaemia
- Not suitable for diagnosing iron deficiency in patients with concomitant inflammatory, neoplastic, or liver disorder.

Soluble Transferrin Receptor (TfR) Assay

Serum transferrin receptors are derived from proteolysis of cell membrane transferrin receptors during red cell maturation. Level of soluble TfR in serum correlates with the number of cellular transferrin receptors. In iron deficiency anaemia, transferrin receptors on erythroid cells increase in number and therefore their serum level also increases. In iron deficiency, elevation of serum TfR follows depletion of iron stores. Unlike serum ferritin, serum TfR is not an acute phase reactant. Therefore its estimation can be helpful in differentiating iron deficiency anaemia from anaemia of chronic disease and in diagnosing iron deficiency anaemia in patients with chronic inflammation. Serum TfR is also elevated in conditions with increased erythropoietic activity (e.g. haemolytic anaemias).

Free Erythrocyte Protoporphyrin (FEP)

Combination of protoporphyrin with iron to form haem occurs in the mitochondria of erythroid precursors. In iron deficiency anaemia this combination fails to occur and the level of **FEP increases.** Increased FEP is also observed in anaemia of chronic disease and lead poisoning. In thalassaemia, however, FEP is normal. Therefore, **this test can be used to differentiate iron deficiency anaemia from thalassaemia.** Determination of FEP can be applied to large-scale screening of iron deficiency in public health surveys.

Diagnostic laboratory features of IDA are shown in Box 3.7.

Investigations to Define Underlying Cause of Iron Deficiency

This may be obvious (e.g. bleeding) or may require tests such as GIT work-up esp. in adults (test for faecal occult blood, endoscopy or radiology), pelvic ultrasound in females (if menorrhagia is present), stool examination for hookworm, etc.

> Diagnosis of iron deficiency anaemia *per se* is not sufficient in itself. It is essential to search for and treat the underlying cause. In adults, cause of iron deficiency anaemia should always be investigated to avoid missing occult gastrointestinal malignancy.

Box 3.7 Diagnosis of iron deficiency anaemia

- Low haemoglobin and packed cell volume
- Low MCV, MCH, and MCHC
- Microcytic hypochromic red cells on blood smear (in late stage)
- Low serum ferritin
- Low serum iron and transferrin saturation, and increased TIBC
- Increased soluble transferrin receptor
- Bone marrow: Micronormoblasts, absence of stainable iron

❑ DIFFERENTIAL DIAGNOSIS

Thalassaemia Minor

Although both iron deficiency anaemia and thalassaemia minor show microcytic and hypochromic red cells, presence of target cells, polychromatic cells, and basophilic stippling on blood smear suggest the diagnosis of thalassaemia minor. Red cell count is normal or raised in thalassaemia minor while it is reduced in iron deficiency anaemia. In thalassaemia, although red cell abnormalities are prominent anaemia is mild or absent. In iron deficiency anaemia, red cell changes correlate with severity of anaemia. MCV and MCH are markedly reduced as compared to the degree of anaemia in thalassaemia minor. A typical feature of thalassaemia minor on haemoglobin electrophoresis is increased proportion of HbA2 (>3.5%). Bone marrow examination for iron stores also distinguishes the two conditions.

Differentiation of iron deficiency anaemia from thalassaemia minor is important as continued iron therapy in the latter condition can cause iron overload.

Anaemia of Chronic Disease

In anaemia of chronic disease, there is defective release of iron from storage sites in reticuloendothelial cells. This leads to insufficient availability of iron for erythropoiesis despite normal iron stores. Anaemia of chronic disease is usually normocytic and normochromic but in some cases it is microcytic and hypochromic. Presence of underlying chronic disease, raised ESR not proportional to reduction in haemoglobin concentration, low serum iron and low TIBC, increased serum ferritin, and normal or increased bone marrow storage iron are helpful in arriving at the correct diagnosis.

Sideroblastic Anaemia

Sideroblastic anaemia may be hereditary or acquired. Typically the peripheral blood smear shows two types of red cells—normocytic normochromic and microcytic hypochromic (dimorphic anaemia). Bone marow examination (Prussian blue stain for iron) reveals increased or normal storage iron with ringed sideroblasts.

Differential diagnosis of iron deficiency anaemia is presented in Table 3.2.

❑ TREATMENT OF IRON DEFICIENCY ANAEMIA

Treatment consists of administration of iron and correction of underlying cause of blood loss (such as worm infestation, bleeding from any site). Either oral or parenteral iron preparation can be used. Rise in haemoglobin is similar with both routes.

Oral iron therapy is preferable as it is safer and cheaper than parenteral therapy.

Ferrous sulphate is the preferred preparation. One tablet of ferrous sulphate (200 mg) contains 60 mg of elemental iron. The usual dose is 1 tablet thrice daily.

Table 3.2: Differential diagnosis of iron deficiency anaemia

Parameter	Iron deficiency anaemia	Anaemia of chronic disease	β thalassaemia
1. MCV	Decreased	Normal or decreased	Markedly decreased
2. RDW	Increased	Increased or normal	Increased or normal
3. Red cell morphology	Microcytic hypochromic, pencil cells, anisocytosis	Normocytic normochromic or microcytic hypochromic	Microcytic hypochromic, basophilic stippling, target cells, polychromasia
4. Red cell count	Decreased	Decreased	Normal
5. Serum iron	Decreased	Decreased	Normal
6. TIBC	Increased	Decreased	Normal
7. Transferrin saturation	Decreased	Decreased or normal	Normal or increased
8. FEP	Increased	Increased	Normal
9. Serum TfR	Increased	Normal	Increased
10. Serum ferritin	Decreased	Increased or normal	Normal
11. Hb electrophoresis	Normal	Normal	HbA2 > 3.5%
12. Marrow haemosiderin	Low or absent	Normal or increased	Normal

Following initiation of therapy, reticulocytosis develops within 3 to 7 days and peaks (to 8–10%) between 8th and 10th days. This is followed by gradual rise in haemoglobin. Haemoglobin should rise by 1 g/dl (or packed cell volume by 3%) in 4 weeks. About 6 to 8 weeks are needed for restoration of haemoglobin level. Treatment is continued for further 4 months (total duration of therapy 6 months) to replace body iron stores. Adverse effects of oral iron are vomiting, constipation, diarrhoea, and abdominal pain.

Causes of poor response to iron replacement therapy are patient non-compliance, inadequate dosage, malabsorption, continued excess bleeding, coexistent vitamin B_{12}/folate deficiency, concurrent infectious, inflammatory, or neoplastic disease, or wrong diagnosis.

Indications for parenteral iron therapy are gastrointestinal intolerance to oral iron, advanced stage of pregnancy with moderate to severe anaemia, non-cooperative patient, and malabsorption of oral iron.

Other indications for parenteral iron are severe anaemia with short time to surgery and use of erythropoietin.

The main parenteral iron preparations include (1) iron dextran and (2) iron sucrose. Iron dextran can be given as a single-dose infusion, but there is a risk of severe life-threatening anaphylactic reaction. A hypersensitivity test is necessary prior to injection of iron dextran. Other side effects of iron dextran are local pain, fever, joint pains, skin rashes, enlargement of lymph nodes, and enlargement of spleen. Iron sucrose is the safest form of parenteral iron but cannot be given as a single dose infusion. It is given in 2 to 3 divided doses every 2 to 3 days to avoid acute iron toxicity. Total iron deficit in mg for treatment is calculated from the formula weight (kg) × (Ideal haemoglobin-

Actual haemoglobin) $\times$ 0.24 + Depot iron. Depot iron is calculated as 15 mg/kg upto 34 kg; maximum is upto 500 mg after 34 kg body weight. Parenteral therapy is expensive and response is no different than oral iron therapy.

MEGALOBLASTIC ANAEMIAS

The megaloblastic anaemias are characterised by defective synthesis of deoxyribonucleic acid (DNA) in all proliferating cells. They most commonly result from lack of folic acid or vitamin (vit) B_{12}.

❑ NORMAL VITAMIN B_{12} METABOLISM

Vitamin B_{12} is composed of (i) a corrin nucleus which has four pyrrole rings bound to a central cobalt atom, and (ii) a 5,6 dimethylbenzimidazole group which is attached to the corrin ring and to the central cobalt atom. The important cobalamins that are distinguished according to the ligand attached to the central cobalt atom are: cyanocobalamin, hydroxocobalamin, adenosylcobalamin, and methyl cobalamin.

Sources of Vitamin B_{12}

Liver, dairy products, and seafish are the major sources. Although bacteria in the large intestine synthesize vitamin B_{12}, it cannot be absorbed from this site. Minimum need of vitamin B_{12} for an adult is 1 to 4 µg per day.

Absorption of Vitamin B_{12}

Vitamin B_{12} is absorbed by two mechanisms—active and passive. About 75% of vitamin B_{12} in the food is absorbed by active mechanism, which requires the presence of intrinsic factor (IF). Intrinsic factor is a glycoprotein produced by parietal cells of gastric mucosa. In passive mechanism, absorption occurs by diffusion and works when pharmacologic doses of vitamin B_{12} are ingested; only about 1% of this amount is absorbed by diffusion.

After entering into the stomach, vitamin B_{12} is freed from proteins by the action of pepsin. The vitamin B_{12}-binding proteins are known as R binders (due to their rapid electrophoretic migration) and are present in body fluids such as saliva, milk, gastric juice, plasma, etc. Initially vitamin B_{12} attaches to R-binder to form R-B_{12} complex. Along with food, R-B_{12} complexes are carried to the duodenum where pancreatic proteases release B_{12} from R-binder. Free B_{12} then binds to intrinsic factor to form IF-B_{12} complex. This complex, which is protease resistant, is transported to the terminal part of ileum where receptors for IF are present on the epithelial cells. After binding to these receptors, the IF-B_{12} complex is internalized into the ileal mucosal cell along with the receptor. Inside the cell, IF is degraded, B_{12} attaches to another transport protein called transcobalamin II (TC II), and the receptor is carried back to the surface

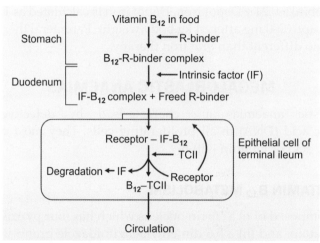

Figure 3.7: Absorption of vitamin B_{12}

of the cell for another cycle of IF-B_{12}. The B_{12} -TC II complex is released into the portal circulation from where it is carried to various organs (Fig. 3.7).

Transport of Vitamin B_{12}

The three vitamin B_{12}-binding proteins in plasma are transcobalamin I (TC I), transcobalamin II (TC II), and transcobalamin III (TC III).

TC II is the main vitamin B_{12} transport protein that is synthesized by different types of cells such as liver cells, macrophages and haematopoietic cells. After absorption vitamin B_{12} circulates bound to TC II and is carried to various organs and tissues. After binding to cell surface receptor, the B_{12}-TC II complex is taken inside the cell. TC II is destroyed, and B_{12} is freed. Congenital absence of TC II causes a severe megaloblastic anaemia due to vitamin B_{12} deficiency.

TC I is synthesised by granulocytes, serves mainly as a storage protein for B_{12} and is not necessary for its transport. Majority of vitamin B_{12} in circulation is bound to TC I rather than TC II; this is so because vitamin B_{12} bound to TC II is rapidly transported to various tissues, while transport of TC I-B_{12} complex needs more time. Absence of TC I is not associated with vitamin B_{12} deficiency.

TC III binds only a very small quantity of vitamin B_{12} in circulation.

Storage Sites

The total amount of vitamin B_{12} in the body is 2 to 5 mg (adequate for 3 years). The major site of storage is the liver.

Vitamin B_{12} is excreted through the bile and shedding of intestinal epithelial cells. Most of the excreted vitamin B_{12} is again absorbed in the intestine (enterohepatic circulation).

Functions of Vitamin B$_{12}$

Synthesis of Methionine from Homocysteine

This reaction is mediated by the enzyme methyl tetrahydrofolate homocysteine methyl transferase and requires a cofactor methylcobalamin. During this reaction, methyl tetrahydrofolate (methyl FH4) is converted to tetrahydrofolate (FH4). FH4 is necessary for the formation of methylene FH4 that is a cofactor in the synthesis of deoxythymidine monophosphate (dTMP) from deoxy uridine monophosphate (dUMP). dTMP is required for DNA synthesis (Fig. 3.8).

The "methyltetrahydrofolate trap" hypothesis has been proposed to explain the cause of impaired DNA synthesis in vitamin B$_{12}$ deficiency. According to this hypothesis, deficiency of methylcobalamin leads to impaired conversion of methyl FH4 to FH4. Methylene FH4 required for the synthesis of dTMP is thus not generated, as most of the folate remains trapped as methyl FH4. This ultimately leads to defective synthesis of DNA.

Conversion of Methyl Malonyl CoA to Succinyl CoA

This reaction requires adenosylcobalamin and methylmalonyl CoA mutase. Deficiency of vitamin B$_{12}$ is associated with increased levels of methylmalonate and propionate. It is thought that this causes synthesis of abnormal myelin lipids with consequent myelin degeneration and neurological abnormalities.

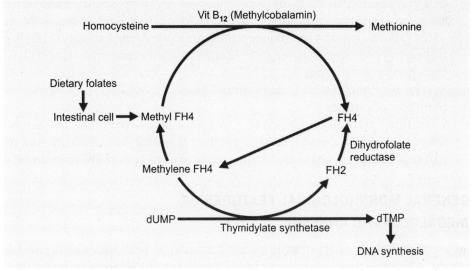

Figure 3.8: Role of vitamin B$_{12}$ and folate in synthesis of DNA

❏ NORMAL FOLATE METABOLISM

The chemical name for folic acid is pteroylmonoglutamic acid. Folic acid is present in nature mostly as polyglutamates. Conversion of polyglutamate to tetrahydrofolate is necessary for folate to participate in metabolic reactions.

1. **Sources of folate:** The major sources are green leafy vegetables, fruits and liver. Folate is easily destroyed by boiling or heating foods in large amounts of water and most of folate in foods can be lost in this manner.

   The average daily requirement for an adult is about 100 µg. The requirement is more during pregnancy and in children during growth.

2. **Absorption:** Dietary folates (polyglutamates) are broken down by intestinal conjugase to monoglutamates. Absorption occurs in proximal jejunum. In the intestinal epithelial cells, monoglutamates are converted to methyl tetrahydrofolate.

3. **Transport:** Folate is released in portal circulation as methyl tetrahydrofolate and is transported to various tissues bound to some unknown protein.

4. **Storage:** Liver is the main site of storage where it is stored mainly as methyl-tetrahydrofolate polyglutamate. The total amount of folate in the body is about 5 mg.

5. **Functions of folate:** The major biological action of tetrahydrofolate is to transfer single carbon substituents (e.g. methylene, methyl or formyl groups) to different compounds. The metabolic reactions in which FH4 acts as a one-carbon donor or acceptor are:

   i.   Synthesis of thymidylate from uridylate: This is biologically the most important reaction mediated by folate since it is necessary for synthesis of DNA (Fig. 3.8). Lack of tetrahydrofolate leads to diminished synthesis of dTMP and consequently of DNA leading to megaloblastic anaemia. In this reaction, methylation of deoxyuridylate monophosphate (dUMP) to deoxythymidylate monophosphate (dTMP) is mediated by methylene tetrahydrofolate. Dihydrofolate (FH2) formed during this process is reduced by FH2 reductase to tetrahydrofolate (FH4) which then re-enters the cycle.

   ii. Synthesis of methionine from homocysteine.

   iii. Synthesis of purines

   iv. Histidine catabolism: Deficiency of folate leads to failure to metabolize formiminoglutamic acid (FIGlu), a product of histidine catabolism. As a result, folate deficiency is associated with excessive excretion of FIGlu in urine.

❏ GENERAL MORPHOLOGICAL FEATURES OF MEGALOBLASTIC ANAEMIA

Following morphological abnormalities are common to both vitamin B₁₂ and folate deficiency. Although they are present in all proliferating cells in the body, they are particularly evident in cells of the haematopoietic system (Figs 3.9 and 3.10).

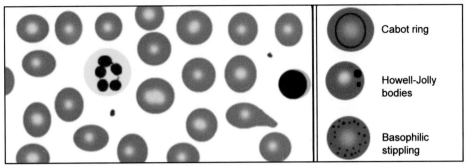

Figure 3.9: Peripheral blood in megaloblastic anaemia showing oval macrocytes, and a hypersegmented neutrophil. A small lymphocyte is shown for comparison of size with red cells. Panel on right shows some morphological abnormalities seen in severe megaloblastic anaemia

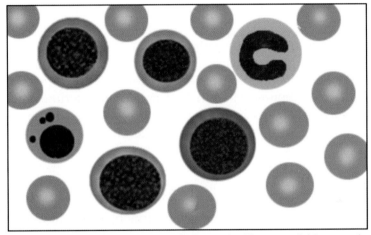

Figure 3.10: Bone marrow in megaloblastic anaemia. Five megaloblasts and one giant band form are seen. Howell-Jolly bodies are seen in the orthochromatic megaloblast

Peripheral Blood

Red Cells

Red blood cells are characteristically large and oval (oval macrocytosis) and normochromic. In vitamin B_{12} or folate deficiency macrocytosis is the earliest sign and can be detected even before the onset of anaemia. Electronic cell counters best detect early macrocytosis. In severe anaemia, in addition to macrocytosis, marked anisopoikilocytosis (variation in size and shape of red cells), basophilic stippling, Howell-Jolly bodies, and Cabot's rings may also be found. Late or intermediate erythroblasts with fine, open nuclear chromatin (megaloblasts) may be seen in peripheral blood in severe anaemia.

(*Note:* Macrocytosis also occurs in alcoholism, hepatic disease, haemolytic states, hypothyroidism and following treatment with chemotherapeutic drugs. Macrocytosis is a normal finding in newborns and during pregnancy. In all these cases however marrow is normoblastic).

White Cells

Total leucocyte count may be normal or decreased. Leucopaenia is more marked in severe anaemia. Hypersegmentation of neutrophils is one of the earliest signs of megaloblastic haematopoiesis and can be detected even in the absence of anaemia. Normally there are 2 to 3 nuclear lobes in a segmented neutrophil. In megaloblastic state, nuclear lobes increase in number. Hypersegmentation of neutrophils is said to be present when more than 5% of neutrophils show 5 or more lobes. (Hypersegmentation also occurs in uraemia and as a congenital abnormality).

Platelets

In severe anaemia, thrombocytopaenia is usual. Morphologic abnormalities of platelets in the form of giant platelets can occur. In advanced cases, bleeding time may be abnormal and sometimes purpura can occur.

Neurologic manifestations of vitamin B_{12} deficiency can occur even in the absence of anaemia; in such cases the diagnostic clues are provided by macrocytosis and hypersegmentation of neutrophils in peripheral blood.

Bone Marrow

Megaloblastic features are present in all erythroid precursors. Megaloblasts are named according to the corresponding stage of normoblast- promegaloblast, and early, intermediate, and late megaloblasts. Morphologic differences between megaloblasts and normoblasts are outlined below:

i. Cell and nuclear size and amount of cytoplasm are increased in megaloblasts.
ii. The nuclear chromatin of megaloblasts is sieve-like or stippled (open) which can be well appreciated at polychromatic stage. Howell-Jolly bodies are common (Fig. 3.10).
iii. The nuclear maturation (progressive condensation of nuclear chromatin) falls behind cytoplasmic maturation (haemoglobinization). This is known as nuclear-cytoplasmic asynchrony or dissociation.
iv. Early precursors of erythroid series (promegaloblasts and early megaloblasts) are increased in number in bone marrow as compared to more mature precursors (intermediate and late megaloblasts). This is known as maturation arrest.
v. Mitotic activity is increased.

Granulocytic series also displays megaloblastic changes. Most prominent changes are seen in metamyelocytes that are large (giant metamyelocytes) with horseshoe-shaped nuclei and finer nuclear chromatin, and in band forms.

Megakaryocytes are often large with multiple nuclear lobes and paucity of cytoplasmic granules.

❑ CAUSES OF MEGALOBLASTIC ANAEMIA

Aetiology of megaloblastic anaemia can be divided into three broad groups: I. Deficiency of folate; II. Deficiency of vitamin B_{12}; III. Miscellaneous causes.

Most common cause of megaloblastic anaemia is deficiency of either folate or vitamin B_{12}. It is worth noting that vitamin B_{12} deficiency most frequently results from defective absorption of the vitamin while folate deficiency is most commonly due to inadequate dietary intake.

About 3 to 5 years are required for development of vitamin B_{12} deficiency after abrupt cessation of availability of vitamin B_{12}; for folate deficiency, this period is about 3 to 4 months. This time interval is related to the daily requirement and the size of the storage compartment.

Severe deficiency of vitamin B_{12} can result secondarily in decreased absorption of folate, and vice versa. This is so because severe lack of either folate or vitamin B_{12} is associated with atrophy of rapidly dividing small intestinal epithelial cells and malabsorption.

Deficiency of Folate

Causes of Folate Deficiency

These are listed in Table 3.3.

Insufficient intake: **The most common cause of folate deficiency is poor dietary intake.** The major aetiological factor in tropical countries is grossly inadequate intake of green leafy vegetables and animal proteins. Improper cooking methods also contribute to the loss of dietary folate.

Folic acid deficiency is very common in **alcoholics** because most of the calories in them are provided by alcohol. Alcohol also interferes with metabolism and probably absorption of folate. It should be noted that apart from folate deficiency, macrocytosis in alcoholics might result from other causes such as direct toxic effect of alcohol on erythroid cells, reticulocytosis secondary to gastrointestinal bleeding or alcohol withdrawal, or hepatic disorder.

Prolonged parenteral fluid therapy in ill patients without vitamin supplements can cause acute megaloblastic anaemia (see later).

Deficient absorption: **Coeliac disease** is due to immunological reaction to gliadin (a product of gluten). Gluten and gliadin are proteins, which are present in certain cereals. Histologically there is atrophy of villi in proximal portion of small intestine

Table 3.3: Causes of folate deficiency

1. **Insufficient dietary intake**—poor diet with lack of green vegetables, chronic alcoholics, prolonged parenteral nutrition.
2. **Deficient absorption**—malabsorption syndromes such as coeliac disease or tropical sprue.
3. **Increased demand**—pregnancy, increased cell turnover (haemolytic anaemia, neoplasia).
4. **Drugs**

with consequent loss of absorptive area. Patient presents clinically with weight loss and steatorrhoea. There is impaired absorption of folate, iron, and other nutrients. D-xylose test for deficient absorption, histopathology, and improvement after diet devoid of gluten are helpful in arriving at the correct diagnosis. Therapy involves gluten-free diet and treatment of associated nutritional deficiencies.

Tropical sprue is endemic in India, West Indies, and Southeast Asia. Infection by enterotoxigenic *E. coli* has been implicated. Tropical sprue affects distal portion of small intestine. Features of tropical and nontropical sprue resemble each other. Inability to deconjugate polyglutamates in the intestine impairs absorption of folate. Due to affection of terminal ileum, vitamin B_{12} deficiency is also usually present. Treatment consists of administration of folic acid, vitamin B_{12} and broad-spectrum antibiotics.

Increased demand: Shunting of folate to the foetus causes upto 5-times increase in folate requirements during **pregnancy.** Megaloblastic anaemia of folate deficiency usually develops during the last trimester. To meet the increased demand and to prevent folate deficiency, pregnant women are routinely given 1 mg folic acid per day. Increased incidence of premature labour, placental abruption, pre-eclampsia, and neural tube defects in foetus has been reported in folate-deficient pregnant women.

Cell turnover and consequently folate requirements are increased in haemolytic states. Patients with myeloproliferative disorders, exfoliative skin disorders, and malignancies also have increased folate requirements.

Clinical Features

Clinical manifestations are related to the severity of anaemia and are non-specific. The common features are pallor and mild icterus (due to ineffective erythropoiesis). Angular stomatitis and glossitis may be present. Cardiac failure can occur in severe cases.

Deficiency of either folate or vitamin B_{12} is associated with increased levels of homocysteine in blood. Hyperhomocysteinaemia has been linked with increased risk of thrombosis. Severe nutritional deficiency of vitamin B_{12} or folate causes megaloblastic anaemia whereas milder deficiencies are associated with increased cardiovascular risk. Insufficient folate during early pregnancy is implicated in the development of neural tube defects in the foetus.

Laboratory Features

Morphologic abnormalities in peripheral blood and bone marrow have been considered earlier. Examination of bone marrow is not indicated in megaloblastic anaemia if diagnosis is unequivocal (from clinical features, blood studies, and vitamin assays).

Estimation of serum folate, red cell folate, and serum vitamin B_{12}: These measurements help in establishing the diagnosis and in differentiating folate and vitamin B_{12} deficiencies from one another. There are two methods of assaying these parameters—microbiological and radioisotopic. Microbiological assays have now largely been replaced by automated methods using radioisotope techniques.

Reduction in serum folate level is an early indicator of folate deficiency. However, low values are also obtained in normal subjects when recent dietary intake is low in folate content. In vitamin B_{12} deficiency, S. folate level is normal or increased in most patients and reduced in a minority of patients. Raised S. folate in vitamin B_{12} deficiency represents accumulation of 5-methyltetrahydrofolate ("folate trap").

Folate is incorporated within red cells during erythropoiesis and its level remains constant throughout the life span of red cells. A low red cell folate indicates megaloblastic anaemia due to folate deficiency. About 50% of patients with vitamin B_{12} deficiency also have reduced red cell folate levels.

Serum vitamin B_{12} levels are thought to reflect tissue stores. S. vitamin B_{12} levels are reduced in megaloblastic anaemia due to vitamin B_{12} deficiency; however low values are also obtained in about 30% of patients with folate deficiency.

Thus in folate deficiency both serum and red cell folate are usually markedly reduced while S. vitamin B_{12} is either normal or mildly decreased. In vitamin B_{12} deficiency, S. vitamin B_{12} and red cell folate are depressed, while S. folate is normal or increased. In combined folate and vitamin B_{12} deficiency, all the values are low (Table 3.5).

Formiminoglutamate (FIGlu) excretion test: FIGlu is excreted in excessive amounts in folate deficiency. In this test, 15 gm oral dose of histidine is given to the patient and urinary excretion of FIGlu is measured spectrophotometrically. Excessive excretion of FIGlu also occurs in vitamin B_{12} deficiency.

Therapeutic trial: Therapeutic trial may be undertaken if nature of deficiency is not evident from clinical data and facilities for vitamin assays are not available. Therapeutic trial should not be undertaken if patient is having severe anaemia, congestive heart failure, angina, neurological manifestations, bleeding tendencies due to thrombocytopaenia, or pregnancy. After obtaining baseline haemoglobin/haematocrit levels and reticulocyte count, patient is given folic acid 200 µg orally or vitamin B_{12} 1 to 2 µg IM every day for 10 days. Reticulocytosis beginning on third day and reaching maximum on sixth or seventh day is the optimal response. If such haematologic response is not obtained or if the response is only partial, then the other vitamin is tried. Suboptimal response to one vitamin may be due to combined deficiency of vitamin B_{12} and folate, concomitant deficiency of iron, or presence of complicating infectious or inflammatory disease.

Other feature: Mild increase in indirect S. bilirubin reflects ineffective erythropoiesis.
See Figure 3.11 for diagnostic approach to megaloblastic anaemias.

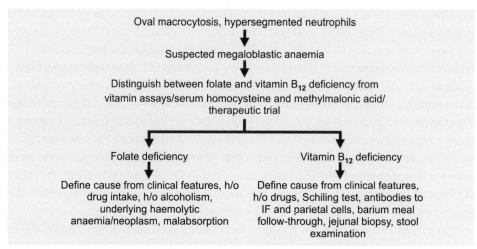

Figure 3.11: Laboratory diagnosis of megaloblastic anaemia

Treatment of Folate Deficiency

Megaloblastic anaemia should never be treated empirically with folic acid alone unless vitamin B$_{12}$ levels are normal. Folate deficiency is treated by 1 to 2 mg folic acid per day orally. Duration of therapy depends on underlying cause. In patients with chronic haemolysis or malabsorption, long-term folate therapy is required.

Treatment with higher doses of folate may partially improve the anaemia of vitamin B$_{12}$ deficiency but not the neurological complications. More dangerously, it can precipitate subacute combined degeneration of spinal cord. Therefore before beginning therapy, vitamin assays should be obtained. If therapy is urgently required then blood samples are first drawn for assays and then both vitamins are administered. Depending upon the vitamin that is deficient, relevant investigations can be carried out to identify the cause of the deficiency.

Deficiency of Vitamin B$_{12}$

Causes of vitamin B$_{12}$ Deficiency

These are listed in Table 3.4.

Insufficient intake: This is a very rare cause of vitamin B$_{12}$ deficiency. It has been reported in rigid vegetarians (vegans) who do not even take milk and other dairy products.

Deficient absorption:
1. *Pernicious anaemia:* This is the most common cause of reduced intestinal absorption of vitamin B$_{12}$. Historical features are presented in Box 3.8.
   This disease occurs in middle and older age groups. (Median age at diagnosis is 60 years). Usual presentation is with anaemia. It is an autoimmune disease characterised by chronic atrophic gastritis, failure of secretion of intrinsic factor, and vitamin B$_{12}$

Table 3.4: Causes of vitamin B_{12} deficiency

1. **Insufficient dietary intake:** Strict vegetarians ('vegans')
2. **Deficient absorption:** Pernicious anaemia, total or partial gastrectomy, prolonged use of proton pump inhibitors or H_2 receptor blockers, diseases of small intestine, fish tapeworm infestation

deficiency. Gastric atrophy is associated with presence of autoantibodies against intrinsic factor and parietal cells. Pathologic changes are infiltration by mononuclear cells in submucosa and lamina propria of fundus and body of stomach, progressive loss of parietal and chief cells, and their replacement by intestinal type mucous cells. Deficiency of intrinsic factor results from destruction of parietal cells and blocking of vitamin B_{12} binding to intrinsic factor by autoantibodies present in gastric juice. Complete absence of intrinsic factor causes failure of absorption of vitamin B_{12} and megaloblastic anaemia. Neurological complications of vitamin B_{12} deficiency may develop. There is association with other autoimmune disorders such as Graves' disease, vitiligo, Hashimoto's thyroiditis, insulin, dependent diabetes mellitus, primary hyperparathyroidism, Addison's disease, and myasthenia gravis.

In addition to morphological signs of megaloblastic anaemia in peripheral blood and bone marrow and reduced S. vitamin B_{12} levels, other laboratory features of pernicious anaemia include abnormal Schilling test (see later), pentagastrin-fast achlorhydria, and anti-IF and anti-parietal cell antibodies in serum. Autoantibodies (IgG) to parietal cells occur in 90% of patients, but are not specific since they also occur in 15% of normal individuals. Antibodies to IF occur in 50% of patients and are diagnostic. These antibodies can also be detected in gastric juice.

Patients with pernicious anaemia have increased risk of gastric cancer and should have regular follow-up examinations by gastric endoscopy. Complete blood count and thyroid function tests should be done annually.

2. *Gastrectomy:* Total gastrectomy is invariably followed by megaloblastic anaemia secondary to vitamin B_{12} deficiency as it removes the site of synthesis of intrinsic factor. These patients should be given prophylactic vitamin B_{12} after surgery.

Patients with partial gastrectomy need regular follow-up after surgery for early detection of vitamin B_{12} deficiency.

Box 3.8 Pernicious anaemia—Historical aspects

- The disease was called as 'pernicious' in old days because it was invariably fatal.
- First described by Thomas Addison, an English physician, in 1849 and therefore also called as Addison's anaemia
- George Minot, William Murphy, and George Whipple jointly shared the Nobel Prize for Physiology or Medicine in 1934 for introduction of raw liver diet for the successful treatment of pernicious anaemia, which was previously uniformly fatal
- Liver extracts were used for treatment till 1948, when specific therapeutic agent (vitamin B_{12}) was isolated
- William B Castle coined the terms 'Intrinsic factor' (which was absent in stomachs of persons of pernicious anaemia) and 'Extrinsic factor' (which corrected pernicious anaemia and was supplied in the diet) in late 1920s. Extrinsic factor was later identified as vitamin B_{12}

3. *Diseases of small intestine:* Diseases of small intestine (e.g. tuberculosis, Whipple's disease, blind loop syndrome) or its resection may interfere with absorption of vitamin B_{12} that occurs in terminal ileum.

   In blind loop syndrome, stasis of small intestinal contents (e.g. by diverticulum or stricture) may predispose to bacterial colonisation and proliferation. Utilisation of most of the ingested vitamin B_{12} by bacteria may lead to reduced or non-availability of vitamin B_{12} for absorption. Treatment consists of parenteral vitamin B_{12}, broad-spectrum antibiotics, and surgical correction of the abnormality.

4. *Infestation by fish tapeworm:* Infestation by fish tapeworm *Diphyllobothrium latum,* due to ingestion of inadequately cooked fish, is observed in Scandinavian countries and the Soviet Republic. The worm produces vitamin B_{12} deficiency by competing with the host for vitamin B_{12} in food. Diagnosis is made by demonstration of ova in stool examination. The infestation can be eradicated by administering niclosamide.

Clinical Features

Clinical features include manifestations of anaemia, mild icterus and sometimes neurologic changes. (Neurologic involvement does not occur in folate deficiency). In vitamin B_{12} deficiency, neurological involvement can occur in the form of:
- Peripheral neuropathy (paraesthesiae and numbness)
- Subacute combined degeneration of spinal cord: Classically vitamin B_{12} deficiency produces degeneration of posterior and lateral columns of spinal cord. This causes loss of position and vibration sense and sensory ataxia
- Cerebral changes (personality changes, dementia, and psychosis).

   In elderly persons, vitamin B_{12} deficiency can present as a neurologic or psychiatric disease without anaemia or haematologic changes. Neurological abnormalities are irreversible in late stages.

   Patients with vitamin B_{12} deficiency can present with only neurological abnormalities without megaloblastic anaemia.

Laboratory Features

Morphologic features of megaloblastic anaemia in peripheral blood and bone marrow have been outlined earlier. Examination of bone marrow is not indicated in megaloblastic anaemia if diagnosis is unequivocal (from clinical features, blood studies, and vitamin assays).

Serum vitamin B_{12} assay: See laboratory features of folate deficiency.

Methylmalonic acid (MMA) and homocysteine in serum: According to some recent reports, measurements of serum methylmalonic acid and serum homocysteine are more sensitive for detection of vitamin B_{12} deficiency than estimation of vitamin B_{12}. They are raised early in tissue deficiency even before the appearance of haematological changes.

Schilling test: This test is used for **evaluation of absorption of vitamin B$_{12}$ in the gastrointestinal tract.** The test can be performed in two parts—part I and part II.

Part I: In part I of the test, 0.5 to 1 μg of radiolabelled vitamin B$_{12}$ is given orally. After two hours, an intramuscular dose (1000 μg) of unlabelled vitamin B$_{12}$ is given. This dose saturates vitamin B$_{12}$-binding sites of transcobalamin I and II and displaces any bound radiolabelled vitamin B$_{12}$ thus permitting urinary excretion of absorbed radiolabelled vitamin B$_{12}$. Radioactivity is measured in subsequently collected 24 hr urine sample and expressed as a percentage of total oral dose.

In normal persons, more than 7% of the oral dose of vitamin B$_{12}$ is excreted in urine. If excretion is less than normal it indicates impaired absorption, which may be due to either lack of intrinsic factor or small intestinal malabsorption. Part II of the test is performed if result of part I is abnormal.

Part II: In part II, patient is orally administered radiolabelled vitamin B$_{12}$ along with intrinsic factor while the remainder of the test is carried out as in part I. If excretion becomes normal, it indicates lack of intrinsic factor. If excretion remains below normal defective absorption in the small intestine is the probable cause.

Abnormal result in part I that is corrected in part II of the test occurs in pernicious anaemia. If both parts yield abnormal results, it indicates malabsorption in small intestine; however such result is also obtained when renal excretion is impaired due to chronic renal disease, commercial intrinsic factor is ineffective or is inactivated by antibodies in stomach, and when absorption of vitamin B$_{12}$ is impaired due to atrophy of ileal epithelial cells secondary to severe vitamin B$_{12}$/folate deficiency. The large parenteral dose of non-radiolabelled vitamin B$_{12}$ in Schilling test is therapeutic and alters the blood levels of the vitamin. Therefore, blood samples for vitamin B$_{12}$ assay should be obtained before Schilling test is performed.

Thus in short (1) reduced vitamin B$_{12}$ absorption corrected by IF occurs in pernicious anaemia and gastrectomy, and (2) reduced vitamin B$_{12}$ absorption not corrected by IF occurs in diseases of terminal ileum and ileal resection (Box 3.9).

Disadvantages of Schilling test:
- Test is tedious and complicated
- It is difficult to procure radiolabelled vitamin B$_{12}$
- Test results are affected by renal function and collection of urine
- Much of the test's relevance is lost due to recent evidence that oral vitamin B$_{12}$ is as effective as parenteral vitamin B$_{12}$ in the treatment of PA.

Intrinsic factor antibodies in serum: Detection of anti-IF antibodies in serum is diagnostic of pernicious anaemia.

Box 3.9	Interpretation of Schilling test

- **Stage I Normal:** Dietary deficiency
- **Stage I Abnormal, Stage II Normal:** Pernicious anaemia, gastrectomy
- **Stage I Abnormal, Stage II Abnormal:** Ileal disease

Table 3.5: Differences between vitamin B_{12} and folate deficiency

Parameter	Vitamin B_{12} deficiency	Folate deficiency
1. Prevalence	Less common	More common
2. Minimum daily requirement of nutrient	1–4 µg	100 µg
3. Effect of cooking on nutrient	No effect	Readily destroyed
4. Time interval between onset of deprivation and manifestations	2–5 years	Few weeks to months
5. Usual cause	Inadequate absorption	Inadequate intake or increased demand
6. Peripheral neuropathy	May be present	Absent
7. Serum vit B_{12}	Low	Normal
8. Serum folate	Normal or Increased	Low
9. Red cell folate	Low	Low
10. Serum homocysteine	Raised	Raised
11. Serum methylmalonic acid	Raised	Normal

Therapeutic trial: See laboratory features of folate deficiency.

See Figure 3.11 for diagnostic approach to megaloblastic anaemias. Differences between vitamin B_{12} deficiency and folate deficiency are outlined in Table 3.5.

Treatment of Vitamin B_{12} Deficiency

In vitamin B_{12} deficiency, administration of only folate will partially correct megaloblastic anaemia; however, neurological disease is precipitated. Therefore, it is necessary to exclude vitamin B_{12} deficiency before beginning folate therapy. Megaloblastic anaemia should never be empirically treated with folate alone. Both vitamins are administered after withdrawing blood samples for vitamin assays. The aims of vitamin B_{12} replacement therapy are correction of haematocrit, to improve neurological abnormalities, and to refill storage pools. Initial therapy consists of 1000 µg of hydroxocobalamin every day for one week. Thereafter patient is given maintenance dosage every 3 months of 1000 µg hydroxocobalamin. Patients of pernicious anaemia require maintenance therapy for indefinite period.

An alternative mechanism independent of IF exists for absorption of vitamin B_{12}. If large amount of vitamin B_{12} is given orally, about 1% of this dose is absorbed. According to some recent observations, oral vitamin B_{12} has been shown to be as effective as parenteral vitamin B_{12} in the treatment of pernicious anaemia.

After initiation of therapy, reticulocyte count begins to increase around third day, reaches peak on 6th or 7th day, and gradually returns to normal by the end of third week. By 24 hours, subjective feeling of well-being develops and erythropoiesis becomes normoblastic. Haematocrit steadily rises and normalises in about 1 to 2 months.

Sudden and severe hypokalaemia can occur immediately after initiation of therapy which may be rapidly fatal (due to cardiac arrhythmias) if untreated. Acute fall in blood potassium level is thought to be due to internalisation of potassium by proliferating cells.

Blood transfusion is indicated in severely anaemic symptomatic patients or in patients with congestive cardiac failure. In such cases one unit of packed red cells may be transfused slowly in view of the risk of circulatory overload.

Miscellaneous Causes of Megaloblastic Anaemia

Drugs

Drug ingestion is a common cause of megaloblastic anaemia, only next in frequency to deficiency of folate or vitamin B_{12}. Methotrexate, and to a lesser extent trimethoprim, pentamidine and pyrimethamine are inhibitors of dihydrofolate reductase, an enzyme required for regeneration of tetrahydrofolate from dihydrofolate. Antimetabolites such as 6-mercaptopurine and 5-fluorouracil inhibit the synthesis of DNA directly. These drugs initially produce mild megaloblastic anaemia, which is eventually followed by marrow hypoplasia if the drug is not discontinued. Some other drugs causing megaloblastic anaemia are cytosine arabinoside, hydroxyurea, zidovudine, antiepileptics, oral contraceptives, and nitrous oxide.

Haematologic Disorders

Megaloblastic features are present in erythroid series in myelodysplastic syndrome and erythroleukaemia. In myelodysplastic syndrome, dysplastic features are present in all the three cell lines (erythroid, granulocytic, and megakaryocytic) along with ringed sideroblasts, increased numbers of immature granulocytic precursors, and abnormal localisation of blasts in bone marrow. In erythroleukaemia, aside from megaloblastic features, erythroblasts are bizarre looking, erythroblastosis is commonly present in peripheral blood, and myeloblasts are increased in bone marrow.

Acute Megaloblastic Anaemia

In this condition there is a sudden and rapid development of megaloblastosis in bone marrow that may be fatal. Nitrous oxide anaesthesia, and total parenteral nutrition without vitamin supplementation in critically ill patients are the usual causes. The patient rapidly develops thrombocytopaenia or leucopaenia or both but anaemia is lacking. Bone marrow shows typical megaloblastic features. Administration of folate and vitamin B_{12} is effective.

Congenital Defects of Metabolism

Congenital defects of metabolism involving either folate or vitamin B_{12} are rare.

APLASTIC ANAEMIA AND RELATED DISORDERS

Aplastic anaemia is a disorder of haematopoiesis in which there are pancytopaenia in peripheral blood and decreased cellularity of bone marrow. By definition, there is no abnormal infiltrate (leukaemic, cancerous, or other) or increase in reticulin in bone marrow. Aplastic anaemia is uncommon in the West; it is more common in East Asia and other developing countries. Causes of aplastic anaemia are listed in Table 3.6.

❑ ACQUIRED APLASTIC ANAEMIA

Causes

Approximately 2/3rds cases of aplastic anaemia are idiopathic. Drugs and chemicals commonly associated with aplastic anaemia are listed in Table 3.7.

Benzene is used as a commercial solvent in many industries. Haematological alterations induced by benzene are hypoplasia of bone marrow, haemolysis, lymphocytopaenia, hyperplasia of bone marrow, and acute myeloid leukaemia.

Bone marrow injury caused by cytotoxic drugs is dose-dependent and transient, being reversible after discontinuation of the drug. In some persons, pancytopaenia with marrow aplasia develops as an idiosyncratic reaction to certain drugs that are normally tolerated by majority of individuals. The idiosyncratic reactions are not dose-dependent, may develop after discontinuation of the drug, and maybe irreversible and life-threatening. Chloramphenicol causes two patterns of bone marrow damage—dose-dependent reversible haematopoietic suppression in about 50% of individuals

Table 3.6: Causes of aplastic anaemia

Acquired	Constitutional
1. Idiopathic	1. Fanconi anaemia
2. Drugs and chemicals	2. Dyskeratosis congenita
3. Ionizing radiation	3. Schwachman-Diamond syndrome
4. Infectious diseases: Viral hepatitis, cytomegalovirus, Epstein-Barr virus	4. Diamond-Blackfan anaemia
5. Paroxysmal nocturnal haemoglobinuria	5. Congenital amegakaryocytic thrombocytopaenia
6. Graft vs host disease	
7. Pregnancy	

Table 3.7: Common drugs and toxins implicated in the aetiology of aplastic anaemia

Drugs	Chemicals
A. Dose-dependent action—Cytotoxic drugs	• Benzene
B. Idiosyncratic action	• Insecticides (Organophosphates, organochlorines)
• Antibacterials (Sulphonamides, Chloramphenicol)	• Pentachlorophenol (an antibacterial, fungicide and a wood-preservative)
• Anti-inflammatory drugs (Phenylbutazone, Indomethacin, Piroxicam, Diclofenac, Naproxen) • Antirheumatics (Gold, Penicillamine) • Antiepileptics (Phenytoin, Carbamazepine) • Antithyroids • Tranquilizers (Chlorpromazine) • Others—Furosemide, Allopurinol	

and idiosyncratic aplastic anaemia in a small number of individuals. The dose-dependent reversible haematopoietic suppression is a more common side effect of chloramphenicol. Usually there is reduction of erythroid precursors that manifests as anaemia and reticulocytopaenia. Less frequently there is suppression of granulocytic and megakaryocytic series. Bone marrow examination shows reduction of erythroid precursors, vacuolisation of nucleus and cytoplasm in premature cells of erythroid and granulocytic series and ringed sideroblasts. Serum iron level is characteristically raised. These changes occur with prolonged high-dose therapy with chloramphenicol and are reversible on cessation of the drug. However continued administration in high dosage may lead to aplastic anaemia. The pathogenesis of this toxic effect appears to be direct inhibition of proliferation and differentiation of precursor cells in bone marrow. More important side effect of chloramphenicol is the development of idiosyncratic aplastic anaemia. It probably occurs due to irreversible genetic damage to the haematopoietic stem cells. It is thought that there is a genetic susceptibility of stem cells to chloramphenicol-induced DNA damage. Patient develops severe pancytopaenia and bone marrow failure, which is often life-threatening. This is not related to the dose or duration of therapy and is reported to occur in 1: 11500 to 1: 40,000 persons taking the drug. Aplastic anaemia may occur days or even weeks after cessation of the drug. Chloramphenicol should be avoided if safer alternative drugs are available and its use for trivial indications should be discouraged.

Bone marrow aplasia has been reported to occur rarely following hepatitis. Serological markers against the known viral agents are often negative. Aplastic anaemia develops about 2 to 3 months following the episode of hepatitis. Post-hepatitis aplastic anaemia is often severe and life-threatening.

There is a strong association between paroxysmal nocturnal haemoglobinuria (PNH) and aplastic anaemia. Aplastic anaemia precedes or follows PNH in a significant proportion of patients.

Transfusion of whole blood to immunodeficient children may lead to aplastic anaemia. This is probably due to immune-mediated destruction of marrow stem cells by immunocompetent donor lymphocytes (graft-versus-host disease).

Pathogenesis

The mechanisms by which various agents produce aplastic anaemia are unknown. Haematopoietic failure can result from various mechanisms:
1. **Reduction in the number of stem cells in bone marrow;**
2. **Defective stem cells** — The causative agent affects the capacity of self-renewal, proliferation, and differentiation of stem cells;
3. **Defective haematopoietic microenvironment** that is not able to sustain normal haematopoiesis;
4. **Deficiency of factors stimulating haematopoiesis;**
5. **Inhibition of haematopoiesis by immunological mechanisms**: Immune-mediated suppression of haematopoiesis is thought to underlie majority of cases of aplastic

anaemia. Response to immunosuppressive therapy supports this concept. Activated T lymphocytes produce cytokines such as γ interferon and tumour necrosis factor α, which have been shown to suppress the growth of haematopoietic stem cells *in vitro*. It is thought that haematopoietic stem cells are first antigenically altered by exposure to the causative agent which is followed by cellular immune response. In addition, Fas receptors on haematopoietic stem cells are upregulated by TNF-α leading to apoptosis of stem cells (Fig. 3.12).

Clinical Features

Aplastic anaemia presents with signs and symptoms related to pancytopaenia. Bleeding is due to thrombocytopaenia and may occur in the form of petechiae, ecchymoses, or nasal or gastrointestinal bleeding. Neutropaenia is associated with infections. Weakness, easy fatiguability, pallor, and breathlessness are related to anaemia. **In aplastic anaemia, lymph nodes, liver, or spleen are not enlarged. If enlarged, diagnosis other than aplastic anaemia should be considered.**

Laboratory Features

Tests to Establish the Diagnosis of Aplastic Anaemia

Peripheral blood examination: Peripheral blood shows pancytopaenia. Anaemia is a constant feature and red cells are usually normocytic and normochromic. Sometimes red cells are mildly macrocytic. The reticulocyte count is low as compared to the degree of reduction in haemoglobin concentration. Granulocytes and monocytes are reduced. If neutrophils are less than 200/cmm, risk of infections is significantly increased.

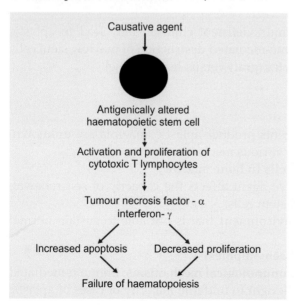

Figure 3.12: Pathogenesis of immune-mediated acquired aplastic anaemia. Antigenically altered haematopoietic stem cells are recognized by cytotoxic T lymphocytes which secrete tumour necrosis factor-α (TNF-α) and interferon-γ (IFN-γ). Both TNF-α and IFN-γ are potent inhibitors of haematopoietic stem cells. Also, Fas receptors on stem cells are upregulated by TNF-α leading to their apoptosis. In addition, cytotoxic T cells can cause direct damage to stem cells

Predominant white cells in the peripheral blood are lymphocytes. Thrombocytopaenia is a consistent finding. Spontaneous bleeding usually occurs when the platelet count is less than 20,000/cmm.

Aplastic anaemia is diagnosed if any two of the following are present in peripheral blood (BCSH, 2003):
- Haemoglobin < 10 g/dl
- Neutrophil count < 1,500/cmm
- Platelet count < 50,000/cmm

Bone marrow examination: In aplastic anaemia, bone marrow fragments are easily obtained by aspiration. In severe cases, cellularity of the marrow is markedly decreased with most of the particles showing predominance of fat cells. Erythroid and myeloid precursor cells are markedly reduced and megakaryocytes are often absent. The surviving erythroid precursors may show megaloblastic features. The predominant cells of white cell series are lymphocytes and plasma cells (Fig. 3.13). Even if bone marrow is hypocellular, at places small foci of active haematopoiesis are often present. Aspirate from such areas may thus appear normocellular. Therefore repeated marrow aspirations are sometimes necessary to make the diagnosis of aplastic anaemia.

Trephine biopsy (at least 2 cm) is essential to assess overall cellularity and morphology of remaining haematopoietic cells, and to rule out abnormal cellular infiltrate and increased reticulin. Biopsy shows hypocellularity with predominance of fat cells and sparse haematopoietic elements.

It is necessary to assess severity of aplastic anaemia from blood and marrow findings. In severe aplastic anaemia there is marked hypocellularity of bone marrow and severe depletion of normal haematopoietic cells. There is marked cytopaenia in

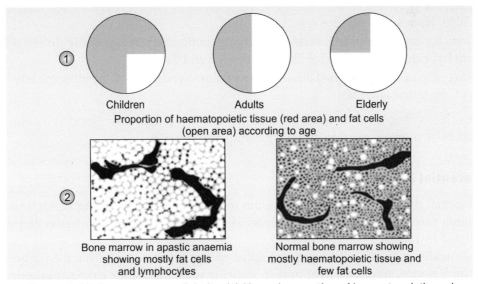

Children   Adults   Elderly
Proportion of haematopoietic tissue (red area) and fat cells
(open area) according to age

Bone marrow in apastic anaemia
showing mostly fat cells
and lymphocytes

Normal bone marrow showing
mostly haematopoietic tissue and
few fat cells

Figure 3.13: Bone marrow cellularity. (1) Normal proportion of haematopoietic and fat cells according to age; (2) Comparison of normal and aplastic bone marrow

Table 3.8: Grading of aplastic anaemia

Severe aplastic anaemia (SAA) (Camitta et al, 1976)	Very severe aplastic anaemia (VSAA) (Bacigalupo et al, 1988)	Non-severe aplastic anaemia
Peripheral blood Any two of the following- • Neutrophils < 500/cmm • Platelets < 20,000/cmm • Reticulocytes (corrected for PCV) < 1% AND **Bone marrow** Any one of the following- • Marrow cellularity < 25% • Marrow cellularity 25–50% with < 30% haematopoietic cells	Criteria similar to SAA except neutrophils < 200/cmm	• Bone marrow cellularity < 25% • Peripheral blood cytopaenia not meeting the criteria for SAA

peripheral blood predisposing the patient to serious infections and bleeding. Defining such patients has therapeutic implications (Table 3.8).

Tests to Determine Cause of Aplastic Anaemia

These tests include:

- Liver function tests and tests for antecedent hepatitis: Hepatitis A antibody, hepatitis B surface antigen, hepatitis C antibody, and for Epstein-Barr virus.
- Tests for autoantibodies: Anti-nuclear antibody, anti-DNA antibody
- Tests for paroxysmal nocturnal haemoglobinuria: Flow cytometry for CD59 and CD55, Ham's test, sucrose lysis test
- Tests for myelodysplastic syndrome: Cytogenetic analysis especially fluorescent *in situ* hybridization (FISH) for chromosomes 5 and 7
- Screening tests for inherited bone marrow failure syndromes: Chromosome breakage test, mutation analysis.

Diagnosis of aplastic anaemia is made by two investigations: Blood cell counts and bone marrow examination (aspiration and biopsy).

Differential Diagnosis

Differential diagnosis of aplastic anaemia includes disorders causing pancytopaenia (anaemia + leucopaenia + thrombocytopaenia). Disorders associated with pancytopaenia are listed in Table 3.9.

Clinically, patients with haematological malignancies usually have enlargement of lymph nodes, spleen or liver and in patients with metastatic carcinoma, primary tumour may be evident. Bone marrow examination shows the presence of abnormal cells.

Table 3.9: Causes of pancytopaenia

Pancytopaenia with hypocellular marrow	Pancytopaenia with cellular marrow
1. Acquired aplastic anaemia	1. Megaloblastic anaemia
2. Inherited bone marrow failure syndromes (Fanconi anaemia, dyskeratosis congenita, Schwachman-Diamond syndrome, congenital amegakaryocytic thrombocytopaenia)	2. Storage disorders
3. Hypocellular myelodysplastic syndrome	3. Paroxysmal nocturnal haemoglobinuria
4. Hypocellular acute leukaemia	4. Hypersplenism
5. Paroxysmal nocturnal haemoglobinuria	5. Acute leukaemia
6. Hairy cell leukaemia	6. Myelodysplastic syndrome
7. Lymphoma	7. Lymphoma
8. Myelofibrosis	8. Autoimmune disorders
9. Mycobacterial infections	9. Overwhelming infections
10. Gelatinous transformation of bone marrow	10. Haemophagocytosis syndrome

Hypersplenism is characterized by enlargement of spleen, peripheral blood cytopaenia, and normal or hypercellular bone marrow. Underlying cause of splenomegaly may be evident.

Pancytopaenia is a common feature of megaloblastic anaemia. Diagnosis however is readily evident from macrocytosis and hypersegmented neutrophils in peripheral blood and megaloblastic erythropoiesis in bone marrow.

Differentiation of hypoplastic anaemia from hypocellular MDS can be difficult. Dysgranulocytic and dysmegakaryocytic features in peripheral blood and bone marrow, and abnormal cytogenetic analysis favour the latter condition. (Dyserythropoietic features are seen in MDS as well as aplastic anaemia). The distinction between hypocellular MDS and hypocellular AML rests on the percentage of blasts in bone marrow.

Diagnosis of PNH is based on demonstration of abnormal sensitivity of red cells to complement (Ham's test) or flow cytometric analysis for CD55 or CD59 antigens.

For systemic lupus erythematosus, tests for anti-nuclear antibody and for anti-DNA antibody are done.

Gelatinous transformation of bone marrow (syn: serous degeneration, serous atrophy) is characterized by replacement of haematopoietic cells and fat cells in bone marrow by amorphous extracellular matrix. Its causes are (1) cachexia due to chronic debilitating illnesses like AIDS, cancer, tuberculosis, etc; (2) anorexia nervosa, and (3) acute infections with multiorgan failure. There is a variable cytopaenia in peripheral blood. Bone marrow examination shows deposition of pink, granular, amorphous matrix material replacing fat and haematopoietic tissue (Fig. 3.14). Matrix material is composed of acid mucopolysaccharides and stains positively with PAS and alcian blue (acid pH).

Haemophagocytosis syndrome (syn: haemophagocytic lymphohistiocytosis) is a potentially fatal disorder characterized by pancytopaenia, phagocytosis

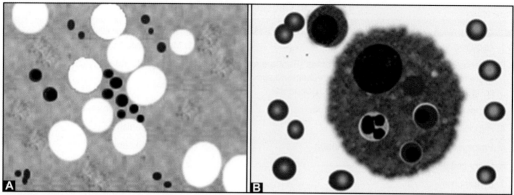

Figure 3.14: (A) Gelatinous transformation of bone marrow showing replacement of marrow by pink amorphous material (B) Haemophagocytosis syndrome showing a macrophage with ingested neutrophil, nucleated red cells and mature red cell

of haematopoietic cells and their progeny (Fig. 3.14), hepatosplenomegaly, and lymphadenopathy. Jaundice, hypofibrinogenaemia, and hypertriglyceridaemia are usual. The main histopathologic feature is lymphohistiocytic proliferation in spleen, liver, lymph nodes, and bone marrow. There is no specific laboratory test for diagnosis. The syndrome may be acquired (secondary to cancer, infections, autoimmune disorders) or familial (autosomal recessive).

Treatment

There are two methods of treatment in severe aplastic anaemia—(1) allogeneic haematopoietic stem cell transplantation that attempts to achieve cure, and (2) immunosuppressive therapy to bring about remission. In patients with less severe aplastic anaemia, the major form of therapy is supportive in the hope of achieving spontaneous recovery.

Haematopoietic Stem Cell Transplantation (HSCT)

This is the ideal treatment in young patients (< 40 years) with severe and very severe aplastic anaemia if HLA-matched sibling donor is available. Patients more than 40 years of age are more likely to develop serious complications such as graft-versus-host disease and tolerate them poorly. Prospective candidates for haematopoietic stem cell transplantation should not be transfused with blood or blood products as far as possible (especially from family members if donor is a sibling) to avoid the risk of alloimmunisation and graft rejection.

Immunosuppressive Therapy

It is thought that a large number of cases of aplastic anaemia are caused by immunological mechanisms. Activated suppressor T cells have been shown to inhibit haematopoiesis.

Antilymphocyte (or antithymocyte) globulin (ALG or ATG) therapy, which is an antibody against T lymphocytes, probably acts by reducing these suppressor cells. ATG is usually combined with cyclosporine that suppresses immune system. This is usually given to patients with severe aplastic anaemia who do not have HLA-matched sibling donor for HSCT and to all other patients of aplastic anaemia. About 30% of patients achieve complete remission while haematopoietic recovery is only partial in majority of patients. Late relapse occurs in some patients. Clonal haematopoietic disorders like paroxysmal nocturnal haemoglobinuria, myelodysplasia, or acute myeloid leukaemia can emerge after a few years.

> Major side effect of HSCT is graft-vs-host disease, while main side effect of immunosuppressive therapy is development of PNH, AML, or myelodysplasia after a few years.

Androgens

Androgens stimulate erythropoiesis in bone marrow. They may be of some benefit in those patients who fail to show desired response to immunosuppressive therapy and who are not suitable for HSCT.

Supportive Measures

Packed red cells should be given when anaemia becomes symptomatic. Platelet transfusions are indicated in the presence of bleeding due to thrombocytopaenia and prophylactically when platelet count falls below 20,000/cmm. Usefulness of granulocyte transfusions is minimal and the chief form of treatment in neutropaenia with infection is antibiotics. Infections should be investigated particularly for opportunistic organisms and vigorously treated.

Prognosis

In the past majority of patients with severe aplastic anaemia used to die within 1 year of diagnosis. Now many patients undergoing marrow transplant can hope to achieve cure; however a proportion of these patients will develop serious complications such as graft-versus-host disease, infections, or graft rejection. Patients receiving immunosuppressive therapy can achieve complete or partial remission; long-term sequelae in these patients are recurrence or evolution of a clonal haematopoietic disorder such as PNH, MDS, or AML.

With supportive therapy, some patients with moderately severe aplastic anaemia can achieve spontaneous remission.

Approach to management of aplastic anaemia is shown in Figure 3.15.

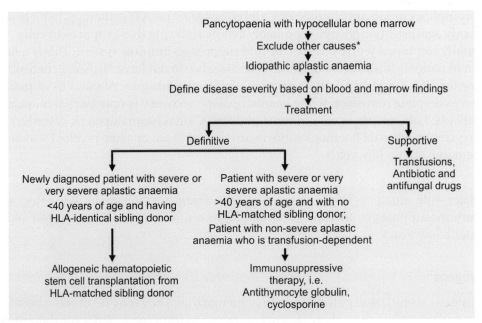

Figure 3.15: Approach to management of aplastic anaemia
*Systemic lupus erythematosus, hypocellular myelodysplastic syndrome/acute leukaemia, myelofibrosis, mycobacterial infections, gelatinous transformation, paroxysmal nocturnal haemoglobinuria, inherited bone marrow failure syndromes

❑ CONSTITUTIONAL APLASTIC ANAEMIA

Inherited bone marrow failure syndromes are a heterogeneous group of disorders characterized by bone marrow failure and somatic abnormalities. They are listed in Table 3.6. Bone marrow failure may involve all cell lines or a single lineage. Presentation is usually in childhood but may sometimes be in adults.

Fanconi's Anaemia

This is a rare disorder with autosomal recessive mode of inheritance, first described in 1927 by a Swiss paediatrician Guido Fanconi. It is associated with short stature, microcephaly, microphthalmia, microstomia, renal aplasia, café au lait spots, generalised hyperpigmentation of skin, mental retardation and hypoplasia of thumbs and of radii. Hypoplastic anaemia develops usually during 5 to 10 years of age. Clinical presentation of Fanconi's anaemia is markedly heterogeneous. In some patients, congenital anomalies are absent.

This disease can result from mutations in any one of 13 different genes.

Cells have increased susceptibility to spontaneous chromosomal breakage. The screening test is chromosomal breakage test (incubation of peripheral blood lymphocytes with diepoxybutane or mitomycin causes chromosomal breaks which can be seen on karyotyping). Definitive diagnosis is made by mutation analysis.

Patients are at increased risk of myelodysplastic syndrome, acute myeloid leukaemia, and solid cancers.

Treatment with anabolic steroids is followed by improvement but side-effects (secondary sexual changes in boys, virilisation in girls, hepatic complications like cholestasis, peliosis hepatis, carcinoma) limit the usefulness of this form of therapy in children. Bone marrow transplantation with marrow obtained from non-affected, HLA-identical sibling donor can establish normal haematopoiesis in most cases.

Dyskeratosis Congenita

This is an inherited bone marrow failure syndrome with diagnostic triad of abnormal skin pigmentation, nail dystrophy and mucosal leucoplakia. In addition to marrow aplasia, other features are pulmonary fibrosis, liver disease, neurologic and eye abnormalities, and increased predisposition to cancer. These patients have short germ line telomeres. Inheritance may be X-linked or autosomal, and mutations in six different genes have been identified. Diagnosis is based on telomere length assay and demonstration of a gene mutation.

Schwachman-Diamond Syndrome

This is a rare autosomal recessive disorder characterized by bone marrow failure, exocrine pancreatic insufficiency, and increased risk of myelodysplasia and leukaemia. It is caused by biallelic mutations in *SBDS* gene on chromosme 7.

Diamond-Blackfan Anaemia

This is a rare autosomal dominant disorder presenting in first year of life with congenital anomalies, severe macrocytic anaemia, reticulocytopaenia, and selective depletion of erythroid precursors in bone marrow. Red cells show elevated foetal haemoglobin and increased erythrocyte adenosine deaminase activity. It is caused by mutations in ribosomal protein genes. Some cases evolve into aplastic anaemia. The disease should be distinguished from transient erythroblastopaenia of childhood in which recovery occurs within 5 to 10 weeks.

Congenital Amegakaryocytic Thrombocytopaenia

This is an autosomal recessive disorder caused by mutations in thrombopoietin (TPO) receptor c-mpl. It presents at birth with severe thrombocytopaenia and absence of megakaryocytes in bone marrow. About 50% of patients develop aplastic anaemia by the age of 5 years. There are no specific congenital malformations.

❑ PURE RED CELL APLASIA

This is characterised by selective depletion of erythroid precursors in the bone marrow with consequent severe normocytic normochromic anaemia and reticulocytopaenia.

Production of leucocytes and platelets is normal. Diagnostic criteria for pure red cell aplasia are (1) severe anaemia, (2) reticulocyte count < 1%, and (3) normocellular marrow with mature erythroblasts <0.5%. Pure red cell aplasia (PRCA) may be divided into two types—constitutional and acquired. Acquired type is further subdivided into primary and secondary forms.

Constitutional Pure Red Cell Aplasia (Diamond-Blackfan syndrome)

This is considered above.

Acquired Pure Red Cell Aplasia

PRCA occurring during the course of chronic haemolytic anaemias in children (such as sickle-cell anaemia, thalassaemia, glucose-6-phosphate dehydrogenase deficiency) has been designated as aplastic crisis. Parvovirus B19 is implicated which has a selective cytopathic effect on erythroid precursors. Patients develop a sudden worsening of their anaemia associated with reticulocytopaenia, and depletion of erythroid precursors in bone marrow. PRCA is transient with recovery usually occurring in 1 to 2 weeks when antibodies against the virus appear. In normal persons cytopathic effect of the virus on erythroid precursors does not manifest as anaemia due to the long life-span of red cells and the transient effect of the virus. In immunocompromised persons, B19 parvovirus causes chronic PRCA since antibody response against the virus is deficient.

It may also be associated with thymoma, collagen vascular disorders, myasthenia gravis, chronic lymphocytic leukaemia, large granular lymphocytic leukaemia, and 5q-myelodysplastic syndrome.

In children PRCA is mostly a self-limited disease while in adults it follows a chronic course. Although immunosuppressive therapy can induce remission, relapses are frequent.

ANAEMIA OF CHRONIC DISORDERS

The anaemia of chronic disorders (ACD) occurs in chronic infections, or inflammatory or neoplastic diseases. Anaemia is normocytic normochromic or microcytic hypochromic and serum iron level is low even though storage iron is adequate.

Anaemia of chronic disorders is the most frequent form of anaemia in hospitalized patients (occurs in 50% of hospitalized patients).

"Big 3" groups of diseases associated with ACD are inflammation, infection, and neoplasm. Diseases associated with anaemia of chronic disease are listed in Table 3.10.

Table 3.10: Diseases associated with ACD

Chronic inflammation	Chronic infections	Neoplasms
• Rheumatoid arthritis	• Tuberculosis	• Carcinoma
• Systemic lupus erythematosus	• Urinary tract infections	• Lymphoma
• Crohn's disease	• Bacterial endocarditis	• Myeloma
	• Deep seated abscess	
	• Pneumonia	

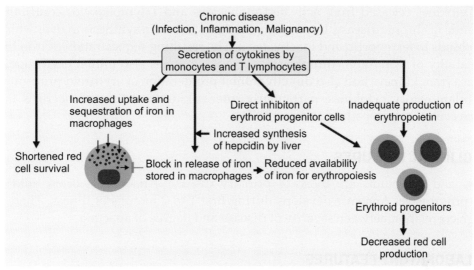

Figure 3.16: Mechanisms underlying anaemia of chronic disease

❏ PATHOGENESIS

Pathogenesis is not clear. Three mechanisms have been proposed—decreased red cell survival, decreased red cell production to compensate for shortened red cell survival, and impairment of iron metabolism (Fig. 3.16).

Decreased Red Cell Survival

Red cell survival is mildly shortened. It is thought that disorders associated with ACD enhance the phagocytic activity of macrophages. These activated macrophages are sensitive to slight alterations in red cells and cause their premature destruction.

Decreased Red Cell Production

This is related to the inappropriately low erythropoietin production for the degree of anaemia. Block in the release of iron for erythropoiesis from storages sites also plays a role.

Impairment of Iron Metabolism

In ACD, amount of storage iron in macrophages of reticuloendothelial system is adequate. However the release of iron from macrophages is inhibited. This leads to hypoferremia (low serum iron) and less iron is made available to erythroid precursors in bone marrow. This causes iron-deficient erythropoiesis despite sufficient storage iron.

Cytokines released from activated monocytes and T lymphocytes contribute to anaemia of chronic disease. Interleukin-6 induces hepcidin synthesis in liver which in turn binds to ferroportin and inactivates it. The resulting sequestration of iron limits availability of iron for erythropoiesis. Certain cytokines also inhibit erythropoietin release from kidneys and also directly inhibit proliferation of erythroid progenitors.

Inflammatory cytokines, particularly interleukin-1 and tumour necrosis factor play a central role in pathogenesis of ACD.

❏ CLINICAL FEATURES

Signs and symptoms are those of primary disease. Anaemia is often mild and non-progressive. Anaemia develops during first 1 to 2 months of illness. There is a rough correlation between severity of disease and degree of anaemia.

❏ LABORATORY FEATURES

Anaemia is mild to moderate (haemoglobin rarely falls below 8–9 g/dl) and is most commonly normocytic and normochronic; less commonly it is microcytic and hypochromic (particularly in rheumatoid arthritis). Reticulocyte count is not increased in proportion with the degree of anaemia.

Decrease in serum iron is a consistent feature and can be detected even before the appearance of anaemia. Total iron binding capacity is decreased. Serum ferritin is normal or raised. As S. ferritin is nonspecifically raised in inflammation (even in the presence of iron deficiency), estimation of serum soluble transferrin receptor and soluble transferrin receptor/S. ferritin index have been advocated for diagnosis (Table 3.11).

Erythrocyte sedimentation rate is increased.

Bone marrow examination shows normal morphology. A characteristic feature is normal or increased storage iron as demonstrated by Prussian blue reaction.

Table 3.11: Differences between iron deficiency anaemia and anaemia of chronic disease

Parameter	Iron deficiency anaemia	Anaemia of chronic disease
1. Degree of anaemia	Variable	Mild
2. Presence of underlying disease	±	Infection, inflammation, neoplasm
3. Mean cell volume	Reduced	Normal or reduced
4. S. iron	Reduced	Reduced or normal
5. Transferrin saturation	Reduced	Reduced or normal
6. TIBC	Increased	Reduced
7. S. ferritin	Reduced	Increased or normal
8. S. transferrin receptor	Increased	Normal
9. S. transferrin receptor/S. ferritin index	High	Low
10. Bone marrow storage iron	Reduced or absent	Normal or increased

> **Box 3.10** Diagnosis of anaemia of chronic disease
>
> - Evidence of chronic disease (raised erythrocyte sedimentation rate, C-reactive protein)
> - Mild to moderate anaemia; red cells normocytic normochromic (in late stage, microcytic hypochromic)
> - Low serum iron, low TIBC, low transferrin saturation
> - Serum ferritin: Normal or increased
> - Serum transferrin receptor/log ferritin ratio <1
> - Serum hepcidin: High

Free erythrocyte protoporphyrin is raised, as there is no sufficient iron available to form haem.

Alterations in leucocytes and platelets are related to the underlying disease.

Diagnostic features of anaemia of chronic disease are shown in Box 3.10.

❑ DIFFERENTIAL DIAGNOSIS

Differentiation of ACD from IDA is given in Table 3.11. As disorders associated with ACD can cause anaemia by other mechanisms such as bleeding, drug-induced haematopoietic suppression, excessive red cell destruction, or infiltration of marrow, these causative factors should be excluded. Anaemias due to renal, liver, or endocrine failure do not come under ACD.

❑ TREATMENT

Iron or vitamin therapy is not indicated in ACD. Effective treatment of underlying disease leads to correction of anaemia. In some cases, administration of recombinant erythropoietin has been found to cause resolution of anaemia of chronic disease.

SIDEROBLASTIC ANAEMIA

❑ SIDEROBLASTS

Sideroblasts are erythroblasts containing aggregates of iron, which are demonstrable by Prussian blue reaction. There are three types of sideroblasts—type I, type II, and type III (Fig. 3.17).

In type I (normal) sideroblasts, iron-containing (siderotic) granules are cytoplasmic, small, and few in number and represent aggregates of ferritin. Such sideroblasts constitute 30 to 50% of erythroblasts in bone marrow in normal subjects. They are reduced in iron deficiency and anaemia of chronic disease. The number of sideroblasts in marrow corresponds with per cent transferrin saturation.

Type II and type III sideroblasts are abnormal. In type II sideroblasts, iron containing granules in cytoplasm are numerous and large. They are observed in haemolytic states and iron overload. In type III or ringed sideroblasts, non-ferritin iron is deposited in mitochondria that are located around the nucleus. In ringed sideroblasts, iron-containing granules are large, multiple, and are distributed in

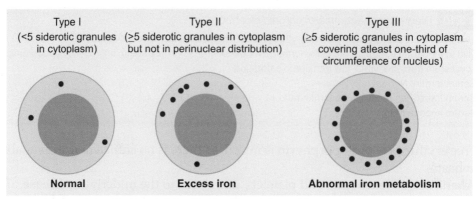

Figure 3.17: Types of sideroblasts. Blue-coloured iron granules are seen in erythroblasts (as seen with Prussian blue staining)

the form of a partial or complete ring surrounding the nucleus. They are present in sideroblastic anaemias. Sideroblastic anaemia is diagnosed if ringed sideroblasts are ≥ 15% of marrow erythroblasts.

❑ TYPES AND CAUSES

Sideroblastic anaemias are characterised by dimorphic or microcytic hypochromic anaemia, ringed sideroblasts in bone marrow, (Fig. 3.18) and ineffective erythropoiesis.
Causes of sideroblastic anaemia are shown in Table 3.12.

❑ PATHOGENESIS

Pathogenesis is not clear; impaired haem synthesis in mitochondria appears to play a significant role. The taking up of iron by erythroblasts is regulated partially by intracellular haem concentration. Defective haem synthesis is associated with increased iron uptake due to the feedback mechanism. Protoporphyrin link-up with iron fails to occur owing to reduced availability of the former and excess iron is deposited in mitochondria.

Hereditary Sideroblastic Anaemia

The mode of transmission is usually X-linked. There is reduced activity of delta aminolevulinic acid synthetase, an enzyme in the haem biosynthetic pathway. Patients present in childhood or early adult life with anaemia. Features of iron overload are often present. Anaemia is moderate to severe and may be microcytic hypochromic or dimorphic (mixture of normocytic normochromic and microcytic hypochromic red cells). S. iron and per cent transferrin saturation are increased. Bone marrow shows erythroid hyperplasia and numerous ringed sideroblasts. Some cases partially respond to pyridoxine given in high doses.

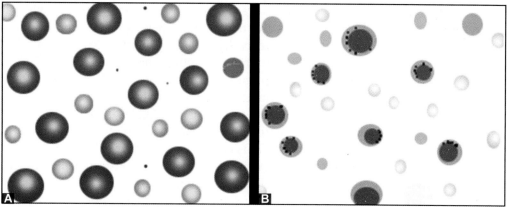

Figure 3.18: (A) Peripheral blood smear in sideroblastic anaemia showing dimorphic population of red cells (one normocytic normochromic and other microcytic hypochromic) (B) Bone marrow aspiration smear stained with iron stain showing ringed sideroblasts containing blue-stained granules of iron in perinuclear distribution

Table 3.12: Causes of sideroblastic anaemia

1. **Hereditary**
2. **Acquired**
   - Primary
     - Refractory anaemia with ringed sideroblasts.
   - Secondary
     - Haematologic malignancies—myeloproliferative disorders, multiple myeloma, acute myeloid leukaemia-M6 type.
     - Drugs—isoniazid, pyrazinamide, cycloserine, chloramphenicol
     - Alcoholism
     - Lead poisoning
     - Other—collagen disorders, carcinoma

Primary Acquired Sideroblastic Anaemia

This is refractory anaemia with ringed sideroblasts (RARS), a form of myelodysplasia. It occurs in middle-aged or elderly subjects. Anaemia is typically dimorphic (microcytic hypochromic and macrocytic). Morphologic abnormalities of neutrophils like Pelger-Huet cells and hypogranular forms are seen. Bone marrow shows variable megaloblastic maturation and dyshaematopoietic features. Prussian blue stain for iron reveals increased storage iron and ringed sideroblasts. Clonal chromosomal abnormalities may be detected. Progression to acute myeloid leukaemia occurs in about 1 to 2% of patients.

Secondary Acquired Sideroblastic Anaemia

Sideroblastic anaemia can occur in severe alcoholics who have malnutrition and deficiency of folate. Morphologic abnormalities are dimorphic anaemia in peripheral blood and megaloblastic erythropoiesis, vacuolisation of erythroblasts, and ringed sideroblasts in bone marrow.

Lead poisoning in adults usually follows industrial inhalation of fumes while in children eating of lead-based paint is the usual cause. The clinical manifestations include abdominal colic and motor neuropathy. Anaemia is mild to moderate and is usually microcytic hypochromic. Basophilic stippling can be striking but is not regularly observed. Stippling is due to aggregation of ribosomes, which are not removed owing to lead-induced deficiency of 5' nucleotidase. Bone marrow reveals erythroid predominance and ringed sideroblasts. The mechanism of anaemia in lead poisoning is not clear. Lead inhibits several enzymes involved in haem synthesis including ALA dehydratase and haem synthetase. This causes raised levels of free erythrocyte protoporphyrin and there is increased urinary excretion of co-proporphyrin and delta-amino-levulinic acid. Apart from defective haem synthesis, there is also some haemolytic component in lead poisoning due to direct injury to red cell membrane. Treatment consists of giving of EDTA.

ANAEMIA OF CHRONIC RENAL FAILURE

Anaemia is a common feature of chronic renal failure (CRF). It refers to anaemia resulting from impaired endocrine and excretory functions of kidney.

❑ PATHOGENESIS

Following mechanisms are involved in the causation of anaemia of CRF:

Loss of Endocrine Function of Kidney

Failure to synthesise erythropoietin plays a major role.

Loss of Excretory Function of Kidney

Inhibition of Erythropoiesis

Retention of toxic products and azotaemia exert direct inhibitory effect on proliferation and differentiation of erythroid precursor cells.

Shortening of Red Cell Survival

The activity of hexose monophosphate shunt has been found to be impaired in CRF. This may make haemoglobin prone to oxidant damage by drugs or chemicals. Activity of the ATPase which fuels the Na^+–K^+ pump of the membrane is also subnormal. Both these functional changes may cause shortening of red cell life-span or haemolysis. The nature of the toxic substance causing these metabolic changes is unknown.

Other factors such as bleeding (secondary to defective platelet function) and microangiopathic haemolytic anaemia (due to deposition of fibrin in arterioles in some renal diseases) may aggravate the anaemia in chronic renal disease but they are not directly responsible for "anaemia of CRF".

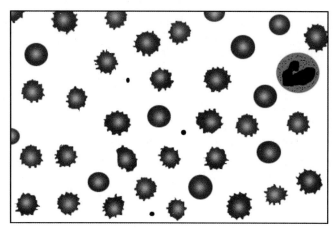

Figure 3.19: Blood smear in chronic renal failure showing numerous burr cells (echinocytes)

❑ CLINICAL AND LABORATORY FEATURES

Usually signs and symptoms of chronic renal failure predominate and anaemia is discovered incidentally. Rarely, manifestations of renal failure are minimal and patient presents with anaemia. Degree of anaemia roughly corresponds with the level of blood urea nitrogen (BUN); the greater concentration of blood urea nitrogen is associated with more severe anaemia. The anaemia is typically normocytic and normochromic with normal reticulocyte count. Burr cells (red cells with many tiny regularly placed projections on surface) are frequent (Fig. 3.19). Platelet function is defective due to uraemia (prolonged bleeding time and impaired platelet aggregation with epinephrine, ADP, and collagen). Bone marrow appears normocellular with normal maturation sequence and there is no or only slight compensatory erythroid hyperplasia in response to anaemia. Concentration of erythropoietin is lower as compared to the degree of anaemia.

❑ TREATMENT

Some improvement in anaemia occurs with haemodialysis. Renal transplantation is followed by rapid correction of anaemia. The effect of androgens (which increase release of erythropoietin from kidneys and also directly stimulate erythropoiesis) is partial in correcting anaemia. Recombinant human erythropoietin has proved to be remarkably effective in anaemia of CRF and is now the treatment of choice.

ANAEMIA OF LIVER DISEASE

"Anaemia of liver disease", which occurs in majority of patients with chronic liver disease, is caused by reduced red cell life-span and impaired red cell production.

The cause of premature red cell destruction is not known but may be related to congestive splenomegaly. Red cell production in chronic liver disease is inadequate for the degree of anaemia. The red cell abnormalities in peripheral blood include round macrocytosis and target cells. Target cells have increased cholesterol and lecithin in the membrane.

Erythropoiesis is normoblastic or macronormoblastic; macronormoblasts are large cells with normal chromatin pattern. Improvement in liver function corrects "anaemia of liver disease." Apart from "anaemia of liver disease," other causes of anaemia in liver disorders are:

i.   Iron deficiency anaemia due to blood loss from anatomical lesions such as oesophageal varices or bleeding secondary to coagulation factor abnormalities;

ii. Acute blood loss anaemia secondary to gastrointestinal haemorrhage;

iii. Spur cell anaemia—Some patients with severe chronic liver disease develop spur cell haemolytic anaemia. Spur cells are red cells with spikes on their surface. Spur cells have increased amount of membrane cholesterol, are rigid, and are prematurely destroyed in the spleen.

iv. Megaloblastic anaemia due to nutritional folate deficiency in alcoholics;

v.   Hypersplenism; and

vi. Aplastic anaemia in viral hepatitis.

MYELOPHTHISIC ANAEMIA

Extensive involvement of bone marrow by neoplastic, infectious, and metabolic (storage) diseases may produce myelophthisic anaemia. The peripheral blood prominently shows nucleated red cells and immature myeloid cells such as metamyelocytes, myelocytes, promyelocytes, or even myeloblasts. This peripheral blood picture is called as leucoerythroblastosis (Fig. 3.20). Underlying disease dominates the clinical presentation. Causes of myelophthisic anaemia are listed in Table 3.13.

Table 3.13: Diseases causing myelophthisic anaemia

1. **Malignant diseases**
   - **Haematological:** Acute and chronic leukaemias, myeloproliferative disorders, multiple myeloma
   - **Non-haematological diseases metastatic to marrow:** Carcinomas of lung, breast, prostate, stomach, etc.
2. **Lipid storage diseases:** Gaucher's disease, Niemann-Pick disease
3. **Disseminated infectious diseases:** Miliary tuberculosis

Anaemia is normocytic normochromic and mild to moderate. Teardrop red cells is a characteristic feature. Total leucocyte count is normal, low or raised. Platelets may be normal or reduced.

Bone marrow biopsy is necessary in all cases for definitive diagnosis. Treatment consists of management of the underlying disorder.

CONGENITAL DYSERYTHROPOIETIC ANAEMIAS (CDA)

These are rare inherited anaemias. The features of CDA are (i) dyserythropoiesis especially presence of erythroblasts with multiple nuclei in bone marrow, (ii) ineffective

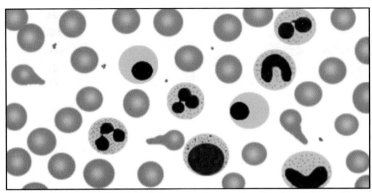

Figure 3.20: Leukoerythroblastic blood picture showing immature white and red blood cells in peripheral blood. Tear drop red cells are also present

erythropoiesis and (iii) presentation usually in infancy or childhood (usually >10 years) with anaemia, splenomegaly and mildly increased indirect S. bilirubin. Morphologic abnormalities in the bone marrow are limited to the erythroid series. There is excessive deposition of iron in tissues. Three types of CDA are distinguished—I, II, and III. Types I and II have autosomal recessive mode of inheritance, while type III is dominantly inherited.

Anaemia with dyserythropoiesis also occurs in association with megaloblastic anaemia, thalassaemia, congenital haemolytic anaemias, certain infections, alcoholism, drugs, myelodysplasia, and acute myeloid leukaemia. However, in CDA, dyserythropoiesis is primary and inborn.

❏ CDA TYPE I

Peripheral blood shows macrocytosis. Bone marrow shows marked erythroid hyperplasia. Morphologic alterations in erythroblasts include megaloblast-like or spongy nuclear chromatin, erythroblasts with incompletely separated nuclei, binucleated erythroblasts, and internuclear chromatin bridges between two erythroblasts.

❏ CDA TYPE II

This is the most frequent type and is also known as HEMPAS (Hereditary erythroblastic multinuclearity with positive acidified serum test).

Bone marrow shows binucleate and multinucleate erythroblasts, pleuripolar mitoses, and karyorrhexis.

The red cells in HEMPAS are haemolysed by acidified normal sera and are thus similar in this character to red cells of paroxysmal nocturnal haemoglobinuria (PNH). However, lysis of red cells in PNH in acidified serum test is due to abnormal sensitivity to complement, and all sera will cause lyses. In HEMPAS there is a unique antigen on the surface of the red cells known as "HEMPAS" antigen which reacts with

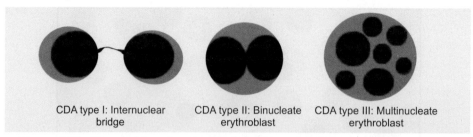

CDA type I: Internuclear   CDA type II: Binucleate   CDA type III: Multinucleate
bridge   erythroblast   erythroblast

Figure 3.21: Abnormalities of erythroblasts in congenital dyserythropoietic anaemias

complement-fixing IgM antibody; only those sera which contain significant amount of anti-HEMPAS antibody cause lysis of red cells.

Cold-reacting anti-I and anti-i antibodies react strongly with HEMPAS cells. Splenectomy is followed by some improvement.

❑ CDA TYPE III

This is the rarest type. It is characterised by red cell macrocytosis in peripheral blood and giant erythroblasts in the bone marrow with multinuclearity (up to 12 nuclei may be present) (Fig. 3.21).

❑ BIBLIOGRAPHY

1. Andrews NC. Disorders of iron metabolism. N Engl J Med. 1999;341: 1986-95.
2. Appelbaum FR, Fefer A. The pathogenesis of aplastic anaemia. Semin Hematol. 1981;4: 241-57.
3. Bacigalupo A, Hows JM, Gluckman E, et al. Bone marrow transplantation (BMT) versus immunosuppression for the treatment of severe aplastic anaemia (SAA): a report of EBMT SAA Working Party. Br J Haematol. 1988;70: 177-82.
4. Beris P, Miescher PA. Hematological complications of infectious agents. Semin Hematol. 1988;25: 123-39.
5. Bottomley SS, Muller-Eberhard V. Pathophysiology of heme synthesis. Semin Hematol. 1988;25: 282-302.
6. British Committee for Standards in Haematology (BCSH) General Haematology Task Force: Guidelines for the diagnosis and management of acquired aplastic anaemia. Br J Haematol. 2003;123: 782-801.
7. Brittenham GM, et al: Clinical consequences of new insights in the pathophysiology of disorders of iron and heme metabolism. American Society of Hematology Education Programme Book. Hematology, 2000.
8. Camitta BM, Donall Thomas E, Nathan DG, Gale RP, Kopecky KJ, Rappeport JM, Santos G, Gordon-Smith EC, Storb R. A prospective study of androgens and bone marrow transplantation for treatment of severe aplastic anemia. Blood. 1979;53: 505-14.
9. Camitta BM, Storb R, Donall Thomas E. Aplastic anemia: Pathogenesis, diagnosis, treatment, and prognosis. N Engl J Med. 1982;306: 645-652, 712-18.
10. Cartwright GE, Deiss A. Sideroblasts, siderocytes, and sideroblastic anemia. N Engl J Med. 1970;292: 185-93.

11. Cartwright GE. The anemia of chronic disorders. Semin Hematol. 1966;3: 351-75.

12. Chanarin I. Megaloblastic anaemia, cobalamin, and folate. J Clin Pathol. 1987;40: 978-84.

13. Chanarin I. The Megaloblastic Anemias. 2nd ed. Oxford. Blackwell Scientific Publications. 1979.

14. Cook JD. Clinical evaluation of iron deficiency. Semin Hematol. 1982;14: 6-18.

15. Cook JD. Iron methodology—An overview. In Cook JD (Ed): Methods in Haematology. Vol 1. Iron. New York. Churchill Livingstone. 1980.

16. Dessypris EN. The biology of pure red cell aplasia. Semin Hematol. 1991;28: 275-84.

17. Eschbach JW, Egrie JC, Downing MR, Browne JK, Adamson JW. Correction of the anemia of end-stage renal disease with recombinant human erythropoietin. Results of a combined phase I and II clinical trial. N Engl J Med. 1987;316: 73-78.

18. Finch C. Regulators of iron balance in humans. Blood. 1994;84: 1697-1702.

19. Ganz T: Hepcidin and iron regulation, 10 years later. Blood. 2011; 117: 4425-4433.

20. Gluckman E, Marmont A, Speck B, Gordon-Smith EC. Immunosuppressive treatment of aplastic anemia as an alternative treatment for bone marrow transplantation. Semin Heamtol. 1984;21: 11-19.

21. Goddard AF, McIntyre AS, Scott BB. Guidelines for the management of iron deficiency anaemia. Gut. 2000;46 (Suppl IV): iv1-iv5.

22. Goodnough LT, Nemeth E, Ganz T: Detection, evaluation, and management of iron-restricted erythropoiesis. Blood. 2010; 116: 4754-4761.

23. Gordon-Smith EC, Rutherford TR. Fanconi anemia: Constitutional aplastic anemia. Semin Hematol. 1991;28: 104-112.

24. Goudsmit R, Beckers D, DeBruijne JI, Engelfrit CP, James J, Morselt AFW, Reynierse E. Congenital dyserythropoietic anaemia type III. Br J Haematol. 1972;23: 97-105.

25. Herbert V. Biology of disease: Megaloblastic anaemias. Lab Invest. 1985;52: 3-19.

26. Hines JD, Grasso JA. The sideroblastic anemias. Semin Hematol. 1970;7: 86-105.

27. Horne III MK: Iton deficiency. In Rodgers GP, Young NS (Eds): Bethesda handbook of clinical hematology. 2nd ed. Philadelphia. Lippincott Williams & Wilkins. 2010.

28. Kumar V, Abbas AK, Fausto N, Aster JC: Robbins and Cotran pathologic basis of disease. 8th Ed. Philadelphia. Saunders Elsevier. 2010.

29. Lee GR. The anemia of chronic disease. Semin Hematol. 1983;20: 61-80.

30. Lewis SM, Nelson DA, Pitcher CS. Clinical and ultrastructural aspects of congenital dyswerythropoietic anaemia type I. Br J Haematol. 1972;23: 113-19.

31. Marsh JCW, Ball SE, Cavenagh J, et al Writing Group British Committee for Standards in Haematology: Guidelines for the diagnosis and management of aplastic anaemia. Br J Haematol. 2009; 147: 47-70.

32. Means Jr. RT and Krantz SB: Progress in understanding the pathogenesis of the anemia of chronic disease. Blood. 1992;80: 1639-47.

33. Mufti GJ, Bennett JM, Goasguen J, et al: Diagnosis and classification of myelodysplastic syndrome: nternational Working Group on morphology of myelodysplastic syndrome (IWGM-MDS) consensus proposals for the definition and enumeration of myeloblasts and ring sideroblasts. Haematologica. 2008; 93: 1712-1717.

34. Nissen C. The pathophysiology of aplastic anaemia. Semin Hematol. 1991;28: 313-8.

35. Oh RC, Brown DL. Vitamin B12 deficiency. Am Fam Physician. 2003;67: 979-86.

36. Provan D, Weatherall DJ. Red cells II: acquired anaemias and polycythaemia. Lancet. 2000;355:1260-68.

37. Sears DA. Anemia of chronic disease. Med Clin North Am. 1992;76: 567-80.

38. Snow CF. Laboratory diagnosis of vitamin B12 and folate deficiency: a guide for the primary care physician. Arch Intern Med. 1999;159: 1289-98.

39. Speck B. Allogenic bone marrow transplantation for severe aplastic anemia. Semin Hematol. 1991;28: 319-21.

40. Stewart FM. Hypoplastic/Aplastic anemia. Role of bone marrow transplantaion. Med Clin North Am. 1992;76: 683-97.

41. Tischkowitz MD, Hodgson SV. Fanconi anaemia. J Med Genetics. 2003;40: 1-10.

42. Toh B, van Driel IR, Gleeson PA. Pernicious anemia. N Engl J Med. 1997;337: 1441-48.

43. Umbriet J: Iron deficiency: A concise review. Am J Hematol. 78: 225-231, 2005.

44. Weiss G, Goodnough LT. Anemia of chronic disease. N Engl J Med. 2005;352: 1011-23.

45. Wickramasinghe SN. Dyserythropoiesis and congenital dyserythropoietic anaemias. Br J Haematol. 1997;98: 785 97.

46. Wong KY, Hug G, Lampkin BC. Congenital dyserythropoietic anaemia type II: Ultrastructural and radioautographic studies of blood and bone marrow. Blood. 1972;39:23-30.

47. Young N. Hematologic and hematopoietic consequences of B19 parvovirus infection. Semin Hematol. 1988;25: 159-72.

48. Young NS, Scheinberg P, Liu JM: Bone marrow failure syndromes: Acquired and constitutional aplastic anaemia, paroxysmal nocturnal hemoglobinuria, pure red blood cell aplasia, and agranulocytosis. In Rodgers GP, Young NS (Eds): Bethesda handbook of clinical hematology. 2nd ed. Philadelphia. Lippincott Williams & Wilkins. 2010.

49. Young NS. Aplastic anaemia. Lancet. 1995;346: 228-32.

CHAPTER

4

Anaemias due to Excessive Red Cell Destruction

HEREDITARY SPHEROCYTOSIS

Hereditary spherocytosis (HS) is a congenital haemolytic disorder characterised by an inherited defect in the red cell membrane cytoskeleton leading to the formation of spherocytic red cells. Spherocytes, being less deformable than normal red cells, are trapped and destroyed in the spleen. Spherocytes have reduced surface area to volume ratio and are osmotically fragile. Although most common mode of inheritance is autosomal dominant, autosomal recessive transmission occurs in some cases. HS occurs in all races but has a high prevalence in people of northern European descent (1:5000). In our country, HS is found mainly in North India.

❑ AETIOPATHOGENESIS

The Basic Lesion

Normally, lipid bilayer of the red cell membrane is anchored to the underlying skeleton by two major linkages. The first linkage involves interaction of ankyrin with spectrin in skeleton and band 3 in the bilayer. The second attachment between skeleton and bilayer is provided by glycophorin C and protein 4.1 (see Fig. 1.13, Chapter 1). Deficiency in any of these interactions causes weakening of contact between lipid bilayer and skeleton. As a result, areas of the lipid bilayer, which are not directly supported by the underlying skeleton, are lost from the cells in the form of small lipid vesicles. This causes decrease in surface area of red cell relative to volume with resultant spherocyte formation.

HS may result from deficiency of following skeletal proteins—spectrin, ankyrin, band 3, and protein 4.2. Ankyrin deficiency is more common.

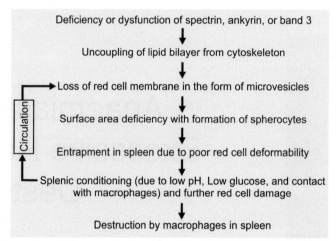

Figure 4.1: Pathogenesis of haemolysis in hereditary spherocytosis

Red Cell Destruction by Spleen

Spherocytes are more rigid and less deformable than normal red cells. This nondeformability prevents the passage of spherocytes from the splenic cords into the splenic sinuses through the slit-like narrow openings. They are retained in the splenic cords for unduly long time. In the splenic cords, red cells encounter unsuitable environment in the form of low glucose and reduced pH. Metabolic deprivation of red cells accentuates membrane loss with release of small vesicles and increase in spherical shape of red cells. Cellular dehydration occurs due to loss of potassium from the red cells. Some of the red cells may escape into the circulation where they appear as dense microspherocytes on blood films. This small population of microspherocytes is osmotically most fragile. Most of the spherocytes are, however, retained in the red pulp where they are destroyed by macrophages. Red cells that escape are retrapped by spleen and phagocytosed (Fig. 4.1).

❑ INHERITANCE

Most of the cases exhibit autosomal dominant pattern of inheritance, while recessive transmission is less common. Usually dominant inheritance is associated with mild to moderate disease while recessively inherited spherocytosis is associated with severe haemolysis.

❑ CLINICAL FEATURES

Heterogeneity

The clinical presentation is markedly heterogeneous. Majority of patients present in childhood with mild to moderate anaemia, intermittent jaundice, and enlarged spleen. Some other member of the family such as a sibling or a parent is similarly affected.

In some patients clinical features are mild or entirely absent. HS may first be detected while investigating a patient who has gallstones or splenomegaly and minimal or no anaemia (well-compensated haemolysis). In still other persons the only abnormality is increased red cell osmotic fragility; such persons come to attention when family members of the affected patient are investigated.

Rarely hereditary spherocytosis may present as a severe haemolytic anaemia requiring regular transfusion support.

Exacerbation of Anaemia

Sometime the steady course of hereditary spherocytosis is punctuated by episodes of exacerbation of anaemia or crises.

In **aplastic crisis**, there is temporary aplasia of erythroid precursors in the bone marrow resulting in sudden worsening of anaemia. Infection by human parvovirus has recently been recognized as the cause. Parvovirus B19 selectively infects erythroblasts and transiently suppresses erythropoiesis. Infection by this virus may be asymptomatic or may manifest with fever, chills, bodyache, and facial rash. Transient suppression of erythropoiesis in persons with normal red cell life-span does not manifest as anaemia. However, in patients with chronic haemolytic anaemia in whom the red cell life-span is markedly shortened, infection is associated with sudden aggravation of anaemia, reticulocytopaenia, and erythroblastopaenia. Treatment consists of transfusion support during the aplastic phase. Increased turnover of erythroid cells due to haemolysis may lead to **megaloblastic crisis** if dietary intake of folate is insufficient. Exacerbation of haemolysis (**haemolytic crisis**) may occur during intercurrent infection due to hyperplasia of monocyte-macrophage system.

Gallstones

Pigment gallstones are common in adolescents or young adults. Sometimes HS is diagnosed incidentally during investigation of a young patient with gallstones.

Chronic Leg Ulcers

These are present in an occasional patient.

❑ LABORATORY FEATURES

Examination of Peripheral Blood

In most patients anaemia is usually mild to moderate. MCHC is increased (due to cell dehydration), MCH is normal, while MCV is slightly low. Reticulocytosis is present.

On blood smear examination, characteristic feature is spherocytosis (Fig. 4.2). A spherocyte is a red cell that is smaller in size, does not have central pallor and appears densely haemoglobinised (hyperchromic). Spherocytes, however, are not unique to

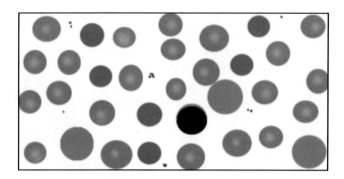

Figure 4.2: Blood smear in hereditary spherocytosis. Spherocytes are small (compare with small lymphocyte), dense cells with no central pallor. Polychromatic cells are also increased due to haemolysis

HS and are also prominently seen in other disorders such as immune haemolytic anaemias, ABO haemolytic disease of the newborn, haemolytic transfusion reactions, and burns.

Bone Marrow Examination

This reveals erythroid hyperplasia. Aplastic and megaloblastic crises can be identified by bone marrow examination.

Osmotic Fragility Test

The osmotic fragility (OF) test is the commonly employed screening test for HS. The incubated variant of OF test (see below) is more sensitive than the unincubated test. This test determines susceptibility of red cells to haemolysis when they are subjected to osmotic stress. The red cells are suspended in decreasing concentrations of hypotonic saline solutions and the amount of haemolysis is measured. Water enters the red cells when they are placed in hypotonic saline solution. Due to their biconcave shape, normal red cells can withstand hypotonicity by increasing their volume; beyond a certain limit increase in swelling is not possible, and cells burst by discharging their haemoglobin into the supernatant. Spherocytes have a decreased surface to volume ratio and therefore, they are able to withstand less swelling than normal and are osmotically fragile, i.e. haemolysis occurs in more concentrated solution than normal cells (Fig. 4.3 and Box 4.1). There are various methods of recording results of osmotic

---

Box 4.1   Osmotic fragility test

- Measures ability of red cells to take up water when kept in hypotonic saline solutions
- Due to their biconcave shape, normal red cells take up more water and increase their volume by up to 70% before lysing. Owing to ↑volume to surface area ratio, spherocytes can take up relatively little water and can withstand very little increase in their volume
- Normally red cells show beginning of haemolysis at 0.5% saline, while spherocytic red cells lyse at higher saline concentration.
- OF is more marked if red cells are incubated at 37°C for 24 hours before the test
- Test is not diagnostic of HS. Positive result (increased fragility) should be interpreted in the light of clinical and other laboratory features

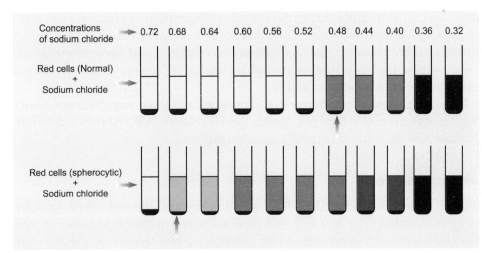

Figure 4.3: Osmotic fragility test. In hereditary spherocytosis (lower set of tubes), haemolysis starts (up arrow) at a higher saline concentration as compared to normal (upper set of tubes)

fragility test: (i) Highest concentration of saline at which haemolysis starts (normal 0.50 g/dl NaCl) and the highest concentration of saline at which it is complete (normal 0.30 g/dl of NaCl); (ii) Concentration of saline showing 50% lysis (Median corpuscular fragility); normal value is 0.40 to 0.45 g/dl NaCl. Higher value denotes increased fragility; (iii) A graph may be plotted with amount of haemolysis on vertical axis and saline concentrations on horizontal axis. Normal osmotic fragility curve is sigmoid-shaped. Shift of the curve to the right indicates increased osmotic fragility.

Limitations of Osmotic Fragility Test

- **Increased osmotic fragility** is due to spherocytosis, which may result from a variety of causes (HS, immune haemolysis, burns, etc.). Therefore, OF test is not specific for diagnosis of HS.
- OF test is **normal in patients with mild HS** having very few spherocytes in their blood. The sensitivity of the test, however, can be increased by performing the test after incubation of cells at 37°C, (see below).
- Test is time-consuming, tedious; and if spherocytes are present on blood smear, adds little to diagnosis.
- **Decreased osmotic fragility** (increased resistance to lysis in hypotonic solutions) is seen in iron deficiency anaemia, thalassaemia, sickle-cell disease, and liver disease. Therefore, the test is falsely negative in the presence of above disorders.
- OF test cannot distinguish between causes of spherocytosis.

Osmotic Fragility Test after Incubation

Sterile blood is incubated at 37°C for 24 hours followed by determination of osmotic fragility in hypotonic saline solutions. During incubation, metabolic deprivation of spherocytes occurs (mainly due to decreased concentration of glucose) with resultant membrane destabilisation, loss of membrane, and enhancement of spherical shape. Failure of membrane pump with accumulation of sodium and water also plays a role. The sensitivity of the test is thus increased. Incubated OF test may, however, be normal in a small number of patients with HS.

It should be noted that osmotic fragility is increased in any disorder associated with spherocytosis and is thus not specific for HS. Normal OF test result does not rule out HS as it may be normal in mildly affected patients.

Autohaemolysis Test

In this test, blood is incubated at 37°C for 48 hours and the degree of spontaneous haemolysis is noted. The test is performed with and without addition of glucose. Amount of haemolysis is estimated in a colorimeter and the result is expressed as a per cent lysis (Normal: <4%; with glucose: <0.5%).

Red cells in hereditary spherocytosis are abnormally permeable to sodium probably because of defect in membrane skeleton. Therefore, there is compensatory increase in sodium extrusion by the membrane pump, which thus requires more ATP than normal. During *in vitro* incubation this causes rapid exhaustion of available red cell ATP and glucose by way of increased glycolysis. Depletion of ATP leads to failure of membrane pump and swelling of red cells as they gain sodium and water. During incubation membrane loss from the red cells is accentuated which increases the volume to surface ratio. Autohaemolysis thus, results with smaller red cell volume. Thus during the 48 hours incubation period in this test, glucose exhaustion occurs due to increased utilisation and autohaemolysis is increased. With the addition of glucose, autohaemolysis is corrected to normal levels.

Autohaemolysis is also increased in deficiency of a glycolytic enzyme such as pyruvate kinase due to a block in the utilisation of glucose. In this case, however, addition of glucose fails to correct the abnormality.

Acidified Glycerol Lysis Time (AGLT)

This test assesses the rate of lysis of red cells and the result is expressed as the length of time needed for 50% lysis ($AGLT_{50}$). Normal blood requires more than 30 minutes for 50% lysis. In HS, the time required for lysis is considerably shortened (25–150 seconds) since spherocytes (due to their high volume to surface area ratio) tolerate swelling for a lesser duration than normal cells. Along with hypotonic saline solution, in the reagent system, glycerol is used which slows the rate of movement of water across the red cell membrane; this allows easier measurement of time required for lysis.

As compared to osmotic fragility test, this test is simple and rapid. But, it is not diagnostic of hereditary spherocytosis since it is also positive in autoimmune haemolytic anaemia, chronic renal insufficiency, leukaemias, and during gestation.

Hypertonic Cryohaemolysis Test

This recently introduced test is reported to be more specific for diagnosis of HS than OF test. In this test, per cent cryohaemolysis is observed after transferring cells from 37° to 0°C for 10 minutes. In HS, per cent cryohaemolysis is more (> 20%) as compared to that in normal (3–15%).

Eosin-5-maleimide (EMA) Binding Test

This is a rapid flow cytometric screening test. EMA binds to band 3, a cytoskeletal protein, on intact red cells. Reduced fluorescence intensity of EMA-labelled red cells is observed in HS.

Identification of Deficient Cytoskeletal Protein

It may be possible to identify the deficiency of a specific red cell membrane protein. The usual method consists of sodium dodecyl sulphate-polyacrylamide gel electrophoresis of red cell membrane proteins followed by quantitation of separated proteins by densitometric tracing. Deficiencies of spectrin, ankyrin, band 3, protein 4.2 and some other membrane proteins can be identified by this method in majority of patients.

More sensitive method of membrane protein quantitation is radioimmunoassay.

❑ DIAGNOSIS OF HEREDITARY SPHEROCYTOSIS

Diagnostic features of HS are shown in Box 4.2.

❑ DIFFERENTIAL DIAGNOSIS

Diagnosis of hereditary spherocytosis is usually easily made on the basis of mild to moderate anaemia with spherocytosis, splenomegaly, jaundice, increased osmotic fragility, and evidence of hereditary spherocytosis in the first-degree relative.

Sometimes anaemia is mild or absent and the patient may first present with isolated splenomegaly, gallstones, or "aplastic crisis". Clinical evaluation and examination of blood film for spherocytes are necessary for correct diagnosis.

Box 4.2 Diagnosis of HS

- Presentation in childhood with anaemia, jaundice, and splenomegaly
- Positive family history (autosomal dominant) of jaundice, gallstones, or of splenectomy
- Spherocytosis on blood smear
- Reticulocytosis
- Red cell indices: ↑MCHC, ↓MCV
- Negative direct antiglobulin test
- Screening test: OF test, AGLT, Cryohaemolysis, EMA binding test
- Confirmatory test: Electrophoretic analysis of red cell membrane proteins

(Diagnosis does not require screening test or confirmatory test if other typical features listed above them are present).

HS may have to be differentiated from other causes of spherocytosis including autoimmune haemolytic anaemia and ABO haemolytic disease of the newborn. Differentiation is made by antiglobulin (Coombs') test and family studies.

❑ TREATMENT

To plan appropriate treatment, it is necessary to grade HS into mild, moderate, and severe forms (based on haemoglobin, reticulocyte count, and serum bilirubin). Treatment of severe HS is **splenectomy.** Splenectomy corrects haemolytic anaemia (though underlying skeletal defect and spherocytosis persist) and prevents complications such as gallstones. Although splenectomy is associated with increased life-long risk of sepsis from pneumococci and other encapsulated bacteria, risk is more in children and for this reason splenectomy is deferred until the child is 6 years old and is carried out only if the disease is severe or moderate. The risk of postsplenectomy infections can be reduced by immunising children with polyvalent pneumococcal, *H. influenzae,* and meningococcal vaccines and by penicillin prophylaxis. Administration of folate is necessary in moderate or severe disease to prevent megaloblastic anaemia due to increased erythrocyte turnover.

HEREDITARY DISORDERS OF HAEMOGLOBIN

❑ GENERAL FEATURES AND APPROACH TO DIAGNOSIS

Inherited disorders of haemoglobin are the commonest genetic disorders in the world. In many countries, they constitute a public health problem.

Classification

These disorders are divided into three broad groups:
- Haemoglobinopathies
- Thalassaemias
- Hereditary persistence of foetal haemoglobin (HPFH)

Inherited disorders of haemoglobin due to structural alteration of the globin poly-peptide chain are called as **haemoglobinopathies.** Majority of haemoglobinopathies result from substitution of a single amino acid in globin chain due to a point mutation in the β globin gene. The most frequent haemoglobinopathies are HbS, HbC, and HbE. Inherited disorders of haemoglobin due to reduced synthesis of one or more globin chains are known as **thalassaemias.** The two common types of thalassaemias are α and β. **HPFH** is characterised by failure of normal neonatal switch from haemoglobin F to haemoglobin A.

Both haemoglobinopathies and thalassaemias are common in India (Box 4.3 and Table 4.1).

Table 4.1: Hereditary disorders of haemoglobin prevalent in India

Disorder	State	Clinical phenotype
A. Haemoglobinopathies		
HbS	Heterozygous	Asymptomatic
	Homozygous	Severe
HbDPunjab	Heterozygous	Asymptomatic
	Homozygous	Mild
HbE	Heterozygous	Asymptomatic
	Homozygous	Asymptomatic
B. Thalassaemias		
β thalassaemia minor	Heterozygous	Asymptomatic
β thalassaemia major	Homozygous	Severe
C. Double heterozygous states		
HbS/β+ thalassaemia		Mild
HbS/β0 thalassaemia		Like sickle-cell anaemia
HbS/HbDPunjab		Like sickle-cell anaemia
HbE/β thalassaemia		Like β thalassaemia major
HbDPunjab/β thalassaemia		Mild

Box 4.3   Hereditary disorders of haemoglobin in India

- **β thalassaemias:** North, West, and East India, with highest prevalence in Sindhis, Punjabis, Gujaratis, and Bengalis
- **HbS:** Central and Southern India
- **HbD:** North India (especially Punjab)
- **HbE:** North East India

Geographic distribution of haemoglobinopathies and thalassaemias parallels the distribution of *Plasmodium falciparum*. Heterozygotes with these disorders are relatively resistant to *P. falciparum* malaria.

It is predicted that frequency of inherited haemoglobin disorders is likely to increase because of following factors: (1) natural selection of heterozygotes due to protection afforded against malaria, (2) practice of consanguineous marriages in some affected ethnic groups, (3) increased survival of affected patients due to improvements in social conditions and public health, and (4) rapidly increasing population size in general in India.

Correct diagnosis of haemoglobin disorders is essential for proper management, for genetic counselling of prospective parents, and for prenatal diagnosis and decision regarding termination of pregnancy.

Different inherited disorders of haemoglobin are as follows:

Haemoglobinopathies

Haemoglobins with reduced solubility: Some point mutations in the β globin gene cause alteration in the solubility of haemoglobin. For example, point mutation GAG → GTG at the 6th codon of β globin gene leads to the formation of sickle haemoglobin

(HbS). Upon deoxygenation HbS polymerises causing formation of sickle cells; these cells are less deformable than normal, cause vascular occlusion and are also phagocytosed in spleen.

Another example is HbC, which is formed by substitution of lysine for glutamic acid at position 6 of globin chain (β^6Glu→ Lys). Crystallisation of HbC increases rigidity of red cells, which are destroyed in spleen.

Unstable haemoglobins: Instability of haemoglobin molecule arises from mutations that interfere with structural relationship between globin chains and haem. Instability results in precipitation of haemoglobin with formation of Heinz bodies that attach to the red cell membrane. The red cells become rigid, and are sequestered and destroyed in the spleen.

Haemoglobins with low oxygen affinity: Some mutations in globin gene stabilise the haemoglobin in deoxygenated state. There is higher than normal oxygen delivery to the tissues so that oxygen demands are met at a lower haemoglobin concentration ("pseudoanaemia"). A large percentage of deoxygenated haemoglobin can cause cyanosis.

Haemoglobins with increased oxygen affinity: An example is Hb Chesapeake in which a mutation at $\alpha_1\beta_2$ interface stabilises the haemoglobin in the oxygenated or relaxed state. Oxygen is not released readily to the tissues resulting in tissue hypoxia and compensatory erythrocytosis.

Haemoglobin M: M haemoglobins arise from mutations that stabilise iron of haem in the nonfunctional ferric state. Such haemoglobins are unable to bind oxygen and produce cyanosis.

Structural haemoglobin variants causing phenotype of thalassaemia: Some mutations produce an abnormal haemoglobin molecule as well as reduced synthesis of globin chains, e.g. haemoglobin E (β^{26} Glu→ Lys) which is associated with the phenotype of β thalassaemia.

Nomenclature of haemoglobinopathies: More than 700 haemoglobinopathies have been reported so far. Majority of them are clinically insignificant. Variant haemoglobins are denoted by various methods like letters, name of the place where first discovered, residence of the prepositus, or family name of the index case. More systematic nomenclature consists of denoting the type of polypeptide chain, position, and the amino acid substitution, e.g. HbS is denoted by $\beta^{6\ \text{Glu-Val}}$, which represents substitution of valine for glutamic acid at position 6 of β globin chain.

Thalassaemias

Molecular lesions in thalassaemias cause reduced or absent synthesis of one or more of the globin chains. Imbalance in globin chain synthesis causes precipitation of unpaired globin chains, ineffective erythropoiesis and haemolysis.

Approach to Diagnosis of Disorders of Haemoglobin

Correct diagnosis can be made if a systematic approach is pursued. This consists of obtaining clinical details including patient's ethnic origin and family history, performing few basic haematological investigations, followed by confirmatory studies, which are guided by clinical data and results of baseline studies. Haemoglobin disorders are widely prevalent among certain population groups and knowledge of this may allow one to make an easier diagnosis in a relevant case, e.g. β thalassaemias are frequent in Mediterranean areas, Middle East, and in parts of North India; sickle-cell disease is common in tropical Africa and in certain tribes in Central and Southern India.

Presence of a similar disease or a relevant positive laboratory test in a close relative is a strong evidence of hereditary nature of the disease and helps in making the diagnosis in doubtful cases.

Various laboratory tests used in the evaluation of haemoglobin disorders are as follows:

(1) Measurement of haemoglobin or haematocrit, red cell count, and red cell indices; (2) Examination of blood smear; (3) Electrophoretic identification of abnormal haemoglobins—cellulose acetate electrophoresis at alkaline pH, citrate agar electrophoresis at acid pH, (4)

Box 4.4	Laboratory diagnosis of disorders of haemoglobin

Presumptive diagnosis
- Haemoglobin electrophoresis
- Isoelectric focusing
- High-performance liquid chromatography
- Capillary electrophoresis

Definitive diagnosis
- DNA analysis
- Protein analysis by mass spectrometry

High-performance liquid chromatography, (5) Immunoassay for haemoglobin variants, (6) Globin chain electrophoresis; (7) Tests for HbS—slide test using reducing agent, solubility test, (8) Quantitation of haemoglobin A2, (9) Quantitation of haemoglobin F, (10) Determination of distribution of HbF in red cells, (11) Tests for inclusion bodies, (12) Globin chain synthesis studies (Fig. 4.4 and Box 4.4).

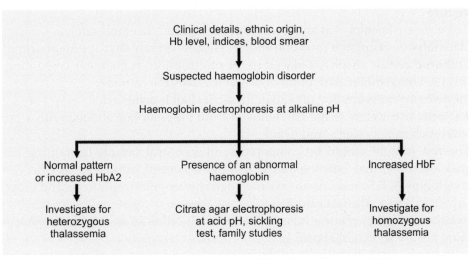

Figure 4.4: Investigations in inherited disorders of haemoglobin

Initial Peripheral Blood Examination

Generally, anaemia is severe in homozygous states whereas in heterozygotes, anaemia may be mild or absent.

Red cell indices are of critical importance in diagnosis of thalassaemias, in which MCV and MCH are characteristically low. Red cell distribution width (RDW, a measure of variation in size of red cells) is increased in iron deficiency anaemia, while it is normal in thalassaemia. Peripheral blood smear will show characteristic morphologic abnormalities such as: permanently sickled cells (sickle-cell diseases), numerous target cells (Haemglobin C disease), etc.

Haemoglobin Electrophoresis at Alkaline pH

The initial screening test in the evaluation of haemoglobinopathies is electrophoresis at alkaline pH (8.5) using a Tris EDTA-borate buffer. Various supporting media are used to achieve separation of haemoglobins such as filter paper, starch gel, or cellulose acetate membranes. Most widely used medium is cellulose acetate because the method is simple, only a small quantity of blood is needed, separation of haemoglobins is rapid, quantitation of different haemoglobins is possible, and strips can be stored permanently.

Principle: The migration of molecules having a net charge in an electric field is known as electrophoresis. Different haemoglobins have different net charge because of variations in their structure. In an alkaline buffer solution, haemoglobins migrate from cathode (-) to anode (+) and various haemoglobins have different rates of migration due to differences in their charge. Haemoglobins having more positive charge than HbA are nearer the cathode while haemoglobins having more negative charge are nearer the anode in relation to HbA. Identification of different haemoglobins is based on their relative positions on cellulose acetate strip.

Procedure
1. Red cells are haemolysed and a solution is prepared (haemolysate).
2. Haemolysate is applied near one end of cellulose acetate strip (point of origin).
3. Cellulose acetate strips are placed in the electrophoresis chamber containing Tris -EDTA-borate buffer with point of origin towards the cathode.
4. Electric current is applied till adequate separation is achieved.
5. The cellulose acetate strips are removed from the chamber, stained with a protein stain such as Ponceau S, and dried.

The test sample should be compared with a control sample containing known normal and abnormal haemoglobins. Usually a control sample known to contain haemoglobins A, F, S, and C is always included in every electrophoresis and is applied to each strip next to the test sample.

Relative mobilities of some haemoglobins using cellulose acetate electrophoresis at alkaline pH are shown in Figure 4.5.

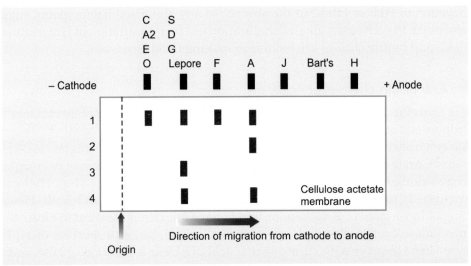

Figure 4.5: Cellulose acetate electrophoresis at alkaline pH. Lane 1: Control (AFSC); control is prepared by mixing blood from normal infant and persons with sickle-cell trait and HbC trait. Lane 2: AA (Normal person); Lane 3: SS (sickle-cell anaemia); Lane 4: AS (sickle-cell trait). Positions of various haemoglobins are shown at the top of cellulose acetate membrane for comparison

Normal electrophoresis pattern in adults is reported as AA. While reporting abnormal haemoglobins, haemoglobin with the highest concentration is written first followed by haemoglobin that is in lesser amount. Thus AC or AS indicate that concentration of HbA is higher than HbC or HbS (i.e. HbC or HbS trait respectively) while CA or SA denote that amount of HbC or HbS exceeds that of HbA (i.e. HbC-β thalassaemia or sickle-cell-β thalassaemia).

Electrophoresis at alkaline pH allows provisional identification from cathode to anode of following haemoglobins—C/A2/E/O-Arab, S/D/G/Lepore, F, A, J, Bart's, H. Thus, haemoglobin variants A2, C, E and O-Arab migrate to the same position on cellulose acetate electrophoresis at alkaline pH. Similarly, haemoglobins S, D, G, and Lepore have identical migration. These co-migrating haemoglobins cannot be differentiated from each other only on the basis of cellulose acetate electrophoresis at alkaline pH. For this purpose, a second procedure is needed. Presence of HbS can be confirmed by sickling test using 2% sodium metabisulphite or solubility test. If test for HbS is positive, then idea about genotype is gained by assessing relative proportions of HbA, HbF, and HbS. If proportion of HbA is more than HbS, it indicates AS genotype (sickle-cell trait). If HbS exceeds HbA, then it is indicative of HbS-β⁺ thalassaemia; and complete absence of HbA in the presence of HbS and HbF occurs in sickle-cell anaemia and HbS β⁰ thalassaemia. Family studies are helpful in arriving at the correct diagnosis.

For differentiating other identically migrating haemoglobins, citrate agar electrophoresis at acid pH needs to be performed.

Elevation of HbF or HbA2 in the absence of any abnormal haemoglobin suggests thalassaemia. In such cases, alkali denaturation test for quantitation of HbF, estimation of HbA2, and family studies are helpful in making the diagnosis.

Citrate Agar Electrophoresis at Acidic pH

This is a useful method for further characterisation of haemoglobin variants after electrophoresis at alkaline pH.

As seen from Figure 4.6, the haemoglobin variants C, S, A, and F migrate to different locations. Citrate agar electrophoresis at acid pH provides separation of haemoglobins that have similar mobilities on cellulose acetate at alkaline pH. Thus HbS can be distinguished from HbD and HbG, and HbC from HbE and HbO-Arab. However, haemoglobin variants D, E, G, Lepore, and H have migration identical to HbA.

In cellulose acetate electrophoresis at alkaline pH, large proportion of HbF can obscure HbS. However with citrate agar at acid pH, clear separation of HbA and HbS from HbF is obtained. Therefore, citrate agar electrophoresis at acid pH is well suited for neonatal screening of sickle-cell anaemia.

High-Performance Liquid Chromatography (HPLC)

This technique is used as a screening test for (1) detection, identification, and quantification of haemoglobin variants, and (2) quantitation of HbA2 and HbF. It is also well suited for neonatal screening since it can detect small amounts of haemoglobin and needs small amount of blood. Various automated HPLC systems are available

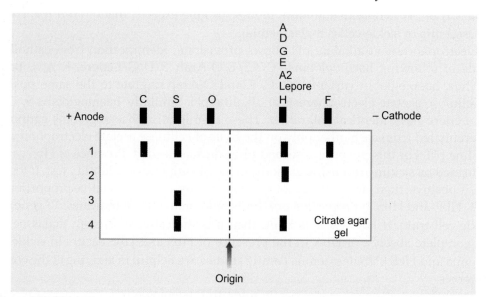

Figure 4.6: Citrate agar gel electrophoresis at acidic pH. Lane 1: Control (A, F, S, C); Lane 2: AA (Normal); Lane 3: SS (Sickle-cell anaemia); Lane 4: AS (Sickle-cell trait). Positions of various haemoglobins are shown above the agar gel for comparison

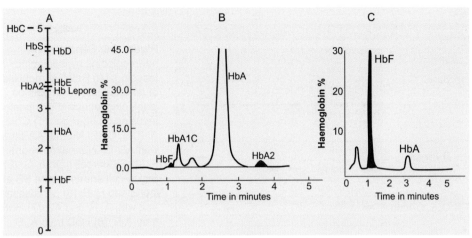

Figure 4.7: High-performance liquid chromatography. (A) Retention time of various haemoglobins (B) HPLC in normal adult (C) HPLC in normal newborn

commercially. Haemoglobins A, F, S, C, E/A2, D^{Punjab}, O-Arab, and D^{Philadelphia} can be separated and identified with HPLC.

In this automated technique, blood sample (haemolysate) is introduced into a column packed with silica gel. Different haemoglobins get adsorbed onto the resin. Elution of different haemoglobins is achieved by changing the pH and ionic strength of the buffer. Haemoglobin fractions are detected as they pass through a detector and recorded by a computer (Fig. 4.7).

Isoelectric focusing: This refers to separation of haemoglobins according to their isoelectric points or pI (i.e. the point at which they do not have a net charge) in an electric field through a pH gradient. Precast polyacrylamide or agarose gels containing ampholytes with varying pI values are available commercially. The ampholytes produce a stable pH gradient (pH 6.0 at anode to pH 8.0 at cathode). When haemolysate is applied near cathode, haemoglobins migrate through the gel and become stationary when their isoelectric points are reached to produce a distinct sharp band. As compared to electrophoresis, the technique has higher resolution and certain haemoglobins which co-migrate on cellulose acetate electrophoresis can be separated. However, quantitation of haemoglobin A2 is not possible and the technique is expensive (Fig. 4.8).

Capillary electrophoresis: This is either zone electrophoresis or isoelectric focusing carried out in a capillary tube. The technique is rapid, needs only a small sample, and quantitation is possible.

Immunoassay for Haemoglobin Variants

Commercial kits are available for detection of haemoglobin variants. These assays use monoclonal antibodies against specific haemoglobin variants. Currently HbS, HbC, HbE, and HbA can be detected by this method.

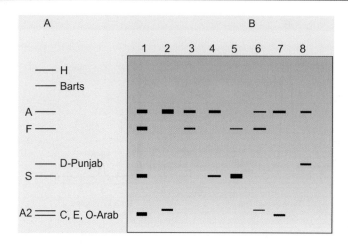

Figure 4.8: Separation of haemoglobins by isoelectric focusing: (A) Relative mobilities of different haemoglobins on isoelectric focusing. (B) Isoelectric focusing on agar gel. (1) Control: A, F, S, C; (2) Normal AA pattern with A2; (3) Normal newborn: A, F: (4) Sickle-cell trait: A, S; (5) Sickle-cell anaemia with SS and increased HbF; (6) β thalassaemia trait with A, F, and A2; (7) HbE trait: A,E; (8) HbD trait: A, D

Globin Chain Electrophoresis

α and β globin chains are separated from each other by the addition of 6 M urea and 2-mercaptoethanol to the buffer. When subjected to electrophoresis these chains migrate differently. The procedure is performed at both acid and alkaline pH and reveals characteristic patterns of migration of abnormal α and β chains.

This method provides a means of identifying abnormal haemoglobin variants that cannot be identified by routine electrophoretic methods (i.e. cellulose acetate at alkaline pH and citrate agar at acid pH.). It is especially helpful when variants other than S and C are present and which have identical migration on both cellulose acetate and citrate agar systems.

Tests for Haemoglobin S

Two types of tests are available:

Sickling test: When red cells containing HbS are subjected to deoxygenation, they become sickle-shaped while cells that do not contain HbS remain normal. Certain reducing chemical agents such as 2% sodium metabisulphite or sodium dithionite can deprive red cells of oxygen.

Blood and a reducing agent are mixed on a glass slide and a cover slip is placed over it that is sealed with petroleum jelly-paraffin wax mixture. Amount of HbS in red cells and degree of deoxygenation influence the speed and extent of sickling. Sickling is usually evident after 30 minutes; if it is not then the slide is re-examined after allowing it to stand overnight. The sickled cells have minimum of two pointed projections (Fig. 4.9).

Causes of false-negative test
- Inactive, outdated reagents (incomplete reduction of oxygen tension)
- Blood samples containing low proportion of HbS (e.g. young infants, some cases of sickle-cell trait).

- Improper sealing of coverslip (in hot climate)

Causes of false-positive test
- High concentration of sodium metabisulphite
- Carryover from positive sample due to inadequate washing of pipette
- Mistaking crenated red cells for sickled cells

Limitations of sickling test
- This test simply detects presence of HbS and does not differentiate sickle-cell anaemia from sickle-cell trait or other sickling syndromes.
- This test cannot be used for mass screening, as an experienced microscopist is required for interpretation.

Solubility test: Small amount of blood is added to a solution that contains high-phosphate buffer, a reducing agent (sodium dithionite) and saponin. Red cells are haemolysed and HbS, if present, is reduced by dithionite. Reduced HbS forms insoluble polymers, which refract light, and solution becomes turbid. A reader scale is held at the back of the tube; in negative test lines will be clearly seen since HbA is soluble in phosphate buffer, while lines will not be seen in positive test due to formation of polymers of HbS (Fig. 4.10). Positive result is also obtained with HbS Travis, and HbC Harlem. The solution remains clear in the presence of HbA, HbF, HbC, HbD, HbG, and HbO-Arab.

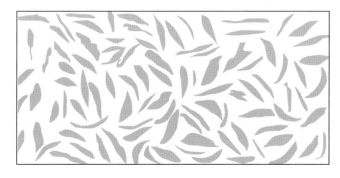

Figure 4.9: Sickling test (Wet preparation)

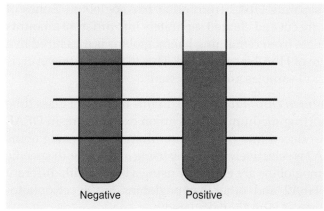

Negative   Positive

Figure 4.10: Sickle-cell solubility test. In negative test, lines of the reader scale kept behind the tubes are clearly visible. In positive test, lines are not seen due to turbidity

For mass scale screening of HbS, solubility test is the most widely used, rapid, reliable, and cost-effective test.

Causes of false-negative test
- Use of old or outdated reagents
- Low concentration of HbS as in young infants or in severe anaemia. (Solubility test should not be performed in infants <6 months to avoid getting misleading results).
- Following blood transfusion

Causes of false-positive test
- Paraproteinaemia
- Hyperlipidaemia
- Polycythaemia
- Leucocytosis

Estimation of HbA2

Normally HbA2 ($\alpha_2\delta_2$) comprises of only a small proportion (1.5–3.0%) of total haemoglobin in adults. A raised HbA2 (3.5–7%) is a characteristic feature of thalassaemia minor. Estimation of HbA2 is also useful for distinguishing sickle-cell anaemia (HbA2 < 4%) from sickle-cell β^0 thalassaemia (HbA2 > 4%).

In some cases of β thalassaemia minor, HbA2 is normal (called as normal HbA2 β thalassaemia). When iron deficiency complicates β thalassaemia minor, HbA2 is usually normal and therefore, it is not possible to make diagnosis of β thalassaemia minor until iron deficiency is adequately treated. HbA2 percentage is normal or low in $\delta\beta$ thalassaemia and in α^0 thalassaemia trait.

There are two methods for estimation of HbA2: elution from cellulose acetate and microcolumn chromatography. A newer method is high-performance liquid chromatography (HPLC).

Estimation of HbA2 by elution from cellulose acetate: Cellulose acetate electrophoresis at pH 8.9 is carried out to separate HbA2 from other haemoglobins. Zones of HbA2 and of other haemoglobins are cut and eluated separately into different amounts of buffer. Absorbance of HbA2 eluate from remaining haemoglobins is measured in a spectrophotometer and percentage of HbA2 is calculated. This technique, however, is labour-intensive if a large number of samples are to be tested.

Estimation of HbA2 by micro-column chromatography: In this method, a glass tube or a column is filled with a supporting medium such as anion exchange resin DEAE cellulose and blood sample is introduced into the column. Mixture of haemoglobins gets adsorbed on to the resin. HbA2 is selectively eluted by using a buffer with specific pH and ionic strength. Other haemoglobins are eluted by using a buffer with different pH and ionic strength. Eluted HbA2 and other haemoglobins are spectrophotometrically measured and percentage of HbA2 is calculated.

Estimation of HbA2 by both the above methods is not possible if a haemoglobin variant which co-migrates with HbA2 at alkaline pH is present (e.g. HbC, E, or O-Arab).

Estimation of Foetal Haemoglobin (HbF)

Foetal haemoglobin ($\alpha_2\gamma_2$) is the predominant form of haemoglobin during foetal life. After birth, HbF level gradually falls and is approximately 25% at 1 month, 5% at 6 months, and less than 2% at 1 year. In adults HbF is less than 1%. **Significant elevation of HbF usually occurs in β thalassaemia major, hereditary persistence of foetal haemoglobin, δβ thalassaemia, and sickle-cell disease; quantitation of HbF is usually done in these disorders.** Mild elevation occurs during pregnancy and in aplastic anaemia, megaloblastic anaemia, paroxysmal nocturnal haemoglobinuria, chronic leukaemias, and erythroleukaemia.

There are various methods for estimation of HbF. (If HbF is >2%, it can be recognised usually on electrophoresis). The commonly used method is the Betke method. In this method, a strong alkali (sodium hydroxide) is added to the haemolysate to denature HbA and after a specified time, saturated ammonium sulphate is added. The denatured haemoglobin is precipitated by ammonium sulphate. Foetal haemoglobin resists denaturation and remains in solution. The amount of haemoglobin remaining in solution (i.e. undenatured haemoglobin or HbF) is measured spectrophotometrically and is calculated as the percentage of the total haemoglobin. Betke's method is reliable for estimation of 2 to 40% of HbF. For higher levels of HbF, method of Jonxis and Visser can be used. In this method, rate of alkali denaturation is measured in a spectrophotometer and extrapolated back to zero time to get the amount of HbF. Other methods are radioimmunoassay and high-performance liquid chromatography.

Intercellular Distribution of HbF

Test for cellular distribution of HbF is employed to distinguish hereditary persistence of foetal haemoglobin (HPFH) from δβ thalassaemias. In HPFH, HbF is distributed evenly in all the red cells (pancellular distribution) whereas in δβ thalassaemias only some of the red cells contain HbF (heterocellular distribution).

The method most commonly employed for evaluation of cellular distribution of HbF is acid elution test of Betke-Kleihauer. In this test, fresh blood films on glass slides are fixed with ethanol. HbA is readily eluted from red cells by acid solution, while HbF resists acid-elution and remains within the cells. After staining, cells containing large amount of HbF appear dark, while cells with no HbF appear unstained and empty ("ghosts"). The acid elution test was originally employed to confirm and quantitate foetomaternal haemorrhage by detecting foetal red cells in maternal circulation (Fig. 4.11).

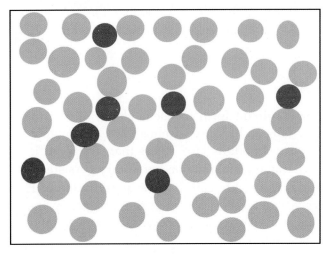

Figure 4.11: Acid elution test for intercellular distribution of HbF. Red cells containing HbF are dark while those without HbF are pale and empty

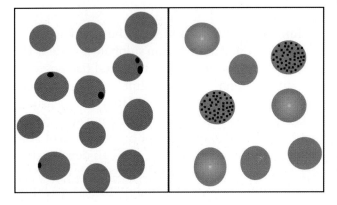

Figure 4.12: Inclusion bodies in red cells: Heinz bodies (left) stained with crystal violet and HbH inclusions stained with brilliant cresyl blue (right)

Tests for Inclusion Bodies

Following types of inclusions are detected in haemoglobinopathies (Fig. 4.12):

HbH inclusions: Due to the redox action of certain dyes (brilliant cresyl blue) HbH may be precipitated in mature or nucleated red cells as multiple, small, ragged inclusions. They are seen in Hb Bart's hydrops foetalis syndrome, HbH disease, and α thalassaemia carrier states.

In splenectomised patients with HbH disease, preformed HbH inclusions can be detected when peripheral blood is incubated with methyl violet.

α chain inclusions: α chain inclusions in homozygous β thalassaemia are seen only in nucleated red cells in bone marrow, but after splenectomy they are also seen in peripheral blood. Peripheral blood or bone marrow sample is incubated with methyl violet, films are prepared and observed under microscope. α chain inclusions appear as single, ragged structures closely attached to the nucleus.

Heinz bodies: Heinz bodies are formed by precipitation of denatured haemoglobin, which can be detected after vital staining with methyl violet. They stain deep purple and are usually attached to the cell membrane. Apart from unstable haemoglobin disease they are also seen in glucose-6-phosphate dehydrogenase (G6PD) deficiency after oxidative denaturation of haemoglobin by drugs or chemicals.

Globin Chain Synthesis Studies

Sometimes electrophoretic and other usual haematological studies fail to diagnose thalassaemias and in these cases globin chain synthesis ratio may be helpful.

Reticulocytes are capable of globin synthesis. Reticulocyte-enriched red cells (obtained by centrifugation) are incubated in a medium, which contains a radioactive amino acid (usually ^{3}H leucine). The cells are then washed and haemolyzed and globin is extracted with acid-acetone. Globin chains are dissociated by CM-cellulose chromatography and their specific radioactivity is determined by counting in a scintillant. The values are expressed as a ratio of α chain to β chain activity.

Normal α/β ratio is about 1.0. It is reduced in α thalassaemia and raised in β thalassaemia and is proportional to the severity of defect.

❑ THE THALASSAEMIAS

The thalassaemias are a heterogeneous group of inherited disorders of haemoglobin characterised by reduced or absent production of one (or rarely more) of the globin chains. They are the commonest single gene disorders in the world.

The disease was termed thalassaemia, derived from the Greek word *thalassa* for sea, since it was formerly thought that the disease occurs only in the Mediterranean population. However, the disease is not restricted to the Mediterranean and is distributed widely in other tropical countries. The disease was first described by Thomas Cooley (a paediatrician from Detroit, USA) in 1925. Homozygous β thalassaemia or thalassaemia major is Cooley anaemia. The thalassaemias constitute a major public health problem in the countries surrounding the Mediterranean and in the Middle and the Far East. Lack of standard medical care and of regular and safe blood supply in some countries is associated with considerable morbidity and mortality from thalassaemias.

Classification of Thalassaemias

The classification of thalassaemias is based on (1) the type of globin chain that is deficiently synthesised, or (2) clinical expression of the disease.

- **Classification according to the type of globin chain which is deficiently synthesised:** The two most common types are α (alpha) and β (beta) thalassaemias. Less common types are $\delta\beta$ (delta beta) thalassaemia and $\gamma\delta\beta$ (gamma-delta-beta) thalassaemia.

- **Classification according to clinical severity:** β **thalassaemias** have been clinically classified on the basis of severity of anaemia into three types—thalassaemia major, thalassaemia intermedia, and thalassaemia minor. Patients with severe transfusion dependent anaemia are said to have thalassaemia major. In thalassaemia minor, affected individuals are usually asymptomatic with mild or no anaemia in spite of prominent red cell abnormalities in peripheral blood. Thalassaemia intermedia is characterised by intermediate degree of severity of anaemia that does not require regular blood transfusions. Each of these clinical types is genetically diverse. Clinical types of α **thalassaemia** are Hb Bart's hydrops foetalis syndrome, HbH disease, thalassaemia trait, and silent carrier.

Molecular Basis of Thalassaemias

Molecular lesions in thalassaemias are complex. Of the two common types, majority of β **thalassaemias are caused by point mutations, while most of the** α **thalassaemias result from gene deletions.**

β Thalassaemias

There is a single β globin locus on each chromosome (number 11) and as humans are diploid there are two β genes. Normal structures of globin genes and globin synthesis have been considered earlier (see chapter on "Overview of physiology of blood").

β thalassaemias are classified into two major types: β^0 thalassaemia and β^+ thalassaemia. β^0 thalassaemia is characterised by complete absence of β chain synthesis (complete deficiency of β chains) while in β^+ thalassaemia β chain synthesis is reduced but not completely lacking (partial deficiency of β chains). Usually individuals having one normal and one abnormal β globin gene have β thalassaemia minor while persons in whom both β globin genes are abnormal have β thalassaemia major.

β thalassaemia displays marked genetic heterogeneity with more than 200 molecular lesions having been reported. It has been observed, however, that in a particular population (e.g. Asian Indians, Mediterranean, Southeast Asian, American Blacks, etc.). Only a few β thalassaemia mutations are consistently and commonly found and account for 90% of the abnormal β thalassaemia genes (Table 4.2). Mutations frequent in Asian Indians are illustrated in Figure 4.13 and also shown in Box 4.5.

Box 4.5   Common β thalassaemia mutations in India
• Intron 1 position 5 (G→C)
• 619 base pair deletion
• Intron 1 position 1 (G→T)
• Frameshift mutation in codon 8–9 (+G)
• Frameshift mutation in codon 41–42 (-CTTT)
• Codon 15 (G→A)

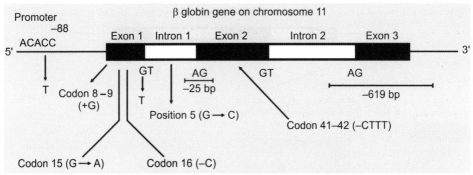

Figure 4.13: Schematic representation of β thalassaemia mutations frequently observed in Asian Indians

Table 4.2: Common mutations causing β thalassaemia in different ethnic groups

Asian Indians
- IVS-1 position 5 (G→C) Consensus splice site mutation
- 619 bp deletion
- Codon 8/9+G Frameshift mutation
- IVS-1 position 1 (G→T) Splice junction mutation
- Codons 41/42 (-TTCT) Frameshift mutation

Southeast Asians
- IVS-2 position 654 (C→T) Cryptic splice site mutation
- Codons 41/42 (-TTCT) Frameshift mutation
- −28 A→G Promoter mutation
- Codon 17 A→T Nonsense codon mutation

Mediterranean
- Codon 39 (CAG→TAG) Nonsense codon mutation
- IVS-1 position 1 (G→A) Splice junction mutation
- IVS-1 position 110 (G→A) Cryptic splice site mutation
- IVS-1 position 6 (T→C) Consensus splice site mutation
- IVS-2 position 745 (C→G) Cryptic splice site mutation

African American
- −88 (C→T) Promoter mutation
- −29 (A→G) Promoter mutation
- Poly-A (AATAAA→AACAAA) RNA cleavage poly-A signal mutation

A brief outline of mutations causing β thalassaemia is given below.

Mutations which affect transcription: Initiation and rate of transcription are regulated by the promoter region which is located immediately in front (upstream or 5' end) of globin genes. Two highly conserved sequences in the promoter region, ATAAA and CACACCC, appear to be essential for efficient initiation of transcription of the β globin gene. Mutations affecting these promoter sequences cause reduction in globin gene transcription. As some amount of β globin is produced, patients develop β⁺ thalassaemia. Some of the mutations that affect transcription are shown in Figure 4.14.

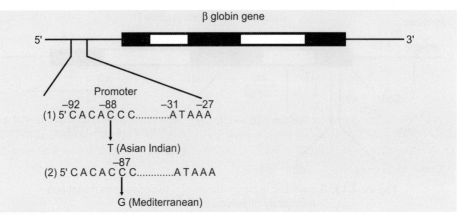

Figure 4.14: Two examples of mutations affecting transcription in selected population groups are shown. Arrows indicate sites where one base is substituted by another (−88C→T and −87 C→G) By convention, nucleotides that are located 5′ to the gene are given minus number from the transcription start nucleotide. Both these mutations cause β⁺ thalassaemia

Mutations that affect splicing of RNA: Mutations that cause abnormal splicing are very common. Majority of them occur within introns but some of them affect exons.

Splicing mutations may alter the normal splice junction or may create alternative splice sites at abnormal locations.

Mutations altering normal splice junction: The GT and AG dinucleotides at the start (5′ splice site) and the end (3′ splice site) of introns respectively are obligatory for normal splicing. If mutations alter these splice sites then splicing fails to occur resulting in absence of β globin synthesis and formation of β⁰ thalassaemia alleles (Fig. 4.15).

Mutations creating alternate splicing sites at abnormal locations. They occur in introns or exons. A mutation in intron or exon produces an alternate splicing site so that some of the messenger RNAs are spliced at mutant site and some are spliced at normal site. As shown in Figure 4.16, a mutation G→A at position 110 of intron 1 produces a new active splicing site AG. It has been shown in this case that 90% of splicing occurs at newly created abnormal site and about 10% at normal site. This results in severe β⁺ thalassaemia as abnormal splicing predominates.

Mutations in exons may also activate cryptic splice sites. An example is substitution G to A in codon 26 (GAG→AAG) of exon 1. This mutation has two effects: activation of cryptic splice site and formation of abnormal haemoglobin, HbE. A cryptic splice site is one, which resembles to some extent the normal splice site but is not used normally for splicing. A mutation in the cryptic site makes it an active splice site. Normal splicing of mRNA containing the G to A substitution in codon 26 of exon 1 leads to the formation of the abnormal haemoglobin, HbE. This mutation is associated with reduced production of mRNA (Fig. 4.17).

Mutations affecting consensus sequences: Apart from AG and GT dinucleotides, sequences surrounding the intron-exon boundaries are markedly similar. These

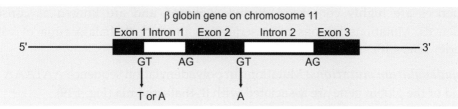

Figure 4.15: Mutations that alter normal splice junctions. Arrows indicate substitutions that alter the normal splice site. The mutations illustrated are intron 1 position 1 G→T (Asian Indians), intron 1 position 1 G→A (Mediterranean), and intron 2 position 1 G→A. All these mutations cause β^0 thalassaemia

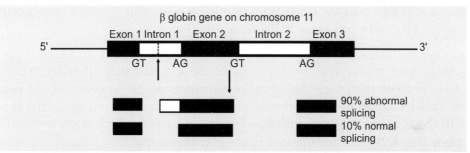

Figure 4.16: Mutation creating alternate splicing site in intron 1. Arrow (↑) shows mutant splicing site in intron 1 due to substitution G→A at position 110

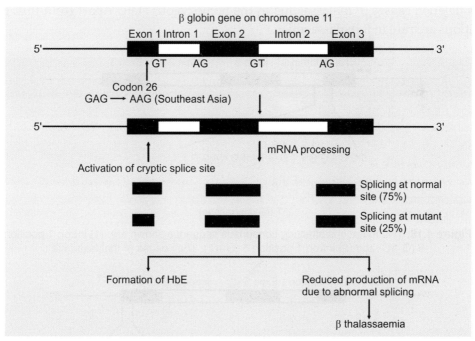

Figure 4.17: Activation of cryptic splice site in exon 1 by mutation G→A in codon 26. This substitution causes (1) formation of an abnormal haemoglobin HbE, and (2) alteration of sequence in exon 1 which activates a cryptic splice site

sequences are highly conserved during evolution and are known as consensus sequences. Mutations in consensus sequences produce β thalassaemia of variable severity (Fig. 4.18).

Polyadenylation mutations: Mutations in polyadenylation sequence AATAAA at the 3' end of the globin gene are associated with β⁺ thalassaemia (Fig. 4.19).

Mutations which lead to the formation of the chain termination codon: UAA, UAG and UGA are chain termination codons in β globin mRNA. Substitution of a single nucleotide in the coding sequence to create chain termination codon (nonsense mutation) will interrupt the translation of mRNA. This will generate non-functional fragments of β globin and cause β⁰ thalassaemia (Fig. 4.20).

Frameshift mutations: Reading frame comprises of sequentially arranged triplets of three bases. Each triplet codes for a specific amino acid. Mutations that delete or insert one, two, or more than three bases cause alteration in the sequence of the reading frame. This results in the formation of incorrect amino acids and secondly, at some place in the sequence, chain termination codon is formed which stops translation at that place (Fig. 4.21). These mutations cause β⁰ thalassaemia.

Deletions: 619-base pair deletion of the β globin gene is common in Asian Indians. It removes part of intron 2, exon 3, and some sequences 3' to the globin gene (Fig. 4.22). This deletion causes β⁰ thalassaemia in the homozygous state. Apart from this, gene deletions are rare in β thalassaemias.

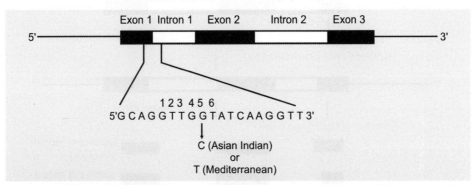

Figure 4.18: Two mutations affecting consensus sequence shown are: (1) intron 1 position 5 (G→C) and (2) intron 1 position 5 (G→T). They cause β⁰ thalassaemia

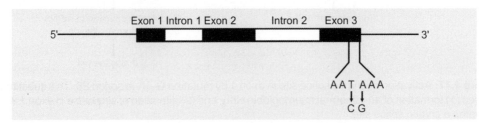

Figure 4.19: Polyadenylation mutations

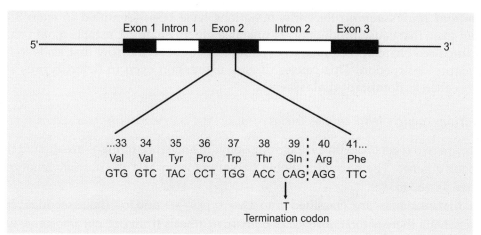

Figure 4.20: Mutation to termination codon. Nonsense mutation in codon 39 (C→T) prevalent in Mediterranean population is shown. This mutation causes formation of a stop codon TAG (UAG in mRNA) at the 39th codon which leads to premature termination of translation

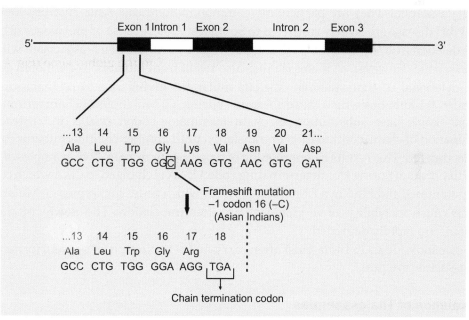

Figure 4.21: Frameshift mutation in codon 16. A deletion C in codon 16 alters the reading frame and also creates a chain termination codon prematurely at codon 18

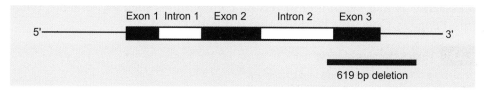

Figure 4.22: The Indian 619 bp deletion

Dominant thalassaemia: Recently, mutations have been identified in exon 3 of β globin gene that cause production of unstable globin chains. Unstable globin chains and unpaired chains precipitate in erythroblasts in bone marrow that leads to their premature destruction. This causes disease expression even in heterozygous state; this is called as **dominant thalassaemia.**

α thalassaemias

There are two α gene loci on each chromosome 16 and since humans are diploid there are four α genes. The normal α globin haplotype is αα and the normal genotype is written as αα/αα.

α thalassaemias are classified into two types—α^0 and α^+ thalassaemias. In α^0 thalassaemia there is total absence of α chain synthesis from one chromosome, while in α^+ thalassaemia α chain synthesis from one chromosome is decreased but not absent.

Most cases of α thalassaemias result from gene deletions. Deletions which remove both α genes cause complete absence of α chain production from the affected chromosome (α^0 thalassaemia). They are particularly common in Southeast Asia. Hydrops foetalis and HbH disease are largely restricted to Southeast Asia because of prevalence of cis α gene deletions (αα/- -). Deletion of one α globin gene out of the two is associated with α^+ thalassaemia. However, α^+ thalassaemias also result from mutations of α globin genes (non-deletional α^+ thalassaemia). Various mutations giving rise to α^+ thalassaemia include: (1) Mutations which cause aberrant splicing; (2) Mutations of chain terminator codon: Single base substitution in chain terminator codon results in, instead of termination of chain, continuation of translation until another chain terminator codon is encountered. This results in lengthening of α polypeptide chain. Two examples of this are Hb Constant Spring (chain terminating codon UAA is changed to CAA which codes for glutamine), and Hb Koya Dora (UAA →UCA which codes for serine); (3) Mutations which cause instability of α globin chain after translation. The newly produced α chains are rapidly degraded.

Since individuals in India most often carry αα/α- haplotype (α^+), severe forms of α thalassaemia are rare.

Prevalence of Thalassaemias

β thalassaemias are prevalent in "β thalassaemia belt" which covers Mediterranean region, Africa, Middle East, some areas of India, Pakistan, and Southeast Asia. In India, β thalassaemia is more common in certain communities such as Punjabis, Lohanas, Sindhis, Bengalis, Gujaratis, Bhanushalis, and Jains (Box 4.6).

Box 4.6 Thalassaemias in India
• β thalassaemia is frequent; α thalassaemia is rare.
• Carrier rate of β thalassaemias is about 3% (Average)
• β thalassaemia is more prevalent in certain communities from North India

α^0 thalassaemias are common in Southeast Asia (China, Thailand, Vietnam, Malaysia, the Phillipines), eastern Mediterranean region, and in Middle East; they are uncommon in Africa and India. α^+ thalassaemia is relatively more common in India.

Thalassaemias (and sickle-cell disease and G6PD deficiency) are prevalent in those parts of the world where malaria has been common. The high frequency of these disorders in certain areas is probably because heterozygotes are protected against falciparum malaria. According to the theory of 'balanced polymorphism', disadvantage of homozygous state is 'balanced' by protection afforded to heterozygotes against malaria. Genetic analysis studies suggest that thalassemic mutations have arisen independently in different parts of the world. Due to natural selection of heterozygotes (who are genetically more 'fit' because of protection against malaria) these genes have achieved high frequency.

The mean prevalence of β thalassaemia heterozygotes in India is reported to be 3.3 per cent. Every year 10,000 to 11,000 children with thalassaemia major are born in India (10% of all thalassaemics in the world).

HbE/β thalassaemia and HbH disease are becoming increasingly more common in many regions of the world due to changing demographics. Clinical phenotype of HbE/β thalassaemia resembles either thalassaemia major or intermedia. HbE/β thalassaemia is the commonest form of severe thalassaemia in eastern India, Bangladesh, and Southeast Asia.

Pathogenesis, Clinical Features, and Laboratory Features of Thalassaemias

β Thalassaemias

There are three clinical forms of β thalassaemias—β thalassaemia major, β thalassaemia intermedia, and β thalassaemia minor.

β Thalassaemia Major

This was first described by Thomas Cooley in 1925 in children of Italian descent and is also known as Cooley's anaemia.

β thalassaemia major is the most severe of the β thalassaemias and is characterised by severe anaemia which requires regular transfusion therapy. It may be produced by following genotypes—β^0/β^0, β^0/β^+, or β^+/β^+.

Pathogenesis

1. *Anaemia:* (i) Normal adult haemoglobin is composed of two α and two β globin chains and haem. In β thalassaemia major, the underlying genetic defect is responsible for inability of erythroid cells to synthesise adequate amounts of β globin chains. This causes excessive accumulation of free α chains since there are no complementary β chains to form a tetramer. The unbound α chains precipitate within erythroblasts and red cells. These α chain inclusions damage the cell membrane leading to the

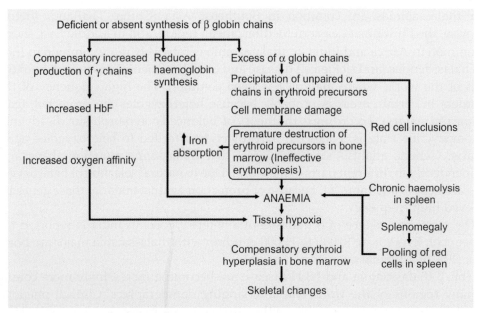

Figure 4.23: Pathogenesis of β thalassaemia major

lysis of erythroblasts and red cells in the bone marrow, i.e. ineffective erythropoiesis (Fig. 4.23). (ii) The red cells containing α chain aggregates have reduced flexibility and are trapped in the spleen. Removal of inclusions by splenic macrophages damages the red cell membranes; such red cells are ultimately destroyed by macrophages in the spleen and liver. Thus in addition to intramedullary destruction, red cells are also destroyed peripherally in the spleen (haemolysis). (iii) Reduced synthesis of haemoglobin due to lack of β globin production leads to the formation of microcytic hypochromic red cells. (iv) Excessive peripheral destruction of red cells invariably leads to splenomegaly. Pooling of considerable proportion of red cells within large spleen further aggravates the anaemia. (v) Haemoglobin F is the predominant haemoglobin in β thalassaemia major and is due to increased proliferation of cells capable of synthesising γ chains. HbF does not release oxygen as readily to the tissues as HbA since it poorly binds 2,3-diphosphoglycerate and thus exacerbates tissue hypoxia.

2. *Skeletal changes:* Severe anaemia and tissue hypoxia stimulate erythropoietic drive and cause extreme bone marrow hyperplasia. Expansion of hyperactive bone marrow causes weakening and deformities of skull and of facial bones. Thinning of cortex may lead to pathological fractures.

3. *Iron overload:* Iron absorption from the intestine is increased in β thalassaemia major due to ineffective erythropoiesis. Chronic regular blood transfusion therapy markedly increases the iron accumulation and causes iron overload (Fig. 4.24). Iron overload may damage parenchymal cells of various organs such as pancreas (diabetes mellitus), liver (cirrhosis), gonads (infertility), and heart (arrhythmias and heart failure).

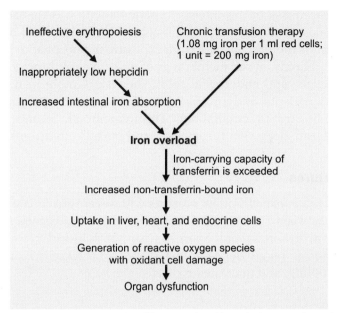

Figure 4.24: Pathogenesis of iron overload in β thalassaemia major

Clinical features: Switch from the synthesis of HbF ($\alpha_2\gamma_2$) to HbA ($\alpha_2\beta_2$) occurs after birth and therefore anaemia develops insidiously during infancy (i.e. around six months of age) and gradually becomes worse. Typically children with β thalassaemia major present with severe anaemia, failure to thrive, retarded growth, hepatosplenomegaly, and skeletal and facial changes. Frontal bossing and overgrowth of maxilla produce thalassemic or "chipmunk" facies. Various radiological changes have been described such as widening of diploe of the skull, "hair on end" appearance, widening of medullary cavity and thinning of cortex of long bones, and pathological fractures. These children suffer from repeated infections; raised serum iron level that favors bacterial proliferation has been implicated. Folate deficiency commonly develops due to increased erythroid turnover. Other complications are hypersplenism, and manifestations related to foci of extramedullary haematopoiesis compressing vital structures, such as spinal cord. Untreated patients usually die from anaemia or infections before five years of age.

Early institution of regular blood transfusion therapy is associated with normal growth and development during the first decade of life. However, iron overload gradually develops during adolescence. Manifestations of iron overload include growth retardation, hyperpigmentation of skin, hepatocellular damage with cirrhosis, insulin-dependent diabetes mellitus, gonadal dysfunction (delayed or absent pubertal development), hypoparathyroidism, hypothyroidism and cardiac failure. Most of the patients die by the end of the twenty or thirty years of life from refractory heart failure and arrhythmias. Chronic transfusion therapy is also associated with risk of transmission of viral infections such as human immunodeficiency virus (HIV), and hepatitis B and C viruses (HBV and HCV).

There is increased risk of thrombosis in patients with β thalassaemia intermedia (and also in β thalassaemia major, α thalassaemia syndromes, and haemoglobin E/β thalassaemia). This is thought to result from exposure of phosphatidylserine and other negatively charged lipids on cell membranes of defective erythrocytes which activate coagulation, platelets, and endothelial cells. The risk is more in non-transfused or under-transfused patients and in splenectomized patients (as more numbers of defective red cells are in circulation). Thromboembolic events include stroke, pulmonary embolism, deep vein thrombosis, and portal vein thrombosis (Fig. 4.25).

Laboratory Features

1. *Peripheral blood examination:* Patient presents with severe anaemia with haemoglobin concentration between 2 and 6 g/dl. Anaemia is typically microcytic and hypochromic. On peripheral blood smear examination, red blood cells show marked anisopoikilocytosis, severe hypochromia, plenty of target cells, Howell-Jolly bodies, basophilic stippling, and nucleated red cells (Fig. 4.26).

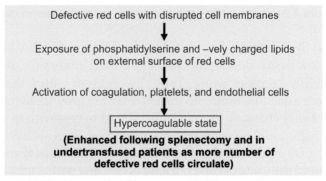

Figure 4.25: Pathogenesis of hypercoagulability state in β thalassaemia

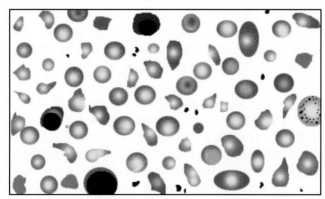

Figure 4.26: Blood smear in thalassaemia major showing microcytic hypochromic red cells, nucleated red cells, anisopoikilocytosis, target cells, basophilic stippling, and polychromasia

Reticulocytosis is modest (5–15%) but is less as compared to the degree of anaemia. The reason for this is ineffective erythropoiesis.

Leucocytes and platelets are usually unremarkable.

2. *Test for inclusion bodies:* Aggregates of unpaired α-chains within erythroblasts in bone marrow may be detected with supravital (methyl violet) staining. After splenectomy they are also demonstrated in red cells in peripheral blood.

3. *Haemoglobin electrophoresis:* This characteristically shows elevated HbF (10–98%) (Fig. 4.27). HbA2 may be normal or increased. In homozygous β^0 thalassaemia, HbA is completely lacking, while in β^0/β^+ and β^+/β^+ thalassaemias, some amount of HbA is present.

4. *Other investigations:* **Bone marrow examination** shows severe erythroid hyperplasia. Storage iron is increased. **Acid elution test** reveals heterogeneous distribution of HbF in red cells.

Unconjugated serum bilirubin and serum iron are increased while osmotic fragility of red cells is decreased.

HPLC findings in thalassaemia major and minor are shown in Figure 4.28.

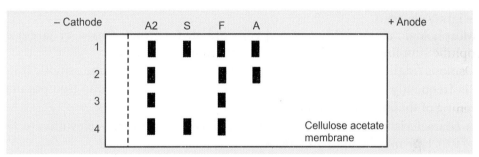

Figure 4.27: Diagrammatic representation of typical electrophoresis findings in β thalassaemia minor (lane 2), β thalassaemia major (lane 3), and sickle-cell β thalassaemia (lane 4). Lane 1 is control

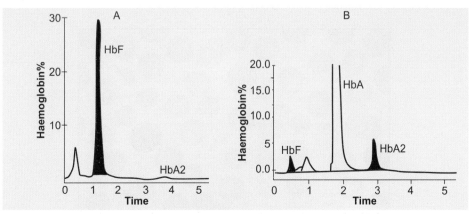

Figure 4.28: High-performance liquid chromatography findings in (A) β thalassaemia major, and (B) β thalassaemia minor

β Thalassaemia Minor

This is the heterozygous carrier state of β thalassaemia characterised by little or no anaemia but prominent morphologic changes of red cells. It results when a person inherits normal β gene from one parent and either $β^0$ or $β^+$ thalassaemia allele from the other. Degree of imbalance of globin chain synthesis and ineffective erythropoiesis are much less as compared to thalassaemia major. These patients are usually asymptomatic but may develop anaemia during demanding situations such as infections or pregnancy.

Detection of β thalassaemia minor is essential for genetic counselling and to distinguish it from iron deficiency anaemia. Long-term administration of iron in these patients can cause iron overload and organ damage.

Laboratory features: Haemoglobin level is either normal or mildly decreased and is generally not less than 9.0 g/dl. Red blood cells characteristically show reduced MCV (< 70 fl) and reduced MCH (< 25 pg). Determination of red cell indices is a commonly employed method for detection of β thalassaemia trait in population screening. MCHC is normal. Red cell count is increased. Reticulocyte count and serum bilirubin are slightly elevated.

Morphologic abnormalities of red cells are striking and consist of target cells, basophilic stippling, microcytosis and hypochromia (Fig. 4.29).

Osmotic fragility test shows resistance to haemolysis. Single tube osmotic fragility test is frequently done to identify heterozygotes of β thalassaemia (see population screening of thalassaemias and Fig. 4.31).

A characteristic laboratory feature of β thalassaemia minor is elevation of HbA2 (3.5–7.0%). HbF may be mildly increased.

Differential diagnosis: The major differential diagnosis is **iron deficiency anaemia** since both exhibit microcytic and hypochromic red cells. This is considered in chapter on iron deficiency anaemia.

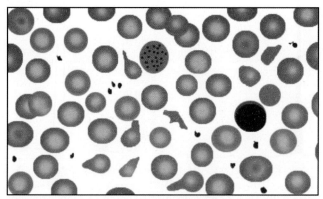

Figure 4.29: Blood smear in thalassaemia minor. Anisopoikilocytosis with microcytic hypochromic red cells and basophilic stippling are seen

Table 4.3: Typical clinical and laboratory features in β thalassaemias

Type	Genotype	Anaemia	Red cell morphology	Hb electrophoresis	Clinical features
β thalassaemia minor	β/β⁺, β/β⁰	Absent or mild (Hb > 10 g/dl)	Microcytic hypochromic; target cells, basophilic stippling	HbA2 > 3.5%; HbF<10%	Asymptomatic
β thalassaemia intermedia	β⁺/β⁺,δβ/δβ, β⁰/δβ; interaction of β⁰/β⁰ or β⁺/β⁺ with α thalassaemia	Moderate (Hb 7–10 g/dl)	Similar to major, but with less severe changes	HbF (10–95%); Absent or little HbA; HbA2 normal or raised	Onset at a later age than major; splenomegaly +; not transfusion-dependent
β thalassaemia major	β⁰/β⁰, β⁰/β⁺, β⁺/β⁺, β⁰/HbE, β⁺/HbE	Severe (Hb <7 g/dl)	Severe aniso-poikilocytosis, microcytosis, hypochromia, many target cells, basophilic stippling, many nucleated red cells	HbF (10–95%); Absent or little HbA; HbA2 normal or raised	Onset in infancy; splenomegaly +++; marked skeletal changes; transfusion-dependent

Typical clinical and laboratory features of β thalassaemias are summarised in Table 4.3.

Inheritance of β Thalassaemia with Structural Haemoglobinopathies

The inheritance of β thalassaemia with structural β globin variants is common. Sickle-cell β thalassaemia is considered below.

Sickle cell β thalassaemia (Micro drepanocytic disease): This disorder occurs when one β gene carries HbS mutation and the other gene carries β thalassaemia mutation (double heterozygous state). It is commonly observed in West Africa, the Mediterranean countries, and India. Clinical manifestations are decided by whether the β thalassaemia gene inherited is β⁰ or β⁺.

i. *Sickle-cell β⁰ thalassaemia:* Clinical manifestations resemble sickle-cell anaemia except splenomegaly that persists into adult life. (In sickle-cell anaemia, spleen characteristically undergoes autoinfarction and is usually not palpable beyond childhood).

Peripheral blood smear shows features of both sickle-cell anaemia and thalassaemia such as sickle cells, microcytic and hypochromic cells, and target cells. MCV and MCH are decreased.

On haemoglobin electrophoresis, HbS is the predominant haemoglobin (70–80%), HbA is absent, and HbA2 (3–5%), and HbF (10–20%) are elevated (see Fig. 4.27). Diagnosis is confirmed by demonstrating that one parent has sickle-cell trait and the other has β thalassaemia trait.

ii. *Sickle-cell β⁺ thalassaemia:* Two clinical phenotypes are distinguished—severe and mild.

Severe form of sickle-cell β⁺ thalassaemia occurs in Mediterranean countries and clinical picture bears resemblance to sickle-cell anaemia. Red cell morphology is typical of thalassaemia. Haemoglobin electrophoresis shows HbS as the major component, some HbA, and mildly raised HbF and HbA2.

Mild sickle-cell β⁺ thalassaemia occurs predominantly in Africa and resembles sickle-cell trait. In sickle-cell β⁺ thalassaemia, HbS is always more than HbA, while reverse is true for sickle-cell trait.

Diagnosis is confirmed by family studies (one parent with sickle-cell trait and the other with β thalassaemia minor).

α Thalassaemias

Humans have four α globin genes, two on each chromosome 16. Defect in any one of the α globin genes produces α thalassaemia. Defect may occur in one, two, three, or all four α globin genes with progressive deficiency of α chain production. Since α chains are present in both foetal and adult haemoglobins, α thalassaemia manifests in both foetal and adult lives. In Punjab, 12% of the population has α^+ thalassaemia. α^0 thalassaemia alleles are rare in India.

There are three main clinical forms of α thalassaemias—Haemoglobin Bart's hydrops foetalis syndrome, haemoglobin H disease, and α thalassaemia carrier state.

Haemoglobin Bart's Hydrops Foetalis Syndrome

This is the most severe form of α thalassaemia and results from homozygous state for α^0 thalassaemia (- -/- -). Since α^0 thalassaemia alleles are prevalent in South East Asia and in eastern Mediterranean countries (Italy, Greece, Cyprus), hydrops foetalis is common in these regions.

Absolute deficiency of α chains in foetal life leads to excess of γ chains that form tetramers (γ_4) or Hb Bart's in foetal red cells. Tetramers of γ chains are more stable than aggregates of α chains in β thalassaemia and therefore, ineffective erythropoiesis is less marked in α thalassaemia. Red cell destruction in spleen and reduced haemoglobin synthesis contribute to anaemia. Hb Bart's is a high oxygen affinity haemoglobin and causes severe tissue hypoxia.

Infants with this disease are either stillborn or die soon after birth. They are severely anaemic, and have massive anasarca and hepatosplenomegaly.

The blood film shows severe anisopoikilocytosis, microcytosis, and erythroblastosis. Haemoglobin level is 5 to 8 g/dl. Large amount of Hb Bart's (approximately 80%) is present in cord blood. Both HbA and HbF are absent since no α chains are synthesised. Globin chain synthesis studies demonstrate complete absence of α chain synthesis (α/β ratio of 0). Both the parents are obligatory carriers of α^0 thalassaemia.

Haemoglobin H Disease

HbH disease most commonly develops when both α^0 and α^+ thalassaemias are inherited (- -/- α), i.e. there is deletion of 3 α genes.

Due to marked deficiency of α chain synthesis, tetramers of β chains (β_4) are formed (HbH). They are more stable and more soluble than tetramers of α chains found in β thalassaemia; ineffective erythropoiesis is therefore not a significant factor in the genesis of anaemia. β chain tetramers precipitate in older red cells and form red cell inclusions; these red cells are destroyed in spleen. HbH is high oxygen affinity haemoglobin and does not readily deliver oxygen to the tissues thus contributing to tissue hypoxia.

These patients have anaemia (haemoglobin 7–10 g/dl), icterus, and hepatosplenomegaly. Transfusions are usually not needed. Blood film shows anisopoikilocytosis, hypochromia, microcytes, and target cells. When blood is incubated with an oxidising dye such as brilliant cresyl blue, inclusion bodies are formed due to precipitation of HbH. If spleen has been removed, preformed HbH inclusions can be shown with methyl violet.

Cord blood of the newborns shows 10 to 40% of Hb Bart's that is slowly replaced by HbH during infancy. In adults, HbH ranges between 5 and 40%. Both Hb Bart's and HbH are fast-migrating haemoglobins at alkaline pH (i.e. they move more rapidly than HbA). Globin chain synthesis studies show α/β ratio of 0.2 to 0.4.

Family study shows that one parent has α^0 thalassaemia trait (- -/$\alpha\alpha$), and the other has α^+ thalassaemia trait (-α/$\alpha\alpha$).

α Thalassaemia Carrier States

These are asymptomatic forms of α thalassaemias. They are of two main forms: α^0 thalassaemia trait (- -/$\alpha\alpha$) and α^+ thalassaemia trait (-α/$\alpha\alpha$).

α^0 thalassaemia trait (- -/$\alpha\alpha$): This results from interaction of α^0 thalassaemia (- -) with normal haplotype ($\alpha\alpha$). Thus, there is deletion of two α genes. Since it is asymptomatic, this condition is usually detected during routine haematological studies or during family studies of a person suffering from thalassaemia.

Persons with this condition have very mild anaemia, microcytic and hypochromic red cells, and decreased MCV and MCH. In adults, haemoglobin electrophoresis is normal (although trace amounts of HbH are present, they are not detectable by electrophoresis). HbH inclusions may be detected in very few red cells after a prolonged and exhaustive search. Globin chain synthesis studies reveal a α/β ratio of approximately 0.7.

5 to 15% of Hb Bart's can be detected by electrophoresis in newborns; it gradually disappears during the first few months of life. α^0 thalassaemia trait may be diagnosed in the newborn period by doing electrophoresis for Hb Bart's.

Table 4.4: Typical clinical and laboratory features in α thalassaemias

Type	Genotype	Anaemia	Red cell changes	Hb electrophoresis		Clinical features
				Newborn	Adult	
1. Silent carrier	αα/α-	Absent	None	1–2% Hb Bart's	Normal	Asymptomatic
2. α thalassaemia trait	α-/α-, αα/- -	Absent or mild	Microcytic hypochromic	5–15% Hb Bart's	Normal	Usually asymptomatic
3. HbH disease	α-/- -	Moderate	Microcytosis, target cells	20–40% Hb Bart's	HbH	Moderate anaemia, hepatosplenomegaly
4. Hydrops foetalis	- -/- -	Severe	Numerous erythroblasts	80–100% Hb Bart's	-	Fatal; death in utero or after birth

Diagnosis is difficult in adults and depends on the exclusion of other causes of microcytic and hypochromic red cells such as iron deficiency, anaemia of chronic disease, sideroblastic anaemia, and β thalassaemia minor. Family studies and ethnic origin of the person may be helpful. Definitive diagnosis requires globin chain synthesis studies and genetic analysis. These persons carry the risk of having a severely affected child if they marry another carrier.

α⁺ thalassaemia trait (-α/αα): This results from interaction of α⁺ thalassaemia (-α) with normal haplotype (αα). Thus there is deletion of one α gene.

Red cell morphology and indices are normal or there may be a slight decrease in MCV or MCH. HbH is not detectable in adults. Globin chain synthesis studies reveal a slight reduction in α/β chain ratio (0.8) which is difficult to interpret in an individual patient.

In some newborns 1 to 2% of Hb Bart's may be detected while in others it is absent. Thus, it is difficult to diagnose α⁺ thalassaemia trait in both newborns and adults and the only definitive way is globin gene analysis that will reveal deletion of one α globin gene.

Salient features of α thalassaemias are summarised in Table 4.4.

Thalassaemia Intermedia

Thalassaemia intermedia is a disorder the clinical expression of which is intermediate between thalassaemia major and thalassaemia minor. These patients do not require transfusions or require them only intermittently.

Thalassaemia intermedia presents in the later age (i.e. 2–5 years) as compared to thalassaemia major. (The age of presentation of thalassaemia major is around six months). These patients have chronic haemolytic anaemia, splenomegaly, and bone changes; growth and development is usually normal and survival into adulthood is common. Haemoglobin level is in the range of 6 to 9 g/dl. Peripheral blood examination shows thalassemic red cell changes: anisopoikilocytosis, microcytosis, hypochromia, target cells, basophilic stippling, and nucleated red cells. Pattern of haemoglobin electrophoresis depends on underlying genotype.

Thalassaemia intermedia is genetically diverse. It can be produced by many different molecular lesions-

1. Inheritance of mild β^+ thalassaemia in homozygous state (β^+/β^+);
2. Homozygous state for $\delta\beta$ thalassaemia ($\delta\beta/\delta\beta$): $\delta\beta$ thalassaemias are characterised by increased synthesis of HbF and therefore homozygous state is milder than β thalassaemia major.
3. In heritance of both β thalassaemia and $\delta\beta$ thalassaemia
4. Coinheritance of α and β thalassaemias. This causes decrease in the globin chain imbalance.
5. Dominant β^+ thalassaemia trait

Prevention of Thalassaemias

Thalassaemias constitute a significant public health problem in some countries. In India, the mean prevalence of β thalassaemia gene is reported to be 3.3% with a much higher frequency in certain communities. Thousands of thalassemic children are born every year in India. The ideal therapy of thalassaemia major consists of regular blood transfusion therapy every 3 to 4 weeks and iron chelation therapy. The cost of such treatment is exorbitant (about Rs. 100,000/- per annum in India) and imposes a considerable strain on economic resources in those countries where thalassaemias are widely prevalent. Therefore, prevention of thalassaemia should receive high priority.

Various Strategies for Prevention of Thalassaemias

1. **Health education:** Education of the people through mass media of communications can create awareness of the disease, its economic load, and desirability of prevention by identifying carriers.
2. **Carrier screening and genetic counselling:** Screening involves identification of heterozygous individuals by some simple tests. Heterozygous persons should not marry another heterozygote for the same gene due to the risk of having affected children. In genetic counselling couples at risk (i.e. when both partners are genetic carriers) are explained various options available such as prenatal diagnosis followed by selective termination of pregnancy and alternative methods of having a child such as artificial insemination, adoption, etc.
3. **Prenatal diagnosis:** Prenatal diagnosis of affected foetus and selective termination of pregnancy is now available at some places. Prenatal diagnosis is carried out in couples who are already having an affected child (retrospective diagnosis) or in couples who are identified as carriers by screening (prospective diagnosis).

Carrier Screening

Screening in thalassaemia consists of detection of genetic carriers or heterozygotes by some rapidly applied tests. Screening is done to identify individuals with β

thalassaemia minor, α^0 thalassaemia trait, $\delta\beta$ thalassaemia trait, or heterozygous state for abnormal haemoglobins such as Hb Lepore or HbS. For the screening programme for the detection of heterozygotes to be successful, following prerequisites should be fulfilled: (i) prevalence of the carrier state should be high in a particular population group; (ii) the screening tests which are employed should be suitable for mass screening; and (iii) facility of genetic counselling and prenatal diagnosis should be available. Heterozygous screening programmes have brought about a remarkable decrease in the incidence of thalassaemia in some Mediterranean countries (Cyprus and Sardinia).

Screening for the carrier state may be conducted in specific caste groups located in particular geographical areas. Those caste groups that are showing a significant prevalence of a haemoglobinopathy should be identified; this information is also obtained from previous public health surveys. Carrier screening can be done during pregnancy in antenatal clinics, after engagement of couples, or during adolescence. One widely used approach is to screen couples just before marriage or before pregnancy. If one partner is found to be a carrier for abnormal gene, then the other partner should be screened. If both are carriers then prenatal diagnosis should be considered to prevent the birth of a thalassemic child (Refer to Fig. 4.37). Screening of pregnant women should be done in first trimester of pregnancy so that prenatal diagnosis by chorionic villus sampling can be offered earlier in pregnancy if required. Limited resources pose an important constraint on large-scale screening programme in India.

Commonly employed methods for screening include the following (Fig. 4.30):

Red cell indices: Determination of red cell indices (MCV, MCH) by electronic counters is a reliable method for assessing microcytosis and hypochromia, a characteristic feature of thalassaemia traits. In these conditions, MCV is less than 76 fl and MCH is less than 27 pg. In α^+ thalassaemia trait, red cell indices may be within normal range.

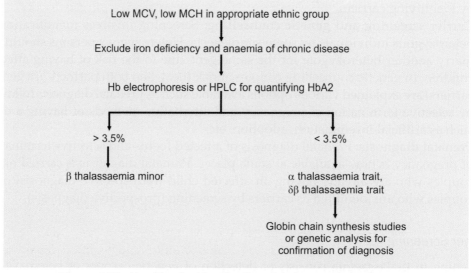

Figure 4.30: Algorithm for identification of thalassaemia carrier state

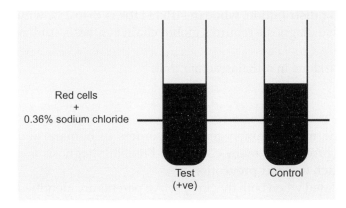

Figure 4.31: Single tube osmotic fragility test. Normal red cells undergo lysis when suspended in 0.36% sodium chloride and the solution becomes clear (line of reader scale visible), while microcytic hypochromic red cells in thalassaemia are resistant to osmotic lysis and solution is turbid (line of reader scale is not visible)

Single tube osmotic fragility test: This test can be performed in small routine-work laboratories, where automated haematology analyser is not available. It is based on the principle that red cells in thalassaemia are more resistant to osmotic haemolysis than normal red cells. Since the usual multiple tube osmotic fragility test is cumbersome, single tube osmotic fragility test has been devised. In this test red cells are suspended in 0.36% buffered saline and haemolysis is looked for either visually (Fig. 4.31) or in a spectrophotometer. This test, however, is not specific for β thalassaemia since positive test is also seen in iron deficiency anaemia, sickle-cell trait, and α^0 thalassaemia trait.

Another measure of resistance to osmotic lysis is **glycerol lysis time** test. This test measures rate of haemolysis of red cells suspended in a solution of glycerol and the result is expressed as the length of time required for 50% lysis. Patients with β thalassaemia trait have increased values.

Estimation of HbA2: If red cell indices show reduced MCH and MCV, and if iron deficiency is ruled out, then quantitation of HbA2 should be carried out. In β thalassaemia trait HbA2 is characteristically raised (3.5–7%). If iron deficiency complicates β thalassaemia trait, then HbA2 quantitation should be repeated after correction of iron deficiency.

HbA2 level is normal in α thalassaemia trait, a specific type of β thalassaemia known as "normal HbA2 β thalassaemia", δβ thalassaemia trait, and Hb Lepore trait. In such cases diagnosis may be suspected when MCV and MCH are reduced and iron status is normal. Definitive diagnosis of carrier state in α thalassaemia trait needs globin chain synthesis studies and DNA analysis.

Haemoglobin electrophoresis at alkaline pH: This should be done in all individuals suspected of having thalassaemia trait. This identifies any abnormal haemoglobin present such as HbS, C, D, E, or Lepore, and also assesses HbF. Further characterisation of some haemoglobin variants can be made by citrate agar electrophoresis at acid pH.

Other tests: HbF, raised in heterozygotes of δβ thalassaemia and of hereditary persistence of foetal haemoglobin (HPFH), can be quantitated by alkali denaturation test and its cellular distribution assessed by acid elution test. In δβ thalassaemia trait,

HbF is 5 to 15% with heterocellular distribution, while in HPFH HbF is 15 to 25% with pancellular distribution. Definitive diagnosis requires globin chain synthesis studies and DNA analysis.

Test for HbH inclusions can be done in α thalassaemia trait.

Prenatal Diagnosis

The haemoglobinopathies are the most common genetic disorders in humans and constitute a major public health problem in many countries. Prenatal diagnosis is a cost-effective and sensible approach for their prevention.

Prenatal diagnosis is contemplated when both the prospective parents are identified as thalassaemia carriers. It is done to prevent birth of a child with β thalassaemia major or Hb Bart's hydrops foetalis syndrome.

There are two major techniques for prenatal diagnosis of thalassaemias:

1. **Globin chain synthesis studies (during second trimester of pregnancy** on foetal blood obtained by cordocentesis**);** and
2. **Foetal DNA analysis (during first trimester of pregnancy** on cells obtained from amniocentesis or chorionic villus biopsy).

1. *Measurement of globin chain synthesis in foetal blood:* This test is done in second trimester of pregnancy because foetal blood can reliably be obtained only after 18 weeks of pregnancy. Foetal blood is aspirated from umbilical cord under ultrasound guidance (cordocentesis). The procedure is as follows:
    i.   Foetal blood sample (reticulocyte-enriched fraction) is incubated with radioactive amino acid (^{3}H leucine) which is incorporated in globin chains during *in vitro* globin synthesis.
    ii. Different types of globin chains are separated on CM-cellulose chromatography.
    iii. Amount of radioactivity incorporated in globin chains is measured in a liquid scintillation counter to assess the rate of synthesis of α, β and γ chains. Whether the foetus is having thalassaemia major or minor is decided on the basis of ratio of β chains to γ and α chains.

    As foetal blood sampling can be carried out only after 18 weeks of gestation, there is a prolonged indecisive period and pregnancy termination, if required, is difficult. The risk of procedure-related foetal loss is 3 to 4%.

    This technique is usually reserved for those cases in which DNA diagnosis is not possible, i.e. if nature of genetic defect is not known and linkage analysis cannot be done.

2. *Analysis of foetal DNA:* Prenatal diagnosis of haemoglobin disorders is most commonly done by foetal DNA analysis. Foetal DNA can be obtained either by amniocentesis or by chorion villus biopsy. In amniocentesis, 20 to 30 ml of amniotic fluid is aspirated at 14 to 20 weeks of gestation and DNA is extracted from amniotic fluid cells after culture. Risk of foetal loss with amniocentesis is 0.5%. Chorion villus biopsy consists of obtaining a small piece of developing placenta under ultrasound guidance at 8 to

12 weeks of gestation. Transcervical route is commonly used to obtain biopsy and with this approach risk of foetal loss is not significantly increased as compared to amniocentesis. Studies on amniotic fluid cells need to be performed relatively late in pregnancy (second trimester). Chorionic villus biopsy can be obtained at 8 to 12 weeks of gestation (first trimester) and it has become the procedure of choice for obtaining foetal cells for DNA analysis.

The nature of the molecular lesion first needs to be determined in both the members of the couple and in other closely related family members. For this, it is necessary to know the ethnic origin of the couple at risk, as only a few specific mutations are prevalent in a particular community.

Method of DNA analysis for prenatal diagnosis in a given case depends on whether mutation remains known or unknown after family studies (both partners and affected child) –

1. *For known mutations:*
   - Amplification refractory mutation system (ARMS)
   - Dot blot using ASO probes
   - Reverse dot blot hybridisation
   - Direct electrophoresis for 619 bp deletion
   - Restriction enzyme analysis of PCR product
2. *For unknown mutations:*
   - Denaturation gradient gel electrophoresis
   - Restriction fragment length polymorphism (RFLP)
   - Direct sequencing of amplified DNA
   - Southern blotting for deletions using specific gene probes.

Techniques of DNA Analysis

For known mutations:

1. *Methods employing DNA amplification:* Polymerase chain reaction (PCR) technology that was introduced in 1985 by Saiki and others has had a remarkable impact on the molecular diagnosis of genetic diseases. PCR can amplify the DNA fragment of interest several million times in a short period. With this technique a specific portion of the patient's DNA can be identified in a few hours even from a very small sample. In PCR, a short segment of DNA (target DNA) is amplified with the help of two primers and a thermostable DNA polymerase. The primers are two short oligonucleotides that hybridise to the sites flanking the region to be amplified. The DNA polymerase is the thermostable Taq polymerase that synthesises the complementary DNA sequence.

   Each cycle of PCR consists of three steps that are performed at different temperatures (Fig. 4.32):

   Denaturation: In this step, double stranded DNA is converted to single stranded DNA by heating at 94° to 96°C. Heating destroys chemical bonds between base pairs.

   Annealing: Temperature is lowered to 50° to 55°C and synthetic primers are allowed to bind to complementary sites flanking the region of interest.

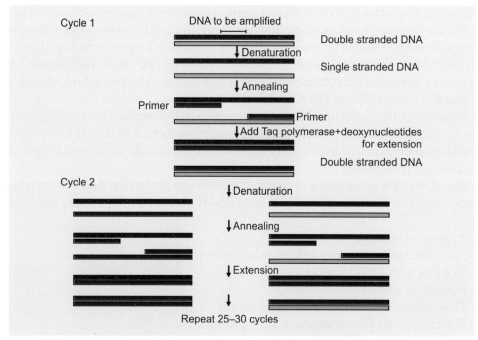

Figure 4.32: Polymerase chain reaction

Extension: The temperature is raised to 72°C. In this step, a thermostable DNA polymerase (Taq polymerase) makes a DNA strand complementary to the DNA that is flanked by the primers. Extension occurs by addition of deoxynucleotides and a copy of the target DNA sequence is made.

Above three steps comprise one cycle and the process is repeated for 25 to 35 cycles. This results in exponential amplification of the target DNA sequence.

Amplified DNA is utilised in various methods for diagnosis of genetic defects. These include restriction enzyme digestion followed by gel electrophoresis, dot-blot analysis using allele-specific oligonucleotide probes, reverse dot hybridisation, and amplification refractory mutation system.

  i. *Restriction enzyme digestion and gel electrophoresis:* This method is used when a mutation affects a restriction site for endonuclease enzyme. DNA sequence of interest is amplified by PCR, cleaved with a restriction enzyme, electrophoresed on agarose gel to separate the fragments according to size, stained with ethidium bromide, and observed under ultraviolet light. When a mutation is present, a fragment of a different size is obtained. An example where this approach is used is detection of codon 39 non-sense mutation (CAG→TAG) by *Mae* I restriction analysis. If this mutation is present, then it creates a restriction site and thus a fragment of smaller size is obtained.

  ii. *Dot blot analysis with allele-specific oligonucleotide probe:* Many mutations can be detected by this method. Genomic DNA of interest is amplified

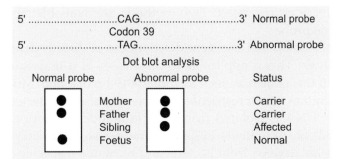

Figure 4.33: Dot blot analysis showing identification of β^0 39 mutation C→T by radiolabelled oligonucleotide probes in a family for prenatal diagnosis. The normal probe consists of normal nucleotide sequence (18–20 bases long) with normal codon CAG at position 39 of β globin gene. The abnormal probe has mutant nucleotide sequence TAG at position 39. The substitution C→T at position 39 causes formation of a chain terminator codon and leads to β^0 thalassaemia. Lower part of the figure shows nylon membrane with blotted amplified DNA that is hybridised with normal and abnormal radiolabelled probes

by PCR, denatured, and applied (dot blotted) on two nylon membranes. Two oligonucleotide probes (each 18–20 bases long), out of which one is complementary to the normal DNA and the other to the abnormal or mutant DNA, are tagged with the radioisotope. After hybridisation of one nylon membrane with normal probe and of other with mutant probe, genotype of a person (normal, heterozygous, or homozygous) can be determined (Fig. 4.33). Oligonucleotide probe can be labelled with horseradish peroxidase (instead of radioactive material) that produces a colour change after hybridisation.

iii. *Reverse dot hybridisation:* This is another PCR-based technique for detection of known genetic mutations. In this method, an oligonucleotide probe complimentary to the mutant sequence is fixed onto a nylon membrane while amplified genomic DNA to be tested is hybridised to the membrane. The primers used for amplification of genomic DNA are biotinylated. Therefore, presence of biotin in dots on the membrane indicates hybridisation of genomic DNA with mutant oligonucleotide probe.

iv. *Amplification refractory mutation system (ARMS):* This technique, based on PCR technology, makes use of two allele specific oligonucleotide primers one of which is complimentary to normal DNA and the other to the mutant DNA sequence. Annealing and subsequent DNA amplification will occur only when nucleotide sequence of primer is identical to that of genomic DNA. A normal primer will not anneal to mutant DNA sequence and thus extension of primer and DNA amplification will not occur. When mutant primer is used, amplification will occur only in the presence of corresponding mutation in genomic DNA. Gel electrophoresis followed by ethidium bromide staining is used for visualisation of amplified DNA.

2. *Direct detection of genetic defect:* Two methods are available: Southern blot and oligonucleotide probe.

   i. *Southern blot analysis:* Large gene deletions can be directly detected by Southern blot analysis. This is applicable to most cases of α thalassaemias and a few cases of β thalassaemias such as Indian 619 bp deletion. Mutations that alter the recognition site for restriction enzymes can also be detected by this method. *Principle:* DNA is isolated from cells (amniotic or chorionic villus) and is separated into fragments by one or more restriction enzymes. Restriction enzymes are derived from bacteria and recognise a specific sequence of base pairs in DNA and cleave the DNA molecule at sites where this sequence is encountered. Multiple fragments of DNA of varying sizes are formed which migrate according to size when electrophoresed (smaller fragments move more rapidly than the larger ones). These double-stranded DNA fragments are then denatured with a strong base into single strands and then blotted onto nitrocellulose membranes. To identify the fragment of interest, a radioactive complementary DNA probe is then hybridised to the nitrocellulose or nylon membrane. (A probe is a radiolabelled DNA sequence used to detect the presence of a complimentary nucleotide sequence in an unknown DNA fragment by molecular hybridisation). The labelled probe and the membrane are then incubated together under conditions that favour the formation of double-stranded DNA molecules. Hybridisation will occur if the probe finds a sequence complementary to the DNA to bind on the nitrocellulose membrane. Since the probe is radioactive, position of the hybridised band can be identified by exposing the membrane to X-ray film (autoradiography) (Fig. 4.34).

   This technique was developed by Edwin Southern and hence the name. This approach is illustrated in prenatal diagnosis of sickle-cell anaemia (see Fig. 4.42).

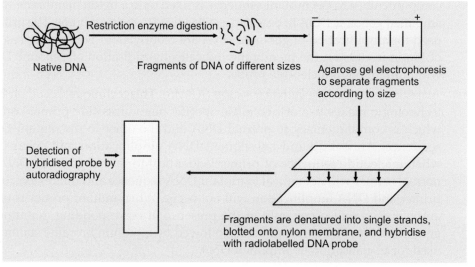

Figure 4.34: Principle of Southern blot analysis

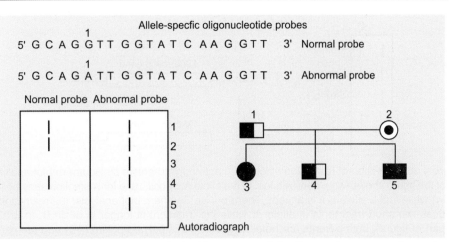

Allele-specfic oligonucleotide probes

1
5' G C A G G TT G G T A T C AA G GTT   3' Normal probe

1
5' G C A G A TT G G T A T C AA G GTT   3' Abnormal probe

Figure 4.35: Oligonucleotide probe analysis: Upper part of the figure shows two oligonucleotide probes. The normal probe represents the sequence near the intron 1 of the normal β globin gene. The abnormal probe represents the point mutation G→A at position 1 of the intron 1 (IVS-1 nt 1 G→A). This mutation alters the splice junction and causes $β^0$ thalassaemia. Lower part of the figure shows autoradiogram of gels used for diagnosis of above mutation in a family. Both normal and abnormal probes are yielding positive signals with DNAs of father (1), mother (2), and child (4) and therefore, they are heterozygous for this mutation. DNA from one child (3) is homozygous for the mutation since it is showing hybridisation only with the abnormal probe. DNA from the foetus (5) is also homozygous for the mutation and termination of pregnancy is advisable

ii. *Oligonucleotide probe analysis:* Majority of point mutations do not change the recognition sequence of restriction enzymes. Here allele-specific oligonucleotide probes may be utilised for direct detection of abnormal genes. The principle of this technique is summarised below:

a. Two oligonucleotide probes (having 18–20 bases), one normal and another abnormal (mutant), are prepared and are radiolabelled. These probes differ from one another by a single base.

b. Foetal DNA is subjected to digestion by a restriction enzyme. Agarose gel electrophoresis is carried out to separate the fragments. This separation can be carried out on two agarose gels (one for each probe). Hybridisation is carried out with normal and abnormal oligonucleotide probes on the respective, identically run gels. This is followed by autoradiography. Under appropriate conditions, these probes hybridise only to complementary (i.e. perfectly matched) sequences in the DNA. The normal probe will hybridise to normal sequence while the abnormal probe will hybridise to mutant sequence. This approach is illustrated in Figure 4.35.

For unknown mutations:

1. *Restriction fragment length polymorphism (RFLP) analysis:* DNA sequence variations which alter cutting site of a restriction enzyme occur frequently in populations and restriction enzyme pattern of all individuals is not alike. These variations that affect restriction sites and produce fragments of different size after digestion of DNA are

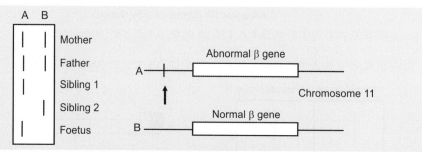

Figure 4.36: Detection of restriction fragment length polymorphism by Southern blot analysis. Right part of the figure shows two β gene alleles. In the allele A, specific site for restriction enzyme is present (arrow) while in the allele B it is absent. Therefore on Southern blot analysis, the restriction enzyme produces two short fragments in allele A, while the fragment is longer in allele B. In this example (left part of figure), both parents are heterozygous for this polymorphism (AB) and are carriers of β thalassaemia gene. Sibling 1 and foetus are homozygous for abnormal β gene (AA) and are affected, while sibling 2 is normal (BB)

known as restriction fragment length polymorphisms (RFLPs). The polymorphic sites can be used as 'markers' for genetic diseases if they are closely linked to an abnormal gene and co-segregate in affected families (Fig. 4.36).

Linkage of the polymorphism to the abnormal gene should be established by studying close family members before attempting prenatal diagnosis. Both the mother and the father should be heterozygous for the polymorphism (i.e. each chromosome should show a different restriction enzyme pattern). The polymorphic site should be closely linked to the abnormal gene so that they are transmitted together during meiosis. If the linkage is not close then the crossing over of chromosomal material between homologous chromosomes during meiosis may 'separate' the polymorphic site from the abnormal gene; this will lead to a false negative result in the foetus. General approach to prenatal diagnosis of thalassaemia is outlined in Figure 4.37.

Principles of Therapy in Thalassaemias

Regular red cell transfusions and chelation therapy for iron overload are the cornerstones of therapy for β thalassaemia major. If faithfully followed this treatment allows the thalassaemia patients to lead a near-normal life.

β thalassaemia major poses a major psychological, financial, and social burden on patients and their families. For them, long-term support is best provided by centers having the necessary expertise in managing these disorders. Societies have been formed by the parents of the affected children that provide guidance and help to newly diagnosed patients.

Blood transfusion: Before the availability of transfusions, patients with β thalassaemia major invariably used to die from severe anaemia and congestive cardiac failure before 2 years of age. Initially transfusions were given to thalassemic patients only when their anaemia became severely symptomatic. With this "on demand transfusion" therapy,

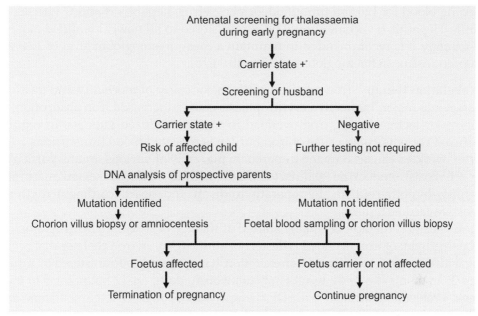

Figure 4.37: Approach to prenatal diagnosis of thalassaemia

although patients could live up to 15–20 years of age, they remained incapacitated and suffered from complications of chronic anaemia and excessive erythroid hyperplasia in bone marrow such as skeletal and facial deformities and hepatosplenomegaly.

"Hypertransfusion programme" was then formulated which consisted of regular transfusion therapy so as to maintain the haemoglobin concentration constantly above 9.5 to 10.0 g/dl. This form of therapy radically improved the quality of life of thalassemic patients and is now widely followed. The aim of this therapy is to prevent anaemia and hypoxia and to suppress endogenous erythropoiesis. If started early in life hypertransfusion programme promotes normal growth and development up to adolescence, prevents disfiguring skeletal deformities as excessive erythropoiesis and consequent marrow expansion are suppressed, limits hepatosplenomegaly by reducing extramedullary haematopoiesis, reduces cardiomegaly by reducing cardiac work, and reduces intestinal iron absorption as endogenous erythropoiesis is suppressed.

Blood transfusion therapy is begun around 6 months of age. Packed red cells should be given. Freshly obtained red cells are preferred to limit *the iron burden* (As each ml of red cells contains 1 mg of iron, only viable red cells should be transfused). Patients are transfused with 11 to 14 ml of red cells per kg every 3 to 4 weeks.

Since these patients are totally dependent on chronic blood transfusion therapy, every effort should be made to minimise transfusion-related complications. Saline-washed red cells can be used to avoid sensitisation to plasma antigens and leucocyte antigens; leucocyte reduction filters reduce alloimmunisation to leucocyte antigens; and the risk of transfusion-transmitted infections is substantially reduced by screening blood for human immunodeficiency virus, hepatitis B and C viruses, and syphilis. Hepatitis B vaccine should be administered to all newly identified patients.

Currently it is recommended to maintain a mean haemoglobin level of 12.0 g/dl, with pretransfusion haemoglobin of 9.5 to 10.0 g/dl.

Iron chelation therapy: Iron overload is the major cause of morbidity and death in β thalassaemia major. Ineffective erythropoiesis causes increased iron absorption; this is the major factor causing iron overload in undertransfused patients. In regularly transfused patients, main cause of iron burden is repeated blood transfusions.

Iron overload causes damage to parenchymal cells of various organs particularly liver (cirrhosis), endocrine glands (diabetes mellitus, delayed sexual maturation, infertility, hypothyroidism, hypoparathyroidism) and heart (cardiac arrhythmias, congestive cardiac failure).

Iron chelation therapy is usually started at the age of 3 years. The drug employed for the treatment of iron overload is desferrioxamine (DF), an iron chelator that is given along with vitamin C to promote iron excretion. It is preferably administered by infusion pump 25 to 60 mg/kg body weight subcutaneously daily for 12 hours for 5 to 6 days a week. Problems associated with DF therapy include high cost, cumbersome mode of administration, noncompliance, and adverse reactions such as convulsions, coma, cataracts, retinal damage, deafness, impairment of growth, and infections by Yersinia.

Due to high cost and difficulties of administration of DF, oral iron chelating drug is needed. Deferiprone (1,2-dimethyl-3-hydroxy-pyridin-4-one or L1) appears to be promising and is being extensively used in India. Major side effects are agranulocytosis, arthropathy, and possible hepatic fibrosis. Another oral iron chelating drug is deferasirox (DFX). Comparison of three main iron chelating drugs in the management of thalassaemia is presented in Table 4.5.

Assessment of body iron load: Methods for assessing body iron burden are:

1. Serum ferritin: This test is widely available, relatively inexpensive, and repeated measurements are possible. However, serum ferritin is elevated during inflammation, infection, and deficiency of ascorbate. Correlation with total body iron is imprecise.

Table 4.5: Properties of iron chelating drugs used in thalassaemia

Parameter	Desferrioxamine	Deferiprone	Deferasirox
1. Molecular weight	657 Da	139 Da	373 Da
2. Iron:chelator binding ratio	1:1	1:3	1:2
3. Plasma ½ life	20–30 min	1.5–3.5 hr	12–18 hr
4. Route of administration	Parenteral (SC/IV)	Oral	Oral
5. Daily dose	25–50 mg/kg 5 days a week	75 mg/kg three times daily	20–30 mg/kg once daily
6. Route of iron excretion	Urine and faeces	Urine	Faeces
7. Side effects	Impaired vision or hearing, growth retardation	Gastrointestinal upset, arthralgia, agranulocytosis	Gastrointestinal upset, rashes, raised serum creatinine

2. Liver biopsy for quantitation of iron: This is considered as the gold standard as it correlates well with body iron stores. Simultaneous assessment of liver histology (fibrosis, inflammation) is possible. The test is invasive with risk of intra-abdominal bleeding. More than 15 mg/g dry weight is associated with high risk of cardiac disease. However, cardiac disease may be present even if liver iron is low.

3. Magnetic resonance imaging (MRI): MRI is gaining popularity for assessment of liver and cardiac iron. The test is non-invasive and correlates well with liver iron and risk of cardiac disease.

4. Superconducting quantum interference device (SQUID) for liver iron load: This test is very expensive and has very limited availability.

Iron chelation therapy and techniques for monitoring iron burden are expensive and majority of patients with thalassaemia major are unable to afford them. In India, only about 5 to 10% of children born with thalassaemia receive optimal treatment.

Splenectomy: Indication for splenectomy is transfusion requirement exceeding 180 to 200 ml of packed red cells/kg/year. Due to the risk of sepsis, splenectomy should be avoided before 5 to 6 years of age. Post-splenectomy, pneumococcal, *H. influenzae*, and meningococcal vaccines and penicillin prophylaxis are necessary.

General measures: These include folic acid supplementation, early treatment of intercurrent infections, hormone replacement therapy in endocrine failure, and treatment of cardiac failure. Patients with HbH disease should refrain from anti-oxidant drugs.

Haematopoietic stem cell transplantation: Regular transfusions and iron chelation therapy have improved the quality of life in thalassaemia. Although bone marrow transplantation is associated with significant morbidity and mortality, it is the only form of therapy that can cure the disease. The decision to transplant bone marrow should be based on assessment of risks and benefits in an individual patient. Results are best if haematopoietic stem cell transplantation is carried out in young patients who have not yet developed complications of disease or of treatment.

Experimental forms of therapy: These include:

- Enhancement of HbF production – Currently hydroxyurea and butyrate are being tried to increase HbF production that will improve haemoglobin level and reduce ineffective erythropoiesis.
- Gene therapy — This consists of introduction of normal gene in stem cells to replace the abnormal gene. Research is in progress for gene therapy.

❏ SICKLE-CELL DISORDERS

Sickle-cell disorders are those conditions in which the red cells become sickle-shaped when they are subjected to low oxygen tension. Herrick first described a case of sickle-cell disease in 1910. Sickle-cell disorders include following conditions:

1. **Sickle-cell diseases (SCD):** Sickled cells are responsible for distinctive clinical manifestations. They can be divided into following types:
   i. *Sickle-cell anaemia (SCA):* This is the homozygous state for haemoglobin S (HbSS) that results when the sickle-cell gene (β^S) is inherited from both parents. The genotype is $\beta^S\beta^S$.
   ii. *Sickle-cell β thalassaemia:* This is the double heterozygous state in which the sickle-cell gene is inherited from one parent and β thalassaemia gene from the other parent. It is divided into two types: Sickle-cell β^0 thalassaemia (genotype $\beta^S\beta^0$) in which normal β chain synthesis is completely lacking, and sickle-cell β^+ thalassaemia (genotype $\beta^S\beta^+$) in which normal β chain synthesis is partially deficient.
   iii. Combination of haemoglobin S (HbS) with other structural haemoglobin variants can produce a double heterozygous state such as HbSD disease, HbSC disease, HbSO-Arab disease, Hb SE disease, etc.
2. **Sickle-cell trait:** This is the heterozygous carrier state for HbS (HbAS) in which sickle-cell gene is inherited from one parent and gene for HbA from the other. The genotype is $\beta^S\beta$.

Sickle-cell Anaemia

Sickle-cell anaemia is the most severe form of sickle-cell disease and is the homozygous state for haemoglobin S (HbSS).

Prevalence of HbS

Haemoglobin S is particularly frequent in Africa, Middle East and Central and Southern India. HbS has a high prevalence in those parts of the world where malaria is common; this relationship is explained by the theory of balanced polymorphism. Young children with sickle-cell trait develop comparatively mild falciparum malaria. Theory of balanced polymorphism proposes that selective advantage gained by sickle-cell heterozygote (i.e. protection against severe falciparum malaria) is balanced by disadvantage of homozygous state (i.e. sickle-cell anaemia). Genetic studies suggest that sickle mutation may have arisen independently in different parts of the world and has achieved high frequency due to natural selection.

Five haplotypes of sickle mutation have been identified by polymorphic sites in 5 regions: Cameroon, Africa (Senegal, Benin, Bantu) and Arab-India. This suggests that sickle mutations has originated independently in 5 regions. sickle-cell anaemia in India is milder than African form. This is due to increased HbF production and co-inheritance of α thalassaemia. Alpha thalassaemia occurs in > 50% of sickle population in India.

The exact mechanism of protective effect in sickle-cell trait is not known. However, it is possible that red cells infected with *P. falciparum* undergo more rapid sickling owing possibly to decreased intracellular pH caused by parasite's chemical reactions and are phagocytosed readily by macrophages of the reticuloendothelial system.

Pathogenesis

The sickle-cell disorders all result from inheritance of sickle-cell gene that codes for abnormal β globin chain. There is change of a single base A→ T in the sixth codon of β globin gene so that there is substitution of thymine for adenine. This in turn results in substitution of valine for glutamic acid at position 6 of β polypeptide chain. The amino acid substitution in HbS is represented as $β^6$ Glu→Val.

Polymerisation of HbS: Polymerisation of HbS molecules inside the red cells is responsible for sickling of red cells. When examined ultrastructurally, sickled cells show bundles of fibres aligned along the long axis of the cell or of the pointed projections. Each fibre consists of 14 filaments arranged in pairs. Each filament is made of HbS molecules stacked in a helical manner.

Polymerisation results only on deoxygenation. It is a time-dependent process. Initially, HbS molecules aggregate to form a polymer of critical size; this is the rate-limiting nucleation phase. Once a critical polymer is formed, aggregation of additional HbS molecules occurs rapidly to form well-aligned fibres. The time between deoxygenation and formation of the polymer of critical size is known as delay time or lag phase. This has significance when sickling and unsickling occurs due to deoxygenation and oxygenation respectively in circulation. Oxygenation in the lungs causes rapid dissociation of aggregated HbS molecules, viscous gel turns into fluid state, and the red cell shape becomes normal (if membrane damage has not occurred.) The red cell remains unsickled in the oxygenated arterial blood. When deoxygenation occurs in capillary circulation, most of the red cells do not sickle since reoxygenation occurs in pulmonary circulation before polymer of sufficient size is formed. However, shortening of delay time (e.g. due to low pH, increased HbS concentration, etc.) will lead to sickling in capillary circulation with resultant vaso-occlusion.

Reversibly and irreversibly sickled cells: Initially sickling of red cells is reversible. The sickle or holly-leaf shape of red cells conforms to the shape of the polymerised haemoglobin. With oxygenation, polymerised HbS (viscous gel state) returns to depolymerised (fluid-liquid) state. When repeated sickling and unsickling of red cells occurs, membrane is damaged and the red cell shape becomes permanently altered leading to the formation of irreversibly sickled cell; even with reoxygenation, shape of the red cell does not return to normal. Thus in sickle-cells disease, two categories of sickle-cells occur-reversibly sickled and irreversibly sickled (Fig. 4.38).

Reversibly sickled cells are those in which polymerisation of HbS and red cell shape alteration can revert back to normal. These cells undergo polymerisation and shape change upon deoxygenation while after reoxygenation in the lungs dissociation of polymers occurs with return of normal cell shape.

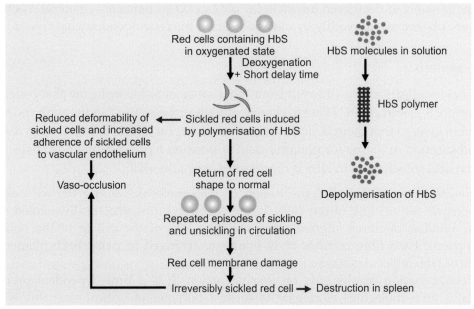

Figure 4.38: Formation of sickled red cells in circulation

In irreversibly sickled cells, red cell shape does not return to normal even after reoxygenation. Although depolymerisation occurs upon reoxygenation red cells remain irreversibly sickled. These cells appear on air-dried blood films as elongated cells one or both ends of which are pointed. The membrane of these cells is damaged which precludes the return of cell shape to normal even after reoxygenation and depolymerisation of HbS. They have rigid cell membranes and are trapped and destroyed in the spleen. The severity of haemolysis correlates with the number of these cells in circulation.

Factors which influence sickling:

i. *Intracellular concentration of HbS and of other haemoglobins:* There is a direct relationship between the amount of HbS in the red cell and propensity of red cells to sickle. In sickle-cell trait due to the predominance of HbA in the cell, sickling is prevented unless the oxygen tension is considerably low. In contrast, in red cells of patients with sickle-cell anaemia, HbS is the predominant form of haemoglobin (80–90%) and sickling occurs readily.

HbF does not participate with HbS in sickling process and therefore, infants do not develop manifestations till the time HbF declines to adult values. In Bedouin Arabs of Saudi Arabia and certain tribes of central India, sickle-cell anaemia is associated with significant elevation of HbF and a less severe disease. Heterozygotes for HbS and HPFH do not have anaemia owing to the high HbF percentage.

ii. *Association with thalassaemias:* In sickle-cell-β⁺ thalassaemia, due to the presence of HbA the disease is milder. Interaction of α thalassaemia with sickle-cell anaemia reduces mean corpuscular haemoglobin concentration and hemolysis; however vaso-occlusive crises remain unchanged.

iii. *Interaction with other abnormal haemoglobins:* HbS interacts less readily with HbC or HbD than with other HbS molecules and therefore, persons with HbSC disease or HbSD disease have milder manifestations (as compared to Hb SS disease).

iv. *Mean corpuscular haemoglobin concentration (MCHC):* Increased MCHC due to cellular dehydration favours the intermolecular contact between HbS and enhances polymerisation. This factor is responsible for sickling of red cells in hyperosmolar milieu of renal medulla.

v. *Decreased oxygen tension:* The most important determinant affecting sickling is deoxygenation. Amount of hypoxia required to induce sickling depends on the proportion of HbS (HbSS red cells: 40 mm Hg whereas HbAS red cells: 15 mm Hg).

vi. *Temperature:* Cold induces vasoconstriction and increases sickling.

vii. *Low pH:* Decrease in pH (acidosis) increases sickling probably by inducing the deoxy state of haemoglobin.

Pathogenesis of vaso-occlusion: Following processes contribute to the development of vaso-occlusion in sickle-cell anaemia: (1) depletion of nitric oxide by free haem released from haemolysis (leading to alteration in vascular tone, slowing of blood flow, and upregulation of adhesion molecules); (2) adhesion of young deformable red cells to vascular endothelium (promoted by leucocyte activation and inflammatory cytokines released during infection/inflammation); and (3) increased blood viscosity from less deformable red cells and sickled forms.

Clinical Features

Clinical manifestations usually develop around 3 to 4 months of age when the level of HbF falls. Clinical expression of sickle-cell anaemia is highly variable. Some patients have a severe disease with early mortality while others experience a near normal life-span with few complications. Main complications are vaso-occlusive crises while anaemia itself poses little problem. Anaemia of variable degree is present in all patients. It is more severe in SCA and sickle-cell β^0 thalassaemia as compared to sickle-cell β^+ thalassaemia. Usually patients adapt well to their anaemia. Anaemia is aggravated in the presence of folate deficiency, aplastic crisis, and splenic sequestration crisis.

Growth and development: These are considerably impaired in children with sickle-cell anaemia.

Splenomegaly: Splenomegaly is present in infants and young children and is caused by reticuloendothelial hyperplasia. In sickle-cell anaemia, in later life, spleen becomes small and fibrotic due to repeated splenic infarctions, and is not palpable. Spleen, however, remains palpable in adults in sickle-cell β thalassaemia.

Infections: Children (esp < 5 years) with sickle-cell anaemia are susceptible to fulminant infections by a variety of organisms especially *Streptococcus pneumoniae* (sepsis, meningitis), *Salmonella* (osteomyelitis), *E. coli, H. influenzae,* and *Shigella.* Increased risk of infections in sickle-cell anaemia is due to impairment of splenic phagocytic function or 'functional splenectomy'.

Vaso-occlusive and haematologic crises: Crises are acute episodic events that interrupt the steady-state course of sickle-cell anaemia. They are of two major types: vaso-occlusive and haematologic.

i.   *Vaso-occlusive crises:* Vaso-occlusive crisis is the most prominent manifestation of sickle-cell anaemia. It results from obstruction of microcirculation by stiff sickled red cells with ischaemia and infarction in the area of distribution of artery. Precipitating factors include infection particularly in children, exposure to cold, and physical and emotional stress; however in many cases precipitating factor is unidentifiable. Presentation is in the form of sudden onset of severe pain, usually in bones (upper or lower limbs or back), joints, chest, or abdomen. In small children, painful crises usually manifest as 'hand foot syndrome' or dactylitis (painful swelling of bones of hand or foot).

ii. *Haematologic crises:* In haematologic crisis, there is an acute aggravation of anaemia that may rapidly lead to cardiac failure and death if untreated. It is of following types:

 a. *Aplastic crisis:* In sickle-cell anaemia, red cell life-span is markedly shortened (average 20 days) due to extravascular haemolysis of abnormal red cells. Therefore any event causing decrease in erythropoiesis will markedly reduce haemoglobin concentration. Aplastic crisis appears to be caused by infection by parvovirus that selectively infects erythroblasts. Suppression of erythropoiesis is usually transient lasting for about 7 to 10 days. Transfusion support is essential during the aplastic phase.

 b. *Megaloblastic crisis:* This results from folate deficiency that may develop during intercurrent illness or during pregnancy.

 c. *Haemolytic ("Hyperhaemolytic") crisis:* Increased rate of red cell destruction over the chronic haemolytic state is called as haemolytic crisis. There is a sudden fall in haemoglobin concentration and levels of icterus and reticulocyte count increase. Haemolytic crisis is uncommon and coexistence of G6PD deficiency with superimposed oxidant stress may be responsible in some cases.

 d. *Splenic sequestration crisis:* Sudden and massive accumulation of blood in spleen causes rapid increase in size of spleen over a period of several hours, with abdominal fullness, decrease in circulatory volume, progressive anaemia, and circulatory failure. This occurs in patients of sickle-cell disease who have splenomegaly, i.e. infants or children (esp 6 months–3 years) with sickle-cell anaemia or adults with sickle-cell β thalassaemia. This is a common cause of death in young children. Recurrence can be avoided by removal of spleen.

Strokes: Ischaemic stroke is one of the most devastating complications of sickle-cell disease and occurs in small children. Cerebral infarction is more common than haemorrhage. It usually manifests with hemiplegia. Strokes are associated with significant morbidity and mortality. Recurrence of stroke is common. Early detection is now possible with the use of transcranial Doppler ultrasonography (which detects cerebral stenoses preceding stroke). If detected early, exchange transfusion reduces the risk of subsequent stroke and brain damage.

Genitourinary system: Renal abnormalities are common in sickle-cell anaemia. Renal medulla is especially vulnerable to ischaemic injury due to its hypertonic, acidotic, and anoxic milieu. Impairment of renal concentrating function is a common and the earliest sign of kidney damage. Ischaemia of renal medulla with papillary necrosis can develop which manifests with sudden onset of haematuria. A few patients develop proteinuria and nephrotic syndrome. Proteinuria and renal failure are increasing in frequency, as patients with sickle-cell anaemia are living longer. In patients with proteinuria due to glomerular sclerosis, administration of angiotensin converting enzyme inhibitor can arrest the progression of disease.

Priapism may be short-lived ('stuttering') or prolonged, painful, and persistent. It is due to obstruction of venous return of corpora cavernosa and is seen in postpubertal males. It may lead to impotence from damage to vascular erectile system.

Pregnancy: During pregnancy there is an increased incidence of spontaneous abortion, prematurity, stillbirth, and intrauterine growth retardation (due to vaso-occlusion of placenta). In the mother, incidence of infections, chest syndrome, and postpartum haemorrhage is increased.

Skeletal system: Apart from vaso-occlusive crises in bone, other skeletal changes in sickle-cell anaemia include widening of medullary cavity due to marrow hyperplasia, dactylitis (hand foot syndrome, i.e. digits are painful, tender and swollen) in small children, avascular necrosis of femoral or humeral heads, and *Salmonella* osteomyelitis.

Respiratory system: Acute onset of fever, cough, pleuritic type of chest pains, and lung infiltrates in sickle-cell anaemia is called as 'acute chest syndrome'. It may be caused by infarction or infection, but the differentiation is difficult. Repeated attacks may lead to chronic lung disease with fibrosis of lung parenchyma. Pulmonary hypertension and cor pulmonale can occur.

Hepatobiliary system: Hepatic damage may result from hepatic infarctions and transfusion-transmitted hepatitis. A significant percentage of patients have bilirubin gallstones (due to persistent elevation of serum bilirubin from chronic haemolysis).

Skin: Chronic leg ulcers are common around ankles on the medial aspect. They do not heal readily and have a tendency to recur.

Proliferative retinopathy: Proliferative retinopathy due to retinal vascular occlusion is an important complication and is more common in patients with HbSC disease (seen in Africa). Arteriovenous communications and neovascularisation may lead to vitreous haemorrhage, detachment of retina, and visual loss.

Laboratory Features

1. *Peripheral blood examination:* Anaemia is usually moderate with haemoglobin concentration ranging between 6 and 9 g/ dl. Anaemia is normocytic and normochromic. Irreversibly sickled cells make up about 5 to 10% of red cells on the blood smear. Their percentage usually parallels the degree of haemolysis (Fig. 4.39). Target

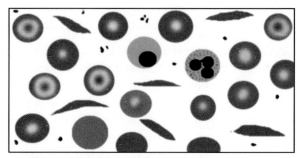

Figure 4.39: Blood smear in sickle-cell anaemia

cells are especially frequent in sickle-cell β thalassaemia. Reticulocyte count is increased. Mild polymorphonuclear leucocytosis is usual. The platelet count is raised as splenic trapping is lacking or is decreased. Thrombocytopaenia occurs during vaso-occlusive crisis.

2. *Other investigations:* Erythrocyte sedimentation rate is low despite reduced haemoglobin concentration. This is because of inability of red cells to form rouleaux. Unconjugated serum bilirubin is increased. Factor VIII and fibrinogen levels are raised.

3. *Identification of HbS:* Sickle haemoglobin or HbS can be detected by slide test using 2% sodium metabisulphite, solubility test, haemoglobin electrophoresis, and high-performance liquid chromatography (HPLC). These tests have been considered earlier. (See "Hereditary disorders of haemoglobin—General features and approach to diagnosis"). A few comments follow.

   Slide test using reducing agent or solubility test merely detect the presence of HbS and cannot distinguish between sickle-cell trait and sickle-cell disease. Diagnosis of the phenotype of the sickle-cell disorder (sickle-cell trait, or a particular type of

Table 4.6: Salient features of sickle-cell disorders

Sickle-cell disease	Genotype	Clinical manifestations	Solubility test	Hb electrophoresis
1. sickle-cell anaemia	β^S/β^S	Moderate to severe anaemia; crises	+	HbS predominant; No HbA; HbA$_2$ normal
2. sickle-cell β^0 thalassaemia	β^S/β^0	Moderate anaemia; splenomegaly persists in adults	+	HbS predominant; No HbA; HbA$_2$ increased
3. sickle-cell trait	β^S/β	No anaemia	+	HbA >HbS
4. sickle-cell β^+ thalassaemia	β^S/β^+	Mild anaemia	+	HbS>HbA; HbA$_2$ increased

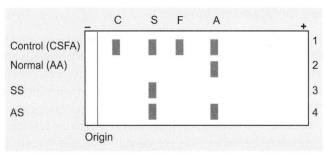

Figure 4.40: Haemoglobin electrophoresis at alkaline pH. Lane 1: Control; Lane 2: Normal or AA pattern; Lane 3: sickle-cell anaemia or SS pattern; Lane 4: sickle-cell trait or AS patern

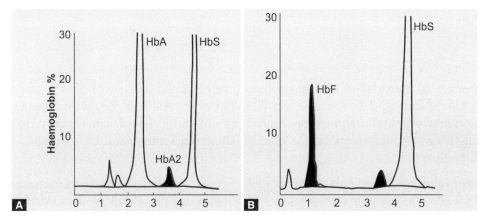

Figure 4.41: High-performance liquid chromatography in (A) sickle-cell trait and (B) sickle-cell anaemia

sickle-cell disease) can be made by haemoglobin electrophoresis at alkaline pH using cellulose acetate or by citrate agar electrophoresis at acid pH. In sickle-cell anaemia, predominant haemoglobin is HbS (80–95%), HbF is variably increased (5–15%), and HbA2 is normal. In sickle-cell β thalassaemia also, HbA is totally absent, but in this condition proportion of HbA2 is increased (>3.5%). Family studies are helpful in making the correct diagnosis (i.e. one parent with sickle-cell trait and the other with β thalassaemia trait). In sickle-cell trait, HbA is about 60% and HbS is 40% (HbA is always more than HbS). In sickle-cell β thalassaemia, HbS is more than HbA and HbA2 is increased (Fig. 4.40 and Table 4.6). Electrophoresis is also necessary for genetic counselling.

HPLC findings in sickle-cell anaemia and sickle-cell trait are shown in Figure 4.41.

4. *Estimation of HbF by alkali denaturation test* is necessary to determine the severity of sickle-cell anaemia and to detect the coinheritance of hereditary persistence of foetal haemoglobin (HPFH).

5. *Estimation of HbA2* is required for the diagnosis of sickle-cell β thalassaemia.

Neonatal Screening for Sickle-cell Anaemia

Screening can be carried out to identify those newborns who will later develop sickle-cell anaemia. The rationale behind this approach is that preventive measures can be taken to avert serious complications and reduce morbidity and mortality in later life. Screening of newborn can be carried out in communities with increased frequency of sickle-cell gene. This approach is used in USA in African Americans.

In newborns, solubility test and sodium metabisulphite test cannot be used for screening since concentration of HbS is very small (< 10%). Widely used test for this purpose is citrate agar gel electrophoresis at acid pH. Haemolysate from cord blood sample is used. Newborns who will develop sickle-cell anaemia show predominance of HbF, some HbS and absent HbA; those with sickle-cell trait have HbF, HbS, and HbA.

Prenatal Diagnosis

Mothers from high-risk ethnic group should be screened in early pregnancy for HbS carrier state. If prospective mother as well as father are positive, they should be offered the option of prenatal diagnosis or of newborn screening. Two distinct approaches are available for prenatal diagnosis of sickle-cell anaemia: foetal blood analysis and foetal DNA analysis.

Foetal blood analysis: This involves globin chain synthesis studies in foetal blood using CM-cellulose chromatography. Abnormal globin chain is separated from normal globin chain and quantitated. Foetal blood sampling (by cordocentesis) can only be done after 18 weeks of gestation. Apart from prolonged waiting period, risk of procedure-related foetal loss is also comparatively greater.

Foetal DNA analysis: Foetal DNA may be obtained either from amniotic fluid cells or from chorionic villi (see prenatal diagnosis of thalassaemias). Chorionic villus biopsy is preferred because, if required, termination of pregnancy can be performed earlier.

Various methods are available for analysis of foetal DNA. Some of them are outlined below. (For details see "Prenatal diagnosis of thalassaemias").

  i. *Southern blot analysis:* A restriction enzyme called *Mst* II recognises three specific sites in normal β globin gene and cleaves DNA at these sites (Fig. 4.42). It produces two fragments of normal β globin gene: one measuring 1.15 kb and the other 0.2 kb. Mutation producing sickle haemoglobin causes a single base change A→T in the sixth codon of β globin gene. This mutation abolishes one cleavage site for *Mst* II in such a manner that only one large fragment 1 .35 kb long is produced after *Mst* II digestion. The technique consists of digestion of extracted DNA with *Mst* II followed by separation of fragments according to size by agarose gel electrophoresis. Fragments are denatured and then transferred onto nitrocellulose membrane. Radiolabelled 1.15 kb probe complementary to 5′ end of normal β globin gene is hybridised. On autoradiography, a single 1.15 kb band indicates normal β

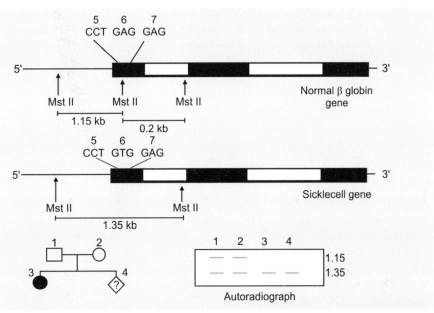

Figure 4.42: Southern blot analysis of β globin gene using restriction enzyme Mst II. Normal β globin gene has three restriction sites for the enzyme Mst II (arrows on upper part of figure) with production of two fragments 1.15 kb and 0.2 kb. Sickle mutation results in abolition of one restriction site with formation of a large fragment 1.35 kb. Lower part of the figure shows Southern blot analysis. Both father (lane 1) and mother (lane 2) are heterozygous for sickle-cell mutation (sickle-cell trait); offspring in lane 3 is affected, while foetus in lane 4 also has sickle-cell anaemia

globin genes on both homologous chromosomes (β/β), and a single 1.35 kb band indicates that both β globin genes have sickle mutation (i.e. βˢ/βˢ or sickle-cell anaemia). Presence of both 1.15 kb and 1.35 kb bands indicate heterozygous state for βˢ gene (i.e. βˢ/β or sickle-cell trait).

ii. *Restriction fragment length polymorphism (RFLP) analysis:* Principle of this technique is already outlined earlier (see "Prenatal diagnosis of thalassaemias"). Normal β globin gene is associated with 7.0 kb fragment while βˢ gene is associated with 13.0 kb fragment in some populations, when restriction enzyme *Hpa* I is used. This polymorphism can be used to track the presence of βˢ gene in a particular family.

iii. *Methods employing DNA amplification:*

a. *Direct detection of mutation with restriction enzymes:* The PCR-amplified DNA is digested with a restriction enzyme (such as *Dde* I). Fragments of different size are produced in normal β globin gene and in βˢ globin gene as mutation abolishes a cleavage site in the latter.

b. *Allele-specific oligonucleotide probe analysis:* Two allele-specific probes are synthesised, one complementary to the normal sequence and the other to the abnormal (sickle mutation) sequence. Amplified DNA is dot blotted on to nylon membranes and probes are applied. Hybridisation occurs if sequences are complementary to each other.

c. *Colour DNA amplification:* Normal β globin gene primer and mutant (β^S) globin gene primer are labeled with different fluorescent dyes. The resulting normal and abnormal amplified gene products are of different colours and can be easily identified.

Treatment

Treatment of sickle-cell anaemia is symptomatic and supportive. Patients with sickle-cell disease are best managed at a comprehensive care centre that has properly trained multidisciplinary staff. Main treatment modalities in sickle-cell anaemia are shown in Box 4.7.

1. Measures to prevent crises include early detection and treatment of infections and avoidance of exposure to extreme cold, stress, hypoxia, and dehydration. All infections should be treated intensively. Pneumococcal vaccine, influenza vaccine and penicillin prophylaxis are indicated during early childhood.

2. Treatment of vaso-occlusive episode involves relieving pain by analgesics, keeping patient warm, maintaining adequate fluid intake, oxygenation, and treatment of infections. Partial exchange transfusion reduces percentage of sickled cells and improves oxygenation; this may limit organ damage during acute vascular episode.

3. During pregnancy in sickle-cell anaemia, due to the increased risk of prematurity and stillbirth in foetus and of maternal vaso-occlusive crisis, close antenatal supervision is required. Folic acid and iron should be given routinely. Regular blood transfusion therapy has been advocated, but usefulness of this approach is not yet proved.

4. Oral contraceptive pill as a means of family planning should be avoided as it poses increased risk of thrombosis.

5. Exchange transfusion has been advised prior to surgery to reduce the risk of vaso-occlusive episodes by decreasing the percentage of HbS (to less than 30%). During operation, hypoxia, dehydration and circulatory stasis and exposure to cold should be avoided.

6. Radiographic contrast media cause dehydration of red cells, increase MCHC and precipitate sickling. Exchange transfusion has been recommended prior to cerebral angiography.

7. Cerebrovascular accidents are managed with prompt exchange transfusion during acute episode to reduce HbS to less than 30%. This limits neurologic damage.

Box 4.7	Main treatment modalities in sickle-cell anaemia

- Penicillin prophylaxis
- Vaccination against *S. pneumoniae, H. influenzae*, influenza virus, and hepatitis B virus
- Folate supplementation
- Hydroxyurea
- Transfusion therapy: chronic or partial exchange
- Iron chelation (if iron overload)

Following this, regular blood transfusion therapy is started to prevent recurrence of strokes by maintaining this HbS level.

8. Acute chest syndrome: Patients with low oxygen saturation level can benefit from exchange transfusion. Patients are given adequate analgesia, incentive spirometry to prevent further infiltrates, and broad-spectrum antibiotics.

9. Role of transfusion therapy in sickle-cell anaemia is summarised in Box 4.8. Regular blood transfusions merely to increase haemoglobin concentration are not indicated since they lead to increase in blood viscosity. Blood transfusions are indicated in certain situations as follows:

    i.   *Packed red cell transfusion* to improve oxygen-carrying capacity are required during symptomatic anaemia (i.e. causing breathlessness, impending CCF) aplastic crisis, acute splenic sequestration crisis, etc.

    ii. *Regular chronic transfusion therapy* is employed to reduce the number of HbS containing cells (to less than 40%). This is indicated to prevent recurrence of strokes in cerebrovascular episodes. Role of this form of therapy prior to major surgery and during pregnancy is being investigated.

    iii. *Partial exchange transfusion* is indicated during acute or impending attack of cerebrovascular episode or vaso-occlusive episode. Exchange transfusion reduces viscocity, avoids hypervolemia and improves oxygen-carrying capacity. The purpose behind this therapy is to limit or prevent the irreversible organ damage.

10. Hydroxyurea: A mainstay of treatment in sickle-cell anaemia is hydroxyurea (now called hydroxycarbamide). It has following benefits in sickle-cell anaemia: (a) it increases production of HbF and reduces number and severity of crises (as HbF does not participate with HbF in sickling process, polymerisation of HbS is retarded); (b) it reduces white cell count thus causing anti-inflammatory effect;

Box 4.8 Blood transfusion in sickle-cell disease

*   In SCD patients, blood for transfusion should be –
    *   Matched for Rh (C, D, E) and Kell antigens since they are responsible for most cases of alloimmunisation
    *   Negative for HbS by sickle solubility test (for correct assessment of sickle-cells post-transfusion)
    *   Leucocyte-depleted (to reduce viral transmission and prevent febrile reactions)
*   Blood transfusion is not indicated in steady state anaemia
*   Main complications are iron overload in adults from chronic transfusion therapy, transmission of infections, and alloimmunisation
*   Packed red cell transfusion (10–15 ml/kg) is indicated in—
    *   Symptomatic anaemia
    *   Aplastic crisis
    *   Splenic sequestration crisis
    *   Before surgery
*   Exchange transfusion is indicated in—
    *   Impending stroke
    *   Acute chest syndrome
*   Chronic transfusion is indicated for –
    *   Prevention of recurrence of stroke.

(c) it increases red cell volume and hydration thus reducing sickling and haemolysis; (d) it decreases adhesiveness of red cells and leucocytes; and (e) it releases nitric oxide that causes vasodilatation.

Hydroxuurea reduces the number of painful crises, transfusion requirements, and incidence of acute chest syndrome. It is indicated in children, adolescents, and adults with sickle-cell anaemia who have frequent pain, severe vaso-occlusive events, and severe anaemia.

11.   Haematopoietic stem cell transplantation is the only form of therapy that can cure the disease. Since it is associated with significant morbidity and mortality, it should be reserved for severely affected patients having HLA- matched sibling donor.

Prognosis

The course of sickle-cell anaemia is highly variable. Some patients have relatively mild disease with survival into adulthood while others die during infancy or early childhood from severe disease. Leading causes of death include severe sepsis, cerebrovascular episode, acute chest syndrome, and splenic sequestration crisis.

Sickle-cell Trait

This is the asymptomatic heterozygous state for sickle-cell gene (β^S/β). In sickle-cell trait, HbS comprises around 40% of total haemoglobin, the remaining 60% being HbA. Since HbA is the predominant haemoglobin, it prevents red cells from sickling at low oxygen tensions occurring physiologically. The red cell life-span is normal.

Persons with sickle-cell trait do not have anaemia and are usually asymptomatic. Some clinical abnormalities, however, have been reported to occur in these persons: deficient urine concentrating ability, infarction of spleen and vaso-occlusive crises at high altitudes, and haematuria (renal papillary necrosis). Instances of sudden death have been reported following strenuous exercise.

Few target cells may be present on blood films (Fig. 4.43). Diagnosis requires demonstration of HbS by sodium metabisulphite slide test or solubility test and

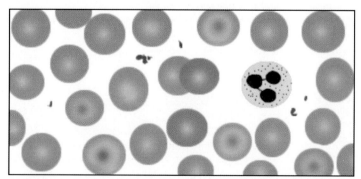

Figure 4.43: Blood smear in sickle-cell trait showing target cells

haemoglobin electrophoresis. Haemoglobin electrophoresis reveals more HbA (60%) than HbS (40%).

No treatment is required and duration of survival of individuals is normal.

DISORDERS OF RED CELL ENZYMES

❑ GLUCOSE-6-PHOSPHATE DEHYDROGENASE DEFICIENCY

Glucose-6-phosphate dehydrogenase (G6PD) deficiency is the most common red cell enzymopathy in humans (affecting about 400 million people worldwide) and is characterised by reduced activity of glucose-6-phosphate dehydrogenase in red cells, and occurrence of haemolysis usually after exposure to oxidant stress (Box 4.9).

More than 400 biochemical variants of G6PD have been identified. The variants are grouped into five classes by World Health Organization Scientific Working Group (Table 4.7).

Polymorphic mutations occur with high frequency in malaria-endemic areas (WHO class II and III) and include G6PD A−(common in Africa) and G6PD Mediterranean (common in Mediterranean countries, Middle East, and India). In such cases, haemolysis develops only following oxidant exposure. **Sporadic mutations** occur anywhere in the world at low frequency and patient develops chronic haemolytic anaemia (WHO class I).

The well-known abnormal G6PD variants associated with G6PD deficiency are G6PD A−(prevalent in Africa; 1/2 life 13 days) and G6PD Mediterranean (1/2 life several hours). G6PD variant with normal enzyme activity is G6PD B (1/2 life 60 days). The deficient variants common in India are G6PD Mediterranean, G6PD Kerala-Kalyan, and G6PD Orissa. Normally enzyme activity decreases with red cell ageing so that young

Table 4.7: Variants of G6PD

Class	G6PD enzyme activity	Clinical manifestations
I	< 5% of normal	Rare; Chronic congenital nonspherocytic haemolytic anaemia
II	< 10% of normal	Episodic acute haemolysis induced by oxidant drugs
III	10–60% of normal	Acute self-limited haemolysis following oxidant drugs or infections
IV	60–100% of normal	—
V	Increased	—

Box 4.9	Prevalence of G6PD deficiency

- Very common, with >7% of the world population having defective gene
- High prevalence in Africa, Middle East, Mediterranean countries, and Asia
- In India, prevalence varies from 0–27% in different castes and ethnic groups
- G6PD Mediterranean, G6PD Kerala-Kalyan, and G6PD Orissa are the variants most prevalent in India
- Especially high prevalence in Parsees and Vatalia Prajapatis.

red cells have the highest enzyme activity and older red cells have relatively lower activity. G6PD A- variant enzyme has decreased stability and therefore, deficiency of enzyme in older red cells is more pronounced. In G6PD deficiency associated with G6PD A- variant, oxidant injury causes haemolysis of only older red cells and therefore, haemolytic episode is mild to moderate in severity and self-limited even if oxidant agent is continued. G6PD Mediterranean is a markedly unstable enzyme and its activity is reduced in red cells of all ages. Therefore in these cases oxidant injury is associated with severe, non-self-limited haemolysis.

Pathogenesis of Haemolysis

G6PD enzyme catalyses the first step in the hexose monophosphate (HMP) shunt. It catalyses the oxidation of glucose-6-phosphate to 6-phosphogluconate, and simultaneously generates NADPH from NADP. The only source of NADPH in red cells is the HMP shunt, which is dependent on the activity of G6PD enzyme. (HMP shunt produces ribose, which is an essential component of DNA and RNA. Ribose, however, can be produced by other pathways that are not G6PD-dependent).

In addition to various biosynthetic reactions, NADPH is required for continuous supply of reduced glutathione (GSH). GSH detoxifies harmful hydrogen peroxide or H_2O_2 (an oxidative metabolite) to water with the help of an enzyme, glutathione peroxidase. In G6PD deficiency, sufficient glutathione is not available to remove H_2O_2 (Fig. 4.44). Accumulation of H_2O_2 causes oxidation of haemoglobin and subsequent denaturation and precipitation of globin chains. This leads to the formation of Heinz bodies that are red cell inclusions bound to red cell membrane and represent

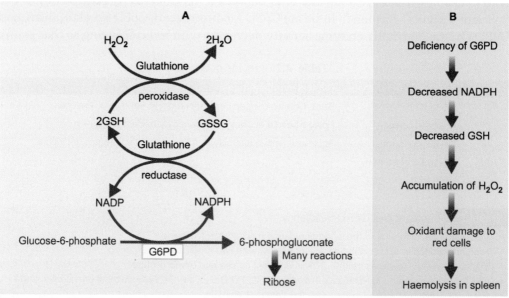

Figure 4.44: (A): Role of G6PD in detoxification of hydrogen peroxide. (B): Effect of G6PD deficiency

precipitated globin. Such red cells are rigid and are trapped in the spleen. Heinz bodies are selectively removed by splenic macrophages ("pitting") with subsequent membrane loss, and formation of spherocytes. Such red cells are susceptible to splenic sequestration and phagocytosis by macrophages. Oxidation of haem also leads to the formation of methaemoglobin; its role in haemolysis, however, is unclear.

Apart from extravascular destruction of red cells in spleen, intravascular haemolysis also occurs and is probably caused by peroxidation of membrane lipids by oxidant injury.

Genetics

G6PD deficiency is an X-linked disorder and therefore, occurs exclusively in males. In female heterozygotes, expression is variable. This is because of the process of random inactivation of one X chromosome (Lyonisation) during embryogenesis. Expression of deficiency in females depends on relative proportions of normal and abnormal chromosomes that are inactivated. Homozygous females showing clinical features of G6PD deficiency have also been reported.

Malaria and G6PD Deficiency

It has been suggested that high frequency of G6PD deficiency in certain parts of the world is probably related to the protection it affords against *P. falciparum* malaria. This protection is largely limited to the female heterozygotes. African heterozygous females have two populations of red cells: G6PD B (normal) and G6PD A—(deficient) —due to random inactivation of chromosomes during embryogenesis. Growth of the parasite is inhibited in the G6PD-deficient red cells. However, it has been shown that the malaria parasite can adapt to this deficiency by synthesising its own G6PD enzyme after 4 to 5 cycles in G6PD-deficient red cells. Therefore, parasite can grow and develop in hemizygous males (in whom all red cells are G6PD-deficient) after a few cycles. In female heterozygotes, the parasite may invade either G6PD- normal or -deficient red cells during successive cycles. Therefore, stimulus to the parasite to adapt by synthesising its own G6PD is considerably diminished. This results in decreased parasitaemia in female heterozygotes and protection against severe disease.

Clinical Features

In G6PD deficiency, haemolysis usually develops after exposure to oxidant stress, such as drugs (Table 4.8) or infection. There is usually sudden development of pallor, jaundice, and dark-coloured urine (due to haemoglobinuria) 1 to 3 days after exposure to the drug. Anaemia is most severe around 7 to 10 days following drug ingestion. Hypotension and acute renal failure may develop in severe cases. In class III variant, haemolysis is mild to moderate and self-restricted, i.e. haemolysis ceases even when patient goes on taking the offending drug. This is due to haemolysis of predominantly

Table 4.8: Common drugs and chemicals causing haemolysis in G6PD deficiency

- **Antimalarials: Primaquine,** Chloroquine, Quinacrine, **Pamaquine**
- **Antibacterials:** Sulphacetamide, **Sulphamethoxazole,** Sulphanilamide, Sulphapyridine, **Nalidixic acid, Nitrofurantoin,** Furazolidone, **Dapsone**
- **Analgesics:** Acetanilid, **Aspirin, Phenacetin**
- **Others:** Phenylhydrazine, Ascorbic acid, Vit K (water-soluble), **Methylene blue**, Naphthalene (moth balls)

Agents marked in bold: Definite risk of haemolysis

older red cells, and resistance of younger red cells to oxidant damage. In class II variant, haemolysis is marked, non-self-limited, and may require blood transfusion; this is because young red cells also have severely deficient G6PD activity.

Haemolysis following infection (pneumonia) develops 1 to 2 days after onset of fever and is usually mild.

Favism (precipitation of haemolysis by ingestion of fava beans) is a unique feature occurring in individuals in Mediterranean and Arab countries. Fava beans contain oxidants that cause haemolysis hours or days following ingestion; it may be fatal.

G6PD deficiency most commonly manifests with neonatal jaundice (Box 4.10). In severe cases, kernicterus and death can occur. It is mainly observed in Asia (including India) and Mediterranean countries.

Box 4.10	Clinical manifestations of G6PD deficiency

- Neonatal jaundice
- Drug-induced haemolytic anaemia
- Chronic haemolytic anaemia
- Favism
- Haemolysis following infection

Individuals with type I variant have chronic haemolytic anaemia. It manifests in infancy or childhood with hepatosplenomegaly and jaundice.

Laboratory Features

Evidence of Haemolysis

During haemolysis, general features of haemolytic anaemia are present. Peripheral blood smear shows: polychromasia, fragmented red cells, spherocytes, bite cells (red cells having bitten out margins due to plucking out of precipitated haemoglobin by splenic macrophages), and half-ghost cells (one half of red cell appears empty, while other half is filled with haemoglobin) (Fig. 4.45). Biochemical investigations reveal unconjugated hyperbilirubinaemia, haemoglobinaemia, haemoglobinuria (Box 4.11), and decreased or absent haptoglobin.

Box 4.11	Causes of haemoglobinuria

- Glucose-6-phosphate dehydrogenase deficiency
- Blackwater fever
- Paroxysmal nocturnal haemoglobinuria
- Paroxysmal cold haemoglobinuria
- Mismatched blood transfusion
- *Clostridium welchii* infection

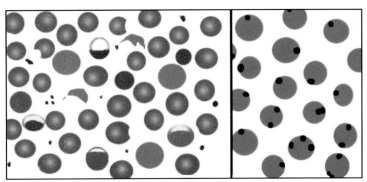

Figure 4.45: (1) Blood smear: half-ghost cells, bite cells, microspherocytes, fragmented cells, and polychromatic cells. (2) Heinz bodies (supravital staining with crystal violet)

Heinz Bodies

They can be detected after vital staining with methyl violet. They are usually seen immediately following haemolysis. Heinz bodies are deep purple small inclusions attached to red cell membrane. In addition to G6PD deficiency, they are also seen in unstable haemoglobin disease.

Tests for Detection of G6PD Deficiency

Diagnosis rests on demonstration of G6PD deficiency by a qualitative or a quantitative test.

Qualitative or Screening tests: Various screening tests are available. The most widely used, inexpensive, and recommended test is fluorescent spot test.

  i. *Fluorescent spot test:* This test is recommended by International Committee for Standardisation in Haematology.

   If G6PD is present in the blood sample, it reduces NADP to NADPH. NADPH fluoresces when exposed to ultraviolet light while NADP fails to do so. The method consists of following steps:

   1. To the reagent mixture that consists of buffered solution of glucose-6-phosphate, NADP, saponin, and oxidised glutathione (GSSG) whole blood is added. Glucose-6-phosphate is substrate for G6PD; saponin is used for lysis of red cells; and GSSG oxidises small amount of NADPH formed and thus renders the test more sensitive for the detection of mild G6PD deficiency.

   2. A drop (spot) of this mixture is applied on to the filter paper and examined under ultraviolet light.

   Following controls should always be run to test the accuracy of results: positive control (known G6PD-deficient sample) and negative control (normal or non-G6PD-deficient sample).

   Result: If G6PD is present in the test sample then NADPH is produced from NADP. NADPH fluoresces under ultraviolet light while NADP fails to do so. Presence of fluorescence indicates normal G6PD activity, while absence of fluorescence indicates G6PD deficiency (< 20% activity).

This test is simple, specific, and requires only small amount of blood. It is used for diagnosis of G6PD deficiency in individual cases and in population surveys.

Limitations:

1. During attack of haemolysis, this test may yield falsely normal result. This is because during haemolysis, preferentially older red cells (which contain the lowest G6PD activity) are destroyed, and the remaining red cells in circulation have more G6PD activity in comparison. Further, a brisk reticulocyte response follows haemolysis. Reticulocytes have high G6PD activity. Therefore, if screening test is performed during this period, normal or increased G6PD activity will be found. In such a case, screening test should be repeated after a few weeks. Another way is to separate older red cells from blood sample by centrifugation (older red cells settle at the bottom) and the test is performed on these cells.

2. Falsely abnormal test may be obtained in severe anaemia from any cause. This is because too few red cells are present in the blood sample.

3. It is difficult to diagnose those female heterozygotes that have small proportion of G6PD-deficient red cells.

ii. *Methaemoglobin reduction test:* Sodium nitrite is an oxidant that converts oxyhaemoglobin to methaemoglobin. Methylene blue is a redox dye that reduces methaemoglobin to haemoglobin in G6PD normal red cells but not in G6PD-deficient red cells. [In methaemoglobin, iron exists in the oxidised or ferric (Fe^{3+}) state]. Presence of methaemoglobinaemia imparts brownish colour to the blood. Brown colour indicates G6PD deficiency; red colour indicates normal G6PD activity, while intermediate colour indicates heterozygous state.

Limitations: Same as in fluorescent spot test.

iii. *Dye decolourisation test:* Haemolysate is incubated with buffered mixture of a dye (such as dichlorophenol indophenol or DPIP), glucose-6-phosphate, and NADP. If G6PD exists in the haemolysate, then it converts NADP to NADPH. NADPH reduces the dye to a colourless compound. In the presence of G6PD deficiency, time taken for dye decolourisation is longer. Advantages of this method include: (1) easy detection of heterozygotes, and (2) suitability for large scale screening since large number of samples can be tested simultaneously.

Quantitative assay of G6PD: This test is available only in reference laboratories. Haemolysate is incubated with glucose-6-phosphate. The rate of reduction of NADP to NADPH depends upon G6PD activity in the lysate. The rate of production of NADPH is measured in a spectrophotometer at 340 nm and G6PD activity is derived.

> During acute haemolytic episode, test for G6PD deficiency may yield negative result due to reticulocytosis (since reticulocytes have high G6PD content). In suspected cases, the test should be repeated about 6 weeks after the haemolytic episode.

Tests for Detection of Heterozygotes

Due to the process of random inactivation of one X chromosome during embryogenesis (Lyonisation), female heterozygotes for G6PD deficiency possess two types of red cells: normal and G6PD-deficient. The proportion of G6PD-deficient and G6PD-normal red cells is therefore, variable. When a screening test is performed which utilises lysate of red cells, or if the proportion of deficient red cells is small then it will give a normal result. Methods that measure enzyme activity in intact red cells are more sensitive in detecting heterozygotes if the proportion of G6PD-deficient red cells is small. Two tests are commonly employed: Methaemoglobin elution test and Tetrazolium-linked cytochemical method.

Methaemoglobin elution method: Blood is incubated with sodium nitrite, and methylene blue (or preferably nile blue sulphate). Sodium nitrite converts oxyhaemoglobin to methaemoglobin. Methylene blue (or nile blue sulphate) changes methaemoglobin to oxyhaemoglobin in G6PD-normal red cells. Potassium cyanide is added which combines with methaemoglobin to form methaemoglobin cyanide. From this blood, smears are prepared on glass slides. After drying, slides are dipped in a solution of hydrogen peroxide. Hydrogen peroxide elutes (or removes) methaemoglobin. The smears are then stained. Red cells containing oxyhaemoglobin (i.e. G6PD -normal red cells) take the stain, while red cells from which methaemoglobin has been removed (i.e. G6PD-deficient red cells) do not stain and appear as 'ghosts'.

Tetrazolium-linked cytochemical method: Methaemoglobin is formed when sodium nitrite is added to blood. In the presence of normal G6PD activity, nile blue sulphate (a redox dye) converts methaemoglobin to oxyhaemoglobin; in G6PD-deficient red cells this conversion does not occur. A tetrazolium compound (MTT) is then added. Oxyhaemoglobin reduces MTT to form coarse purplish-black granules of monoformazan. MTT is not reduced by methaemoglobin. In heterozygotes two populations of red cells can be distinguished: one containing granules (normal red cells) and one without granules (G6PD-deficient red cells).

Differential Diagnosis

Some cases of unstable haemoglobinopathy resemble G6PD deficiency in causing haemolysis of red cells on exposure to oxidant stress. Diagnosis of unstable haemoglobins requires heat instability test and isopropanol precipitation test.

Treatment

Patients should be instructed to avoid oxidant drugs that precipitate haemolysis. Prompt treatment of infections is essential.

Treatment during haemolytic attack is supportive. Blood transfusion may be indicated in severe cases. Adequate urinary output should be maintained to prevent renal damage due to haemoglobinuria.

IMMUNE HAEMOLYTIC ANAEMIAS

❑ CLASSIFICATION

Haemolysis due to immune mechanism occurs when antibody and/or complement bind to red cell membrane. In immunologically mediated haemolysis, destruction of red cells usually occurs by type II (cytotoxic) hypersensitivity reaction. The antigen is on the surface of the red cells. The specific antibody in the circulation binds with the antigen. This causes extravascular or intravascular red cell destruction.

Immune haemolytic anaemias are classified into three types—autoimmune, iso (or allo-) immune, and drug-induced (Box 4.12).

In autoimmune haemolytic anaemia (AIHA), haemolysis occurs when antibodies and/or complement in patient's circulation react with and cause destruction of patient's own red cells. Classification of AIHA (Table 4.9) is based on thermal characteristics of the antibody and presence or absence of underlying disease. In AIHA, autoantibodies may be of IgG, IgM, or IgA class. Generally, IgG and IgM antibodies are respectively of warm and cold types; however in paroxysmal cold haemoglobinuria, IgG antibodies are of cold-reactive type.

In alloimmune haemolytic anaemia, haemolysis occurs due to reaction between red cells (antigen) from one individual with antibody from another individual. Alloantibodies are usually of IgG class.

Table 4.9: Classification of autoimmune haemolytic anaemias

Warm antibody type (antibody maximally active at 37°C and mostly IgG)
- Primary (Idiopathic)
- Secondary:
    - Autoimmune disorders (e.g. systemic lupus erythematosus)
    - Neoplastic disorders (lymphoproliferative disorders like chronic lymphocytic leukaemia and malignant lymphoma, ovarian teratoma)
    - Drugs

Cold antibody type (antibody maximally active at 0 to 4°C)
- Cold agglutinin disease (cold-reactive antibody is IgM)
    - Primary
    - Secondary (Infections like *Mycoplasma pneumoniae*, EBV, CMV, malaria, etc; Lymphoproliferative disorders)
- Paroxysmal cold haemoglobinuria (cold-reactive antibody is IgG)
    - Primary
    - Secondary (Infection by *T. pallidum*, viruses)

Box 4.12 Classification of immune haemolytic anaemias
- Autoimmune
    - Warm-reactive antibody type
    - Cold-reactive antibody type
- Alloimmune
    - Haemolytic disease of newborn—Rh or ABO
    - Haemolytic transfusion reactions
- Drug-induced

Autoimmune Haemolytic Anaemias due to Warm-reacting Autoantibodies

This is the most common form of AIHA. In this type, IgG antibodies or complement (C3b) bind to red cell membrane and are recognised by specific receptors on macrophages. IgG-coated red cells are trapped in the spleen. Macrophages may completely phagocytose the red cell or may remove a small part of the membrane; in the latter case, loss of surface area causes formation of a microspherocyte. Some such red cells escape into the circulation and can be recognised on peripheral blood smear. Spherocytes are rigid and are sequestered and destroyed during subsequent passages through spleen (Fig. 4.46). There is a direct relationship between severity of haemolysis and number of spherocytes.

Clinical Features

Most patients have mild anaemia, icterus, and splenomegaly. Occasionally onset may be sudden with severe manifestations. In secondary AIHA, clinical features of underlying disease predominate. Association of haemolytic anaemia with thrombocytopaenia can occur in children and is known as Evans' syndrome.

Laboratory Features

Peripheral blood examination: This shows variable degree of anaemia depending on severity of haemolysis, microspherocytosis of red cells, and reticulocytosis. A spherocyte is smaller in size than normal red cell, lacks central area of pallor, and appears densely haemoglobinised. Fragmented red cells, polychromasia, and nucleated red cells may be present (Fig. 4.47). Mild neutrophilic leucocytosis is usual. Platelet count is normal. In the presence of thrombocytopaenia, Evans' syndrome should be considered. In this condition, antibodies against both red cells and platelets are present.

Antiglobulin (Coombs') test: This test determines whether haemolysis has an immunological basis. There are two types of antiglobulin test—direct and indirect. Direct antiglobulin test (DAT) is used to demonstrate antibodies or the complement

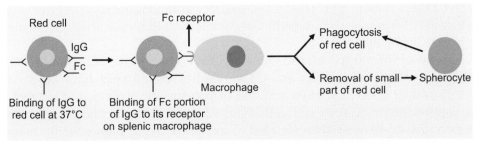

Figure 4.46: Mechanism of haemolysis in warm-type AIHA

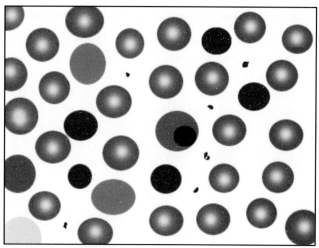

Figure 4.47: Blood smear in autoimmune haemolytic anaemia. Spherocytes, polychromatic cells and a normoblast are seen

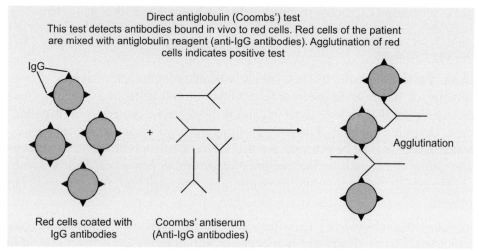

Direct antiglobulin (Coombs') test
This test detects antibodies bound in vivo to red cells. Red cells of the patient are mixed with antiglobulin reagent (anti-IgG antibodies). Agglutination of red cells indicates positive test

IgG

Agglutination

Red cells coated with
IgG antibodies

Coombs' antiserum
(Anti-IgG antibodies)

Figure 4.48: Principle of direct antiglobulin test

attached to red cells *in vivo* (Fig. 4.48). Indirect antiglobulin test (IAT) is used to demonstrate the presence of antibodies or complement in serum after sensitising red cells *in vitro* (Fig. 4.49).

Diagnosis of warm type AIHA is based on DAT. Polyspecific antiglobulin reagent consists of anti-IgG as well as anti-C3 antibodies. If red cells have been coated with IgG and/or C3 *in vivo*, then addition of polyspecific antiglobulin reagent will cause agglutination of such red cells (Fig. 4.50). If red cells show agglutination with polyspecific reagent then the test is repeated using monospecific reagents. The monospecific antisera react selectively with anti-IgG or specific complement

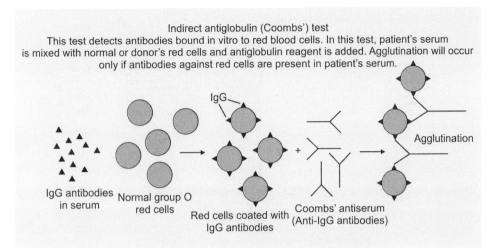

Figure 4.49: Principle of indirect antiglobulin test

components and thus the nature of the antibody can be identified. A negative DAT does not rule out the diagnosis of AIHA. Causes of positive DAT are shown in Box 4.13. Antiglobulin antibodies give a positive reaction when about 300 IgG molecules are bound to each red cell; if less, a negative result will be obtained. More sensitive tests that can detect smaller number of antibodies are available.

Laboratory diagnosis of AIHA is presented in Box 4.14.

Other investigations: Search should be made for underlying disorder. Osmotic fragility of red cells is increased and correlates with number of spherocytes. Unconjugated Serum bilirubin is elevated.

Differential Diagnosis

AIHA should be distinguished from hereditary spherocytosis that may present for the first time during adult life (positive family history and negative antiglobulin test), drug

Box 4.13 Causes of positive direct antiglobulin test

- Autoimmune haemolytic anaemia
- Immune haemolytic transfusion reaction (immediate or delayed)
- Haemolytic disease of foetus and newborn
- Drug-induced immune haemolytic anaemia
- Haematopoietic stem cell transplantation
- Administration of intravenous immunoglobulin, antilymphocyte globulin, or Rh immunoglobulin

Box 4.14 Laboratory diagnosis of autoimmune haemolytic anaemias

- Evidence of haemolytic anaemia: normocytic or macrocytic anaemia, reticulocytosis, decreased serum haptoglobin, increased serum lactate dehydrogenase, increased serum bilirubin (indirect)
- Warm AIHA: Direct antiglobulin test positive with IgG or IgG+C3d
- Cold AIHA: Direct antiglobulin test positive with C3d only

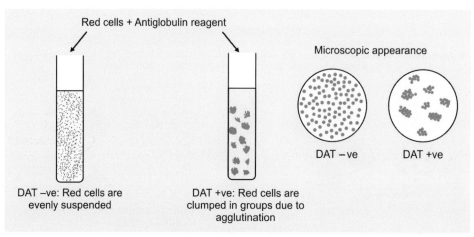

Figure 4.50: Interpretation of antiglobulin test

induced immune haemolytic anaemia (h/o recent drug exposure) and microangiopathic haemolytic anaemia (schistocytes, thrombocytopaenia, and evidence of intravascular coagulation).

Treatment

1. Underlying disease should be found and appropriately treated.
2. Majority of patients respond to corticosteroids (1 mg/kg body weight/day). Steroids inhibit macrophage phagocytosis and reduce synthesis of antibodies by spleen.
3. Splenectomy is indicated when improvement does not occur with corticosteroids. Splenectomy removes the major site of red cell destruction in AIHA.
4. Rituximab (monoclonal antibody against CD20 antigen of B lymphocytes) is another option for unresponsive cases. Other forms of treatment which may be of benefit are azathioprine, cyclophosphamide, and cyclosporine.
5. Blood transfusion: Blood transfusion is given only when absolutely essential. It is difficult to obtain serologically compatible blood because antibody in the patient's serum is a 'panagglutinin' and reacts with red cells from most donors. Therefore on cross matching all the blood units are found to be incompatible.

If the patient has developed alloantibody due to previous transfusion or pregnancy then autoantibodies may conceal this alloantibody during cross matching. This may induce haemolytic transfusion reaction in the recipient. For detection of alloantibodies, autoadsorption technique is employed in which autoantibodies in the serum are removed by adsorbing them with patient's own red cells and the serum is then tested for alloantibodies.

If the autoantibody is found to have specificity against a particular blood group antigen, then blood that is deficient in the particular antigen should be used for transfusion. If specificity against a particular antigen is not detected, then a large number of group-specific blood units should be tested and the unit that is most compatible should be transfused. Smallest volume of blood necessary for maintaining oxygen carrying capacity should be transfused at a slow rate.

Autoimmune Haemolytic Anaemias due to Cold-reacting Autoantibodies

This is caused by those autoantibodies which react with red cells maximally in cold (0–4°C) and which also retain immunologic reactivity at higher temperatures (30°C). It is of two types—cold agglutinin disease (CAD) and paroxysmal cold haemoglobinuria (PCH). The two types differ from each other in antibody class, nature of the red cell antigen, and clinical features.

Cold Agglutinin Disease

Cold-reactive antibodies or agglutinins are usually of IgM class. Polyclonal IgM cold agglutinins are present in all normal human sera in low titer and are probably formed as a result of immunologic response to infection by certain microorganisms. Since they are present at low level, they are clinically insignificant. Increased production of polyclonal IgM cold agglutinins occurs in Epstein-Barr virus and mycoplasma infections commonly. Occasionally in large cell lymphoma, monoclonal IgM cold agglutinins are increased. In primary CAD, monoclonal (kappa) IgM cold agglutinins are found in the absence of any underlying disease. It occurs in older persons and some such patients subsequently develop B cell lymphoproliferative disorder.

Most cold agglutinins are directed against I and i antigens on red cells.

The ability of the cold agglutinins to cause significant haemolysis depends on its titer and thermal amplitude (i.e. highest temperature at which antibody can cause red cell agglutination). If the antibody is having high titer and high thermal amplitude, it will cause significant haemolysis.

In CAD, cold agglutinins having high thermal amplitude react with red cell antigens in cooler peripheral circulation. This leads to (i) aggregation of red cells in peripheral circulation with acrocyanosis, and (ii) activation of complement via classical pathway. Complement activation stops at C3b stage due to the presence of regulatory inhibitors on red cell surface. IgM cold agglutinins dissociate from red cells in central warmer circulation, but C3b remains bound to red cells. Haemolysis of C3b-coated red cells occurs mostly in liver (Fig. 4.51). Cell-bound C3b is rapidly converted to C3dg by C3b inactivator. C3dg coated red cells are resistant to haemolysis since macrophages do not have receptors for C3dg. In addition complement pathway is terminated once C3dg is formed and membrane attack complex is not generated. Haemolysis in CAD therefore, is of extravascular type, and intravascular haemolysis by membrane attack complex is rare.

Clinical features: In idiopathic and lymphoma-associated CAD, two types of presentation are seen depending on thermal amplitude of the antibody. Autoantibody

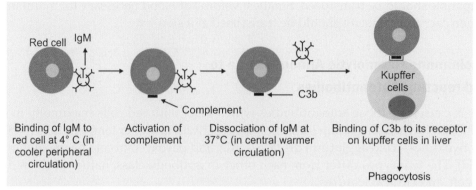

Figure 4.51: Mechanism of haemolysis in cold type AIHA (cold agglutinin disease)

with high thermal amplitude causes chronic haemolysis; with low thermal amplitude autoantibody acute haemolysis develops during exposure to cold. Raynaud's phenomenon and acrocyanosis may result from blockage of cooler peripheral microvasculature by agglutination of red cells.

CAD associated with infectious disease usually develops 2 to 3 weeks after onset and causes mild and short-lived haemolysis.

Laboratory features: Anaemia is commonly mild to moderate but may be severe during acute episode. Autoagglutination of red cells is a characteristic feature. It can be observed on peripheral blood smear (Fig. 4.52) and also in anticoagulated blood kept at room temperature. On warming autoagglutination disappears.

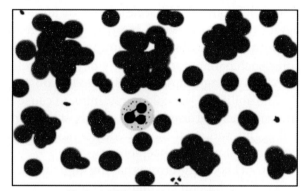

Figure 4.52: Blood smear showing autoagglutination of red cells

Red blood cell autoagglutination is also observed in paroxysmal cold haemoglobinuria, IgM paraproteinaemia, and presence of cold agglutinins in blood.

The DAT employing anticomplement (anti-C3) reagent is positive and detects C3dg-coated red cells.

Cold-reactive autoantibodies agglutinate all red cells and therefore may cause error in blood grouping. For cell grouping blood sample should be kept at 37°C and should be washed with normal saline before testing to remove IgM autoantibodies coating red cells. A diluent control (red cells + 6% albumin in saline) must be included. Sometimes it may be necessary to inactivate IgM molecules by 2 mercaptoethanol before doing cell grouping. Serum grouping is usually done at 37°C or autoadsorbed serum may be employed.

IgM autoantibodies may mask the presence of alloantibody during antibody screening test and crossmatching. Alloantibody screening should be carried out at 37°C; red cells should be washed with pre-warmed saline and mono-specific anti-IgG reagent is used. Agglutination-potentiating reagent (such as albumin) should not be used during the test procedure. Alternatively, autoadsorbed serum may be employed for identification of alloantibody.

Treatment

i. Underlying cause should be identified and treated (e.g. lymphoma).
ii. Exposure to cold should be avoided.
iii. Corticosteroids and splenectomy are not helpful.
iv. In primary disease, mainstay of treatment is rituximab.
v. Plasmapheresis to reduce circulating antibody level is a temporary measure.
vi. Transfused red cells are destroyed by cold antibodies in the same manner as patient's red cells and may sometimes precipitate acute renal failure. Therefore transfusions should be given only when absolutely essential.

Paroxysmal Cold Haemoglobinuria (PCH)

In this rare type of AIHA, there is a sudden onset of acute intravascular haemolysis with abdominal pain, backache, pallor and haemoglobinuria. Association with cold is usual but is not always present.

In children the haemolytic episode usually follows a viral infection, is self-limited and is not related to exposure to cold. In older people the condition is idiopathic, follows a chronic course and is precipitated by cold. Association with syphilis is nowadays rare.

The antibody is a polyclonal IgG with specificity against P red cell antigen. IgG antibodies react with red cells and bind complement in colder peripheral circulation. On return of red cells to central warmer circulation, IgG antibodies dissociate. Formation of membrane attack complex causes lysis of red cells.

DAT is positive during haemolytic attack due to coating of red cells with C3. Diagnosis is made by Donath-Landsteiner test. In this test, patient's serum (containing IgG antibodies and complement) is incubated with normal red cells in cold (4°C). IgG autoantibodies bind to red cells and cause haemolysis of coated red cells when temperature is raised to 37°C. The IgG autoantibody in PCH is also called as biphasic haemolysin because of this property.

Secondary PCH is self-limited and exposure to cold should be avoided. Steroids and cytotoxic therapy may be of benefit in idiopathic chronic cases.

Differences between warm type and cold type AIHA are listed in Table 4.10.

Table 4.10: Differences between warm type AIHA, cold agglutinin disease, and paroxysmal cold haemoglobinuria

Parameter	Warm-type AIHA	Cold agglutinin disease	Paroxysmal cold haemoglobinuria
1. Nature of antibody	IgG	IgM	IgG
2. Temperature at which antibody is maximally active	37°C	4°C	4°C
3. Mechanism of haemolysis	Opsonisation	Complement-mediated	Complement-mediated
4. Site of haemolysis	Extravascular	Extravascular	Intravascular
5. Blood smear	Spherocytes	Agglutination	Agglutination, spherocytes, erythrophagocytosis
6. Direct antiglobulin test	Positive with IgG or IgG+C3d	Positive with C3d only	Positive with C3d only
7. Donath-Landsteiner test	Negative	Negative	Positive
8. Target red cell antigen	Panagglutinin	I, i	P
9. Underlying diseases	B-lymphoproliferative disorders, autoimmune disorders	B-lymphoproliferative disorders, viral infections	Syphilis, viral infections
10. Main forms of treatment in idiopathic cases	Corticosteroids, splenectomy, rituximab	Protection from cold, rituximab, chlorambucil	Supportive, rituximab

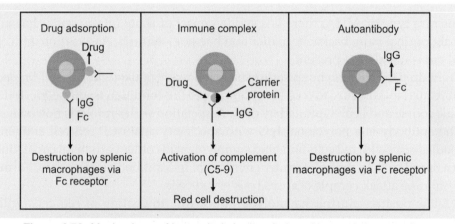

Figure 4.53: Mechanisms of haemolysis in drug-induced haemolytic anaemias

Drug-induced Immune Haemolytic Anaemias

Drug-induced immune haemolytic anaemia may result from three mechanisms:
- Drug adsorption on red cell membrane
- Immune complex or "innocent bystander" mechanism
- Production of autoantibodies against red cell antigens.

Mechanisms of haemolysis in drug-induced immune haemolytic anaemia are shown in Figure 4.53. Selected drugs causing drug-induced immune haemolytic anaemia are shown in Box 4.15.

> **Box 4.15**   Selected drugs causing immune haemolytic anaemia
> - Drug adsorption: Penicillin, ampicillin, methicillin, carbenecillin, cephalosporins
> - Immune complex: Quinidine, quinine, phenacetin, hydrochlorothiazide, rifampicin, isoniazid.
> - Autoantibody formation: Methyldopa, mefenamic acid, L-dopa, procainamide, diclofenac, ibuprofen.

Drug Adsorption on Red Cell Membrane

When penicillin is given in very high doses, it binds tightly to red cell membrane proteins. If the patient has developed IgG antibody against penicillin, it reacts with the penicillin bound to the red cell membrane. The red cells to which penicillin and its IgG antibody are bound are destroyed by macrophages via Fc receptors (extravascular haemolysis). Although typically seen with penicillin, it also occurs with cephalosporins. Mild to moderate haemolysis of insidious onset usually occurs.

Direct antiglobulin test is positive with anti-IgG reagent. Antibodies in the serum and eluted from patient's red cells react *in vitro* only with red cells which are preincubated with the drug.

Immune Complex or "Innocent Bystander" Mechanism

The offending drug when introduced into the body serves as a hapten and binds to a plasma protein carrier to form hapten-protein carrier complex. This elicits formation of antibodies (IgM or IgG). When re-exposure to the drug occurs, antigen-antibody immune complexes are formed. These immune complexes non-specifically bind to the erythrocyte membranes, activate complement and cause red cell destruction.

Patient usually experiences a severe haemolytic episode with haemoglobinaemia and haemoglobinuria; renal failure may occur. Direct antiglobulin test is positive with anticomplement reagent. Indirect antiglobulin test is positive only when patient's serum is preincubated with the drug in solution (to allow formation of immune complexes) and then tested against normal red cells. Eluate from the red cells is non-reactive. The prototype drug causing haemolysis by this mechanism is quinidine; other less commonly implicated drugs include—quinine, phenacetin, hydrochlorothiazide, etc.

Production of Autoantibodies Against Red Cell Antigens

α methyldopa (an antihypertensive drug) induces the formation of autoantibodies reactive against the red cell antigens (but not against the drug). Possibly the drug in some manner alters the red cell membrane antigen so that it is recognised as foreign. Alternatively, the drug may inhibit the suppressor T lymphocytes resulting in loss of control over B-lymphocytes and production of autoantibodies. About 10 to 15% of patients who are receiving α methyldopa develop autoantibodies and 0.5 to 1% develop haemolytic anaemia. Direct antiglobulin test is positive due to coating of red cells with IgG antibodies; complement is rarely demonstrated on red cells. IgG antibodies in serum react with red cells in the absence of the drug. The results of direct and indirect antiglobulin tests resemble those seen in warm antibody autoimmune haemolytic anaemia.

Mild to moderate haemolytic anaemia usually develops due to destruction of red cells coated with IgG in spleen. Other drugs that are implicated are L-dopa, mefenamic acid, procainamide, diclofenac, etc.

Treatment: The responsible drug should be stopped. Red cell transfusions may be required if anaemia is severe.

HAEMOLYTIC DISEASE OF THE NEWBORN

Haemolytic disease of the newborn (HDN) is a disease in which destruction of red cells of the foetus or newborn occurs due to the passage of maternal antibodies across the placenta into the foetal circulation. The production of these maternal antibodies is stimulated due to blood group incompatibility between mother and the foetus.

This disease develops if the red cell antigens inherited by the foetus from father are foreign to the mother. Leakage of foetal red cells into the maternal circulation induces formation of antibodies; these antibodies pass across the placenta into the foetal circulation and cause haemolysis of foetal red cells. Only IgG antibodies against red cell antigens can cause HDN since antibodies only of IgG class can traverse the placental barrier. The main red cell antigens responsible for HDN are:

- Rh D
- Rh c
- Kell
- A and B

HDN due to anti-RhD, anti-c, and anti-Kell can cause severe foetal haemolytic anaemia. HDN due to ABO incompatibility is usually a mild disease.

Maternal and foetal blood group incompatibilities associated with HDN are shown in Table 4.11.

Table 4.11: Maternal and foetal blood group incompatibilities associated with HDN

Blood group system	Maternal blood group	Foetal blood group	Severity of HDN
1. ABO	O	A	Mild
	O	B	Mild
2. Rh	C-	C+	Mild to severe
	D-	D+	Mild to severe
	E-	E+	Mild to severe
	c-	c+	Mild to severe
	e-	e+	Mild to severe
3. Kell	K-	K+	Mild to severe
4. Kidd	Jk(a-)	Jk(a+)	Mild to severe
	Jk(b-)	Jk(b+)	Mild to severe
5. Duffy	Fy(a-)	Fy(a+)	Mild to severe
6. MNS	M-	M+	Moderate to severe
	S-	S+	Moderate to severe

Note: Most cases of severe HDN are associated with D, c, and K alloantibodies.

❑ Rh HAEMOLYTIC DISEASE OF THE NEWBORN

Pathogenesis

Rh HDN develops when a Rh-negative mother who is previously sensitised to the RhD antigen carries a RhD-positive foetus. The usual causes of sensitisation of Rh-negative mother to D antigen are previous pregnancy or past RhD-positive blood transfusion. During pregnancy most common cause of maternal immunisation is foetomaternal haemorrhage that occurs at the time of separation of placenta during delivery. Other causes of primary immunisation during pregnancy are listed in Table 4.12.

Foetomaternal haemorrhage induces primary immune response consisting of IgM antibodies. Because IgM antibodies do not cross the placenta and sensitisation occurs during labor, Rh HDN does not develop during first pregnancy. During the second and following pregnancies with Rh-positive foetus, a slight foetomaternal leak can induce a strong and rapid secondary IgG immune response. IgG anti-D antibodies cross the placenta and bind to RhD-positive red cells of the foetus. The IgG-coated red cells are destroyed by macrophages in the spleen (opsonisation) (Fig. 4.54). Excessive destruction of red cells leads to anaemia, compensatory erythroid hyperplasia in bone marrow, erythroblastosis in peripheral blood, and extramedullary erythropoiesis in liver and spleen. Unconjugated bilirubin in the foetal circulation crosses the placenta and is metabolised by maternal liver. After birth, unconjugated bilirubin in the neonate increases markedly due to immaturity of the glucuronyl transferase enzyme, and may cross the blood-brain barrier and damage the basal ganglia (kernicterus).

Some factors influence the production of anti-D antibodies by the RhD-negative mother. One of the major factors is **amount of foetomaternal haemorrhage**. The larger the foetomaternal bleed, the greater the risk of sensitisation. For induction of secondary immune response, a very small leak may be sufficient. **ABO incompatibility** between mother and foetus reduces the risk of sensitisation to RhD antigen. This is because when ABO incompatible foetal red cells enter the maternal circulation they are rapidly coated by maternal anti-A or anti-B and removed by macrophages before sensitisation to RhD can occur.

Zygosity of the father decides the Rh status of the child. If father is homozygous (DD) then all his offsprings will be RhD-positive; if he is a heterozygous (Dd), then there is a 50% chance in every pregnancy of child being Rh-positive or Rh-negative.

Table 4.12: Causes of primary immunisation to blood group antigens in females of reproductive age group

• Previous pregnancy	• Ruptured ectopic pregnancy
• Abortion	• Accidental haemorrhage
• Medical termination of pregnancy	• Abdominal trauma
• Amniocentesis	• Lower segment caesarean section
• Chorion villus biopsy	• External cephalic version
• Cordocentesis	• Previous blood transfusion

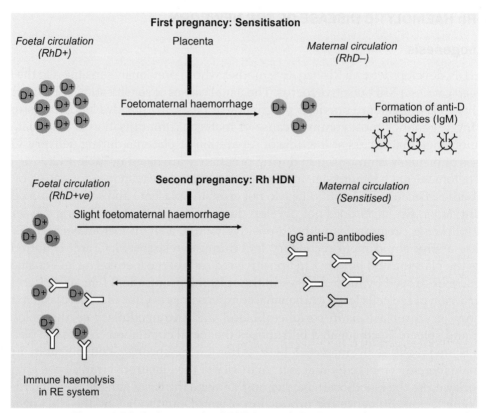

Figure 4.54: Pathogenesis of RhD haemolytic disease of newborn

Clinical Features

Clinical presentation is variable. There may be only mild anaemia and jaundice. In some cases, there is severe unconjugated hyperbilirubinaemia (icterus gravis neonatorum). Jaundice is rapidly progressive and develops within 24 hours of birth. Damage to basal ganglia leads to kernicterus, which may be fatal or may cause neurological deficit. In its most severe form, Rh HDN manifests as fresh stillbirth or as hydrops foetalis. Most of the hydropic foetuses perish *in utero*; if the hydropic infant has live birth, it shows severe anaemia, hepatosplenomegaly, ascitis, and anasarca.

The disease should be differentiated from haemolytic anaemias that manifest in the newborns (Box 4.16).

Laboratory Features

Antenatal Investigations

Antenatal investigations are carried out to detect pregnant women with high risk of haemolytic disease developing in the foetus.

Box 4.16	Haemolytic anaemias manifesting in the newborn period

- Haemolytic disease of newborn
- Infections
- Microangiopathic haemolytic anaemia in disseminated intravascular coagulation
- Glucose-6-phosphate dehydrogenase deficiency
- Hereditary spherocytosis
- Hereditary elliptocytosis, pyropoikilocytosis
- Haemoglobin H disease
- Homozygous α thalassaemia

A. *Maternal investigations*
1. Clinical history: Mothers having similar previous childbirth need careful supervision. Various possible causes of previous sensitisation should be identified such as Rh-positive blood transfusion, medical termination of pregnancy, abortion, ectopic pregnancy, etc.
2. Blood grouping: ABO and Rh typing should be done. If red cells of the mother test negative for D antigen, then test for a weaker form of D (i.e. D^u) should be carried out.
3. Antibody detection: This needs to be performed in all pregnant women on first antenatal check-up irrespective of their Rh status. This is because apart from anti-D antibodies, certain other IgG antibodies listed earlier can also cause HDN. Indirect Coombs' test employing two different group O screening cell panels should be used for antibody screening. If antibodies are detected, then they should be identified with the help of cells, the antigen make-up of which is known. Antibody titre should be checked every month. A titre of 1:32 or more and an increasing titre on subsequent testing are reasons for amniocentesis.
B. *Blood grouping of the father:* Father's ABO and Rh grouping should be done. ABO grouping helps in knowing the likely blood group of the foetus and also the chance of ABO incompatibility between the mother and the foetus. If the foetus is ABO-compatible then the risk of alloimmunisation of the mother is more.
   Whether father is homozygous or heterozygous for the D antigen may be ascertained provided he has a previous Rh-negative child. This is helpful in counselling if anti-D antibodies are present in the mother.
C. *Foetal investigations:* Severity of haemolysis in the foetus is assessed by measuring the concentration of bilirubin in amniotic fluid or in foetal blood. Severity of haemolysis is also judged from previous obstetric history and maternal anti-D titre. This will help identify at risk RhD+ve foetus early in pregnancy.
   i. Amniocentesis: Amniocentesis is indicated in following situations:
      - *Maternal anti-D titre of 1:32*
      - *Rising anti-D titre on follow-up testing*
      - *Bad obstetric history in Rh-negative mother (previous severely affected offspring).*
      Amniotic fluid is obtained under ultrasound guidance by introducing a long needle through the abdominal wall into the uterine cavity. It is done between 28 and 32 weeks of pregnancy if there is no history of previously affected baby.

If such previous history is present, then it should be done 10 weeks prior to the date of previous foetal or neonatal death. Repeat amniocentesis may be done after 2 weeks to establish whether bilirubin is rising.

Amniotic fluid bilirubin is measured spectrophotometrically and shows peak absorbance at 450 nm. The degree of absorption at 450 nm (i.e. difference in optical density between baseline and peak of elevation) is a precise reflection of the amount of bilirubin; it is denoted as Δ A 450.

Level of bilirubin in amniotic fluid depends on the period of gestation. Liley's chart relates degree of absorption at 450 nm (Δ A 450) to gestational age on a semilogarithmic graph paper. This chart is used for prediction of severity of HDN and is divided into three zones: I (Low), II (Middle), and III (High). Values falling within zone III indicate severely affected foetus with imminent death. Therapy is based on gestational age or foetal maturity: intrauterine transfusion (<34 weeks) or delivery (>34 weeks). Values within zone II need observation in the form of repeated amniocentesis. Depending on the result, foetus may need intrauterine transfusion or early delivery. Values in zone I indicate unaffected foetus and pregnancy may be continued till term.

ii. Cordocentesis: Foetal blood obtained from cord blood vessel is used for assessing severity of haemolysis by estimating haemoglobin and bilirubin concentrations. Blood grouping and direct antiglobulin test can also be done.

iii. Other techniques for foetal monitoring are foetal ultrasound (for determining foetal size and organomegaly) and Doppler ultrasonography of foetal middle cerebral artery peak systolic velocity or MCA-PSV (for predicting foetal haemoglobin or anaemia). With increasing foetal anaemia, blood flow velocity (MCV-PSV) increases due to the rise in cardiac output and vasodilatation; this measurement is specific for gestational age. This technique is replacing the amniotic fluid spectrophotometry for foetal monitoring.

Investigations of Newborn

Following investigations are done on the cord blood of the newborn:

1. *Blood grouping:* ABO grouping in the newborn rests solely on cell grouping since antibodies in the blood are passively acquired from the mother. Wharton's jelly of the umbilical cord may cause agglutination of red cells and therefore red cells should be washed thoroughly to avoid erroneous result.

2. *Blood smear:* In Rh HDN, blood smear will show markedly increased number of nucleated red cells (erythroblastosis) and polychromasia (reticulocytosis) (Fig. 4.55).

3. *Direct antiglobulin test:* This is strongly reactive in the newborn. Positive DAT is indicative of incompatibility between red cell antigens of the foetus and antibodies in the mother. If DAT is positive, specificity of the antibody can be determined using mother's serum.

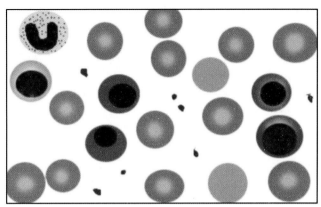

Figure 4.55: Blood smear in Rh haemolytic disease of newborn showing many erythroblasts and polychromatic cells

4. *Determination of haemoglobin and bilirubin concentrations:* These parameters are helpful in assessing the severity of the disease. Cord blood haemoglobin value of less than 12.0 g/dl or indirect bilirubin more than 5 mg/dl is an indication for immediate exchange transfusion.

Post-delivery Maternal Investigations

After delivery, maternal investigations include repeat ABO and RhD grouping, antibody screening (by indirect antiglobulin test), and Betke-Kleihauer test (see below) to assess amount of foetomaternal haemorrhage.

Treatment

Foetus

If measurement of Δ A 450 indicates a severely affected foetus, then nature of treatment depends upon the maturity of the foetus. Foetal lung maturity is most commonly assessed by measuring lecithin/sphingomyelin (L/S) ratio in the amniotic fluid. L/S ratio more than 2:1 indicates foetal lung maturity. In severely affected foetus with L/S ratio >2:1, prompt delivery is indicated; if L/S ratio indicates foetal lung immaturity, then intrauterine foetal transfusions should be given. Intrauterine foetal transfusion may be either intraperitoneal or intravascular. Packed red cells of O Rh-negative blood group, which are compatible with mother's serum, are given. Blood to be transfused should be fresh (<5 days old). Leucocyte-poor and irradiated blood is preferred to prevent the development of alloantibodies against leucocytes and platelets in the mother, and for prevention of cytomegalovirus infection and graft-versus-host disease in the foetus. Severely affected foetuses may be transfused at 2 to 4 weeks intervals. Following this treatment, delivery is carried out at 36 weeks.

Neonate

Exchange transfusion: Rapidly rising bilirubin concentration in the neonate is associated with the danger of kernicterus. In newborns (especially in premature infants), breakdown products of haemolysis cannot be metabolised due to immaturity of the liver. Kernicterus is more likely in the presence of prematurity, septicaemia, hypoxia, acidosis, hypoglycaemia and hypoproteinaemia. Exchange transfusion removes antibody-coated red cells, bilirubin and IgG anti-D antibodies from the plasma, and also corrects anaemia. An exchange transfusion equal to twice the newborn's blood volume is ideal. In exchange transfusion, a small amount of patient's blood is withdrawn and replaced by equal amount of donor blood at a time (2–3 ml/kg/min). Blood for exchange transfusion should be fresh (<5 days old). Donor red cells should be cross-matched against mother's serum because any alloantibodies in the neonatal serum are derived from the mother and in the mother's serum they are more in number. If ABO blood groups of the mother and baby are identical then RhD-negative blood of the same ABO group is used. If blood groups of the mother and baby are different then O Rh-negative blood should be used.

At birth, cord blood haemoglobin concentration less than 12 g/dl and cord blood unconjugated bilirubin more than 5 mg/dl are indications for exchange transfusion. Rate of rise of unconjugated bilirubin more than 0.5 mg/dl/hr is also considered by some as an indication for exchange transfusion.

Adjunctive therapy: **Phototherapy** causes unconjugated bilirubin to be converted into a soluble form that is excreted in urine and bile. **Infusion of albumin** binds free bilirubin in plasma and thus decreases the risk of kernicterus. Both phototherapy and albumin help in reducing the need for exchange transfusion.

Prevention of Rh Immunisation

For prevention of immunisation of Rh-negative mother against D antigen, Rh immune globulin (RhIg) is administered. It must be given before primary immunisation has occurred. The mode of action of RhIg is not known. IgG anti-D in RhIg coat the D-positive foetal red cells that may have entered maternal circulation and probably blocks the antigen recognition by the immune system.

RhIg consists of IgG anti-D antibodies and is prepared from pooled plasma of donors who have high levels of anti-D antibodies. For prevention of Rh HDN, it can be administered in different ways:

- *After delivery:* All Rh D-ve women are given RhIg within 72 hours of delivery of Rh D+ve infant. The usual dose is 300 mcg given intramuscularly which neutralises up to 15 ml of foetal red cells (which is the usual amount of foetomaternal haemorrhage). If a larger foetomaternal leak is suspected, a maternal blood sample is taken within 1 to 2 hours of delivery to determine the amount of foetal red cells by acid elution test of Betke-Kleihauer. Principle of this test is outlined earlier in "Disorders of haemoglobin—General features and approach to diagnosis." Rh D+ve red cells can also be quantitated by flow cytometry. Depending on the amount of foetomaternal haemorrhage, further RhIg (125 IU/ml of foetal red cells) can be administered.

- *During antenatal period*: All Rh D-ve pregnant women are given 300 mcg of RhIg intramuscularly at 28 and 34 weeks of gestation. If infant is Rh D+ve, anti-RhIg is also given following delivery.
- *Following sensitising event during pregnancy*: RhIg is given to Rh-ve women if there is a potentially sensitising event such as abortion, antepartum haemorrhage, abdominal trauma, external cephalic version, stillbirth, caesarean section, ectopic pregnancy, multiple pregnancy, amniocentesis, cordocentesis, and chorion villus biopsy. RhIg is given in the dose of 50 mcg intramuscularly (before 20 weeks of gestation) or 100 mcg intramuscularly (after 20 weeks).

❑ ABO HAEMOLYTIC DISEASE OF NEWBORN

Haemolytic disease of newborn due to ABO incompatibility is more common than Rh HDN (because of low frequency of Rh D-ve women in the population) and is usually a mild disease. Unlike Rh HDN, ABO HDN does not present *in utero* and does not cause hydrops foetalis. There is no correlation between the titre of antibodies in the mother and occurrence of HDN. Therefore, monitoring of anti-ABO antibodies during pregnancy is not necessary. It usually develops when blood group of the mother is O and that of the foetus is A or B and when maternal high titre IgG anti-A and anti-B antibodies are present (>1:64 titre). Less commonly it results when blood group of the mother is A or B and that of the foetus is respectively B or A.

IgG anti-A and anti-B antibodies are naturally occurring and therefore ABO HDN can occur in first as well as in subsequent pregnancies. The mild nature of ABO HDN is probably related to the neutralisation of anti-A and anti-B antibodies by tissue A and B antigens and also by soluble A or B substances. Incomplete expression of A and B antigens on foetal red cells also plays a role.

Differences between Rh and ABO haemolytic disease of the newborn are outlined in Table 4.13. The usual clinical manifestations are mild anaemia and jaundice within 24 hours of birth. Severe anaemia and kernicterus are rare.

Peripheral blood smear examination shows spherocytosis in ABO HDN (but not in Rh HDN) (Fig. 4.56). Blood group of the mother is O and that of the infant is A or B. Direct antiglobulin test in the infant is either negative or weakly positive. This is because of (1) weak expres-

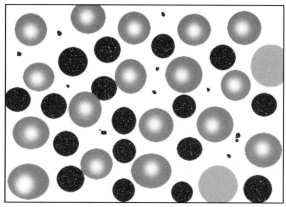

Figure 4.56: Blood smear in ABO haemolytic disease of newborn showing numerous microspherocytes

Table 4.13: Differences between Rh and ABO haemolytic disease of the newborn

Parameter	Rh HDN	ABO HDN
1. Frequency	Less common	More common
2. Blood group • Mother • Foetus	Rh negative Rh positive	O A or B
3. Pregnancy affected	Usually second	Usually first
4. Severity	Usually severe	Usually mild
5. Blood smear	Erythroblastosis	Spherocytosis
6. Direct antiglobulin test	Strongly positive	Weakly positive or negative
7. Prevention	Rh immune globulin	Not available
8. Stillbirth or hydrops	Common	Rare
9. Jaundice	Marked	Mild
10. Hepatosplenomegaly	Marked	Mild
11. Antenatal monitoring	Required	Not required

sion of ABO antigens on red cells of newborn, and (2) neutralisation of most of the IgG antibodies by tissue A and B antigens and by soluble A and B substances in the foetus so that very few antibodies remain for binding to red cells. Eluate from cord red cells will react against A or B red cells (but not against O cells) in indirect antiglobulin test.

Blood haemoglobin and bilirubin should be estimated to assess the severity of haemolysis and need for exchange transfusion.

Management usually consists of phototherapy and supportive measures. In severe hyperbilirubinaemia, exchange transfusion may be necessary to prevent development of kernicterus. For exchange transfusion, group O blood with same Rh D type as the neonate and which is lacking in high titre haemolytic IgG antibodies should be selected. It should be cross-matched against mother's serum.

PAROXYSMAL NOCTURNAL HAEMOGLOBINURIA

Paroxysmal nocturnal haemoglobinuria (PNH) is a rare acquired haematopoietic stem cell disorder characterised by abnormal sensitivity of red cells to haemolytic action of complement. White cells and platelets also show similar defect. Typically red cell destruction occurs at night so that haemoglobinuria is noticed in the first-voided urine in the morning. However presentation is varied, e.g. iron deficiency anaemia due to haemosiderinuria, pancytopaenia, aplastic anaemia, chronic intravascular haemolytic anaemia, or repeated venous thromboses.

❑ PATHOGENESIS

PNH is a clonal disorder characterised by expansion of defective haematopoietic stem cell. The defective stem cell in PNH gives rise to red cells, white cells, and platelets, which are abnormally sensitive to complement. The defective stem cell can arise on the background of abnormal marrow such as aplastic anaemia. Both the defective and the normal clones coexist in varying proportions. Depending on the degree of sensitivity to complement, three different types of red cells are found in PNH:

- **PNH I:** Red cells with normal sensitivity to complement;
- **PNH II:** Red cells with intermediate sensitivity to complement-mediated lysis
- **PNH III:** Red cells with marked sensitivity to complement-mediated lysis.

Many patients have both PNH II and PNH III red cells. The severity of haemolysis depends on the number of PNH III red cells: mild haemolysis occurs when less than 20% PNH III red cells are present, and chronic haemolysis results when these exceed 50%.

In PNH, the abnormal sensitivity of red cells to the lytic action of complement is due to an intrinsic abnormality of red cells. In PNH, many cell membrane proteins are deficient; the most significant being (1) decay accelerating factor (DAF, CD 55) and (2) membrane inhibitor of reactive lysis (MIRL, CD 59). DAF is an inhibitor of C3 convertase, while MIRL inhibits the membrane attack complex (C5–9). Normally *in vivo*, small amount of C3b is being continuously generated via alternate complement pathway by C3 convertase (C3bBb), some of which also binds to red cell membranes. In the presence of DAF, C3bBb is inactivated and subsequent formation of membrane attack complex does not occur. Thus, in PNH, due to the deficiency of DAF and especially of MIRL, cells are more susceptible to the lytic action of the complement.

In addition to the deficiencies of CD 55 and CD 59, deficiencies of some other proteins also occur in PNH. These include acetylcholinesterase, neutrophil alkaline phosphatase, and 5'-nucleotidase. Normally all these proteins are anchored to the cell membrane by a phospholipid called as glycosylphosphatidylinositol (GPI) (Fig. 4.57). In PNH, GPI anchor is nonfunctional because of an acquired somatic mutation of the X-linked gene called as phosphatidylinositol glycan class A (PIG-A) in a haematopoietic stem cell. This leads to the deficiency of multiple proteins on cell membrane. About 200 different mutations of PIG-A gene have been reported.

Classification of PNH proposed by International PNH Interest Group is shown in Table 4.14.

Table 4.14: Classification of paroxysmal nocturnal haemoglobinuria
(International PNH Interest Group, 2005)

Classic PNH	Severe intravascular haemolysis; cellular marrow with erythroid hyperplasia; large PNH clones
PNH in the setting of another specific bone marrow disorder	Mild to moderate intravascular haemolysis; evidence of another specific bone marrow disorder (aplastic anaemia, myelodysplastic syndrome); moderate sized PNH clones
Subclinical PNH	No evidence of intravascular haemolysis; evidence of another specific bone marrow disorder (aplastic anaemia, myelodysplastic syndrome); small PNH clones detected by flow cytometry

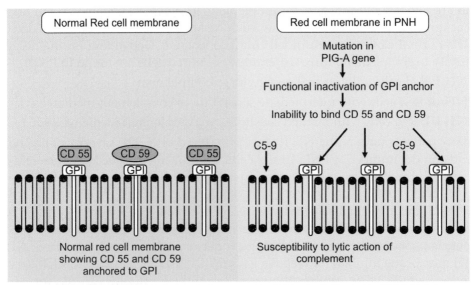

Figure 4.57: Red cell membrane in normal individuals (left) and in PNH (right)

❏ CLINICAL FEATURES

PNH usually presents during the 3rd or 4th decade of life with features of chronic haemolytic anaemia: weakness, pallor, and mild jaundice. Mild to moderate splenomegaly is present in some cases. Nocturnal haemoglobinuria (passage of reddish-brown urine after getting up in the morning) occurs in only a minority of the cases; it is due to increased haemolysis during sleep and is not related to the time of the day. Haemosiderinuria, however, is a constant feature and leads to iron deficiency anaemia.

Recurrent venous thrombosis is a common feature and probably results from activation of platelets due to complement-mediated damage with subsequent aggregation. Budd-Chiari syndrome due to hepatic vein thrombosis is a classical feature and runs a rapidly fatal course. Abdominal pain is a common complaint and may be related to thrombosis of mesenteric veins. Thrombosis of deep veins of limbs can occur.

Bleeding (due to thrombocytopaenia) and infections (due to neutropaenia or impaired chemotaxis) are other common features.

Some cases of PNH terminate in acute myeloblastic leukaemia.

Clinical features in PNH result from intravascular haemolysis, anaemia, bone marrow failure, and thrombosis.

❏ LABORATORY FEATURES

Peripheral Blood Examination

The usual manifestation of PNH is pancytopaenia. Anaemia is moderate to severe. If iron deficiency is present, red cells are microcytic and hypochromic. Reticulocyte count is raised.

Urine Examination

Haemoglobinuria (excretion of free haemoglobin in urine) develops when plasma haptoglobin cannot bind any more haemoglobin. Some amount of haemoglobin is reabsorbed in proximal renal tubular epithelial cells where haemoglobin iron is stored as ferritin or haemosiderin. When these cells are shed in urine, haemosiderinuria results. Haemoglobinuria is detected by benzidine or orthotoluidine test on urine sample and haemosiderinuria by Prussian blue staining of urinary sediment (Fig. 4.58).

Serological Studies

These demonstrate unusual sensitivity of PNH red cells to the haemolytic action of complement.

Sucrose Haemolysis Test

This is the standard screening test. In this test, red cells from the patient are added to the mixture of fresh ABO-compatible normal serum and isotonic sucrose solution. Sucrose is the low ionic strength medium and favours the attachment of IgG and complement to red cells (alternate pathway activation). After incubation at 37°C and centrifugation, amount of haemolysis is quantified in a spectrophotometer. If it is more than 10%, it is indicative of PNH.

Acidified Serum Test (Ham Test)

This is the confirmatory test for PNH. Acidification of serum (to pH 6.5) activates complement via alternate pathway and causes haemolysis of red cells if they are abnormally sensitive to complement.

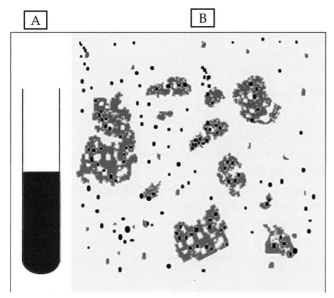

Figure 4.58: (A) Gross appearance of urine in PNH (haemoglobinuria) (B) Urine microscopy showing haemosiderinuria

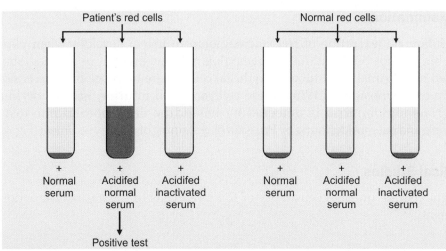

Figure 4.59: Principle of Ham's test in PNH. Patient's red cells are haemolysed in the presence of complement (provided by normal serum) and acid (activates complement). Inactivated serum (heated at 56°C) is devoid of complement

In this test, fresh normal ABO-compatible serum (source of complement) is acidified and red cells from the patient are added to it (Although patient's serum may also be used, it may be exhausted of complement). Per cent haemolysis is noted. PNH red cells show 10 to 50% lysis (Fig. 4.59).

Acidified serum test is the confirmatory test for PNH and is usually performed if sucrose haemolysis test is positive. Although acidified serum test is positive in another condition called as congenital dyserythropoietic anaemia type II (hereditary erythroid multinuclearity with positive acidified serum or HEMPAS), it can be differentiated from PNH on the basis of clinical history, abnormal morphology of erythroblasts in bone marrow, and negative sucrose haemolysis test. (See "Congenital dyserythropoietic anaemia"). Ham's test has largely been superseded by flow cytometric analysis for CD 55 and CD 59.

Flow Cytometric Analysis of GPI-linked Proteins

The analysis of CD 55 and CD 59 proteins on blood cells by flow cytometry has recently replaced Ham's test as the definitive test for diagnosis of PNH. In PNH, a population of red cells, which is deficient in more than one GPI-anchored protein, is present. Size of the PNH clone can also be estimated by flow cytometry.

A fluorescein-labelled proaerolysin (FLAER) is commonly being used for diagnosis of PNH. It binds selectively and with high affinity to the GPI anchor on granulocytes and provides more accurate assessment of GPI anchor deficiency in PNH than anti-CD55 and anti-CD59.

Red cell analysis by CD59 fluorescence histogram is shown in Figure 4.60.

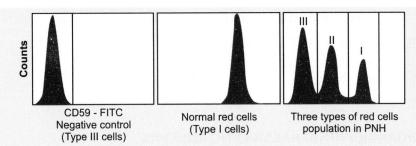

Figure 4.60: Red cell analysis by CD59 fluorescence histogram. Figure on left shows negative control which corresponds to red cells deficient in CD59 (type III red cells); figure in middle shows normal red cells which correspond to type I red cells; while figure on right shows histogram from a patient with PNH showing three distinct populations of red cells: type I (normal red cells), type II (red cells partially deficient in CD59), and type III (red cells completely deficient in CD59).

❑ TREATMENT

Eculizumab (a humanised monoclonal antibody directed against C5 complement thus blocking terminal complement activation) is highly effective in reducing intravascular haemolysis. It is especially helpful in classic PNH. It decreases or eliminates need for blood transfusion, reduces the risk of thrombosis, and improves quality of life. However, it is very expensive and life-long treatment is required as it does not eradicate the PNH clone. It also does not have any effect on associated bone marrow failure. Since it increases the risk of infection with encapsulated organisms (due to complement inhibition), vaccination against *N. meningitidis* is necessary.

Allogeneic bone marrow transplantation is the only curative therapy but is associated with significant morbidity and mortality. It is indicated in patients with severe aplastic anaemia or in patients not responding to eculizumab.

Supportive treatment measures include (1) blood transfusion to maintain haemoglobin level, (2) anticoagulant therapy for venous thrombosis, (3) iron supplementation, and (4) corticosteroids to reduce haemolysis.

❑ PROGNOSIS

The median life expectancy is about 10 years. Course of PNH is variable. Patients may remain stable with chronic haemolytic anaemia for many years. In some patients abnormal PNH clone may spontaneously disappear. Evolution of PNH to aplastic anaemia or acute myeloblastic leukaemia can occur. There is a close relationship between PNH and bone marrow failure. PNH develops in about 10% of patients with aplastic anaemia and about 25% patients with PNH progress to aplastic anaemia. Venous thrombosis is a major cause of morbidity and mortality.

MECHANICAL HAEMOLYTIC ANAEMIAS

The mechanical haemolytic anaemias include:
- Microangiopathic haemolytic anaemia
- March haemoglobinuria
- Cardiac haemolytic anaemia.

☐ MICROANGIOPATHIC HAEMOLYTIC ANAEMIA

This refers to haemolytic anaemia resulting from intravascular fragmentation and lysis of red cells due to alteration in small blood vessels. Usually direct damage to red cells occurs when they pass through the fibrin strands deposited in the microcirculation.

Common causes of microangiopathic haemolytic anaemia are given in Table 4.15.

Clinical features are related to the underlying disease. Severity of anaemia is variable.

The characeristic feature on peripheral blood smear is fragmented red cells or schistocytes. Schistocytes include small red cell fragments with 1 to 3 sharp spicules as well as large helmet-shaped red cells from which fragments have been split off (Fig. 4.61). Evidence of intravascular haemolysis and consumptive coagulopathy is often present.

Primary treatment consists of correction of underlying cause.

Table 4.15: Common causes of microangiopathic haemolytic anaemia

1. Thrombotic thrombocytopaenic purpura
2. Haemolytic uraemic syndrome
3. Disseminated intravascular coagulation
4. Malignant hypertension
5. Eclampsia
6. Disseminated malignancy, e.g. mucin secreting adenocarcinomas
7. Severe infections
8. Generalised vasculitis due to immunologic diseases, e.g. systemic lupus erythematosus.

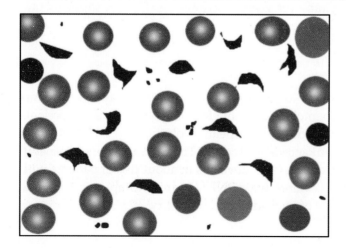

Figure 4.61: Blood smear in microangiopathic haemolytic anaemia showing many fragmented cells (schistocytes)

❑ MARCH HAEMOGLOBINURIA

Intravascular haemolysis may result following physical exercise such as marching or running on a hard surface for prolonged period (e.g. long-distance runners). Traumatic destruction of red cells occurs within vessels of the feet. The usual complaint is of passing reddish-brown urine following physical exertion. Haemoglobinuria is transient in most cases. The degree of haemolysis is usually mild and does not cause anaemia.

❑ CARDIAC HAEMOLYTIC ANAEMIA

Prosthetic cardiac valves may be associated with chronic intravascular haemolysis. This may be related to turbulent blood flow resulting from leaking valve and presence of artificial surface in bloodstream. Degree of anaemia depends upon severity of mechanical damage to red cells.

HAEMOLYTIC ANAEMIA DUE TO DIRECT ACTION OF PHYSICAL, CHEMICAL, OR INFECTIOUS AGENTS

❑ PHYSICAL AGENTS

Acute intravascular haemolysis follows extensive burns and its degree depends on body surface area involved. Haemolysis usually occurs within 1 to 2 days of burn injury and is due to direct action of heat on red cells.

❑ CHEMICAL AGENTS

Haemolysis can occur due to direct toxic action of some chemicals such as lead (discussed earlier under "Sideroblastic anaemia"), arsenic chloride (workers in galvanising or soldering industries), distilled water (introduction of large quantity of distilled water in circulation may follow intravenous injection or irrigation during surgery), and some insect venoms.

❑ INFECTIOUS AGENTS

Malaria

Malaria is caused by four species of Plasmodia: *P. vivax, P. falciparum, P. malariae,* and *P. ovale*. Infected female Anopheles mosquitoes transmit the disease. Recurrent high-grade fever with chills and rigors, and splenomegaly are the characteristic features. Icterus may be present. In *P. vivax* infection fever occurs on alternate days, while in *P. falciparum* infection it occurs daily.

In malaria, anaemia is usually mild and is caused mainly by excessive destruction of parasitised red cells by spleen. Other factors in the pathogenesis of anaemia are suppression of erythropoiesis by inflammatory cytokines, decreased production of erythropoietin, and shunting of iron from erythroblasts to macrophage stores.

Acute intravascular haemolysis (blackwater fever) occurs with *P. falciparum* infection and is characterised by fever, prostration, and marked haemoglobinuria. It may lead to acute renal failure. Pathogenesis is not known. It usually occurs in those patients who have had chronic malaria and were treated with quinine irregularly.

Acute intravascular haemolysis in *P. falciparum* malaria should be distinguished from drug-induced acute haemolytic episode in G6PD deficiency.

Diagnosis is based on demonstration of the parasite in blood film. Recently, immunochromatographic strip tests have been introduced that have high sensitivity and specificity.

Clostridium welchii

Clostridium welchii sepsis usually follows septic abortion and frequently causes marked intravascular haemolytic anaemia. *Clostridium welchii* liberates a lecithinase that acts on red cell membranes to form lysolecithins; lysolecithins have strong haemolytic activity. Prognosis is usually serious.

HYPERSPLENISM

❑ NORMAL STRUCTURE AND FUNCTION OF SPLEEN

The spleen is organised into two areas—white pulp and red pulp. The white pulp consists of malpighian or splenic follicles that are collections of lymphocytes around centrally located arterioles. Periarteriolar lymphocytes are mainly T lymphocytes. Adjacent to this is the area of B lymphocytes which exhibits prominent germinal centres upon antigenic stimulation. Red pulp is composed of anastomosing cords and vascular sinuses. The splenic cords are made of a meshwork of macrophages. The vascular sinuses are lined by a discontinuous layer of endothelial cells, i.e. small pores or slits occur between endothelial cells which permit blood cells to traverse between sinusoids and cords.

Most of the blood supply from the splenic artery passes from the smaller branches and arterioles into the capillaries and then into the splenic veins (closed circulation). A small proportion of the capillary blood supply passes slowly into the splenic cords; the blood from the cords then enters the sinuses through narrow slits between endothelial cells and then passes into the veins (open circulation).

Spleen plays a principle role in removal of undesirable elements from blood. As the blood passes slowly through the splenic cords, macrophages recognise and phagocytose micro-organisms, defective or damaged red cells occurring in various haemolytic anaemias, senescent red cells and IgG-coated blood cells. Splenic macrophages also excise inclusions such as Howell-Jolly bodies or Heinz bodies from red cells and the remainder of the red cell is returned to the circulation.

Spleen plays a role in both B-cell mediated (humoral) and T-cell mediated (cell-mediated) immune responses.

Spleen also functions as a haematopoietic organ during foetal life. Postnatally, however, bone marrow is the sole site of blood cell production. In some disorders such as thalassaemia major and myelofibrosis, extramedullary haematopoiesis may become re-established in the spleen.

❑ CAUSES OF SPLENOMEGALY

See Table 4.16.

❑ DIAGNOSTIC CRITERIA

The clinical syndrome of hypersplenism occurs in only some of the cases of splenomegaly. The diagnostic criteria for hypersplenism are:
- Enlargement of spleen
- Peripheral blood cytopaenia (anaemia, leucopaenia, thrombocytopaenia), either isolated or in combination
- Normal or hypercellular bone marrow with normal maturation
- Normalisation of blood cell count after splenectomy.

Cytopaenia in hypersplenism results from sequestration of blood cells in enlarged spleen. Normally about one-third of total platelets in the body are pooled in the spleen; enlarged spleen can sequester large number of platelets to induce thrombocytopaenia. A massively enlarged spleen can also trap a considerable proportion of red cells and granulocytes to cause anaemia and neutropaenia, respectively.

Table 4.16: Common causes of splenomegaly

Infectious diseases
- Viral: Infectious mononucleosis
- Bacterial: Typhoid fever, miliary tuberculosis, subacute bacterial endocarditis
- Protozoal: Malaria*, kala-azar*

Inflammatory diseases
- Felty's syndrome
- Systemic lupus erythematosus

Haematological disorders
- Disorders of red cells: Hereditary spherocytosis, thalassaemia major*
- Disorders of white cells: Chronic myeloid leukaemia*, acute leukaemias, chronic lymphocytic leukaemia, hairy cell leukaemia*, myelofibrosis*, lymphomas

Cirrhosis of liver
Storage disorders
- Gaucher's disease*
- Niemann-Pick disease
* Disorders marked with asterisk can cause massive splenomegaly.

❏ BIBLIOGRAPHY

1. Agarwal R, Deorari AK. Unconjugated hyperbilirubinaemia in newborns: Current perspective. Indian Pediatrics. 2002;39: 30-42.
2. Beris P, Darbellay R, Exterman P. Prevention of β thalassaemia major and Hb Bart's hydrops fetalis syndrome. Semin Hematol. 1995;32: 244-61.
3. Beutler E, Blume KG, Kaplan JC, et al. International Committee for Standardization in Haematology. Recommended screening test for glucose-6-phosphate dehydrogenase (G6PD) deficiency. Br J Haematol. 1979;43: 465-67.
4. Beutler E. G6PD deficiency. Blood. 1994;84: 3613-36.
5. Bolton-Maggs PHB. Hereditary spherocytosis: new guidelines. Arch Dis Child. 2004;89: 809-12.
6. Brewer GJ, Tarlov AR, Alving AS. The methemoglobin reduction test for primaquine type sensitivity of erythrocytes. A simplified procedure for detecting a specific hypersusceptibility to drug hemolysis. JAMA. 1962;180: 386-88.
7. Brodsky RA. How I treat paroxysmal nocturnal hemoglobinuria. Blood. 2009; 113: 6522-27.
8. Bunn HF. Pathogenesis and treatment of sickle-cell disease. N Engl J Med. 1997;337: 762-69.
9. Cao A, et al. Prenatal diagnosis of inherited haemoglobinopathies. Indian J Pediatr. 1989;56: 707-17.
10. Cao A, Galanello R, Rosatelli MC, et al. Clinical experience of management of thalassaemia: The Sardinian experience. Semin Hematol. 1996;33:66-75.
11. Carrell RW, Lehman H. The hemoglobinopathies. In Dawson AM, Compston ND, Besser GM (Eds): Recent advances in medicine. No. 19. Edinburgh. Churchill Livingstone. 1984.
12. Chang JC, Kan YW. A sensitive new prenatal test for sickle-cell anaemia. N Engl J Med. 1982;307:30.
13. Chehab FF, Kan YW. Detection of sickle-cell anaemia mutation by colour DNA amplification. Lancet. 1990;335: 15-17.
14. Clarke GM, Higgins TN. Laboratory investigation of hemoglobinopathies and thalassaemias: Review and update. Clin Chem. 2000;46: 1284-1290.
15. Claster S, Vichinsky EP. Managing sickle-cell disease. BMJ. 2003;327: 1151-55.
16. Colah RB. Prenatal diagnosis. Ind J Haematol and Blood Transf. 1992;10: 55-62.
17. Dacie J. Historical review. The immune haemolytic anaemias. A century of exciting progress in understanding. Br J Haematol. 2001;114:770-85.
18. Dhaliwal G, Cornett PA, Tierney LM, Jr. Hemolytic anemia. Am Fam Physician. 2004;69:2599-2606.
19. Eaton WA, Hofrichter J. Hemoglobin S gelation and sickle-cell disease. Blood. 1987;70: 1245-66.
20. Embury S. The clinical pathophysiology of sickle-cell disease. Ann Rev Med. 1986;37: 361-76.
21. Engelfriet CP, Overbeeke MAM, vondem Borne AEG. Autoimmune hemolytic anemia. Semin Hematol. 1992;29:3 12.
22. Fairbanks VF, Lampe LT. A tetrazolium-linked cytochemical method for estimation of glucose-6-phosphate dehydrogenase activity in individual erythrocytes: Application in the study of heterozygous for glucose-6-phosphate dehydrogenase deficiency. Blood. 1968;31: 589-603.
23. Festa RS. Current concepts in the management of thalassaemia. Indian J Pediatr. 1987;4: 379-89.
24. Fixler J, Styles L: sickle-cell disease. Pediatr Clin North Am. 2002;49: 1193-1210.
25. Fosburg MT, Nathan DG. Treatment of Cooley's anemia. Blood. 1990;76: 435-44.
26. Gangakhedkar RR. Primary prevention. Ind J Haematol and Blood Transf. 1992;10: 50-55.

27. Garewal G. Alpha thalassaemia in India: Diagnosis and interaction with beta thalassaemia. In Madan N (Moderator): APCON 2000 Preconference CME-Thalassaemia. Safdarjang Hospital, New Delhi.

28. Garraty G, Petz LD. Drug-induced immune hemolytic anemia. Am J Med. 1975;58:398-407.

29. Gehrs BC, Friedberg RC. Autoimmune hemolytic anemia. Am J Hematol. 2002; 69:258-71.

30. Globin Gene Disorder Working Party of the BCSH General Haematology Task Force: Guidelines for the fetal diagniosis of globin gene disorders. J Clin Pathol. 1994;47:199-204.

31. Higgs DR, Vickers MA, Wilkie AOM, et al. A review of the molecular genetics of human α-globin gene cluster. Blood. 1989;73:1081-1104.

32. International Committee for Standardization in Hematology: Recommendations of a system for identifying abnormal hemoglobins. Blood. 1978;52:1065-67.

33. Kan YW, Dozy M. Antenatal diagnosis of sickle-cell anaemia by DNA analysis of amniotic fluid cells. Lancet. 1979;2:910-12.

34. Kaufman RE. Analysis of abnormal hemoglobins. In Koepke JE (Ed): Practical Laboratory Hematology. New York. Churchil Livingstone. 1991.

35. Kazazian HH, Boehm Corinne D. Molecular basis and prenatal diagnosis of β thalassaemia. Blood. 1988;72:1107-16.

36. Kazazian HH, Jr. The thalassaemia syndromes: Molecular basis and prenatal diagnosis in 1990. Semin Hematol. 1990;27:209-28.

37. Kramer MS, et al. Accuracy of cord blood screening for sickle hemoglobinopathies. Three-to-five year follow-up. JAMA. 1979;241:481-86.

38. Krauss JS. Laboratory diagnosis of paroxysmal nocturnal hemoglobinuria. Ann Clin Lab Science. 2003;33:401-6.

39. Kwiatkowski JL. Oral iron chelators. Hematol Oncol Clin N Am. 2010;24:229-48.

40. Lechner K, Jager U. How I treat autoimmune hemolytic anemia in adults. Blood. 2010;116:1831-38.

41. Lee AI, Kaufman RM. Transfusion medicine and the pregnant patient. Hematol Oncol Clin N Am. 2011;25:393-413.

42. Lo L, Singer ST. Thalassaemia: Current approach to an old disease. Pediatr Clin North Am. 2002;49:1165-91.

43. Luzzatto L. Malaria and the red cell. In Hoffbrand AV (Ed): Recent Advances in Haematology. No. 4. Edinburgh. Churchill Livingstone. 1985.

44. Luzzatto L. Pathophysiology of paroxysmal haemoglobinuria. Fifth Congress of the European Haematology Association. Educational Book. Birminghham, UK. 2000.

45. Maheshwari M, Arora S, Kabra M, Menon PSN. Carrier screening and prenatal diagnosis of beta thalassaemia. Indian Pediatrics. 1999;36:1119-25.

46. Mehta BC. Geographical variation in blood disease: India. In Weatherall DJ, Ledingham JGG, Warrell DA (Eds.): Oxford Textbook of Medicine. 2nd ed. Oxford. Oxford University Press. 1987.

47. Mehta BC. Thalassaemia management. Ind J Haematol and Blood Transf. 1992;10:43-50.

48. Mohanty D, Mukherjee MB, Colah RB. Glucose-6-phosphate dehydrogenase deficiency in India. Indian J Pediatr. 2004;71:525-9.

49. Nagel RL, Roth EF Jr. Malaria and red cell genetic defects. Blood. 1989;74:1213-21.

50. Newland AC, Evans TGJR. ABC of clinical haematology: Haematological disorders at the extremes of life. BMJ. 1997;314:1262.

51. Nydegger UE, Kazatchkine MD, Miescher PA. Immunopatholic and clinical features of hemolytic anemia due to cold agglutinins. Semin Hematol. 1991;28:66-67.

52. Old JM, Varawalla NY, Weatherall DJ. Rapid detection and prenatal diagnosis of β thalassaemia: Studies in Indian and Cypriot populations in the UK. Lancet. 1990;336:834-37.

53. Olivieri NF. The β thalassaemias. N Engl J Med. 1999;341:99-109.

54. Orskin SH. Prenatal diagnosis of hemoglobin disorders by DNA analysis. Blood. 1984;63: 249-59.

55. Palek J, Jarolim P. Clinical expression and laboratory detection of red cell membrane protein mutation. Semin Hematol. 1993; 30: 249-283.

56. Palek J, Lambert S. Genetics of the red cell membrane skeleton. Semin Hematol. 1990;27: 290-332.

57. Palek J, Lux S. Red cell membrane skeletal defects in hereditary and acquired hemolytic anemias. Semin Hematol. 1983;20: 189-224.

58. Parker C, Omine M, Richards S, et al. Diagnosis and management of paroxysmal nocturnal hemoglobinuria. Blood. 2005; 106: 3699-703.

59. Parker CJ. Bone marrow failure syndromes: Paroxysmal nocturnal hemoglobinuria. Hematol Oncol Clin N Am. 2009; 23: 333-46.

60. Pearson HA, et al. Routine screening of umbilical cord blood for sickle-cell diseases. JAMA. 1974;227: 420-22.

61. Piomelli S. The management of patients with Cooley's anemia: Transfusions and splenectomy. Semin Hematol. 1995;32: 262-68.

62. Rachmilewitz EA, Giardina PJ. How I treat thalassemia. Blood. 2011; 118: 3479-88.

63. Richards SJ, Barnett D. The role of flow cytometry in the diagnosis of paroxysmal nocturnal hemoglobinuria in the clinical laboratory. Clin Lab Med .2007; 27: 577-90.

64. Rosse WF. The control of complement activation by the blood cells in paroxysmal nocturnal hemoglobinuria. Blood. 1986:67: 268-69.

65. Rosse WF. Variations in the complement sensitive cells in paroxysmal nocturnal haemoglobinuria. Br J Haematol. 1973;24: 327-42.

66. Rotoli B, Luzzatto L. Paroxysmal nocturnal hemoglobinuria. Semin Hematol. 1989;26: 201-07.

67. Ryan K, Bain BJ, Worthington D, et al On behalf of the British Committee for Standards in Haematology: Significant haemoglobinopathies: guidelines for screening and diagnosis. Br J Haematol. 2010;149: 35-49.

68. Schmidt RM. Laboratory diagnosis of hemoglobinopathies. JAMA. 1973;224: 1276-80.

69. Schwartz RS. Black mornings, yellow sunsets - A day with paroxysmal nocturnal hemoglobinuria. N Engl J Med. 2004;350: 537-38.

70. Serjeant GR. sickle-cell disease. In Hoffbrand AV (Ed): Recent Advances in Haematology. No. 4. Edinburgh. Churchill Livingstone. 1985.

71. Serjeant GR: sickle-cell disease. Lancet. 1997;350: 725-30.

72. Shah D, Choudhury P, Dubey AP. Current trends in the management of beta thalassaemia. Indian Pediatrics. 1999;36:1229-42.

73. Sokol RJ, Booker DJ, Stamps R. Investigations of patients with autoimmune haemolytic anemia and provision of blood for transfusion. J Clin Pathol. 1995;48:602-10

74. Steensma DP, Hoyer JD, Fairbanks VF. Hereditary red blood cell disorders in middle eastern patients. Mayo Clin Proc. 2001;76: 285-93.

75. Steinberg MH. Management of sickle-cell disease. N Engl J Med. 1999;340: 1021-30.

76. Steingart R. Management of patients with sickle-cell disease. Med Clin North Am. 1992;76: 669-82.

77. The Thalassaemia Working Party of the BCSH General Haematology Task Force: Guidelines for investigation of the α and β thalassaemia traits. J Clin Pathol. 1994;47: 289-95.

78. Thein SL. β thalassaemia. In Green AR (Ed): Fifth congress of the European Haematology Association. Educational Book, Birmingham. 2000;132-37.

79. Valentine WN (Moderator). Hemolytic anemia and erythrocyte enzymopathies. Ann Intern Med. 1987;103: 245-57.

80. Verma IC, Choudhry VP, Jain PK. Prevention of thalassaemia: A necessity in India. Indian J Pediatr. 1992;59: 649-54.

81. Ware RE. How I use hydroxyurea to treat young patients with sickle-cell anemia. Blood. 2010; 115: 5300-11.

82. Wasi P. Population screening. In Weatherall DJ (Ed): Methods in Hematology. The thalassaemias. Edinburgh. Churchill Livingstone. 1983.

83. Weatherall DJ, Provan B. Inherited anaemias. Lancet. 2000;355: 1169-75.

84. Weatherall DJ, Wainscoat JS. The molecular pathology of thalassaemia. In Hoffbrand AV (Ed): Recent advances in hematology. No. 4. Edinburgh. Churchill Livingstone. 1985.

85. Weatherall DJ. Hematologic methods. In Weatherall DJ (Ed): Methods in Hematology. The thalassaemias. Edinburgh. Churchill Livingstone. 1983.

86. Weatherall DJ. The diagnostic features of different forms of thalassaemia. In Weatherall DJ (Ed): Methods in Hematology. The thalassaemias. Edinburgh. Churchill Livingstone. 1983.

87. Weatherall DJ: The challenge of haemoglobinopathies in resource-poor countries. Br J Haematol. 2011; 154: 736-44.

88. Working Party of the General Haematology Task Force of the British Committee for Standards in Haematology: The laboratory diagnosis of haemoglobinopathies. Br J Haematol. 1998;101: 783-92.

CHAPTER

5

Acute Leukaemias

❑ DIAGNOSIS AND CLASSIFICATION

Acute leukaemias are malignant clonal disorders originating in haematopoietic stem cells characterised by the proliferation of poorly-differentiated blast (immature) cells in the bone marrow and a rapidly progressive fatal course if untreated (survival < 6 months without treatment).

Acute leukaemias primarily originate in the bone marrow. Proliferating leukaemic blasts replace normal bone marrow cells and subsequently enter into the peripheral blood. They are clonal disorders that arise from malignant transformation of a single haematopoietic progenitor cell followed by proliferation and accumulation of abnormal clone. There is an arrest in the differentiation of immature cells into functionally mature cells (Fig. 5.1).

Acute leukaemias comprise about 50% of all cases of leukaemias. Approximate frequencies of different types of leukaemias in India are shown in Box 5.1.

Box 5.1 Leukaemias in India
• Chronic myeloid leukaemia: 40%
• Acute lymphoblastic leukaemia: 35%
• Acute myeloid leukaemia: 15%
• Chronic lymphocytic leukaemia: 10%

Predisposing Factors

Various factors associated with increased risk of acute leukaemias are as follows:

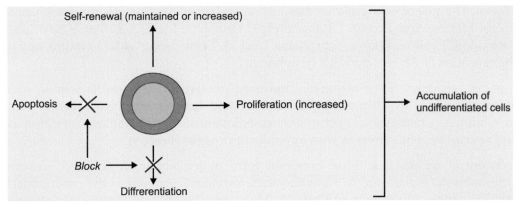

Figure 5.1: In acute leukaemia, genetic lesions in haematopoietic stem cell or its committed progenitor lead to dysregulation of processes that control proliferation, apoptosis, self-renewal, and differentiation. These leukaemic cells have proliferative and survival advantage with a block in differentiation and in apoptosis

Hereditary Factors

Some congenital disorders are associated with increased predisposition to acute leukaemia, e.g. Down's syndrome (20 times increased incidence), Fanconi's anaemia, Bloom's syndrome, ataxia telangiectasia, Klinefelter's syndrome, Diamond-Blackfan syndrome, Wiskott-Aldrich syndrome and Kostmann's syndrome.

Acquired Factors

Ionising radiation:
1. Nuclear fall-out: Following nuclear explosions in Hiroshima and Nagasaki, increased incidence of leukaemias (particularly acute and chronic myeloid leukaemias, and less commonly acute lymphoblastic leukaemia) was observed in survivors.
2. Therapeutic irradiation: Patients treated with irradiation for treatment of disorders such as ankylosing spondylitis, Hodgkin's lymphoma, and polycythaemia vera have an increased risk of development of acute myeloid leukaemia. Acute myeloid leukaemia (AML) is usually preceded by myelodysplastic syndrome in these patients.
3. Diagnostic X-rays: Intra-uterine foetal exposure to low-dose radiation (for X-ray pelvimetry) has been found to increase the risk of subsequent occurrence of acute leukaemia in childhood.

Chemical agents: Occupational exposure to benzene is associated with increased risk of acute myeloid leukaemia and aplastic anaemia.

Alkylating agents used for cytotoxic chemotherapy of neoplasms may induce acute myeloid leukaemia. Such secondary leukaemias develop about 5 to 6 years after chemotherapy, are usually preceded by myelodysplastic syndrome, have high incidence of clonal cytogenetic abnormalities, and are resistant to treatment.

Treatment with drugs that inhibit topoisomerase II (such as epipodophyllotoxins or etoposide) are implicated in causation of AML.

Viruses: The role of oncogenic viruses in human leukaemogenesis is not established, except for one virus human T lymphotropic virus type I (HTLV-I) that is associated with adult T cell leukaemia/lymphoma (ATLL). Epstein-Barr virus is implicated in the causation of African Burkitt's lymphoma.

Acquired conditions: Some acquired conditions predispose to acute leukaemia such as myeloproliferative disorders (chronic myeloid leukaemia, polycythaemia vera, myelofibrosis), paroxysmal nocturnal haemoglobinuria, myelodysplastic syndromes, and aplastic anaemia (treated with immunosuppressive therapy).

Influence of age and sex: Most common form of leukaemia in children is acute lymphoblastic leukaemia (ALL), while acute myeloid leukaemia is the predominant form in adults, adolescents and infants. Males are slightly more frequently affected than females in ALL, while AML has equal sex incidence.

Mechanisms of Oncogenesis in Acute Leukaemias

Leukaemias are biologically a diverse group of disorders. This is evident from differences in their morphology, antigen expression, chromosomal and molecular abnormalities, response to treatment, and prognosis.

Like all other malignant tumours, leukaemia is a clonal disorder (i.e. it originates from a single haematopoietic stem cell or its committed progenitor) and evolves through more than one mutation. Interactions between exogenous factors (listed under 'Predisposing factors'), endogenous factors, and genetic susceptibility are involved in its pathogenesis.

Current evidence indicates that the initiating event in acute leukaemias is an acquired genetic abnormality in a haematopoietic progenitor cell. Chromosomal translocations occurring in specific types of leukaemias play a major role in leukaemogenesis. These genetic abnormalities (shown in Table 5.1) are associated with a unique disease phenotype, responsiveness to therapy, and prognosis.

Table 5.1: Genetic abnormalities in acute leukaemias

Type of leukaemia	Chromosomal abnormality	Genetic alteration	Mechanism of oncogenesis	Prognosis
Acute myeloid leukaemia (AML)				
1. AML M2	t(8;21)(q22;q22)	*AML1/ETO*	Chimeric transcription factor	Favourable
2. AML M3	t(15;17)(q22;q12)	*PML/RARα*	Chimeric transcription factor	Favourable
3. AML M4	inv(16)(p13q22) or t(16;16)(p13;q22)	*CBFβ/MYH11*	Chimeric transcription factor	Favourable
Acute lymphoblastic leukaemia (ALL)				
1. ALL L3	t(8;14)(q24;q32)	*MYC/IgH*	Activation of proto-oncogene	No effect
2. ALL L1, L2	t(1;19)(q23;p13.3)	*PBX/E2A*	Chimeric transcription factor	Unfavourable
	t(12;21)(p13;q22)	*TEL/AML1*	Chimeric transcription factor	Favourable
	t(9;22)(q34;q11)	*BCR/ABL*	Increased tyrosine kinase activity	Unfavourable

Different Mechanisms of Leukaemogenesis

1. **Activation of a proto-oncogene to an oncogene when it is translocated to a transcriptionally active site:** Translocation may cause a proto-oncogene to be brought closer to a transcriptionally active gene; this can cause activation of proto-oncogene and neoplastic transformation. An example is translocation between chromosomes 8 and 14 that occurs in pre B-cell acute lymphoblastic leukaemias. Normally the proto-oncogene *C-MYC* is located at chromosome 8q24, and immunoglobulin heavy chain gene at 14q32. The translocation (8;14)(q24;q32) places *C-MYC* close to transcriptionally active immunoglobulin locus; this causes activation and increased transcription of *C-MYC* and abnormal cellular proliferation.

2. **Formation of a chimeric transcription factor:** This is the major mechanism in pathogenesis of AML. The classical example is translocation between chromosomes 15 and 17 in acute promyelocytic leukaemia that leads to fusion of gene for retinoic acid receptor α *(RARα)* on chromosome 15 with the promyelocytic leukaemia *(PML)* gene on chromosome 17. Normally, RARα can interact with both transcriptional co-activators and repressors on target gene. However, PML/RARα fusion protein favours recruitment of transcriptional repressors. This causes block in differentiation at promyelocyte stage. Administration of all-trans-retinoic acid normalises RARα signalling by releasing the transcription repressors and allowing normal maturation and differentiation of promyelocytes.

3. **Formation of a fusion protein with enhanced tyrosine kinase activity:** The translocation between chromosomes 9 and 22 in precursor B-ALL causes formation of a fusion protein BCR/ABL that has enhanced tyrosine kinase activity.

   These genetic abnormalities are insufficient by themselves to induce leukaemia. Additional genetic alterations are required to cause leukaemic transformation. Examples of these second mutations are as follows:

1. **Activation of FLT3 receptor:** Constitutive activation of FLT3, a receptor tyrosine kinase, occurs after certain acquired mutations in both ALL and AML. Constant activation of this receptor turns on signal transduction pathways and contributes to neoplastic transformation.

2. **Inactivation of tumour suppressor gene pathway** controlled by *RB1*or *p53* occurs in a proportion of cases of ALL.

Foetal origin of ALL: Evidence indicates that some cases of ALL may arise *in utero*. Leukaemia-specific fusion gene sequences (*MLL/AF4, TEL/AML1*) have been identified in archived blood spots from neonates who subsequently developed ALL after a variable latent period and their leukaemic cells contained the identical fusion gene sequences. Probably, exposure of the foetus to a mutagen induces a pre-malignant clone that requires subsequent additional genetic alterations ('hits') afterbirth to develop into full-blown ALL. Transplacental exposure to various compounds is implicated including some antimosquito agents, dipyrone (NSAID), and topoisomerase II inhibitors. It is thought that all cases of leukaemias presenting during infancy originate in foetal life.

Classification of Acute Leukaemias

There are two major forms of acute leukaemias—acute lymphoblastic leukaemia (ALL) and acute myeloid leukaemia (AML). The distinction between ALL and AML is important because of the differences in the treatment of these two types of leukaemias. In 1976, haematologists from France, America, and Britain proposed a classification of acute leukaemias that was designated as French-American-British (FAB) Classification. In subsequent years, FAB classification was modified and newer entities were added (like M0 and M7). This classification is based on well-defined morphological criteria, cytochemical reactions, and in some cases, immunophenotyping. In this classification, AML is subclassified into 8 categories (designated from M0 to M7) based on the lineage of leukaemic cells (granulocytic, monocytic, erythroid, and megakaryocytic) and their level of differentiation. ALL is classified into 3 groups (designated as L1, L2, and L3) based on morphology of lymphoblasts. FAB classification is easy to use with well-defined cytological criteria, reproducible, and majority of acute leukaemias can be placed in one of the categories (Table 5.2).

In recent years, several distinct categories of acute leukaemias have been identified by genetic (cytogenetic and molecular genetic) studies that correlate closely with biologic behaviour, treatment responsiveness, and prognosis. These features do not always correlate with FAB categories. Cytogenetic and molecular genetic studies have become vitally important in defining optimum treatment protocols.

In 2001 (revised in 2008), World Health Organization (WHO) proposed a classification of haematological malignancies in which distinct diseases have been defined according to a combination of clinical syndromes, morphology, immunophenotype, and genetic features. This classification has clinical, therapeutic, and prognostic relevance (Tables 5.3 and 5.4).

Table 5.2: The French-American-British (FAB) Co-operative Group classification of acute leukaemias

Acute lymphoblastic leukaemias (ALL)

- ALL-L1 type
- ALL- L2 type
- ALL- L3 type

Acute myeloid leukaemia (AML)

- Acute myeloblastic leukaemia minimally differentiated (M0)
- Acute myeloblastic leukaemia without maturation (M1)
- Acute myeloblastic leukaemia with maturation (M2)
- Hypergranular promyelocytic leukaemia (M3)
  - Hypo-or micro-granular promyelocytic leukaemia (M3 variant)
- Acute myelomonocytic leukaemia (M4)
  - Acute myelomonocytic leukaemia with bone marrow eosinophilia (M4 Eo)
- Acute monocytic leukaemia (M5)
  - Undifferentiated (monoblastic) (M5a)
  - Well-differentiated (promonocytic-monocytic) (M5b)
- Acute erythroleukaemia (M6)
- Acute megakaryocytic leukaemia (M7)

Table 5.3: World Health Organization (WHO) classification of acute myeloid leukaemia (AML) and related precursor neoplasms, 2008

Acute myeloid leukaemia with recurrent genetic abnormalities

- AML with t(8;21)(q22;q22); *RUNX1-RUNX1T1*
- AML with inv(16)(p13.1q22) or t(16;16)(p13.1q22); *CBFB-MYH11*
- Acute promyelocytic leukaemia with t(15;17)(q22;q12) *PML-RARA*
- AML with t(9;11)(p22;q23); *MLLT3-MLL*
- AML with t(6;9)(p23;q34); *DEK-NUP214*
- AML with inv(3)(q21;q26.2) or t(3;3)(q21;q26.2); *RPN1-EVI1*
- AML (megakaryoblastic) with t(1;22)(p13;q13); *RBM15-MKL1*
- AML with mutated *NPM1*
- AML with mutated *CEBPA*

Acute myeloid leukaemia with myelodysplasia-related changes

Therapy-related myeloid neoplasms

Acute myeloid leukaemia, not otherwise specified

- AML with minimal differentiation
- AML without maturation
- AML with maturation
- Acute myelomonocytic leukaemia
- Acute monoblastic and monocytic leukaemia
- Acute erythroid leukaemia
- Acute megakaryoblastic leukaemia
- Acute basophilic leukaemia
- Acute panmyelosis with myelofibrosis

Myeloid sarcoma

Myeloid proliferations related to Down syndrome

Blastic plasmacytoid dendritic cell neoplasm

Salient Features of WHO Classification

Acute myeloid leukaemia:
- Blast count for diagnosis of AML is ≥20% in blood smear or bone marrow (In previous FAB classification, this cut off was ≥30%). It has been demonstrated that survival pattern of patients with 20 to 30% blasts is similar to those with ≥30% blasts.
- AML is divided into following major categories.
  - AML with recurrent genetic abnormalities: Each of these categories has distinctive morphologic and clinical features, and high correlation with response to therapy and prognosis. There is some correlation with FAB categories.
  - AML with myelodysplasia-related changes: This type is seen in older age and has poor response to treatment and unfavourable prognosis.

Table 5.4: World Health Organization classification of precursor lymphoid neoplasms, 2008

B lymphoblastic leukemia/lymphoma

* **B lymphoblastic leukaemia/lymphoma, NOS**
* **B lymphoblastic leukaemia/lymphoma with recurrent genetic abnormalities**
    - B lymphoblastic leukaemia/lymphoma with (9;22)(q34;q11.2);*BCR-ABL1*
    - B lymphoblastic leukaemia/lymphoma with t(v11q23);*MLL* rearranged
    - B lymphoblastic leukaemia/lymphoma with t(12;21)(p13;q22) *TEL-AML1 (ETV6-RUNX1)*
    - B lymphoblastic leukaemia/lymphoma with hyperdiploidy
    - B lymphoblastic leukaemia/lymphoma with hypodiploidy
    - B lymphoblastic leukaemia/lymphoma with t(5;14)(q31;q32) *IL3-IGH*
    - B lymphoblastic leukaemia/lymphoma with t(1;19)(q23;p13.3);*TCF3-PBX1*

T lymphoblastic leukaemia/lymphoma

- AML therapy-related: AML following alkylating therapy has distinctive cytogenetic abnormalities and has worse prognosis as compared to *de novo* AML.
- AML not otherwise categorised: This category is similar to FAB classification, with some modifications.

Acute Lymphoblastic Leukaemia

Classification of ALL is presented in Table 5.4. According to WHO classification, lymphoblastic lymphoma and ALL are biologically the same disease with different clinical presentations. FAB categories L1, L2, and L3 do not correlate with immunophenotype, genetic abnormalities, and clinical behaviour. ALL L3 is equivalent to Burkitt lymphoma/leukaemia.

Clinical Features of Acute Leukaemias

Due to Bone Marrow Failure

Replacement of marrow and suppression of normal haemopoiesis by leukaemic blasts is responsible for bone marrow failure. The main clinical features are due to lack of red cells, white cells and platelets.
* Anaemia which manifests as pallor, dyspnoea, CCF
* Infections are due to neutropaenia
* Bleeding due to thrombocytopaenia or disseminated intravascular coagulation.

Due to Organ Infiltration

* Organomegaly (lymph nodes, spleen, liver, other)
* Bone pain and tenderness (common with ALL)
* CNS (meningeal) disease (common with ALL)
* Gum hypertrophy (common in monocytic leukaemia)

- Chloromas (Localised proliferation of myeloblasts outside marrow producing solid tumours): Common sites are soft tissues and bones of head and neck area. Chloroma may precede or occur concurrently with overt AML.

Other

- Hyperleucocytosis (very high TLC, i. e. > 1 lac/cmm can increase blood viscosity and cause sludging of blood flow with headache, neurologic and visual changes, and respiratory distress).
- Disseminated intravascular coagulation (Release of procoagulant substances from leukaemic cells may induce DIC. Common in AML M3).

Diagnosis of Acute Leukaemias

The first aim of laboratory investigations is to establish the diagnosis of acute leukaemia by peripheral blood and bone marrow examinations. This is followed by investigations to identify the type of acute leukaemia, i.e. ALL or AML and its subtype (Box 5.2). This is essential because of differences in their management. Laboratory studies in acute leukaemias are:
- Morphological examination of peripheral blood and bone marrow aspiration smears
- Cytochemistry
- Immunophenotyping
- Cytogenetic analysis
- Molecular genetic analysis.

Morphology

The laboratory diagnosis of acute leukaemias is based mainly on morphology and cytochemistry. Morphological examination is done on both peripheral blood, and bone marrow aspiration smears stained with one of the Romanowsky stains (e.g. Giemsa's, Leishman's, etc.). Bone marrow aspiration smears are necessary for confirmation of diagnosis and for morphological subclassification of acute leukaemias (Fig. 5.2). Morphology of different types of blasts (myeloblast, monoblast, megakaryoblast, and lymphoblast) and blast equivalents (promyelocytes and promonocytes) is shown in Figure 5.3.

Box 5.2   Diagnosis of acute leukaemias

1. Establish the presence of acute leukaemia and distinguish it from other neoplastic and reactive conditions. Acute leukaemia should be differentiated from infectious mononucleosis, myelodysplastic syndrome, non-Hodgkin's lymphoma infiltrating the bone marrow, haematogones, and transient myeloproliferative disorder in Down's syndrome.
2. Distinguish between AML and ALL.
3. Classification of AML or ALL into a specific subtype that has clinical (therapeutic and prognostic) relevance.

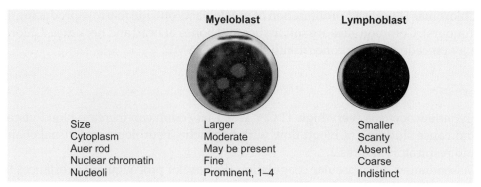

	Myeloblast	Lymphoblast
Size	Larger	Smaller
Cytoplasm	Moderate	Scanty
Auer rod	May be present	Absent
Nuclear chromatin	Fine	Coarse
Nucleoli	Prominent, 1–4	Indistinct

Figure 5.2: Morphological comparison of myeloblast and lymphoblast

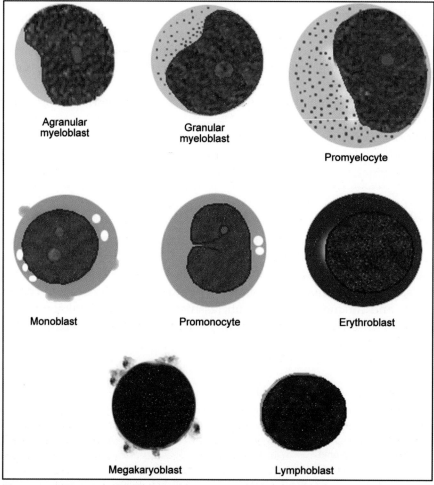

Figure 5.3: Morphology of different types of blasts and blast equivalents in acute leukaemias

In peripheral blood, total leucocyte count is elevated (in most cases), normal, or low. The characteristic feature is presence of blast cells. In subleukaemic leukaemia, total leucocyte count is normal or low but blasts are demonstrable in peripheral blood. In aleukaemic leukaemia, blasts are not demonstrable in peripheral smear but are present in the bone marrow; however, if buffy coat preparation is examined then some blasts will usually be seen in peripheral blood. (In buffy coat preparation, small amount of anticoagulated blood is centrifuged, smear is prepared from white cell layer, and examined).

Bone marrow aspiration smears reveal hypercellular marrow with almost complete replacement of marrow by blast cells. Normal haematopoietic cells are reduced. Morphological features of various leukaemias are considered later under respective chapters.

Role of morphology in diagnosis of AML is shown in Box 5.3.

Cytochemistry

In many cases it is difficult to differentiate between various types of blasts only on the basis of morphology on Romanowsky-stained smears. Various cytochemical procedures are employed to aid in this differentiation. When morphology and cytochemistry are combined together, 80 to 90% of acute leukaemias can be correctly categorised. Diagnostic accuracy increases to 95 to 99% with immunophenotyping.

By cytochemical techniques, certain enzymes, fat, glycogen, or other substances are identified in blast cells. The main aim of cytochemical studies in acute leukaemias is to distinguish ALL from AML. In AML, cytochemical stains allow delineation of granulocytic lineage (AML M1, M2, M3), mixed myeloid and monocytic leukaemia (AML M4), and erythroid leukaemia (AML M6). The cytochemical stains, which are employed in acute leukaemias (Table 5.5), are:

- **Myeloperoxidase**, Sudan black B, Chloroacetate esterase: Positive in granulocytic lineage (AML M0, M1, M2, M3).
- **Non-specific esterase**: Alpha naphthyl acetate esterase (ANAE), Alpha naphthyl butyrate esterase (ANBE), Naphthol AS acetate esterase (NASA), Naphthol AS-D acetate esterase (NASDA): Positive in monocyte lineage (AML M4, M5)
- **Periodic acid Schiff's (PAS) reaction**: Positive in B-ALL (block-like), and in erythroblasts in AML M6.
- **Acid phosphatase:** Positive (focal) in T-ALL.

Box 5.3	Role of morphology in AML

- Diagnosis of AML requires blast count ≥20%; [except t(8;21), inv(16), t(16;16) or t(15;17)]
- Identification of (i) myeloblasts especially of AML M2 (blast cells with abundant, large, pink granules and slightly basophilic cytoplasm), (ii) promyelocytes of AML M3 (folded, bilobed nuclei, abundant, small, azurophilic granules and numerous Auer rods), (iii) abnormal eosinophils (containing basophilic granules) in AML M4 Eo, (iv) promonocytes and monocytes in AML M4 and AML M5, and (v) multilineage dysplasia
- Provides a basis for ordering further studies, e.g. tests for disseminated intravascular coagulation in acute promyelocytic leukaemia.

Table 5.5: Cytochemical reactions in acute leukaemias

Type	MPO	NSE	PAS	AP
1. AML M0	- (+ on EM)	-	-	-
2. AML M1–M3	+	-	-	-
3. AML M4	+	+	-	-
4. AML M5	±	+	-	-
5. AML M6	±	-	+	-
6. AML M7	-	-	-	-
7. B-ALL	-	-	+ (blocks)	-
8. T-ALL	-	-	-	+ (focal)

MPO: Myeloperoxidase; NSE: Non-specific esterase; PAS: Periodic acid Schiff; AP: Acid phosphatase; EM: Electron microscopy.

Principles and Applications of Cytochemical Reactions

Myeloperoxidase (MPO): Myeloperoxidase is an enzyme located in the azurophil (primary) granules of myeloid cells. MPO positivity appears as coloured granules in the cytoplasm of cells mainly at the site of enzyme activity (Golgi zone). All the stages of neutrophil series show MPO positivity. In monocyte series azurophil granules are smaller and MPO activity stains less strongly and appears late during maturation. MPO is never seen in lymphoblasts. Therefore, positive MPO stain in leukaemic blasts differentiates between AML and ALL.

The main use of MPO is to distinguish AML from ALL. The blasts in AML show granular positivity while blasts in ALL are negative for MPO. MPO is positive in AML subtypes M1, M2, M3, and M4 (Figs 5.4 and 5.5), and permits diagnosis of these leukaemias. In AML M0, peroxidase activity is not visible on light microscopy, but can be demonstrated by electron microscopy. Megakaryoblasts are MPO-negative.

Sudan black B (SBB): Phospholipids in the membrane of neutrophil granules are stained by SBB. SBB positivity parallels that of MPO in neutrophil series.

Chloroacetate esterase (CAE): The reaction is present in all cells of neutrophil series (though less sensitive than MPO and SBB) and is negative in monocyte series. It is commonly used in combination with non-specific esterase (NSE) for diagnosis of leukaemia with both myeloid and monocyte components (AML M4). Both esterases (CAE for myeloid and NSE for monocytic components) can be demonstrated in the same blood film; this is called as combined or double esterase reaction.

Non-specific esterase (NSE) reaction (usually demonstrated by ANAE or ANBE): α-naphthyl acetate esterase is an enzyme that is present in large quantities in monocytic cells. It is present in small amounts in myeloid and lymphoid cells. The non-specific esterase reaction is intensely and diffusely positive in monocyte series and is sensitive to sodium fluoride. In T lymphocytes it is focally positive and is resistant to sodium fluoride.

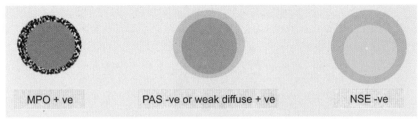

Figure 5.4: Cytochemical reactions in AML M1, M2, and M3

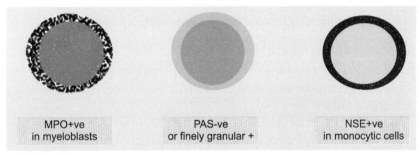

Figure 5.5: Cytochemical reactions in AML M4. There is both granulocytic (MPO+ve blasts) and monocytic (NSE+ve cells) differentiation

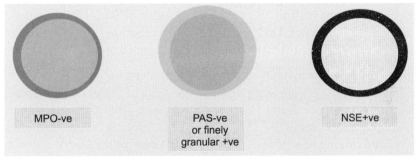

Figure 5.6: Cytochemical reactions in AML M5

In AML M4, ANAE allows identification of blasts with monocytic differentiation (Fig. 5.5). In AML M5, reaction is strongly and diffusely positive (Fig. 5.6), while in erythroblasts in M6 and in megakaryoblasts in M7 it is focally positive. The reaction is strongly and focally positive also in T-ALL.

In acute leukaemias, the principal role of NSE is to differentiate neutrophilic cells, i.e. myeloblasts and promyelocytes (negative reaction) from monocytic cells, i.e. monoblasts and promonocytes (positive reaction).

Periodic acid Schiff's reaction (PAS): Periodic acid is an oxidising agent that transforms glycols and related compounds to aldehydes. The aldehyde groups then along with Schiff's reagent form an insoluble red-or magenta-coloured compound. In haematopoietic cells, positive reaction is due to the abundance of glycogen in cytoplasm.

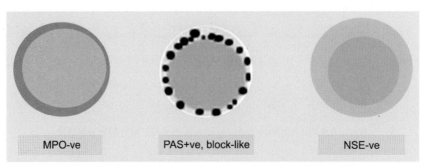

Figure 5.7: Cytochemical reactions in ALL (70% cases)

All stages in neutrophil series show a diffuse positive reaction. Monocytes show a fine, scattered, and faint staining positivity. A few small or coarse granules are present in the cytoplasm of lymphocytes. Red cell precursors do not show positive granules. Platelets are PAS-positive.

In L1 and L2 subtypes of ALL (B cell-ALL), PAS-positive 'blocks' are present in lymphoblasts on a clear cytoplasmic background (Fig. 5.7). In T cell-ALL and in L3 subtype of ALL, PAS reaction is negative. PAS positivity is also seen in monoblasts (in AML M5) and in erythroblasts (in AML-M6); however, in these cells small blocks of positive material are present against a diffusely positive cytoplasmic background.

When MPO, SBB, and NSE are negative and PAS shows block-like positivity in blasts, there is a strong possibility of ALL. However such a reaction can occur in certain other cell types and therefore definitive diagnosis of ALL is made by immunophenotyping.

Acid phosphatase (AP): Strong focal acid phosphatase activity is observed in T cell ALL. However, focal activity is also seen in AML M6 and M7. Monoblasts show a strong and diffuse reaction. Since aside from T cells, certain other cells also show strongly positive reaction, diagnosis of T-ALL requires confirmation by immunophenotyping. If tartrate is used during reaction, then it inhibits AP in most cells; however, abnormal cells in hairy cell leukaemia are resistant to tartrate inhibition. The tartrate-resistant acid phosphatase (TRAP) activity is a characteristic feature of hairy cell leukaemia.

Immunological Cell Marker Analysis (Immunophenotyping)

In immunophenotyping, various antigens on the surface (or in the cytoplasm or nucleus) of the leukaemic cells are identified using antigen-specific antibodies. Cell surface antigens are named according to the internationally accepted CD (cluster of differentiation) system in which each cell surface antigen is ascribed a unique number (e.g. CD1, CD2, etc.). This analysis gives information about lineage and stage of development of the particular cell. Methods employed for immunophenotyping are immunofluorescence or immunoenzyme method (such as peroxidase-antiperoxidase) and flow cytometric analysis. Since blood and marrow cells are in fluid suspension, flow cytometric analysis is the method of choice. Multiple monoclonal antibodies are commercially available for this technique.

Normal haematopoietic cells have a characteristic pattern of antigen expression at different stages of maturation. A panel consisting of a combination of different antibodies is commonly employed to determine the immunophenotypic profile of a sample. The antibodies are labelled with a fluorescent marker and the reactivity of the cell to various antibodies can be detected.

Applications of immunophenotyping in acute leukaemias are shown in Box 5.4 and in Tables 5.6 and 5.7.

In acute leukaemias, immunophenotyping is essential in those cases that cannot be diagnosed as ALL or AML on the basis of morphology and cytochemistry.

Acute myeloid leukaemia: In AML, immunophenotyping is invaluable for diagnosis of certain subtypes such as AML M0, M6, and M7. The designation M0 is used for those cases of AML which have negative cytochemistry (myeloperoxidase, Sudan black B) on light microscopy, but cell surface marker studies show myeloid differentiation antigens (CD 13 or CD 33); T or B lymphoid markers are absent.

Table 5.6: Monoclonal antibodies used for diagnosis of acute leukaemias by immunophenotyping

Lineage	Primary panel*	Secondary panel**
1. Myeloid	CD13, CD33, CD117, MPO (cyt)	CD14, CD64, lysozyme, glycophorin A, CD41, CD61
2. B-lymphoid	CD19, CD79a (cyt), CD22 (cyt), CD10	Cyt IgM, surface Ig (κ/λ)
3. T-lymphoid	CD3 (cyt), CD2, CD7	CD1a, membrane CD3, CD5, CD4, CD8
4. Non-lineage restricted (primitive stem cell)	HLA DR, TdT (Nuclear), CD34	

* Primary panel: To distinguish AML from ALL, and to further classify B-ALL and T-ALL.
** Secondary panel: (1) To diagnose AML of monocytic, erythroid, and megakaryocytic lines, and (2) further subtyping of B- and T-ALL.

Table 5.7: Cell antigens detected by monoclonal antibodies for characterisation of acute leukaemias
- **Myeloid:** CD13, CD 33, MPO, CD117, CD41, CD61, glycophorin A, CD14, CD15, CD36, lysozyme
- **B lymphoid:** CD19, CD20, CD22, CD79a, surface Ig, cytoplasmic Ig, CD38
- **T lymphoid:** CD2, CD3, CD5, CD7

Box 5.4   Applications of immunophenotyping in acute leukaemias

- Diagnosis and classification
  - Distinction between ALL and AML
  - Diagnosis of specific types of AML: AML M0, AML M6, and AML M7
  - Distinction between B-ALL and T-ALL and further immunological subtyping of B- and T-ALL
- Assessment of prognosis
- Detection of aberrant antigen expression that corresponds with certain specific subtypes and also helps in monitoring minimal residual disease
- Monitoring of minimal residual disease (detection of the unique leukaemia phenotype on a single cell amongst numerous cells allows early detection of residual disease following treatment and thus earlier institution of further treatment)
- To monitor effectiveness of monoclonal antibody therapy directed against antigens present on leukaemic cells (e.g. rituximab directed against CD20 antigen).

In AML M6, diagnosis is based on typical morphological features and demonstration of glycophorin A on surface.

Morphologically, megakaryoblasts (AML M7) resemble lymphoblasts. Diagnosis requires demonstration of CD41 (GpIIb/IIIa) or CD 61 (Gp IIIa) by immunophenotyping, or platelet peroxidase by electron microscopy.

Acute lymphoblastic leukaemia: Definitive identification of lymphoblasts is based on immunological cell marker studies.

Immunologically ALL is divided into B cell ALL and T cell ALL. Immunophenotyping is helpful in differentiating B cell ALL from T cell ALL and is invaluable for further subclassification of these leukaemias. Immunological classification of ALL has utmost therapeutic and prognostic relevance (see chapter on "Acute Lymphoblastic Leukaemia").
Bilineage and biphenotypic acute leukaemias: In bilineage acute leukaemia, two abnormal blast cell populations exist with phenotypes of two different lineages; e.g. co-existence of acute lymphoblastic and myeloblastic leukaemias.

In biphenotypic leukaemia, a single abnormal blast cell population exists which demonstrates surface markers of two different lineages (e.g. blast cell exhibiting both myeloid and lymphoid antigens). Bilineage or biphenotypic leukaemias are usually seen in blast crisis of chronic myelogenous leukaemia. In such cases treatment may have to be directed towards both lineages.

Small round cell malignancies: Immunophenotyping permits distinction of small round cell malignancies and leukaemic phase of non-Hodgkin's lymphoma from acute leukaemia.

Cytogenetic Studies (Karyotyping) and DNA Ploidy Studies

Applications of cytogenetic analysis in acute leukaemias are shown in Box 5.5.

Due to the consistent association of certain chromosomal abnormalities with particular types of leukaemias, specific subtypes of AML can be diagnosed with certainty by cytogenetic studies (e.g. t(15;17) is characteristic of AML M3). Certain cytogenetic abnormalities are associated with favourable or unfavourable prognosis (Tables 5.8 and 5.9). Clonal cytogenetic abnormalities are observed in about 80% cases of AML and ALL. Detection of a specific cytogenetic abnormality in all the abnormal cells establishes the clonal or neoplastic nature of the disease.

Cytogenetic analysis is also helpful in detection of remission and relapse.

DNA ploidy studies: In ploidy studies, number of chromosomes is determined, either by karyotyping or by measuring cellular DNA content. Cellular DNA content

---

Box 5.5   Cytogenetic analysis in acute leukaemias

- Confirmation of diagnosis of specific subtypes of leukaemias (acute leukaemias with recurrent genetic abnormalities)
- Assessment of prognosis
- Assessment of response to therapy
- Assessment of clonality, e.g. distinguishing hypoplastic AML from aplastic anaemia
- Detection of minimal residual disease.

Table 5.8: Chromosomal abnormalities in AML

Chromosomal abnormality	Type of AML	Prognosis
1. t(8;21)(q22;q22)	M2	Favourable
2. t(15;17)(q22;q12)	M3	Favourable
3. inv(16)(p13;q22) or t(16;16)(p13;q22)	M4 Eo	Favourable
4. Abnormalities of 11q23	Monocytic	Intermediate
5. −7, del(7q), −5, del(5q), +8, +9, del(11q)	AML with multilineage dysplasia, therapy-related AML	Unfavourable

Table 5.9: Chromosomal abnormalities in precursor B ALL

Type of ALL	Chromosomal abnormality	Prognosis
Precursor B ALL	t(9;22) (q34; q11.2)	Unfavourable
	t(4;11)(q21;q23)	Unfavourable
	t(1;19)((q23;p13.3)	Unfavourable
	t(12;21)((p13;q22)	Favourable
	Hyperdiploidy >50	Favourable
	Hypodiploidy	Unfavourable

is measured by flow cytometry. Ploidy studies are especially important in childhood ALL; hyperdiploid (chromosome number >50) ALL has better prognosis as compared to diploid (46 chromosomes) and hypodiploid (<46 chromosomes) ALL. DNA index >1.16 is associated with favourable prognosis and therapeutic response.

Molecular Genetic Studies

Applications of molecular genetic studies in acute leukaemia are shown in Box 5.6. Methods of molecular genetic analysis are Southern blot analysis, polymerase chain reaction-based techniques, and fluorescent *in situ* hybridisation (FISH).

Principle of Southern blot analysis is given elsewhere in this book. In a clonal disorder like acute leukaemia, cleaving of DNA by restriction enzyme will produce DNA fragments of same size (since all the cells of a clone will have identical gene rearrangement), which can be detected by electrophoresis of DNA. In a non-malignant or reactive condition, due to the presence of multiple clones, fragments of DNA produced after restriction enzyme digestion are of different size.

Immunoglobulin and T cell receptor gene rearrangements occur during B and T lymphocyte development respectively. The rearrangement of immunoglobulin genes

---

Box 5.6   Applications of molecular genetic analysis in acute leukaemias

- Diagnosis of specific types through identification of unique fusion genes formed due to genetic rearrangements
- Early detection of minimal residual disease and relapse
- Identification of lineage of leukaemic cells
- Detection of clonality.

occurs in a specific sequence: μ heavy chain followed by kappa (κ) light chain that in turn is followed by lambda (λ) light chain. T gamma (Tγ) and T beta (Tβ) chain genes are rearranged earlier than T alpha (Tα) chain genes during T cell ontogeny. These rearrangements are detected by Southern blot analysis using labelled cDNA probes. The usefulness of gene rearrangement studies in acute leukaemias as a lineage-specific marker is limited. This is because immunoglobulin heavy chain gene rearrangement, which occurs during B cell ontogeny, has also been observed in some cases of T-ALL and AML. Similarly T cell receptor gene rearrangements have been detected in some cases of B-ALL and AML. However, light chain gene rearrangements occur only in B cells and are lineage specific.

Identification of fusion genes (which are formed after translocations) such as *PML/RARα* gene in AML M3, and *BCR-ABL* and *TEL-AML1* fusion genes in ALL has prognostic and therapeutic importance.

Algorithmic approach to diagnosis of acute leukaemias is shown in Figure 5.8.

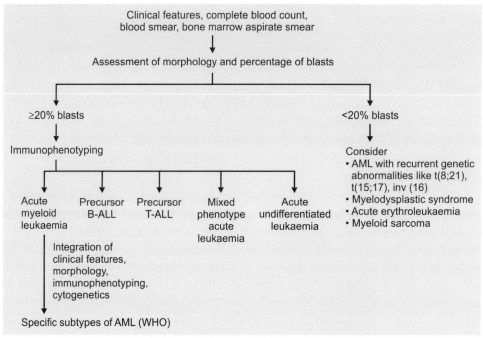

Figure 5.8: Algorithmic approach for diagnosis of acute leukaemia. Integration of clinical, morphologic, immunophenotypic, cytogenetic, and molecular genetic information is required for proper diagnosis and classification. In some cases, based on patient demographics, clinical features, and blast morphology, a specifically-directed panel for immunophenotyping can be used. If blast differentiation is not apparent, then an initial full screening panel followed by specific additional markers for assignment of blast lineage need to be used. An example of screening panel is CD45 (haematopoietic), CD34 (blast), CD117 (myeloblast), CD79a or PAX-5 (B lymphoid), and CD3 (T lymphoid). Specific markers: AML-M0 (CD13+, CD33+), Acute promyelocytic leukaemia (HLADR-), Acute myelomonocytic leukaemia (MPO+, CD68+), Acute monoblastic leukaemia (MPO-, CD68+), Acute erythroleukaemia (CD71+, glycophorin+, HbA+), Acute megakaryoblastic leukaemia (CD41+, CD61+), T-ALL (TdT, CD2, CD5, CD4, CD8), B-ALL (TdT, CD22, CD10).

❑ ACUTE LYMPHOBLASTIC LEUKAEMIA

Syn: Acute lymphatic leukaemia

Acute lymphoblastic leukaemia (ALL) is a malignant neoplasm of haematopoietic stem cells of lymphoid lineage arising in the bone marrow. It is the commonest form of malignancy in childhood.

Clinical Features

ALL occurs predominantly during childhood with a peak incidence at 4 to 5 years of age. Onset is acute with history of short duration. Children usually present with manifestations related to bone marrow and organ infiltration by leukaemic cells. These include pallor, fatigue (due to anaemia), bleeding in the form of bruising and petechiae (due to thrombocytopaenia), and persistent fever (due to neutropaenia). Enlargement of lymph nodes, spleen, and liver commonly occurs. Bone and joint pains are due to periosteal and bone involvement. Extramedullary disease can also occur in central nervous system, testis, eye, gastrointestinal tract, and kidneys.

Classification

There are two classification schemes for ALL as follows:

Morphological Classification of ALL (FAB Co-operative Group, 1976)

According to FAB classification, there are three morphological subtypes of ALL: L1, L2, and L3 (Table 5.10). The approximate frequencies of the three subtypes in childhood ALL are: L1: 80%, L2: 15–20%, and L3: 1–2%. In adults with ALL, L2 subtype is most common. Although this classification is simple, it does not correlate adequately with immunophenotype, genetic abnormalities, clinical behaviour, and response to treatment.

Although ALL-L3 is fairly easy to recognise, it was observed that morphological differentiation between L1 and L2 was not clear-cut. The FAB group, in 1981, introduced a scoring system to distinguish between L 1 and L2. According to this scoring system, high nuclear/cytoplasmic ratio in >75% cells, and 0 to 1 small nucleoli in >75% of cells are each given a + score, while low nuclear/cytoplasmic ratio in >25% of cells, one

Table 5.10: FAB classification of ALL

Morphology	L1	L2	L3
1. Size of blast	Small	Large, heterogeneous	Large, homogeneous
2. Cytoplasm	Scanty	Moderate	Moderate, intensely basophilic
3. N/C ratio	High	Lower	Lower
4. Cytoplasmic vacuoles	±	±	Prominent
5. Nuclear membrane	Regular	Irregular with clefting	Regular
6. Nucleoli	Invisible or indistinct	Prominent, 1–2	Prominent, 1–2

or more prominent nucleoli in >25% cells, irregular nuclear membrane in >25% of cells, and large cells (double the size of small lymphocytes) in >50% of cells are each assigned a score of –. Positive score (0 to +2) is obtained in L1 while negative score (–1 to –4) is obtained in L2.

World Health Organization Classification (2008)

In WHO Classification, there are following categories of ALL (Table 5.4):
- B lymphoblastic leukaemia/lymphoma, not otherwise specified
- B lymphoblastic leukaemia/lymphoma with recurrent genetic abnormalities
- T lymphoblastic leukaemia/lymphoma

In children, majority of cases are of B-cell type. Within the category of B-cell ALL, several subtypes are defined according to the genetic abnormalities. These have prognostic and therapeutic significance. There is no correlation between WHO categories and FAB subtypes L1 and L2. Leukaemic phase of Burkitt's lymphoma corresponds with L3 subgroup which is now considered as a separate entity. Patients with Burkitt lymphoma who have bulky disease present with leukaemic phase; pure Burkitt leukaemia is rare.

The lymphoblastic lymphoma and lymphoblastic leukaemia are considered as a single disease with different clinical presentations. Majority of lymphoblastic leukaemias/lymphomas present as leukaemia (blasts in bone marrow >25%).

Laboratory Features

Peripheral Blood Examination

Anaemia, which may be severe, is present in all patients. It is normocytic and normochromic.

Total leucocyte count may be raised, normal, or low. Patients with T-ALL have very high leucocyte count at presentation. Proportion of lymphoblasts is variable (Fig. 5.9). Absolute granulocytopaenia and thrombocytopaenia are commonly present.

Bone Marrow Examination

Bone marrow is hypercellular due to proliferation of leukaemic blasts. Normal haematopoietic elements are diminished. Bone marrow aspiration smears are necessary for diagnosis and subclassification of ALL into L1, L2, and L3 subtypes.

Rarely ALL may present with hypocellular marrow (aplastic anaemia) that after a few months is followed by overt manifestations of ALL.

Cytochemistry

Cytochemical stains are an adjunct to the morphological examination of the bone marrow.

By conventional definition, lymphoblasts in ALL are negative for myeloperoxidase. Other stains which are negative in ALL are Sudan black B, chloroacetate esterase, and alpha naphthyl acetate esterase.

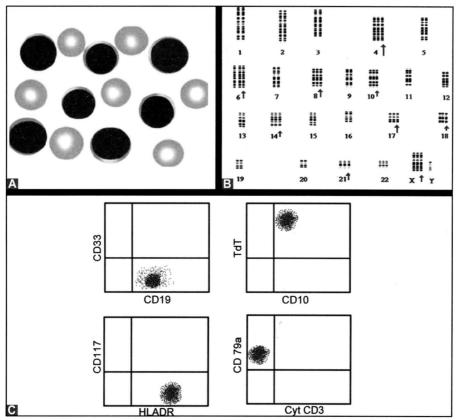

Figure 5.9: (A) Bone marrow aspiration smear in ALL; (B) Karyotyping showing hyperdiploidy; (C) Flow cytometry shows common ALL phenotype: HLADR+, TdT+, CD10+, and CD79a+ and CD33-, CD117-, and cytCD3-

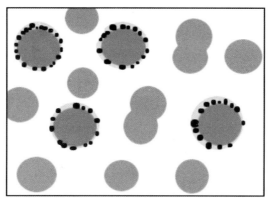

Figure 5.10: Periodic acid Schiff stain in ALL showing block-like positivity

In leukaemic lymphoblasts, PAS stain is positive in a characteristic manner and has been used for the diagnosis of ALL (Fig. 5.10). PAS-positive material (glycogen) in leukaemic lymphoblasts is typically large and block-like, surrounds the nucleus, and is present against a clear cytoplasmic background. PAS stain is positive in L1 and L2 subtypes but is negative in L3 subtype. PAS stain is not specific for leukaemic lymphoblasts. Also in many cases of ALL (~30% of L1 and L2), PAS stain is negative; furthermore, PAS positivity may also be observed in leukaemic myeloblasts (diffuse positivity) and in monoblasts and erythroblasts (small block-like on a diffusely positive background). No cytochemical stain is specific for lymphoblasts. Therefore, morphologic features and immunologic markers are necessary for definitive identification of lymphoblasts.

In T-ALL, acid phosphatase stain is positive in a focal paranuclear manner. In ALL L3, cytoplasmic vacuoles are positive for oil red O stain, while cytoplasm is methyl green pyronine positive.

Immunophenotyping

By immunophenotypic analysis, various subtypes of ALL have been identified.

B-ALL: accounts for 80% of all cases of ALL.
- Pro-B ALL (Early precursor B-ALL) (8–10%): TdT (terminal deoxynucleotidyl transferase) +, HLADR+, **CD19+**, cytoCD79a+, CD22+. This correlates with FAB subtypes L1 and L2. This type has been found to be more common in infants and children.
- 'Common' ALL (50%): TdT+, HLADR+, CD19+, cytoCD79a+, CD22+, **CD10 (common ALL antigen or CALLA)+**, CD20+. This subtype is the most common form of ALL in children, and is associated with best prognosis. It correlates with FAB L1 and L2 morphological subtypes.
- Pre-B ALL (20%): TdT+, HLADR+, CD19+, cytoCD79a+, CD22+, CD10+, CD20+, **Cyt μ (cytoplasmic μ chain)+.**
- B ALL (1–2%): HLA DR+, CD19+, cytoCD79a+, CD22+, CD10+, CD20+, **SmIg (surface membrane immunoglobulin) +.** This subtype correlates with L3 morphology, is considered as a leukaemic phase of Burkitt's lymphoma, and is associated with poor prognosis.

T-ALL: accounts for 15–20% cases of ALL.
- **Pro–T ALL: CD7+, CytCD3+**
- **Pre–T ALL:** CD7+, CytCD3+, **CD5+and/or CD2+**
- **Cortical T-ALL:** CD7+, CytCD3+, CD5+, **CD1a+**
- **Mature T-ALL:** CD7+, CytCD3+, CD1a+, **membrane CD3+.**

Cytogenetic Analysis

This is one of the most important investigations in ALL that has a great impact on selection of therapy in childhood ALL. Clonal chromosomal abnormalities occur in 80%

Table 5.11: Cytogenetic abnormalities in B cell ALL

Chromosomal abnormality	Molecular abnormality	Prognosis
1. Hyperdiploidy (>50)	-	Favourable
2. Hypodiploidy	-	Unfavourable
3. t(12;21)(p13;q22)*	TEL/AML1	Favourable
4. t(1;19)(q23;p13.3)	PBX/E2A	Unfavourable
5. t(9;22)(q34;q11.2)	BCR/ABL	Unfavourable
6. t(v;11)(v;q23)	Commonly MLL/AF4	Unfavourable
7. t(8;14)(q24;q32)	MYC/IGH	No effect
* Identified only by molecular analysis. v: variable		

cases of ALL (Table 5.11). Certain chromosomal abnormalities are consistently observed in specific types of ALL. Thus, cytogenetic analysis improves the diagnostic efficiency. Secondly, chromosomal abnormalities have prognostic and therapeutic importance. Chromosomal abnormalities in ALL include both numerical and structural alterations.

Hyperdiploidy with >50 chromosomes is the most frequent abnormality in childhood precursor B ALL. It is associated with high sensitivity to chemotherapy, complete remission rate of 100%, and long-term disease-free survival of 90%.

Patients with t(9;22)(q34;q11) and abnormalities of 11q23 have unfavourable prognosis with increased risk of relapse, lower remission rate, and poor long-term survival. In these patients, allogeneic haematopoietic stem cell transplantation should be considered in first remission.

Molecular Genetic Studies

Applications of molecular genetic analysis in ALL include:
- Establishment of lineage: In those cases in which immunophenotyping fails to conclusively identify the lineage of leukaemic cells, DNA analysis (Southern blot) may be carried out to detect rearrangement of heavy and light chain genes and T cell receptor genes. However, gene rearrangement studies should be interpreted carefully for reasons outlined earlier (see chapter on "Acute leukaemias"). Rearrangement of light chain genes is specific for B lineage cells.
- Establishment of clonality
- Identification of translocations that cannot be identified by cytogenetic analysis, e.g. t(12;21)(p13;q22) is identified only by molecular analysis.
- Detection of minimal residual disease
- Early detection of relapse.

Other Investigations

Lumbar puncture: Not all patients with CNS involvement have clinical features of raised intracranial tension. Therefore, cerebrospinal fluid should be examined for lymphoblasts at the time of diagnosis in all patients with ALL.

Testicular biopsy: Testis is a frequent organ of relapse in ALL. Therefore before stopping treatment, testicular biopsy may be performed to rule out residual disease.

X-ray chest: Chest X-ray examination may reveal mediastinal widening especially in T-ALL.

Differential Diagnosis of ALL

Diagnosis of ALL is usually obvious in the presence of fever, anaemia, thrombocytopaenia, lymphadenopathy, hepatosplenomegaly, and diffuse replacement of bone marrow by lymphoblasts. However, ALL should be differentiated from following conditions:

Reactive Lymphocytosis due to Infections

Infections such as by Epstein-Barr virus or cytomegalovirus can produce fever, lymphadenopathy, splenomegaly and reactive lymphocytosis and mimick ALL. Absence of anaemia and thrombocytopaenia, positive serological tests (e.g. Paul-Bunnell test in infectious mononucleosis, raised IgM viral antibody titres) and morphology of reactive lymphocytes (relatively more amount of cytoplasm, coarse chromatin, scalloping and skirting of borders) are helpful in differentiating infectious lymphocytosis from ALL. Chromosomal studies and immunophenotyping can help in difficult cases.

Acute Myeloid Leukaemia

Differences between ALL and AML are outlined in Table 5.12 and Figure 5.2.

Table 5.12: Differences between ALL and AML

Parameter	ALL	AML
1. Age	More common in children	More common in infants, adolescents, and adults
2. Significant lymphadenopathy in more than one location	Common	Uncommon
3. Meningeal disease	More common	Less common
4. Mediastinal lymphadenopathy	Seen in T-ALL	Rare
5. Morphology of blasts		
• Size	Small to medium	Large
• Cytoplasm	Scanty	Moderately abundant
• Auer rod	Absent	Pathognomonic if present
• Nuclear chromatin	Coarse	Fine
• Nucleoli	Indistinct, 0–2	Prominent, 1–4
6. Myelodysplasia	Absent	May be present
7. Cytochemistry		
• Myeloperoxidase	Negative	Positive
• PAS	Block-like positive in 70% cases	Diffuse
8. Immunophenotyping	B lineage: CD19, CD22, TdT; T lineage: CD7, cCD3, CD2, TdT	Granulocytic: CD13, CD33, CD117; Monocytic: CD14, CD64; Erythroid: Glycophorin A; Megakaryocytic: CD41
9. Ig or TCR gene rearrangement	B-ALL: Clonal Ig; T-ALL: Clonal TCR	Germline configuration

Leukaemic Phase of Non-Hodgkin's Lymphoma

Bone marrow and peripheral blood involvement by non-Hodgkin's lymphoma may be difficult to distinguish from acute leukaemia, particularly when prior history of lymphomatous stage is absent. Lymphoblastic lymphoma, small lymphocytic lymphoma, mantle cell lymphoma, and small cleaved cell lymphoma have a high incidence of bone marrow involvement.

Peripheral blood involvement in small-cleaved cell lymphoma has in the past been referred to as lymphosarcoma cell leukaemia. Characteristically the cells show irregular and clefted nuclei and bone marrow shows focal and paratrabecular pattern of involvement.

Leukaemic phase of lymphoblastic lymphoma is morphologically indistinguishable from ALL.

Metastatic Tumours in Bone Marrow

In children, metastasis of neuroblastoma and in adolescents and adults, Ewing's sarcoma and small cell carcinoma of lung may have to be differentiated from ALL. Metastatic tumour in bone marrow occurs as clumps (or clusters) rather than as diffuse sheets. Demonstration of primary tumour, immunocytochemical studies, and electron microscopy are helpful in determining the cell of origin.

Haematogones

Haematogones are normal B lymphocyte precursors, which increase in bone marrow in marrow regenerative states and immune cytopaenias. Morphologically they may be mistaken for lymphoblasts of ALL. Cell surface analysis of haematogones shows a spectrum of immature to mature cells (with normal antigenic evolution of B cell precursors). Lymphoblasts in ALL show predominance of immature cells and aberrant antigen expression.

Prognostic Factors in ALL

At the time of diagnosis a number of factors affect prognosis (Table 5.13).

Total Leucocyte Count

This is one of the most important prognostic variables. TLC <50,000/cmm is associated with good prognosis while high TLC (>50,000/cmm) is associated with poor prognosis.

Age

Children between 1 and 10 years of age have the best prognosis with about 70% of them achieving long-term remission with current methods of treatment. Children <1 year, >10 years, and adults have relatively poor outlook.

Table 5.13: Prognostic factors in ALL

Parameter	Unfavourable	Favourable
1. Age	<1 year, >10 year	1–10 years
2. Sex	Male (testicular relapse)	Female
3. TLC	>50,000/cmm	<50,000/cmm
4. Immunophenotype	T-ALL, early B-ALL (SmIg+)	'Common' ALL (CALLA+, Cμ-)
5. CNS disease	Presence of blasts in CSF	Absence of blasts in CSF
6. Cytogenetic or molecular genetic abnormalities	Hypodiploidy; t(9;22) or *BCR/ABL* fusion; t(4;11)(q21;q23) or *MLL/AF4* fusion.	Hyperdiploidy (>50); t(12;21) (p13;q22), i.e. *TEL/AML1* fusion
7. Remission after first induction	Failure to remit	Early achievement of remission

Immunophenotype

Best prognosis is associated with 'common' ALL (CALLA +, Cμ-) while poorest prognosis is with T-ALL and early B-ALL (SmIg+). The order (favourable to unfavourable) is as follows: 'common' ALL (CALLA+, Cμ-) – Pre-B ALL (Cμ+) – Pro-B ALL -T-ALL and -Early B-ALL (SmIg+).

Cytogenetics

Hyperdiploidy (>50 chromosomes) has better prognosis, while prognosis is unfavourable with translocations especially Ph' chromosome.

Other Bad Prognostic Indicators

These are massive tumour burden (hepatosplenomegaly, lymphadenopathy, mediastinal mass), early CNS disease, and slow response for achieving remission. The most favourable prognostic group is of children between 1 and 10 years of age who have 'common' ALL (CALLA+, Cμ-) phenotype and have hyperdiploidy (>50 chromosomes). With current modes of treatment, most of these children will achieve long-term remission and many of them are probably cured.

It should be noted, however, that with successful and effective chemotherapy significance of the various prognostic factors is lost.

Risk Categorisation in ALL

Different workers have defined different risk groups on the basis of various features. One such scheme is presented in Table 5.14. According to a recent National Cancer Institute-sponsored workshop, in children with precursor B ALL, age 1–9 years and TLC <50,000/cmm should be defined as low-risk. All other patients should be categorised as high-risk.

Table 5.14: Risk categories in ALL

Low-risk	Intermediate risk	High-risk	Very high-risk
1. Hyperdiploidy	Age 1–10 years and	1. *E2A/PBX* fusion	1. *BCR/ABL* fusion with high TLC
2. *TEL/AML1* fusion	TLC<50,000/cmm without genetic risk factors	2. T-ALL	2. *MLL* rearrangement
		3. Age<1 year, >10 years and TLC >50,000/cmm without genetic risk factors	3. Induction failure

Treatment

Major success has been achieved in the treatment of ALL with modern chemotherapy. In Western countries, with current methods of treatment more than 90% of children with ALL achieve complete remission (CR) and majority of them are probably cured. However, in adults with ALL, complete remission is achieved only in a minority of patients.

The average duration of therapy in ALL is 2 to 2½ years.

Phases of Treatment in ALL (Box 5.7)

Remission induction: In this phase systemic chemotherapy is given to reduce the leukaemic cell load below the level of detection and to restore haematopoiesis and health. Remission induction is achieved in 90% of patients by combination of vincristine and prednisone.

Box 5.7 Phases of treatment in ALL
• Remission induction
• CNS prophylaxis
• Consolidation (Intensification)
• Maintenance

Addition of anthracycline (daunorubicin or doxorubicin) or L-asparaginase or both can induce remission in even more number of patients. Remission is usually induced in 4 to 6 weeks.

In complete remission, there is no clinical or laboratory evidence of leukaemia. Complete remission is defined as presence of less than 5% blasts in bone marrow and normalisation of peripheral blood cell counts.

Central nervous system prophylaxis: After achieving CR, prophylactic therapy to CNS is necessary in ALL. Leukaemic lymphoblasts infiltrate the CNS and CSF in the initial period of the disease. CNS is the sanctuary site in ALL in that the drugs used for remission induction are unable to pass through the blood-brain barrier and thus leukaemic cells are protected from chemotherapeutic drugs. Subsequently these cells may cause leukaemic meningitis and relapse. If CNS prophylaxis is administered soon after completion of remission induction, risk of CNS relapse is markedly decreased.

CNS prophylaxis is achieved by combination of cranial irradiation (1800 cGy for children, 2400 cGy for adults) plus intrathecal methotrexate. However, with this treatment, children often subsequently develop neuropsychological problems and

CNS tumours. Therefore, many investigators omit cranial irradiation, and reserve it for high-risk cases such as T-ALL, TLC >50,000/cmm, and translocation between chromosomes 9 and 22.

Consolidation treatment: This is the high dose intensive chemotherapy administered immediately after remission induction to eradicate the residual blast cells and reduce the potentially resistant leukaemic cell mass. In this regime, alternative drugs not used for remission induction are employed. Different protocols have been used for this purpose by different centres. The commonly used drugs are anthracycline, cytarabine, cyclophosphamide, asparagine, and thioguanine.

Recently, it has been demonstrated that addition of another block of consolidation therapy at approximately 35 weeks improves the long-term survival in intermediate risk and high-risk patients; this is called as double-delayed intensification.

Maintenance therapy: After achieving complete remission, treatment is continued for further 2 to 2½ years. Chemotherapeutic drugs are administered for 2 to 2½ years to maintain the remission and prevent or delay the occurrence of relapse by eradicating residual leukaemic cells. The usual drugs for this purpose are 6-mercaptopurine (daily) along with methotrexate (weekly). Careful monitoring is necessary for toxic side effects and compliance.

Supportive Care

1. Appropriate blood product replacement therapy includes packed red cell transfusions for anaemia and platelet transfusions to maintain platelet count above 20,000/cmm to reduce the risk of spontaneous haemorrhage.

2. Infections: Viral infections such as measles (interstitial pneumonitis and encephalitis) and disseminated chickenpox are particularly common. Varicella-zoster immune globulin and gammaglobulin for prevention of chickenpox and measles respectively are recommended. For established chickenpox infection, acyclovir is used.

   Co-trimoxazole is the standard form of prophylactic treatment for prevention of *Pneumocystis carinii* pneumonia.

   Empiric antibiotic treatment is indicated in febrile neutropaenic patients until definitive cause is identified.

3. For prevention of uric acid nephropathy, allopurinol should be given and fluid and electrolyte balance should be maintained.

4. Tumour lysis syndrome: This is a potentially life-threatening metabolic disorder resulting from destruction (spontaneous or post-treatment) of rapidly proliferating neoplastic cells. It is characterised by hyperuricaemia, hyperkalaemia, hyperphosphataemia, and hypocalcaemia. Acute renal failure can develop. For prevention, adequate hydration should be maintained during induction chemotherapy and patient should be closely monitored (urine output, renal function, and serum chemistry studies).

Treatment of Relapse

Despite achieving remission, relapse occurs in 25 to 30% of patients. Relapse may occur in bone marrow, central nervous system, or testis. If relapse occurs during maintenance therapy, then possibility of achieving second remission is remote as it indicates refractoriness to therapy. However, if relapse occurs sometimes after maintenance therapy is stopped, then prognosis is better and second remission can be achieved in most patients. Treatment of relapse needs to be more aggressive with induction of new drugs (podophyllins, anthracycline analogues, and fludarabine).

Long-term Side Effects of Intensive Therapy

These include:
- Deficit in intellectual and cognitive functions (in children who receive cranial irradiation at young age)
- Increased risk of CNS tumours
- Therapy-related AML (with epipodophyllotoxin and alkylating drug therapy)
- Cardiac toxicity (with anthracyclines)
- Thyroid dysfunction (with cranial and neck irradiation, chemotherapy).

Haematopoietic Stem Cell Transplantation (HSCT)

Many children achieve long-term clinical remission and probably cure with modern chemotherapy. Secondly, allogeneic HSCT is associated with risk of graft-versus-host disease, opportunistic infections, and considerable morbidity and mortality. Therefore, HSCT is reserved for children with ALL in second or subsequent remission; in these cases survival with HSCT is superior as compared to chemotherapy. HSCT in first remission can be considered in those cases resistant to conventional chemotherapy and in high-risk cases such as Philadelphia chromosome-positive ALL and ALL with TLC > 50,000/cmm at diagnosis.

Risk-adapted Therapy in ALL

The aim of risk-adapted therapy in ALL is to administer therapy according to the risk category of the patient (Table 5.14). The goal is to achieve cure with as little toxicity as possible (especially in low-risk patients). Low-risk patients should be treated with less intensive therapy (to limit the toxic effects of therapy), while high-risk patients are treated with more aggressive treatment (to improve survival).

Minimal Residual Disease (MRD) in ALL

Although more than 95% of children achieve complete remission (i.e. presence of <5% of blast cells in marrow on microscopy) after treatment, relapse occurs in 20% of low-risk and 70% of high-risk patients. This is due to the presence of a small number of viable leukaemic cells which survive the cytotoxic chemotherapy and which cannot be detected by the conventional method. This submicroscopic persistence of disease following treatment is called as minimal residual disease. Aim of estimation of MRD following remission induction is to assess initial response to treatment, prognosis, and risk categorisation so that further treatment can be individualised (less intensive, more aggressive, or stem cell transplantation) to increase the chance of cure. Various methods available for detection of MRD include cytogenetic analysis, fluorescent *in situ* hybridisation, immunophenotyping, and molecular genetic analysis (like Southern blotting or RT-PCR).

Experience in India

Currently, the 5-year survival rate of ALL in children following therapy reported from major centres in India is 45 to 55%. Poor outcome in Indian children as compared to those in the Western countries appears to be due to various reasons including (1) T-ALL and molecular abnormalities associated with unfavourable prognosis (such as *BCR/ABL*, *E2A/PBX*) are more common in Indian children; (2) Non-compliance due to financial burden; and (3) Poor tolerance to cytotoxic chemotherapy due to malnourishment.

❑ ACUTE MYELOID LEUKAEMIA

Synonyms: Acute myelogenous leukaemia, Acute nonlymphocytic leukaemia
Acute myeloid leukaemia (AML) is a malignant neoplasm of haematopoietic stem cells originating in bone marrow and characterised by proliferation of blast cells of myeloid lineage. AML is genotypically and phenotypically extremely heterogeneous. Since last 30 years, AML is being treated with the same induction regimen (cytosine arabinoside + anthracycline). With the recent identification of specific types in WHO classification (2008), individualisation of treatment is possible.

Clinical Features

Acute myeloid leukaemia is the commonest form of acute leukaemia in adults and becomes increasingly more common as age advances. Median age at diagnosis is 65 years. It is also the predominant form of leukaemia before 1 year of age. It is much less frequent in children as compared to ALL.

AML can arise from pre-existing disorders such as myelodysplastic syndrome, myeloproliferative diseases (chronic myeloid leukaemia, polycythaemia vera, myelofibrosis), and paroxysmal nocturnal haemoglobinuria. Alkylating drugs, epipodophyllotoxins, and radiotherapy given for treatment of other neoplasms can induce AML. Genetic diseases with increased predisposition to AML include Down's syndrome, Bloom's syndrome and Fanconi's anaemia.

Clinical features are mainly due to bone marrow failure caused by infiltration by neoplastic cells, i.e. anaemia (weakness, fatigue), granulocytopaenia (infections), and thrombocytopaenia (bleeding tendencies). As compared to ALL, AML is equally common between sexes and more commonly occurs in adults; bone pain, hepatomegaly, and splenomegaly are less common, and lymphadenopathy is rare. Skin infiltration (leukaemia cutis) and gum hypertrophy occur in 50% of patients with monocytic leukaemia (AML M4 and M5). About 10% of patients present with hyperleucocytosis (TLC >1,00,000/cmm); these patients belong to the poor prognostic category and have increased risk of leucostasis due to intravascular clumping of blasts. Sludging of blood flow can cause pulmonary manifestations (severe dyspnoea and diffuse lung shadowing), retinal haemorrhages, or neurological manifestations (altered mental status, ocular muscle palsy, etc.). Rarely, a patient may present with an isolated mass of leukaemic cells in an extramedullary site called as chloroma or myeloid sarcoma. The common sites are bones (skull, sternum, ribs, vertebrae, pelvis, paranasal sinuses), skin, and lymph nodes. Myeloid sarcoma may precede or occur simultaneously with AML.

Disseminated intravascular coagulation (DIC) is especially likely to occur in AML M3 due to release of thromboplastin-like material from primary granules of abnormal promyelocytes. DIC can also occur in monocytic leukaemias (AML M4 or M5) due to the release of lysozyme.

Rapid response to chemotherapy may induce 'tumour lysis syndrome' which is characterised by hyperuricaemia with renal insufficiency, hyperphosphataemia, hypocalcaemia, and acidosis.

Classification

There are two classification systems for AML
- French-American-British Co-operative Group Classification (1976)
- World Health Organization Classification (2008)

The French-American-British (FAB) Co-operative Group Classification

The French-American-British (FAB) Co-operative Group classification is outlined in Table 5.2.

The FAB Co-operative Group has defined eight types of AML: M0 to M7. These include leukaemias of granulocytic (M0, M1, M2, M3), monocytic (M4 and M5), erythroid (M6), and megakaryocytic (M7) lineages. The name 'myeloid' is given because these lineages arise from the pleuripotent myeloid stem cell.

This classification is based on morphological and cytochemical features. Diagnosis of AML is made when 30% or more of nucleated cells in bone marrow are blasts. (If less than 30% of all nucleated cells are blasts, then diagnosis of myelodysplastic syndrome is considered). Percentages of granulocytic and monocytic components are assessed in non-erythroid cells for classifying M1 to M5 types. Percentage of erythroblasts should be less than 50% of all nucleated cells in bone marrow. If >50% of all nucleated cells in bone marrow are erythroblasts and >30% of non-erythroid cells are blasts then diagnosis is AML-M6. (If erythroblasts are >50% of all nucleated cells and <30% of non-erythroid cells are blasts, then diagnosis is myelodysplastic syndrome).

World Health Organization Classification

This classification is listed in Table 5.3. The new WHO classification retains the categories of FAB classification, and also creates some new categories. The blast count for diagnosis of AML is reduced to 20% from previous FAB standard of 30%. This is because recent studies have indicated that patients with 20 to 30% blasts (classified as 'refractory anaemia with excess blasts in transformation' or RAEB-T in FAB classification) have prognosis similar to patients with ≥30% blasts. A brief description of WHO classification follows.

AML with recurrent genetic abnormalities: This subgroup recognises the importance of certain genetic abnormalities that correlate with response to treatment and prognosis. This type of AML occurs in young patients and is associated with relatively favourable response to therapy and longer survival. The chromosomal rearrangement leads to the formation of a fusion gene that is linked with the pathogenesis of leukaemia. For detection of genetic abnormalities, reverse transcriptase-polymerase chain reaction (RT-PCR) is more sensitive than conventional techniques. Cases with specific clonal recurrent genetic abnormalities but with low blast count (<20%) are also categorised as AML.

- AML with t(8;21)(q22;q22) *(RUNX1-RUNX1T1):* In most cases, blasts are large with moderately abundant basophilic cytoplasm which contains many azurophil granules. Auer rods are frequent. Although morphology correlates with AML M2 (FAB), some cases show evidence of maturation or monocytic differentiation. Immunophenotyping shows positivity for myeloid markers (CD13, CD33, MPO), lymphoid marker (CD19), and haematopoietic stem cell marker (CD34).
- AML with inv(16)(p13.1q22) or t(16;16)(p13.1;q22)*(CBFβ/MYH11):* There is evidence of both granulocytic and monocytic differentiation similar to acute myelomonocytic leukaemia with abnormal eosinophils (FAB: AML M4 with Eo). However, some cases do not show eosinophils or monocytic differentiation. Immunophenotyping shows both myeloid antigens (CD13, CD33, MPO) and monocytic differentiation antigens (CD14, lysozyme).
- Acute promyelocytic leukaemia (AML with t(15;17)(q22;q12)*(PML/RARA)* and variants: There is predominance of abnormal promyelocytes. In the hypergranular or 'typical' type, promyelocytes show innumerable, large azurophil granules in the cytoplasm. Auer rods are often arranged as bundles ('faggots'). Pancytopaenia in peripheral blood is typical.

In the 'microgranular' variant cytoplasm contains very fine granules that are difficult to recognise and the nucleus is typically bilobed. Total leucocyte count is markedly elevated in this variant.

Myeloperoxidase stain is strongly positive. There is formation of a fusion gene RARα/PML due to t(15;17) translocation that leads to arrest in maturation at promyelocyte stage.

A unique feature is abnormal promyelocytes can be induced to differentiate to more mature granulocytes following treatment with all-trans retinoic acid.

- AML with t(9;11)(p22;q23);MLLT3-MLL: Genetic abnormalities involving chromosome 11q23 usually (but not invariably) correlate with monocytic or myelomonocytic leukaemias.

AML with myelodysplasia-related changes: Multilineage dysplasia is defined as dysplasia present in ≥50% of cells in 2 or more myeloid cell lines. AML (≥20% blasts in blood or marrow) with multilineage dysplasia occurs usually in elderly persons with or without prior history of myelodysplastic syndrome (MDS) and is associated with poor prognosis and chromosomal abnormalities similar to those seen in MDS.

Therapy-related myeloid neoplasms: Therapy-related AML following alkylating therapy is different from *de novo* AML in that it is associated with characteristic cytogenetic abnormalities (esp of chromosomes 5 or 7, and complex abnormalities), multilineage dysplasia, refractoriness to therapy, and short survival.

Acute leukaemia following topoisomerase II inhibitor therapy may be myeloid or lymphoid.

AML not otherwise categorised: This category consists of those cases of AML that do not belong to any of the previous categories. Most of these subtypes are similar to FAB categories, with some modifications. The various subtypes are defined on the basis of morphology, cytochemistry, immunophenotyping, and degree of maturation.

- *Acute myeloblastic leukaemia, minimally differentiated (FAB synonym- AML M0):* This designation is applied to those cases of AML that appear undifferentiated by light microscopy (i.e. absence of myeloid differentiation and negative MPO reaction). However, myeloid nature is evident on electron microscopy (peroxidase positive granules) or immunological cell marker studies (presence of one or more myeloid antigens like CD13, CD 33, CD117). B or T lymphoid markers are absent. Primitive haematopoietic stem cell markers are present (CD34, HLADR). Immunophenotyping is essential for differentiation from ALL.

- *Acute myeloblastic leukaemia without maturation (FAB synonym: AML M1):* There is no or minimal maturation along granulocytic pathway. Cell population is predominantly composed of myeloblasts. There are two types of blasts: one type does not show any cytoplasmic azurophil granules, while another type shows few granules. Cytochemically, ≥3% of blasts are peroxidase positive. Immunologic cell marker studies reveal expression of at least two myeloid antigens (CD13, CD33, CD117, MPO).

- *Acute myeloblastic leukaemia with maturation (FAB synonym: AML M2):* This is the most frequent subtype (30–45% of AML cases). There is clear evidence of maturation to promyelocyte stage and beyond. Auer rods, which represent aggregates of azurophil granules in lysosomes, are commonly seen. Blasts are 20% or more (20–89%) of all nucleated cells in bone marrow. Mature cells (promyelocytes to granulocytes) are ≥10%. Monocytic cells should be less than 20%. Some cases of AML M2 show increased basophils. Myeloperoxidase reaction is strongly positive. Immunophenotyping shows one or more myeloid associated antigens.

- *Acute myelomonocytic leukaemia (FAB synonym: AML M4):* Along with granulocytic series, a significant proportion of cells of monocytic series are also present. In bone marrow, blasts are ≥20%, and monocytic cells and their precursors and neutrophils and their precursors each are 20% or more. Nonspecific esterase reaction is positive in cells of monocytic lineage. Myeloperoxidase is positive in ≥3% blasts. Leukaemic cells express myeloid associated antigens (CD13, CD33) and markers of monocytic differentiation (CD14, lysozyme).

- *Acute monoblastic leukaemia and acute monocytic leukaemia (FAB synonym: AML M5):* In this type, monocytic differentiation is readily apparent with 80% or more of leukaemic cells in bone marrow being monocytic (monoblasts, promonocytes, and monocytes). In acute monoblastic leukaemia, 80% or more of all monocytic cells are monoblasts. In monocytic leukaemia, predominant monocytic cells are promonocytes. There is intense nonspecific esterase activity. There is variable expression of myeloid antigens (CD33, CD13, CD117). Markers of monocytic differentiation (CD14, CD36, CD64, CD11c) are positive.

- *Acute erythroid leukaemia (FAB synonym: AML M6):* These are characterised by predominant population of erythroblasts. There are two subtypes - *erythroleukaemia* (≥20% of nonerythroid cells are myeloblasts, and ≥50% of all nucleated cells are erythroblasts) and *pure erythroid leukaemia* (predominant, i.e. ≥80% of marrow cells are erythroblasts, with no significant myeloblastic component). In erythroleukaemia, erythroblasts are bizarre-looking with bi-and tri-nucleate forms and megaloblastic nuclear features. Cytoplasmic vacuoles are frequently seen. Erythroblasts are commonly observed in peripheral blood. Cytochemically, PAS stain is positive in erythroblasts (in a diffuse or block-like manner), iron stain may show ring sideroblasts and MPO stain is positive in myeloblasts. Erythroblasts react with monoclonal antibodies against glycophorin A.

- *Acute megakaryoblastic leukaemia (FAB synonym: AML M7):* In this type, megakaryoblasts are 20% or more in bone marrow. This type is usually characterised by marked bone marrow fibrosis and therefore marrow aspiration is difficult to obtain. Bone marrow biopsy is often necessary. Megakaryoblasts are either small or round with scanty cytoplasm and coarse chromatin (resembling lymphoblasts) or are medium-to-large with fine chromatin and prominent 1 to 3 nucleoli. Blasts may show distinct cytoplasmic blebs or pseudopod formation. In peripheral blood, fragments of megakaryoblasts, micromegakaryocytes, or dysplastic large platelets are seen. Cytochemically, blasts are negative for myeloperoxidase. The specific cytochemical stain is platelet peroxidase that needs electron microscopy for its demonstration. Immunologic markers for platelet glycoprotein IIb/IIIa and Factor VIII-related antigen are positive. The megakaryoblasts express CD41 (glycoprotein IIb/IIIa) and/or CD61 (glycoprotein IIIa).

- *Acute basophilic leukaemia:* This is a very rare type with basophilic differentiation. Blasts contain basophilic granules and characteristically show positive metachromatic staining with toluidine blue.
- *Acute panmyelosis with myelofibrosis:* This is a very rare type characterised by proliferation of all the major myeloid cell lines (granulocytic, erythroid, and megakaryocytic) with predominance of immature cells along with fibrosis of bone marrow.
- *Myeloid sarcoma:* This is an isolated tumour mass composed of myeloblasts or immature myeloid cells occurring in an extramedullary site. It may precede or occur simultaneously with AML, myeloproliferative disorder, or myelodysplastic syndrome. It may be a sign of relapse in a treated case of AML.

Laboratory Features of AML

Peripheral Blood Examination

Anaemia is common and is normocytic and normochromic with low reticulocytes. Total leucocyte count may be low or markedly raised. Blasts are usually present in peripheral blood (Fig. 5.11). Absolute granulocyte count is always low. Morphologic abnormalities of neutrophils such as Pelger-Huet cells and hypogranular forms may be seen. Thromobocytopaenia is commonly present. Platelets are often large and bizarre.

Bone Marrow Examination

Bone marrow examination is necessary for diagnosis and classification of AML. The diagnosis of AML requires 20% or more blasts in all nucleated cells in bone marrow. Bone marrow is hypercellular. However, older patients with AML may present with hypocellular marrow; in these cases interstitium of bone marrow shows blast cells. Normal haematopoietic elements are severely reduced.

Cytochemistry
(See also "Acute Leukaemias—Diagnosis and Classification")

With careful morphological examination of blood and bone marrow aspirations smears, many cases of AML and ALL can be correctly diagnosed. Comparative morphological features of myeloblasts and lymphoblasts are shown in Figure 5.2 and Table 5.12. Additional studies (cytochemistry and immunophenotyping) are required if morphological features are equivocal.

Myeloperoxidase stain is used for identification of primary granules in myeloid precursors and is an important stain for diagnosis of AML M1, M2, M3, and M4 (Fig. 5.4). In the early stage, myeloperoxidase is formed in perinuclear area which needs ultrastructural examination for its demonstration.

The staining reactions with Sudan black B and chloroacetate esterase are mostly similar to myeloperoxidase.

Nonspecific esterase activity (using alpha naphthyl acetate esterase) is positive in AML M4 and M5 (monocytic component) and is sensitive to sodium fluoride (see Figs 5.5 and 5.6).

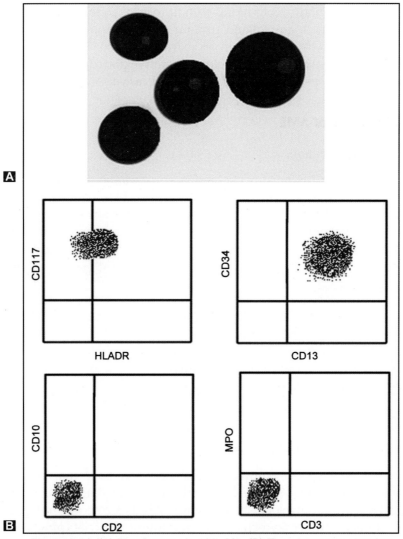

Figure 5.11: (A) Blood smear in AML M0, (B) Flow cytometry showing HLADR+, CD117+, CD13+. CD34+, CD10-, CD2-, MPO-, and CD3-blasts

In AML M6, erythroblasts show granular positivity with PAS. Iron stain usually reveals ringed sideroblasts. Myeloperoxidase is positive in myeloblastic component.

Demonstration of platelet peroxidase in AML M7 requires electron microscopic examination.

Cytochemical reactions in different types of AML are listed in Table 5.5.

Immunophenotyping (Table 5.15)

See also under "Acute Leukaemias—Diagnosis and Classification")

In AML, immunophenotyping is mainly necessary for (1) diagnosis of AML M0, M6, and M7; and (2) for distinction of AML M0 from ALL.

Cytogenetic Analysis

Cytogenetic abnormalities are common in AML (Table 5.16). In the recent WHO classification, syndromes of AML have been characterised with recurrent genetic abnormalities that correlate with clinical features, morphology, response to therapy, and overall prognosis. Two main types of cytogenetic abnormalities are observed in AML: (1) structural rearrangements (translocations or inversions), and (2) gain or loss of whole or part of a chromosome. Genetic analysis by a sensitive method (like reverse transcriptase-polymerase chain reaction) should be carried out in all newly diagnosed cases before beginning therapy because of their prognostic and therapeutic relevance.

The genetic abnormalities play a major role in the pathogenesis of AML.

Table 5.15: Immunophenotyping in AML

Antigen	AML subtype (FAB)							
	M0	M1	M2	M3	M4	M5	M6	M7
1. Primitive stem cell								
• CD34	+	+	±	−	−	−	−	±
• HLADR	+	+	±	−	+	+	±	±
2. Myeloid								
• CD13	+	+	+	+	+	+	+	±
• CD33	+	+	+	+	+	+	+	±
3. Monocytic								
• CD14	−	−	−	−	+	+	−	−
• CD64	−	−	−	−	+	+	−	−
4. Erythroid								
• Glycophorin A	−	−	−	−	−	−	+	−
5. Megakaryocytic								
• CD41, CD61	−	−	−	−	−	−	−	+

Table 5.16: Genetic abnormalities in AML

Chromosomal abnormality	Prognosis	WHO subtype	FAB subtype
1. t(8;21)(q22;q22)	Favourable	AML with t(8;21)(q22;q22); *(RUNX1-RUNX1T1)*	AML M2
2. inv(16)(p13q22) or t(16;16) (p13;q22)	Favourable	AML with abnormal bone marrow eosinophils inv(16)(p13q22) or t(16;16) (p13;q22)*(CBFβ/MYH11)*	AML M4 Eo
3. t(15;17)(q22;q12)	Favourable	Acute promyelocyte leukaemia t(15;17) (q22;q12)*(PML/RARα)*	AML M3
4. Abnormalities of 11q23	Unfavourable	AML with t(9;11)(p22;q23);*MLLT3-MLL*	AML M4, M5
5. -5, 5q-,-7, 7q-, +8, +9, +11, 11q-, 12p-	Unfavourable	1. AML with multilineage dysplasia 2. AML, therapy related	-

Cytogenetically normal AML (CN AML): A significant proportion of patients (45%) with AML have normal cytogenetics. This is called as CN AML. Such patients commonly show following gene mutations: *NPM1* (favourable prognosis), *FLT3* (poor prognosis with *FLT3-ITD*) and *CEBPA* (favourable prognosis). It should be noted that patients with favourable cytogenetic risk category may still harbour mutations like *FLT3-ITD* which impart adverse prognosis.

Morphology, immunophenotyping and genetic features of different types of AML are shown in Figures 5.11 to 5.14.

Differential Diagnosis

Leukaemoid Reaction

Presence of immature white blood cells in peripheral blood may be due to non-leukaemic causes, e.g. infections, acute haemolysis, or other infiltrative diseases of the bone marrow. In leukaemoid reaction, total leucocyte count is moderately increased and blast cells rarely exceed 5%. The whole range of granulocytic maturation is seen. In infections, toxic changes in neutrophils are evident. Clinical features of the causative disorder may be obvious. In difficult cases, cytogenetic analysis may be helpful.

Myelodysplastic Syndrome (MDS)

Differentiation of AML from MDS depends on proportion of myeloblasts in the bone marrow. In AML, myeloblasts are ≥20%, while in MDS they are <20%. (See classification of AML).

Acute Lymphoblastic Leukaemia

AML M0 and AML M7 should be differentiated from ALL (Table 5.12).

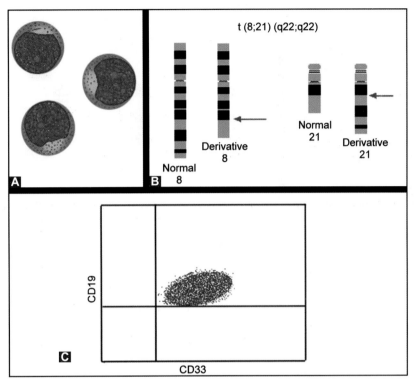

Figure 5.12: AML with t(8;21)(q22;q22). (A) Blood smear showing blasts with abundant large pink granules, basophilic cytoplasm, perinuclear hof, and thin Auer rod; (B) Diagrammatic representation of t(8;21)(q22;q22); (C) Flow cytometry showing expression of CD33 and aberrant expression of CD19. Other markers that are positive but not shown are CD13 and CD34

Blast Crisis of Chronic Myelogenous Leukaemia (CML)

It may be difficult to differentiate AML from blast crisis of CML if previous history is absent. Marked splenomegaly, basophilia, and Philadelphia chromosome are suggestive of chronic myelogenous leukaemia.

Prognostic Factors in AML

In AML, cytogenetic abnormalities and age are the major prognostic determinants. Depending on the risk of relapse, three prognostic categories are defined in AML as shown in Box 5.8.

Box 5.8   Risk groups of AML according to karyotype
• **Favourable:** t(8;21), t(15;17), inv(16)t(16;16)
• **Intermediate:** Normal karyotype, +8, +21, -Y, t(9;11)
• **Unfavourable:** -5, -7, 5q-, 7q-, inv(3), t(6;9), t(9;22), complex karyotype (3 or more chromosomal abnormalities).

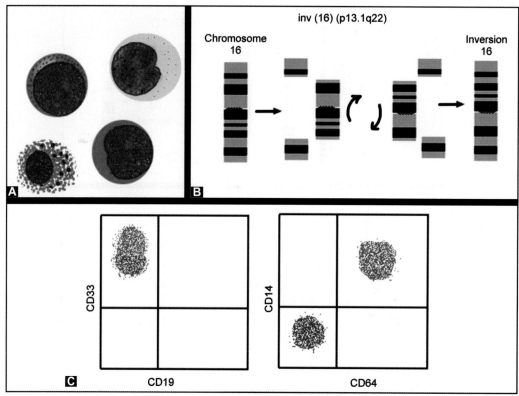

Figure 5.13: AML with inv(16)(p13.1q22). (A) Blood smear showing myelomonocytic appearance and abnormal eosinophils containing large, basophilic granules. (B) Diagrammatic representation of inv(16) (p13.1q22). (C) Representative flow cytometry graphs showing myeloblasts (orange) positive for CD33 and negative for CD19, CD14 and CD64; and monocytic cells (blue) positive for CD33, CD14, and CD64

Poor prognostic factors in AML are age >60 years; chromosomal abnormalities such as monosomies of chromosomes 5 or 7, deletion of long arm of chrosome 5, and complex chromosomal abnormalities; elevated lactate dehydrogenase; hyperleucocytosis (TLC>1,00,000/cmm); secondary AML; and AML with myelodysplasia.

Treatment

Forms of therapy in AML are listed in Box 5.9.

Box 5.9   Forms of therapy in AML

- Remission induction (Daunorubicin + Cytosine arabinoside)
- Post-remission therapy- Options:
  - Consolidation therapy (High dose cytosine arabinoside)
  - Intensive chemo- or chemoradio-therapy followed by haematopoietic stem cell transplantation (autologous or allogeneic).

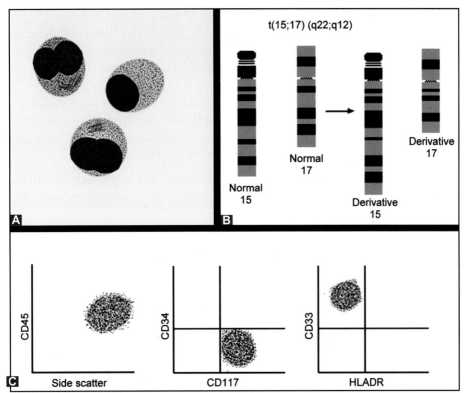

Figure 5.14: (A) Promyelocytes showing numerous azurophil granules, multiple Auer rods, and typical bilobed nucleus; (B) Diagrammatic representation of t(15;17)(q22;q12); (C) Dot plots of flow cytometry showing positivity for CD117, CD33 and negativity for CD34 and HLADR

Chemotherapy

Remission induction: The aim of therapy in AML is induction of complete remission (i.e. to eradicate the leukaemic cells and restore normal haematopoiesis). Criteria for complete remission are shown in Box 5.10.

The drug combination most commonly employed for this purpose is daunorubicin (3 daily infusions) and cytosine arabinoside (continuous infusion for 7 days); this regimen is commonly called as "7 and 3" regimen. Complete remission is usually

---

Box 5.10   Criteria for complete remission (CR)

- <5% of blasts in a normocellular bone marrow
- Return of peripheral blood counts to normal
  - Neutrophils>1500/cmm
  - Platelets>1,00,000/cmm
  - Haemoglobin>10.0 g/dl
- Disappearance of signs and symptoms

(Note: The term 'complete remission' is not synonymous with cure and blast cells may be demonstrated by a sensitive molecular technique).

achieved in about 70% of patients who are below 60 years of age. However, significant number of leukaemic cells persist (which are below the level of detection by conventional methods) that cause subsequent relapse if post-remission therapy is not administered. Due to persistent toxicity of induction therapy, many patients may not be able to receive post-remission therapy.

In addition to "7 and 3" therapy, additional (initial) therapy in acute promyelocytic leukaemia is all-trans retinoic acid that induces differentiation of abnormal promyelocytes to mature cells and reduces risk of early death from bleeding. Newer agent for acute promyelocytic leukaemia is arsenic trioxide.

Post-remission therapy: After achieving remission, further intensive therapy is essential for eradication of residual leukaemic cells and to prevent relapse. Options for post-remission therapy are:

a. *Intensive consolidation therapy:* High dose cytosine arabinoside is commonly used.
b. *Haematopoietic stem cell transplantation:* Disease-free survival of 40 to 60% is reported with allogeneic haematopoietic stem cell transplantation (HSCT) from a sibling donor in young patients during first remission. As compared to conventional chemotherapy, the risk of relapse is reduced to about 20%. High-dose marrow ablative therapy and graft-versus-leukaemia effect (eradication of residual leukaemic cells by donor T lymphocytes) are responsible for low-risk of subsequent relapse, as compared to other forms of therapy. Long-term survival is reported in about 30% of patients with AML who are treated with HSCT during second remission or first relapse. Therefore in AML, HSCT during first remission is a better option. However, high-dose cytotoxic chemotherapy used for marrow ablation is extremely toxic, and procedure-related mortality can occur due to severe infections (due to immunosuppression) and graft versus-host disease. Therefore, allogeneic BMT is usually reserved for younger patients.

With marrow ablative therapy followed by autologous HSCT, relapse remains a major problem (due to contamination of autograft by leukaemic cells and lack of graft versus leukaemia effect).

Patients with favourable cytogenetic abnormalities are treated with intensive consolidation therapy following remission induction, while in younger patients with unfavourable cytogenetic abnormalities, more aggressive remission induction therapy followed by haematopoietic stem cell transplantation should be considered (Box 5.11).

Treatment of acute promyelocytic leukaemia: All-trans retinoid acid (ATRA) along with concurrent anthracycline appears to be the safest treatment for acute promyelocytic

---

Box 5.11 Principles of therapy in AML

- t(8;21): Induction therapy followed by consolidation
- t(15;17): All-trans retinoic acid and induction therapy, followed by consolidation
- inv(16) or t(16;16): Induction therapy followed by consolidation
- Unfavourable cytogenetic abnormalities: Aggressive or newer therapies; haematopoietic stem cell transplantation in first remission.

leukaemia. Maintenance therapy is given with either ATRA or chemotherapy. Arsenic trioxide is helpful in patients who relapse or are refractory to ATRA.

The major toxic effect of ATRA is ATRA syndrome characterised by fever, fluid overload, hypoxia, and lung infiltrates. It is due to neutrophilic leukocytosis resulting from differentiation of promyelocytes followed by adhesion of differentiated cells to vascular endothelium of lung. Tratment is intravascular dexamethasone.

Supportive Therapy

Supportive therapy mainly consists of blood component replacement as required and management of infections. Platelet transfusions are indicated in treatment of haemorrhages due to thrombocytopaenia and for prevention of bleeding when platelet count falls below 20,000/cmm. Packed red cell transfusion should be given for symptomatic anaemia. Measures for prevention of infections include reverse isolation for neutropaenic patients, oral non-absorbable antibiotics for suppression of gastrointestinal organisms, etc. For fever in a neutropaenic patient, empiric broad-spectrum antibiotic should be initiated until underlying cause is identified. In patients with hyperleucocytosis, intensive hydration and alkalinisation of urine are indicated to prevent tumour lysis syndrome.

❑ BIBLIOGRAPHY

1. Arya LS. Acute lymphoblastic leukaemia: Current treatment concepts. Indian Pediatrics. 2000;37: 397-406.
2. Bennett JM, Catovsky D, Daniel MT, Flandrin G, Galton DAG, Gralnick HR, Sultan C. (FAB Cooperative Group): Proposals for the classification of the acute leukaemias. Br J Haematol. 1976;33: 451-58.
3. Bennett JM, Catovsky D, Daniel MT, Flandrin G, Galton DAG, Gralnick HR, Sultan C. (FAB Cooperative Group): The morphological classification of acute lymphoblastic leukaemia: Concordance among observers and clinical correlations. Br J Haematol. 1981;47: 553-61.
4. Bennett JM, Catovsky D, Daniel MT, Flandrin G, Galton DAG, Gralnick HR, Sultan C. A variant form of hypergranular promyelocytic leukaemia. Ann Intern Med. 1980;92: 261.
5. Bennett JM, Catovsky D, Daniel MT, Flandrin G, Galton DAG, Gralnick HR, Sultan C. Criteria for diagnosis of acute leukaemia of megakaryocytic lineage (M7): A report of the French-American-British Co-operative Group. Ann Intern Med. 1985;103: 460-62.
6. Bennett JM, Catovsky D, Daniel MT, Flandrin G, Galton DAG, Gralnick HR, Sultan C. Proposal for the recognition of minimally differentiated acute myeloid leukaemia (AML M0). The FAB Cooperative Group. Br J Haematol. 1991;789: 325-29.
7. Betz BL, Hess JL. Acute myeloid leukemia diagnosis in the 21st century. Arch Pathol Lab Med. 2010; 134: 1427-33.
8. Devine SM, Larson RA. Acute leukemia in adults: Recent developments in diagnosis and treatment. CA. Cancer J Clin. 1994;44:326-52.
9. Devine SM, Larson RA. Acute leukemia in adults: Recent developments in diagnosis and treatment. CA: Cancer J Clin. 1994;44:326-52.
10. Greaves M. Science, medicine, and the future: Childhood leukaemia. BMJ. 2002;324:283-87.

11. Jaffe ES, Harris NL, Stein H, Vardiman JW (Eds). World Health Organization Classification of Tumours. Pathology and Genetics of Tumours of Hamatopoietic and Lymphoid Tissues. Lyon: IARC Press, 2001.

12. Liesner RJ, Goldstone AH. ABC of clinical haematology: The acute leukaemias. BMJ. 1997;314: 733.

13. Lowenberg B, Downing JR, Burnett A. Acute myeloid leukemia. N Engl J Med. 1999;341: 1051-62.

14. McKenna RW. Multifaceted approach to the diagnosis and classification of acute leukemia. Clin Chem. 2000; 46: 1252-59.

15. Pui C, Relling MV, Downing JR. Mechanisms of disease. Acute lymphoblastic leukemia. N Engl J Med. 2004;350; 1535-48.

16. Pui CH, Evans WE. Acute lymphoblastic leukemia. N Engl J Med. 1998;339:605-15.

17. Pui CH, Relling MV, Downinig JR. Acute lymphoblastic leukemia. N Engl J Med. 2004;350: 1535-48.

18. Rubnitz JE, Crist WM. Molecular genetics of childhood cancer: Implications for pathogenesis, diagnosis, and treatment. Pediatrics. 1997; 100: 101-8.

19. Rubnitz JE, Crist WM. Molecular genetics of childhood cancer: Implication for pathogenesis, diagnosis, and treatment. Pediatrics. 1997;100: 101-8.

20. Rubnitz JE, Pui CH. Childhood acute lymphoblastic leukemia. The Oncologist. 1997;2: 374-380.

21. Schrappe M. Prognostic factors in childhood acute lymphoblastic leukaemia. Indian J Pediatr. 2003;70: 817-24.

22. Swerdlow SH, Campo E, Harris NL, Jaffe ES, Pileri SA, Stein H, Thiele J, Vardiman JW (Eds): WHO classification of tumours of haematopoietic and lymphoid tissues. 4th Ed. Lyon. International Agency for Research on Cancer. 2008.

CHAPTER 6

Myelodysplastic Syndromes

Myelodysplastic syndromes (MDS) are a heterogeneous group of acquired, clonal stem cell disorders characterised by:
- Occurrence mainly in elderly individuals
- Dysplasia of one or more haematopoietic cell lines with resultant characteristic morphological abnormalities
- Ineffective erythropoiesis due to increased apoptosis, causing cytopaenia of one or more cell lines in peripheral blood, and
- Increased risk of transformation to acute myeloid leukaemia.

MDS was previously called as dysmyelopoietic syndrome, preleukaemic syndrome, smoldering acute leukemia, and oligoblastic leukaemia.

❏ PATHOGENESIS

MDS is a clonal disorder, which originates in a pleuripotent haematopoietic stem cell (Fig. 6.1).

Evolution of MDS appears to be a multistep process. The initial event is a somatic mutation at the level of stem cell that results in the formation of functionally and structurally defective blood cells having shortened survival. Increased blood cell proliferation in marrow together with enhanced apoptosis lead to ineffective erythropoiesis and peripheral cytopaenia. The defective clone in MDS has growth advantage over the normal haematopoietic cells so that it expands gradually and suppresses normal haematopoiesis. The phenotypic expression of the pathologic clone is variable and can manifest as abnormalities of erythrocytic, granulocytic, monocytic, or megakaryocytic cell lines.

Table 6.1: Causes of myelodysplastic syndrome

1. Primary (Idiopathic)
2. Secondary
   - Prior radiotherapy
   - Prior alkylating drug or epipodophyllotoxin therapy
   - Exposure to chemicals, e.g. benzene, organic solvents
   - Genetic predisposition, e.g. Down's syndrome, Fanconi's anaemia, neurofibromatosis type I.

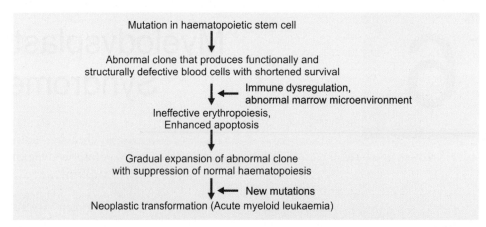

Figure 6.1: Pathogenesis of myelodysplastic syndrome

The pathological clone is unstable; new (second) genetic insults can superimpose on the original clone and initiate neoplastic transformation (acute myeloid leukaemia). With leukaemic transformation, ability of the stem cell to differentiate into mature cells is lost though it is capable of proliferation.

Previously, these disorders were called as "Preleukaemia". However, MDS are not considered as preleukaemic but as qualitative haematopoietic stem cell disorders. This is because many cases of MDS do not evolve into acute leukaemia. As the disease can be called as preleukaemic only retrospectively after its transformation to acute leukaemia, the term myelodysplastic syndrome appears to be more appropriate.

MDS may be primary (*de novo*) or secondary (e.g. occurring following exposure to chemo-or radio-therapy) (Table 6.1).

❑ CLASSIFICATION OF MDS

There are two classification systems for MDS:
- French-American-British (FAB) Classification (1982)
- World Health Organization Classification (2008)

French-American-British (FAB) Classification

In 1982, French-American-British (FAB) Co-operative Group proposed classification of MDS. The basis of this classification is type and degree of dysplasia, and percentage of ringed sideroblasts and of blast cells in bone marrow. According to FAB classification myelodysplastic syndromes are divided into five groups (Table 6.2).

World Health Organization (WHO) Classification

This classification is presented in Table 6.3. The WHO classification has set the dividing line between MDS and AML at 20% of blasts. In FAB classification, this demarcation is 30%. Also, chronic myelomonocytic leukaemia (included in FAB classification) is placed under the category of "Myelodysplastic/Myeloproliferative disorders" since it shares features of both the disorders.

❏ CLINICAL FEATURES

MDS usually occurs in elderly persons >60 years of age (median age at diagnosis being 70 years) and is more common in males. It is uncommon in children. Patients present with symptoms related to peripheral cytopaenias. These are fatigue, weakness, and dyspnoea due to anaemia; fever and infections due to neutropaenia; and easy bruising, petechiae, and other bleeding tendencies due to thrombocytopaenia. Hepatosplenomegaly is usually seen in chronic myelomonocytic leukaemia. A significant proportion of patients do not have clinical manifestations and are discovered incidentally on blood examination (as unexplained macrocytosis or cytopaenia).

History of treatment with chemotherapy (alkylating drugs) and/or radiotherapy for malignancies is obtained in secondary MDS.

❏ LABORATORY FEATURES

Peripheral Blood Examination

Cytopaenia such as anaemia, neutropaenia or thrombocytopaenia, either singly or in combination, is present in majority of patients.

Red Blood Cells

Anaemia is present in majority (80%) of patients. Oval macrocytosis is a typical feature. Reticulocyte count is low in relation to the level of anaemia. Other red cell abnormalities include basophilic stippling, hypochromia, dimorphic red cells, and megaloblastoid erythroblasts.

White Blood Cells

Neutropaenia is seen in 60% of patients. Both immature and abnormal granulocytes are present. Neutrophils are typically hypogranular and hypolobated (pseudo Pelger-Huet abnormality). Type I (non-granular) and type II (granular) blasts may be seen.

Table 6.2: FAB Classification and laboratory features of primary myelodysplastic syndromes

Category	Blasts (blood)	Blasts (marrow)	Ringed sideroblasts	Comments
1. Refractory anaemia (RA)	<1%	<5%	<15%	Anaemia with dyserythropoiesis predominant; macrocytosis
2. Refractory anaemia with ringed sideroblasts (RARS)	<1%	<5%	≥15%	Dimorphic anaemia
3. Refractory anaemia with excess blasts (RAEB)	<5%	5–20%	Variable	Bi- or tri-cytopaenia, trilineage dysplasia
4. Refractory anaemia with excess of blasts in transformation (RAEB-T)	≥5%	21–30%	Variable	Auer rods± (in the presence of Auer rods, diagnosis is RAEB-T even if blasts are <20%
5. Chronic myelomonocytic leukaemia	<5%	1–20%	Variable	Monocytosis>1000/cmm, hepatosplenomegaly

Table 6.3: World Health Organization classification of myelodysplastic syndromes, 2008

Type	Cytopaenia	Blast % (Blood)	Blast % (Marrow)	Dysplasia	Other
1. Refractory cytopaenia with unilineage dysplasia (Refractory anaemia, refractory neutropaenia, refractory thrombocytopaenia)	Unicytopaenia or bicytopaenia	<1	<5	Erythroid, granulocytic, or megakaryocytic	<15% ringed sideroblasts
2. Refractory anaemia with ringed sideroblasts	Anaemia	<1	<5	Erythroid	≥15%
3. Refractory cytopaenia with multilineage dysplasia	Bi- or pan-cytopaenia	<1	<5	≥2 myeloid lineages	No auer rods; ringed sideroblasts < or ≥15%; <1×10⁹/L monocytes
4. Refractory anaemia with excess blasts-1	≥1 cell line	2–4	5–9	Uni- or multi-lineage	No auer rods; <1×10⁹/L monocytes
5. Refractory anaemia with excess blasts-2	≥1 cell line	5–19	10–19	Uni- or multi-lineage	Auer rods±; <1×10⁹/L monocytes
6. Myelodysplastic syndrome-unclassifiable	Cytopaenia(s)	≤1	<5	≥1 myeloid lineages but in <10% of cells of each lineage	Specific MDS-related cytogenetic abnormality present
7. MDS associated with isolated del(5q)	Anaemia	<1	<5	Hypolobated megakaryocytes	Deletion of 5q

Notes: (1) ≥10% of cells of at least one myeloid lineage (erythroid, granulocytic, megakaryocytic) should show dysplasia for diagnosis of MDS; (2) Ringed sideroblasts are defined as erythroblasts showing ≥10% iron granules encircling at least one-third diameter nucleus (Prussian blue stain)

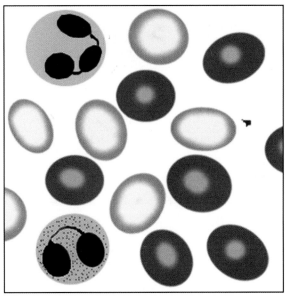

Figure 6.2: Peripheral blood smear from a patient with myelodysplastic syndrome showing dimorphic population of red cells (one normochromic and other hypochromic), a pseudo-Pelger-Huet cell on lower left, and a hypogranulated neutrophil on upper left

Platelets

Thrombocytopaenia is seen in one half of patients. Bleeding time is prolonged despite normal platelet count (due to platelet function defect). Other abnormalities include agranular platelets, giant platelets, micromegakaryocytes, and megakaryocyte fragments.

Blood smear in a case of myelodysplastic syndrome is shown in Figure 6.2.

Bone Marrow Examination

Bone Marrow Aspiration

Haematopoietic dysplasia is characteristic of MDS (Fig. 6.3). Erythroid hyperplasia with megaloblastoid maturation is a typical feature. Other dyserythropoietic features in erythroblasts include nuclear budding, multinuclearity, nuclear fragmentation, internuclear bridging, bizarre shapes, multilobation of nuclei, Howell-Jolly bodies, and cytoplasmic changes like PAS-positivity and uneven cytoplasmic staining. Iron stain (Prussian blue reaction) may reveal ringed sideroblasts (iron granules are present in mitochondria surrounding the nucleus). In granulocytic series, myeloid precursors are increased in number. Other abnormalities include—small size, nuclear hyposegmentation (pseudo-Pelger-Huet anomaly) or hypersegmentation (ring nuclei), hypogranulation, and deficiency of myeloperoxidase. Abnormalities in megakaryocytes include micromegakaryocytes, megakaryocytes with non-lobulated nuclei, and megakaryocytes with multiple separate nuclei.

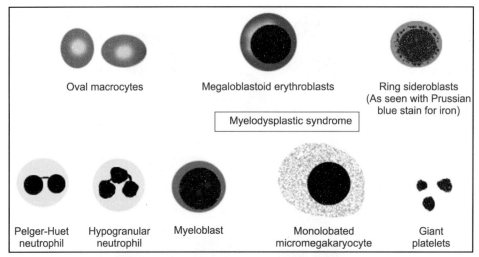

Figure 6.3: Some characteristic morphological abnormalities in MDS

Bone Marrow Biopsy

a. Bone marrow biopsy is necessary for assessment of cellularity. Bone marrow is hypercellular or normocellular in majority of patients. Some patients have hypocellular bone marrow. Hypocellularity is often seen in secondary MDS following cytotoxic chemotherapy.

b. Immature cells such as myeloblasts and promyelocytes are present in the centre of the marrow spaces away from the vascular structures rather than along the endosteum. This has been called as abnormal localisation of immature precursors (ALIP). ALIP is positive if three or more foci of immature precursors are present. ALIP is a feature of high-grade lesion such as RAEB. ALIP is associated with increased risk of progression to AML.

c. Bone marrow fibrosis, which is more common in secondary MDS, is assessed on bone marrow biopsy.

Cytogenetic Analysis

Non-random, clonal chromosomal abnormalities are observed in 50% of patients with primary MDS and in 80% of patients with secondary MDS. In contrast to AML, chromosomal abnormalities in MDS are numerical (i.e. loss or gain of chromosomal material) rather than structural (i.e. translocations). Common cytogenetic abnormalities in MDS include: -5, 5q-,-7,7q-, 20q-, +8, loss of X or Y chromosome, and 17p-.

Presence of a clonal chromosomal abnormality strongly favours the diagnosis of MDS over reactive conditions (Box 6.1). Patients of MDS who have complex chromosomal abnormalities (i.e. abnormality of >3 chromosomes) have poor prognosis with increased risk of progression to AML. Patients with normal or near-normal karyotype have better survival. Certain cytogenetic abnormalities are associated with

> **Box 6.1**   Role of cytogenetics in myelodysplastic syndrome
>
> - Confirmation of clonal nature of the disorder, thus distinguishing MDS from reactive disorders
> - Presumptive diagnosis of MDS in the presence of persistent unexplained cytopaenia but in the absence of conclusive morphologic features if a specific cytogenetic abnormality listed below is present:
>   - Unbalanced: -7 or del 7q, -5 or del 5q, i(17q) or t(17p), -13 or del 13q, del 11q, del 12p or t(12p), del 9q, idic (X)(q13)
>   - Balanced: t(11;16)(q23;p13.3), t(3;21)(q26.2;q22.1), t(1;3)(p36.3;q21.2), t(2;11)(p21;q23), inv(3) (q21q26.2), t(6;9)(p23;q34)
>   - Complex: ≥3 of above abnormalities
> - Prognosis and selection of optimal treatment
> - Documentation of additional cytogenetic abnormalities (in addition to existing) may indicate evolution to AML.

> **Box 6.2**   Typical diagnostic features of myelodysplastic syndromes
>
> - Persistent unexplained cytopaenia in an older adult
> - Dysplasia in ≥ 10% of cells in at least one myeloid lineage (erythroid, granulocytic, megakaryocytic)
> - Blasts < 20% in blood or bone marrow
> - Presence of a typical cytogenetic abnormality
> - Monocyte count $<1 \times 10^9/L$ (for exclusion of chronic myelomonocytic leukaemia).

distinctive clinical and haematological features. The 5q- abnormality is associated with a distinctive clinical syndrome; this entity is characterised by occurrence mainly in elderly women, presence of monolobulated megakaryocytes in bone marrow, increased platelets with giant forms, macrocytic anaemia, and favourable prognosis. In addition, some cytogenetic abnormalities are more consistently observed in specific FAB subgroups. Although loss of chromosomal material is frequent, the genes affected have not been identified so far.

❑ DIFFERENTIAL DIAGNOSIS

Typical diagnostic features of MDS are shown in Box 6.2.

In elderly subjects with RA, megaloblastic anaemia due to nutritional deficiency (vit B_{12} or folate) should be excluded since morphological features in both the conditions are similar. A therapeutic trial should always be given even if vitamin levels are normal. Other causes of dyshaematopoiesis which should be distinguished are exposure to toxic chemicals, heavy metals, or chemotherapy; inflammatory or neoplastic disease; alcohol-induced sideroblastic anaemia; and HIV infection.

Differentiation from AML has been considered earlier under AML.

MDS should also be distinguished from aplastic anaemia if bone marrow is hypocellular, congenital dyserythropoietic anaemia in children, and acute myelomonocytic leukaemia.

❑ PROGNOSIS

All patients with MDS have reduced life expectancy as compared to age- and sex-matched controls. Median survival and progression to AML are affected by FAB (Table 6.4) or WHO subtype. High-grade lesion such as RAEB has the worst prognosis with poor median survival and high-risk of progression to AML. A scoring system based on number of blasts in bone marrow, karyotype, and cytopaenias has been introduced recently that has prognostic importance (Table 6.5).

Apart from transformation to AML, patients may die from complications of cytopaenias (infections, bleeding) or from unrelated disease.

❑ TREATMENT

No safe and effective form of therapy is available for MDS as yet. Patients with RA and RARS have low incidence, while patients with RAEB-1 and RAEB-2 have higher incidence of transformation to AML. However, even in the absence of progression to AML, patients have increased morbidity and mortality due to complications related to various cytopaenias. Treatment in MDS should be individualised. Treatment options in MDS are summarised below.

Table 6.4: Median survival and risk of AML in MDS

WHO subtype	Median survival (months)	Transformation to AML (%)
RA	69	6
RARS	69	1–2
RCMD	33	11
RCMD-RS	32	11
RAEB-1	16	25
RAEB-2	9	33
MDS-U	Unknown	Unknown
5q-	145	<10

Table 6.5: International Prognostic Scoring System for myelodysplastic syndromes

Score	Bone marrow blasts%	Cytogenetics	Cytopaenia (Hb < 10 g/dl, neutrophils < 1500/µl, platelets < 1 lac/µl)
0	<5	Good (normal, -Y, 5q-, 20q-)	Absent or unilineage
0.5	5–10	Intermediate (other)	≥2 lineages
1.0	-	Poor (complex, chromosome 7 anomalies)	-
1.5	11–20	-	-
2.0	21–30*	-	-

Based on FAB classification of MDS; Risk groups: 0:Low; 0.5–1.0: Intermediate-1; 1.5–2.0:Intermediate-2; ≥2.5:High.
*: Considered as AML in WHO classification

1. Supportive therapy: This consists of red cell transfusions, platelet transfusions and antibiotic as required. Iron chelating therapy is instituted in multiply transfused patients as ineffective erythropoiesis and frequent red cell transfusions will cause iron overload and parenchymal damage. Recently haematopoietic growth factors (erythropoietin and G-CSF) are being tried to improve cytopaenias in MDS patients. Supportive therapy is indicated as an adjunctive therapy for all risk groups, elderly patients with severe co-morbidities, and low risk disease, and in patients not willing for aggressive forms of therapy.

2. Hypomethylating agents (5-azacytidine, decitabine) are indicated in intermediate-1 or high-risk disease.

3. Lenalidomide is useful in MDS with 5q- abnormality.

4. Immuosuppressive therapy: Antilymphocyte globulin and/or cyclosporine is indicated in hypocellular MDS with normal cytogenetics and no excess blasts.

5. High dose AML-like chemotherapy: This may be tried in young patients with high-risk MDS with good performance status and non-availability of HLA-identical sibling donor. Some of the patients treated with chemotherapy can achieve remission.

6. Haematopoietic stem cell transplantation: The only curative form of therapy is haematopoietic stem cell transplantation. Transplantation may be considered in younger patients who have high-risk disease, good performance status, no co-morbidities, and HLA-identical sibling donor; this form of therapy may result in long-term disease-free survival and cure.

❑ BIBLIOGRAPHY

1. Bennett JM, Catovsky D, Daniel MT, Flandrin G, Gralnick HR, Sultan C. Proposals for the classification of myelodysplastic syndromes. Br J Haematol. 1982;51: 189-199.

2. Beris P. Primary clonal myelodysplastic syndromes. Semin Hemato.l 1989;26: 216-233.

3. Besa EG. Myelodysplastic syndromes (Refractory anemia). A perspective of the biologic, clinical, and therapeutic uses. Med Clin North Am. 1992;76: 599-617.

4. British Committee for Standards in Haematology: Guidelines for the diagnosis and therapy of adult myelodysplastic syndromes. Br J Haematol. 2003;120:187-200.

5. Cheson BD. The myelodysplastic syndromes. The Oncologist. 1997;2:28-39.

6. Greenberg P, Cox C, LeBeau MM, et al. International scoring system for evaluating prognosis in myelodysplastic syndromes. Blood. 1997; 89: 2079-2088.

7. Heaney ML, Golde DW. Medical Progress. Myelodysplasia. N Engl J Med. 1999;340:1649.

8. Jaffe ES, Harris NL, Stein H, Vardiman JW (Eds). World Health Organisation Classification of Tumours. Pathology and Genetics of Tumours of Haematopoietic and Lymphoid Tissues. Lyon: IARC Press, 2001.

9. Koeffler HP. Introduction: Myelodysplastic syndromes. Semin Hematol. 1996;33: 87-94.

10. Koeffler HP. Myelodysplastic syndromes (pre-leukaemia). Semin Hematol. 1986;23: 284-299.

11. Kouides PA and Bennett JM. Morphology and classification of the myelodysplastic syndromes and their pathologic variants. Semin Hematol. 1996;33: 95-110.

12. Nimer SD. Myelodysplastic syndromes. Blood. 2008; 111: 4841-4851.

13. Swerdlow SH, Campo E, Harris NL, Jaffe ES, Pileri SA, Stein H, Thiele J, Vardiman JW (Eds): WHO classification of tumours of haematopoietic and lymphoid tissues. 4th ed. Lyon. International Agency for Research on Cancer. 2008.

14. Tefferi A, Vardiman JW. Myelodysplastic syndromes. N Engl J Med. 2009; 361: 1872-85.

15. Tricot G, Dewolf-Peeters C, Vlietinck R, Verwilghen RL. Bone marrow histology in myelodysplastic syndromes II. Prognostic value of abnormal localization of immature precursors in MDS. Br J Haematol. 1984;58:217-225.

16. Zoumbos NC. The pathogenesis of myelodysplastic syndromes. Haema. 2001;4:151-157.

CHAPTER

7

Myeloproliferative Neoplasms

These are clonal neoplastic disorders of pluripotent haematapoietic stem cell characterised by excessive proliferation of one or more of the myeloid cell lines like granulocytic, erythroid, and megakaryocytic. The WHO classification of myeloproliferative neoplasms is presented in Table 7.1.

The characteristic features of myeloproliferative neoplasms are:

- They are clonal haematopoietic stem cell disorders with origin from a single stem cell
- Usually one cell line predominates in a given disorder
- There is a close relationship between different disorders with interconversions, overlapping manifestations, and progression to myelofibrosis and acute leukaemia
- Maturation of blood cells is relatively normal, so that mature cells (red cells, granulocytes, or platelets) are increased in number
- Enlargements of spleen and liver are common.

Myeloproliferative neoplasms should be distinguished from one another because of different treatment approaches of each.

Table 7.1: World Health Organization classification of myeloproliferative neoplasms (2008)

1. Chronic myelogenous leukaemia, *BCR-ABL* positive
2. Chronic neutrophilic leukaemia
3. Polycythaemia vera
4. Primary myelofibrosis
5. Essential thrombocythaemia
6. Chronic eosinophilc leukaemia, not otherwise specified
7. Mastocytosis
8. Myeloproliferative neoplasm, unclassifiable

❑ PATHOGENESIS

The myeloproliferation is the result of a genetic abnormality in a haematopoietic stem cell. Clonal nature of these disorders is established by glucose-6-phosphate dehydrogenase (G6PD) isoenzyme studies in female heterozygotes and cytogenetic analysis.

Gene for G6PD enzyme is located on X chromosome. Various isoenzymes of G6PD exist of which most common is G6PD B. G6PD A variant is more common in Africa. About one-third of black women are heterozygous for G6PD B or G6PD A. During embryogenesis there is random inactivation of one X chromosome so that heterozygous females have two populations of cells—one with G6PD B and the other with G6PD A. As clonal disorders arise from a single stem cell, all the neoplastic cells contain either G6PD A or G6PD B enzyme. In myeloproliferative disorders, erythroid, myeloid, and megakaryocytic elements all contain a single G6PD enzyme (Fig. 7.1). This indicates that myeloproliferative disorders originate from a single pluripotent stem cell capable of producing erythroid, myeloid, and megakaryocytic cells. Fibroblasts are not part of the neoplastic clone in myeloproliferative disorders and their proliferation is reactive.

Non-random chromosomal abnormalities in myeloproliferative disorders, if present, are observed in all the haematopoietic cell lines (erythroid, myeloid, megakaryocytic, and B lymphocytic) but not in fibroblasts and other non-haematopoietic tissues.

At the molecular level, neoplastic transformation results from activation of tyrosine kinase signal transduction pathway. This is exemplified in chapter on chronic myeloid leukaemia.

❑ CHRONIC MYELOID LEUKAEMIA

Chronic myeloid leukaemia (CML) is a myeloproliferative neoplasm characterised by predominant proliferation of granulocytic cells. It is a clonal neoplastic haematopoietic

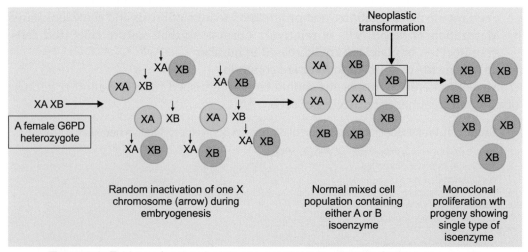

Figure 7.1: Evidence for clonal origin of a neoplasm in a female G6PD heterozygote

stem cell disorder as evidenced by involvement of all haematopoietic cell lines. The defining characteristic of CML is presence of Philadelphia chromosome and/ or *BCR/ABL* fusion gene in all the neoplastic cells. It is the most common of the myeloproliferative diseases.

Pathogenesis

CML is a clonal disorder and evidence for its origin from a single pluripotent haematopoietic stem cell is as follows:

i. A single G6PD isoenzyme is present in erythroid, granulocytic, and megakaryocytic elements, but not in fibroblasts or other somatic cells in females with CML who are heterozygous for G6PD enzyme;

ii. Presence of Philadelphia chromosome in granulocytic, monocytic, erythroid, and megakaryocytic cell lines, and sometimes also in lymphoid cells.

iii. Occurrence of lymphoid blast crisis in CML.

The characteristic cytogenetic abnormality in CML is Philadelphia (Ph') chromosome, which results from reciprocal translocation between chromosomes 9 and 22, i.e. t(9;22) (q34; q11). The Philadelphia chromosome refers to shortened chromosome 22; this was first described by investigators in Philadelphia and hence the name (Fig. 7.2). This translocation results in the fusion of *ABL* (Abelson leukaemia virus) gene on chromosome 9 with *BCR* (breakpoint cluster region) gene on chromosome 22. Ph' chromosome is present in 95% of patients with CML. However, abnormality of chromosome 22 at the molecular level (i.e. *BCR/ABL* gene rearrangement) is present in almost all patients with CML.

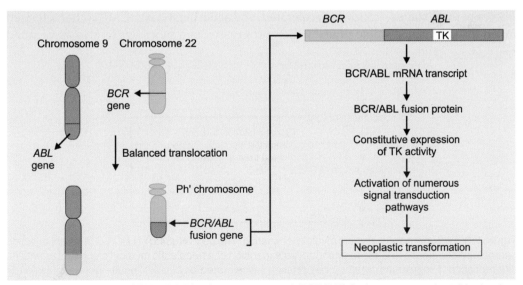

Figure 7.2: Formation of Philadelphia chromosome and *BCR/ABL* fusion gene product. Mechanism of leukaemogenesis is shown on right side. TK: tyrosine kinase

The tyrosine kinase activity resides in ABL protein; with juxtaposition of BCR sequences next to ABL, tyrosine kinase activity is constitutively activated. The site of breakpoint in *BCR* gene is variable, and therefore the size of BCR/ABL protein varies from 185 kDa to 230 kDa. Most patients with typical CML have 210 kDa fusion protein. The *BCR/ABL* fusion gene plays a central role in the pathogenesis of CML. The resultant BCR/ABL fusion protein is constitutively active tyrosine kinase, which is confined to the cytoplasm. The BCR/ABL protein activates a number of cytoplasmic and nuclear signal transduction pathways affecting cell growth and differentiation. The uncontrolled activity of BCR/ABL tyrosine kinase ultimately results in deregulation of cellular proliferation, decreased apoptosis, and poor adherence of leukaemic cells to bone marrow stroma (which causes CML cell to escape negative regulatory influences exerted by stromal cells).

During evolution to blast crisis, additional nonrandom chromosomal abnormalities occur (such as duplication of Ph' chromosome, +8, etc.) which are responsible for arrest in maturation and transformation to acute leukaemia.

Pathogenesis of CML is presented in Figure 7.3.

Incidence

CML accounts for 40% of all leukaemias in the Indian population. It is slightly more common in males, with median age at diagnosis being in the fifth and sixth decades of life.

Stages of CML

There are three stages—chronic, accelerated, and acute blast crisis. CML is characterised by an initial chronic stable phase which progresses to a more aggressive accelerated

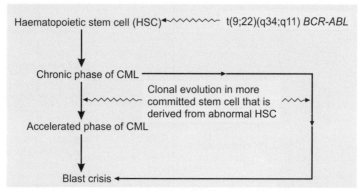

Figure 7.3: Pathogenesis of chronic myeloid leukaemia. The t(9;22)(q34;q11) *BCR-ABL* event affecting haematopoietic stem cell leads to uncontrolled expansion of a neoplastic myeloid clone that maintains differentiation. Progression to advanced phases (accelerated or blastic) results from acquisition of additional genetic abnormalities like additional Ph', +8, i(17), or +19 (termed clonal evolution). The additional genetic lesions in advanced stages cause arrest in maturation and expansion of blast population

phase and eventually to blast crisis within 3 to 5 years. In a significant proportion of patients, direct transformation from chronic phase to blastic phase occurs. In contrast to chronic phase, cells fail to mature in blast crisis. In some patients presentation is in the form of blast crisis without preceding chronic or accelerated phase.

1. **Chronic phase:** In this phase, leukaemic cells retain the capacity for differentiation and maturation and are largely able to function normally. The disease is responsive to chemotherapy and remains stable for variable period. The duration of this stage is 3 to 5 years.

2. **Accelerated phase:** In 70% of patients, chronic phase gradually evolves into accelerated phase. In this phase, leukaemic cells show increasing loss of differentiation and maturation, increased proliferation, and resistance to chemotherapy that controlled the chronic phase. Patient's disease becomes more aggressive and signs and symptoms of disease progression appear; majority of patients in this phase eventually progress to blast crisis within a span of few months.

3. **Blast crisis:** This occurs when there is transformation to acute leukaemia and the disease becomes extremely resistant to chemotherapy. Median survival is 2 to 6 months. About 30% of patients progress to blastic phase without intervening accelerated phase.

Chronic Phase of CML

Clinical features: Majority (85%) of patients with CML present in chronic phase. Median age at presentation is 50 years. Patient usually presents with generalised weakness, weight loss, night sweats and abdominal fullness (due to splenomegaly). Easy bruisability, and spontaneous bleeding such as purpura, petechiae, and mucous membrane bleeding can occur. The principal finding on physical examination is splenomegaly, which ranges in size from being just palpable to massive. Hepatomegaly is present in about half the patients. About 40% of patients are asymptomatic and are detected incidentally (abnormal white blood cell count).

Laboratory features:
   i. *Peripheral blood examination:* Anaemia is present in virtually all patients at diagnosis, and is usually mild to moderate in degree, and normocytic normochromic. There is minimal variation in size and shape of red cells. A few nucleated red cells are present in peripheral blood.
   Total leucocyte count is moderately to markedly raised and is commonly more than 1,00,000/cmm. Height of total leucocyte count is usually directly proportional to the size of spleen, basophil count, percentage of blast cells, and degree of anaemia. All stages of maturation from myeloblast to segmented neutrophils are present with 'peaks' of myelocytes and segmented neutrophils. In chronic phase, blast cells are less than 10%. Basophils and eosinophils are mildly increased. Basophilia is important for diagnosis of CML since it is rarely seen in any other disorder.

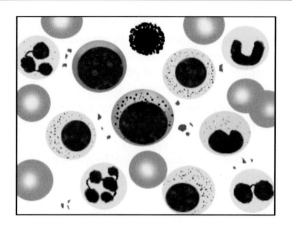

Figure 7.4: Blood smear in chronic myeloid leukaemia. All stages from myeloblast to segmented neutrophil are present. A basophil is present at the top

Mild to moderate thrombocytosis is present in most patients (Fig. 7.4).

ii. *Bone marrow examination:* Bone marrow aspiration reveals hypercellular marrow with markedly increased granulopoiesis. Cells of erythroid series are usually reduced in percentage. Myeloid : erythroid ratio is 10:1 to 50:1 (normal ratio is 2:1 to 4:1). Myeloblasts constitute less than 10%. Basophils, eosinophils, and monocytes are increased as in peripheral blood. Megakaryocytes are frequently increased in number and are typically smaller in size with hypolobated nuclei. Pseudo-Gaucher cells and sea-blue histiocytes may be observed due to increased turnover of cells.

Bone marrow aspiration is not essential for diagnosis of CML; however it is needed to exclude accelerated or blastic phase. Also, cytogenetic analysis for Ph' chromosome is more satisfactorily done on marrow cells than on peripheral blood. Bone marrow biopsy is helpful for assessment of myelofibrosis. Increased fibrosis is associated with severe anaemia, increase in the number of blast cells, and more rapid clinical course.

iii. *Neutrophil alkaline phosphatase (NAP) score:* Alkaline phosphatase is present in metamyelocytes, band cells, and segmented neutrophils. In this test naphthol AS phosphate (substrate) is converted by alkaline phosphatase in neutrophils to aryl naphtholamide which in turn combines with diazonium salt to form insoluble coloured precipitate. Intensity of colour reaction in neutrophils is graded 0 to 4+ in 100 neutrophils and values are added together to get the NAP score. Normal NAP score is 40 to 100. In chronic phase of CML, NAP in mature neutrophils is markedly decreased or absent. Increased NAP score is observed in leukaemoid reaction due to infections, polycythaemia vera, and agnogenic myeloid metaplasia with myelofibrosis. Therefore, NAP score can be used for differentiating CML from these conditions.

iv. *Cytogenetic analysis:* Cytogenetic analysis in CML serves to confirm the diagnosis. It also has prognostic importance. Cytogenetic analysis of bone marrow and peripheral blood shows a characteristic abnormality, the Ph' chromosome, in more than 95% of patients with CML (Fig. 7.5). Ph' chromosome is present in all haematopoietic cell lines, i.e. erythroid, granulocytic, monocytic, megakaryocytic, B lymphocytic, and in some cases T lymphocytic. In accelerated phase or blast crisis more chromosomal changes often develop such as duplication of Ph' chromosome, +8, +19, and –Y.

In some cases of CML, Ph' chromosome cannot be demonstrated by cytogenetic analysis. However, in most such patients rearrangement of *BCR/ABL* can be demonstrated by Southern blot analysis, fluorescent *in situ* hybridisation (Fig. 7.6), or polymerase chain reaction. Patients without Ph' chromosome but with *BCR/ABL* gene rearrangement have clinical and haematological features similar to Ph'-positive CML.

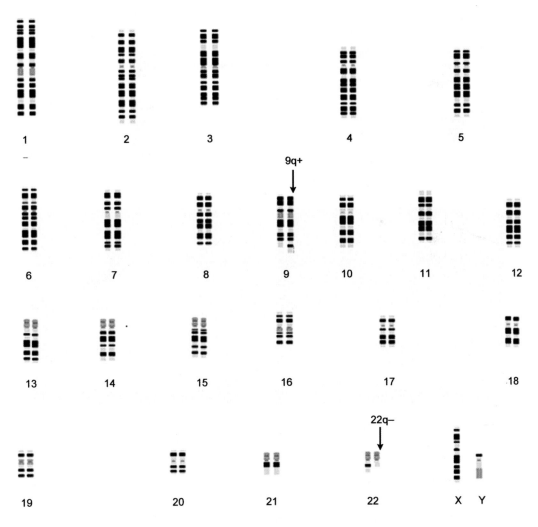

Figure 7.5: Karyogram of a patient with chronic myeloid leukaemia depicting t(9;22)(q34;q11.2). The shortened chromosme 22 (22q-) is Philadelphia chromosome

Accelerated Phase of CML

In this phase, blood cell counts and organomegaly become increasingly resistant to chemotherapy. According to WHO classification, accelerated phase is characterised by presence of one or more of the following features:

- Increased percentages of blast cells (10–19%) in peripheral blood and/or bone marrow

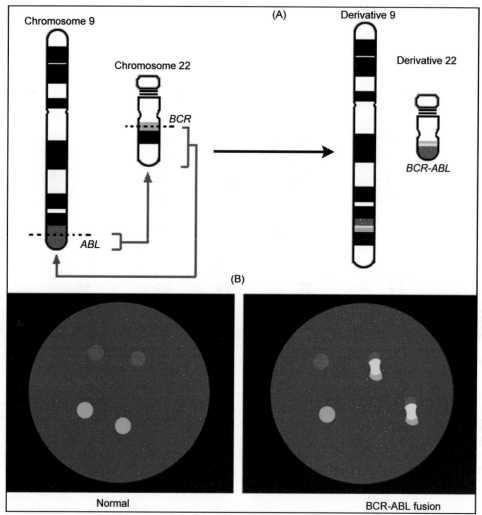

Figure 7.6: Fluorescent in situ hybridisation in chronic myeloid leukaemia. (A) Upper part of figure shows diagrammatic representation of t(9;22)(q34;q11) *BCR-ABL*. (B) Fluorescently labeled DNA probes (*ABL* on chromosome 9, *BCR* on chromosome 22) are hybridised onto interphase cells that have been attached to a glass slide. In the commonly used dual colour, dual fusion method, ABL probe is labeled with a red fluorophore and BCR with a green fluorophore. In a fusion gene product, both probes overlap and produce a yellow colour. The typical pattern seen in CML is 1R1G2F. 1R1G represents normal chromosome 9 (1 red) and 22 (1 green), respectively; 2F represents reciprocal exchange of material between *ABL* and *BCR* portions of genome

- Peripheral blood basophilia ≥20%
- Persistence of thrombocytopaenia (<1 lac/cmm) unrelated to therapy or persistent thrombocytosis (>10 lac/cmm) not responsive to therapy
- Progressive splenomegaly and increase in leucocyte count despite adequate treatment
- Cytogenetic evidence of clonal evolution, i.e. cytogenetic changes in addition to Ph' chromosome such as duplication of Ph' chromosome, trisomy 8, etc.

   Most of these patients eventually progress to blast crisis or acute leukaemia.

Blast Crisis

This represents acute leukaemic transformation. According to WHO classification, blast phase is diagnosed in the presence of one or more of the following:

- Blasts in peripheral blood or bone marrow ≥20%
- Blast proliferation at a site other than bone marrow
- Focal clustering of blasts in bone marrow.

   Blast crisis in CML may be myeloid (70%) or lymphoid (30%). Differentiation between myeloid and lymphoid blast crisis is important because of different treatment considerations.

   Typical laboratory features of CML are shown in Box 7.1. Differences between chronic, accelerated, and blast phases of CML are shown in Table 7.2.

Box 7.1 Typical laboratory features of chronic myelogenous leukaemia

Chronic phase
- Blood: Leucocytosis with granulocytes of all stages of maturation, myelocyte 'peak', basophilia, blasts<10%
- Bone marrow: Hypercellular; myeloid: erythroid ratio 10:1 to 20:1; granulocytic hyperplasia; dwarf megakaryocytes; blasts<10%; basophilia
- Laboratory features: Low LAP score; Increased vitamin B_{12}
- Cytogenetic analysis on marrow: t(9;22) in >95% cases
- Molecular analysis on marrow: *BCR-ABL* by FISH or PCR in 100% cases

Accelerated phase (WHO, 2008 criteria)
Any one of following:
- Blasts in blood or marrow: 10–19%
- Basophils in blood: ≥ 20%
- Persistent thrombocytosis not responding to therapy
- Persistent thrombocytopaenia not due to therapy
- Cytogenetic evolution: Additional Ph' chromosome, +8, i(17)
- Increasing TLC and/or splenomegaly not responding to therapy

Blast crisis (WHO, 2008)
Any one of following:
- Blasts in blood or bone marrow ≥20%
- Extramedullary blast proliferation.

Differential Diagnosis of CML

Chronic Phase

Diagnosis of CML is based on presence of splenomegaly, moderate to marked granulocytosis (TLC usually>1 lac per cmm) with presence of all stages of maturation, basophilia, decreased NAP score, and Ph' chromosome or *BCR/ABL* gene rearrangement on chromosome 22.

Chronic phase of CML should be distinguished from following conditions:

Leukaemoid reaction: Leukaemoid reaction can occur in infections, inflammation, and malignancy. In leukaemoid reactions due to infections or haemolysis, leucocytosis is usually modest and shift to left is usually up to metamyelocyte or myelocyte stage; however occasional blast may be seen. Underlying cause is frequently obvious. Other features favouring leukaemoid reaction are absence of splenomegaly or basophilia, presence of toxic granules in neutrophils (in infections), normal or increased NAP score, and absence of Ph' chromosome (Table 7.3).

Table 7.2: Differences between chronic, accelerated, and blast phases of chronic myelogenous leukaemia

Parameter	Chronic phase	Accelerated phase	Blast phase
1. Blast%	<10%	10–19%	≥20%
2. Basophils	<20%	≥20%	Variable
3. Leucocytosis, thrombocytosis, splenomegaly	Responsive to therapy	Not responsive to therapy	-
4. LAP score	Low	Increased	Increased
5. Extramedullary blast proliferation	Absent	Absent	May be present
6. Clonal evolution	-	Yes	-
7. First line therapy	Imatinib	Allogeneic stem cell transplantation preceded by tyrosine kinase inhibitor therapy	

Table 7.3: Differences between chronic myeloid leukaemia and leukaemoid reaction

Parameter	Chronic myeloid leukaemia	Leukaemoid reaction
1. Clinical features	Splenomegaly	As per underlying disease
2. Peripheral blood a. Leucocyte count b. Myelocyte and neutrophil 'peaks' c. Basophilia, eosinophilia, monocytosis d. 'Toxic' granules	 Usually >1,00,000/cmm Present Present Absent	 Usually <50,000/cmm Absent Absent Present
3. NAP score	Low	Normal or increased
4. Bone marrow examination	Trilineage hyperplasia	Myeloid hyperplasia
5. Genetic analysis	Ph' chromosome or *BCR/ABL* gene rearrangement	Normal

Other myeloproliferative disorders: In polycythaemia vera and myelofibrosis, in contrast to CML, leucocyte count is moderately raised, NAP score is normal or increased, and Ph' chromosome or *BCR/ABL* gene rearrangement is absent. Packed cell volume is markedly increased in polycythaemia vera while in CML it is normal or low. In myelofibrosis, peripheral blood smear shows marked anisopoikilocytosis, numerous nucleated red cells and tear-drop red cells; bone marrow shows marked myelofibrosis at diagnosis. Comparative features of common myeloproliferative neoplasms are shown in Table 7.4.

Chronic myelomonocytic leukaemia (CMML): In the WHO classification, this is included under myeloproliferative/myelodysplastic disorders. Clinically CMML usually presents with anaemia and splenomegaly in elderly persons. There is moderate leucocytosis, neutrophils and band forms are increased, and monocyte count is in excess of 1000/cmm. Bone marrow typically shows trilineage dysplasia and increase in monocytic cells that can be demonstrated by non-specific esterase reaction. Serum/urinary lysozyme is increased. Basophilia, Ph' chromosome, or *BCR/ABL* gene rearrangement are absent.

Table 7.4: Comparative features of common myeloproliferative neoplasms

Parameter	Chronic myelogenous leukaemia	Polycythaemia vera	Essential thrombocythaemia	Primary myelofibrosis
Age	40–60 yrs	50–70 yrs	50–60 yrs (second peak 30 years)	60–70 years
Sex	M>F	M>F	50–60 yrs: M=F 30 years: F>M	M>F
Splenomegaly	Moderate to massive	Mild to moderate	Absent or mild	Massive
Haemoglobin	Low	Raised	Normal	Low
Platelets	N, raised or low	Often raised	Persistently raised (>4.5 lac/µl)	Raised or low
LAP score	Low	Raised	Raised	Raised
Blood smear	Granulocytosis with cells of all stages in chronic phase; basophilia; neutrophil and myelocyte peak	Thick smear due to erythrocytosis	Thrombocytosis with marked variation in size	Leucoerythroblastic reaction
Bone marrow examination	Trilineage hyperplasia with granulocytic predominance; small and hypolobated megakaryocytes	Trilineage hyperplasia with erythroid predominance	Numerous dispersed, large, mature hyperlobated megakaryocytes	Predominant granulocytic hyperplasia; highly bizarre megakaryocytes in tight clusters
Bone marrow fibrosis	Variable	Increased in spent phase	Minimal or absent	Marked
Predominant cell line affected	Granulocytic	Erythroid	Megakaryocytic	Granulocytic and megakaryocytic
Mutation	*BCR-ABL* fusion	*JAK2V617F* (>95%)	*JAK2V617F* (50%); *MPL*	*JAK2V617F* (50%); *MPL*

Blast Crisis

Sometimes CML may present for the first time as blast crisis, in which case it may be difficult to distinguish it from acute leukaemia. Evidence favouring the former includes large spleen, basophilia, and Ph' chromosome or *BCR/ABL* gene rearrangement. It should be noted that Ph' chromosome can occur in some acute lymphoblastic leukaemias.

Course and Prognosis of CML

The chronic phase runs a stable course with a median duration of about 3.5 years, although the range is wide. The natural history of CML is progression from chronic phase to accelerated and blastic phases and development of increasing refractoriness to previous chemotherapy. The median survival of blast crisis is 2 to 6 months. Currently used cytotoxic chemotherapy (busulfan or hydroxyurea) does not affect the duration of survival or basic evolution of CML. With newer forms of treatment like IFN α, median survival times of 5 to 7 years have been reported. At diagnosis, prognostic factors associated with shorter duration of survival are – older age, large spleen and liver size, increased number of blasts, increased number of basophils, and fibrosis of bone marrow.

Treatment

CML was the first malignancy to be associated with a chromosomal abnormality and the first malignancy for which targeted molecular therapy became available as the treatment of choice.

The treatment of CML was revolutionised in 1998 when imatinib mesylate, a potent and specific inhibitor of tyrosine kinase, became available. It is the standard first-line treatment for newly diagnosed chronic phase CML. Eighty per cent of patients with CML present in chronic phase. Majority of patients achieve a complete haematologic response at 3 months and complete cytogenetic response at 6, 12, or 24 months. A complete haematologic response refers to (1) disappearance of all signs and symptoms of CML, (2) disappearance of palpable splenomegaly, (3) normalisation of total leucocyte count and platelet count, and (4) no immature cells (myelocytes, promyelocytes, blasts) on differential count. A complete cytogenetic response refers to no Philadelphia chromosome positive metaphases. Patients should be monitored for response at 3, 6, 12, and 18 months. Some patients taking imatinib may possibly be cured. The most common side effects of imatinib are nausea, periorbital swelling, oedema, rash, and myalgia.

For patients showing suboptimal response, options include imatinib dose escalation or alternate tyrosine kinase inhibitors like dasatinib or nilotinib.

Second line drugs for patients who cannot take imatinib include hydroxyurea and α-interferon.

For accelerated phase, dasatinib or nilotinib are recommended. For blast phase, tyrosine kinase inhibitor therapy either alone or in combination with chemotherapy followed by allogeneic haematopoietic transplantation is recommended.

Alllogeneic haematopoietic transplantation is the only curative form of therapy. Considering the risks of significant morbidity and mortality, it is reserved for young patients with an HLA-matched sibling donor and who show inadequate response to imatinib or who show disease progression to accelerated or blast phase.

❏ POLYCYTHAEMIA VERA

Syn: Polycythaemia rubra vera

Polycythaemia vera (PV) is a myeloproliferative neoplasm characterised by trilineage (granulocytic, erythroid, and megakaryocytic) hyperplasia in bone marrow with predominant involvement of erythroid series (erythrocytosis or increased red cell mass). Increased erythropoiesis in PV is independent of normal regulatory mechanisms.

Distinction should be made between primary, secondary, and apparent polycythaemias (Fig. 7.7 and Table 7.5).

Recently it has been found that mutation in tyrosine kinase *JAK2V617F* occurs in 95% of cases and a mutation in another exon of gene (exon 12) occurs in another 4% of cases of PV. The *JAK2* mutation also occurs in a significant proportion of patients with primary myelofibrosis and essential thrombocythaemia. Role of this mutation in the pathogenesis of PV and other myeloproliferative neoplasms is presented in Figure 7.8.

Erythropoietin production is reduced in PV and abnormal erythroid stem cells require very small amounts of erythropoietin for their differentiation. The neoplastic clone suppresses normal haematopoietic stem cells as well as erythropoietin production.

There are two phases of PV:

• Proliferative or polycythaemic phase (initial phase characterised by proliferation of erythroid cells leading to increased red cell mass)

Table 7.5: Causes of polycythaemia

Absolute polycythaemia (Increased red cell mass)
1. Primary - Polycythaemia vera
2. Secondary-
   • Hypoxia with decreased arterial oxygen saturation (physiologically appropriate, increased erythropoietin): high altitude, chronic obstructive pulmonary disease, congenital cyanotic heart disease with right to left shunt, haemoglobins with increased oxygen affinity, heavy smoking.
   • Neoplasms (physiologically inappropriate, pathologic production of erythropoietin): renal cell carcinoma, hepatocellular carcinoma, cerebellar haemangioblastoma, uterine leiomyoma
   • Familial erythrocytosis
   • Truncated erythropoietin receptor due to mutation

Apparent polycythaemia (Normal red cell mass)
1. Stress or spurious polycythaemia
2. Dehydration

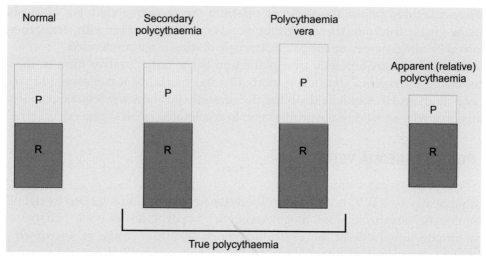

Figure 7.7: Red cell mass and plasma volume in different types of polycythaemia. P= plasma volume, R= red cell mass. In true polycythaemia, red cell mass is increased and may result from PV or secondary causes. Apparent polycythaemia is due to lowering of plasma volume relative to red cell mass

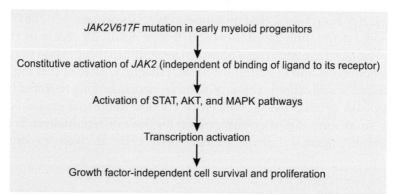

Figure 7.8: Pathogenesis of polycythaemia vera. Role of *JAK2V617F* mutation in myeloproliferative neoplasms. Normally, JAK2 molecules are associated with cytoplasmic domains of cell surface receptors (e.g. erythropoietin receptors). After binding of ligand to its receptor, the receptor-associated JAKs get phosphorylated and in turn activate or phosphorylate tyrosine residues in receptor cytoplasmic tail. Activation of various pathways and signalling proteins send signals for survival, proliferation, and differentiation of erythroid progenitors

- "Spent" or post-polycythaemic phase (characterised by cytopaenias and myelofibrosis).
  Progression to acute myeloid leukaemia occurs in a proportion of patients.

Clinical Features

PV is an uncommon disease occurring between 50 and 60 years of age. Males are affected more commonly.

Increased blood viscosity and volume related to erythrocytosis may lead to decreased blood flow and dilatation of blood vessels. This may cause headache, vertigo, facial plethora, blurring of vision, and congestion of conjunctiva and mucosa. Thrombosis can occur in cerebrovascular, coronary, or peripheral arteries and in deep veins of legs. Thrombosis at unusual locations such as mesenteric, portal, or hepatic veins should prompt investigations for PV. Spontaneous mucous membrane bleeding can occur such as epistaxis and gastrointestinal bleeding (due to platelet dysfunction). Incidence of peptic ulcer is higher than normal in PV. Erythromelalgia (painful and burning sensation of hands and feet associated with increased skin temperature and redness) can occur. Pruritus occurs in 30% of patients and is increased by warm bath. Moderate splenomegaly is usual and its presence virtually rules out secondary polycythaemia. With progression to "spent" phase, marked enlargement of spleen occurs.

Laboratory Features

Peripheral Blood Examination

After collection, blood appears thick and viscous. The red cell count, haemoglobin concentration, and packed cell volume are raised. Initially at presentation, red cells are normocytic and normochromic; with progression to spent phase (myelofibrosis), anisopoikilocytosis, tear drop cells, and nucleated red cells appear (leucoerythroblastic smear).

There is usually mild to moderate leucocytosis with shift to left up to myelocyte stage. Basophils, eosinophils, and monocytes are often increased.

Platelet count is increased in 50% of patients and is usually >5 lac/cmm. Giant platelets are often seen.

Bone Marrow Examination

In the polycythaemic stage, bone marrow aspiration smears show hypercellular marrow with trilineage hyperplasia, especially involving erythroid series. Megakaryocytes are increased and often occur in clusters and show abnormal morphology such as giant forms and pleomorphism.

Bone marrow biopsy in polycythaemic phase usually reveals normal reticulin fibre network. With progression of the disease to spent phase, marked myelofibrosis develops.

Other Investigations

- Serum erythropoietin level: Low erythropoietin level in the presence of increased red cell mass is highly suggestive of PV
- Cytogenetic analysis reveals abnormalities at diagnosis in about 15% of patients such as +8, +9, and 20q-

- Neutrophil alkaline phosphatase (NAP) score is increased or normal
- Arterial oxygen saturation is normal
- Red cell mass is elevated as determined with ^{51}Cr-labelled red cells
- Spontaneous or endogenous erythroid colony formation *in vitro* without added erythropoietin is an important feature.

Important features necessary for diagnosis of PV are presented in Box 7.2.

Differential Diagnosis

1. *Secondary polycythaemia:* Various causes of polycythaemia are listed in Table 7.5. Differences between them are presented in Table 7.6.
2. *Other myeloproliferative disorders:*

Differentiation from other myeloproliferative disorders is considered under chronic myeloid leukaemia.

Diagnosis of polycythaemia vera: Criteria for diagnosis of polycythaemia vera by World Health Organisation (2008) require presence of 2 major plus one minor OR first major and two minor criteria given below:

Table 7.6: Differences between polycythaemia vera (PV), secondary polycythaemia (SP), and relative polycythaemia (RP)

Parameter	PV	SP	RP
1. Nature of disease	Clonal, myeloproliferative neoplasm	Hypoxia or increased erythropoietin level	Relative lowering of plasma volume
2. Red cell mass	Increased	Increased	Normal
3. Plasma volume	Increased	Normal	Decreased
4. Splenomegaly	Present	Absent	Absent
5. White blood cells	Increased, immature forms+	Normal	Normal
6. Platelets	Increased	Normal	Normal
7. Bone marrow	Trilineage hyperplasia	Erythroid hyperplasia	Normal
8. Arterial O$_2$ saturation	Normal	Decreased or normal	Normal
9. Erythropoietin	Decreased	Increased	Normal
10. NAP score	Increased	Normal	Normal
11. Cytogenetic abnormality	May be present	Absent	Absent

Box 7.2 Diagnosis of polycythaemia vera

Diagnosis of PV should be considered in the presence of following features:
- Adult patient presenting with plethora and splenomegaly
- Raised haemoglobin and PCV above normal
- Exclusion of causes of secondary polycythaemia
- Erythrocytosis, leucocytosis, and thrombocytosis in blood
- Bone marrow showing trilineage proliferation along with prominent hyperplasia of erythroid and megakaryocytic series
- Low or normal serum erythropoietin level.

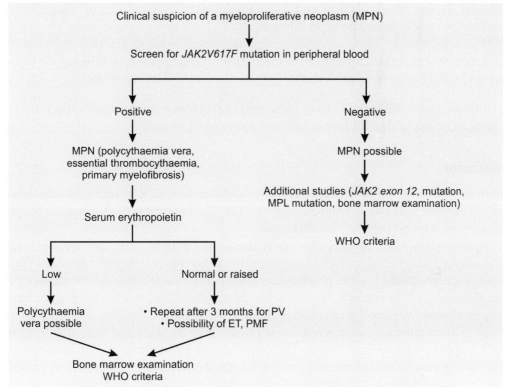

Figure 7.9: Algorithm for diagnosis of myeloproliferative neoplasms
(polycythaemia vera, essential thrombocythaemia, and primary myelofibrosis)

Major criteria
1. Haemoglobin >18.5 g/dl (men) or >16.5 g/dl (women)
2. *JAK2V617F* or other functionally similar mutation

Minor criteria
• Trilineage hyperplasia in bone marrow
• Low serum erythropoietin
• Endogenous erythroid colony formation *in vitro*
Algorithm for diagnosis of myeloproliferative neoplasms is shown in Figure 7.9.

Course and Prognosis

Without treatment, patients with PV have a median survival of about 18 months with death occurring most commonly from thrombotic complications (myocardial infarction, stroke, venous thromboembolism). With recent modes of therapy, survival is approximately 10 to 15 years.

The course of PV consists of proliferative and spent phases. In the proliferative phase, trilineage proliferation with predominance of erythroid series occurs in the bone marrow. This is followed by gradual progression to a spent phase (15–20% of patients) during which clinical and haematological manifestations of myelofibrosis develop (postpolycythaemic myelofibrosis).

Transformation to acute myeloid leukaemia occurs in about 5% of patients of PV. Incidence of leukaemia in patients treated with myelosuppression (chemo- or radio-therapy) is higher as compared to those treated with phlebotomy alone.

> Untreated patients with PV have increased risk of thrombotic complications and long-term risk of myelofibrosis and acute myeloid leukaemia.

Treatment

There are two modes of therapy in PV: (i) phlebotomy that aims to rapidly lower the packed cell volume or haematocrit, and (ii) myelosuppressive therapy to control production of blood cells in bone marrow.

Treatment in PV should be individualised. Patient can be treated with myelosuppressive therapy, phlebotomy plus myelosuppressive therapy, or phlebotomy alone. Patients treated with phlebotomy alone have increased risk of thrombotic complications, while patients treated with chlorambucil or radioactive phosphorous have increased incidence of developing AML.

All patients usually require repeated phlebotomy as an initial measure to lower the haematocrit to normal levels. This reduces the immediate risk of thrombosis. Myelosuppressive therapy, often combined with phlebotomy, is indicated in patients with previous history of thrombosis, systemic symptoms, and thrombocytosis. Radioactive phosphorous is usually reserved for patients older than 70 years of age (to reduce the problems of treatment compliance and regular follow-up) while in younger patients hydroxyurea or interferon α is employed (to reduce the risk of transformation to acute leukaemia).

Post-polycythaemic myelofibrosis and AML respond poorly to therapy.

❑ PRIMARY MYELOFIBROSIS (PMF)

Syn: Idiopathic myelofibrosis with agnogenic myeloid metaplasia
Primary myelofibrosis (PMF) is a clonal, myeloproliferative neoplasm characterised by trilineage proliferation in bone marrow (with predominance of granulocytic and megakaryocytic lines), reactive bone marrow fibrosis, and extramedullary haematopoiesis mainly in spleen. (Extramedullary haematopoiesis or 'myeloid metaplasia' refers to ectopic haematopoiesis occurring in organs other than bone marrow like spleen and liver). There is a gradual progression of disease from initial pre-fibrotic stage to fibrotic stage.

Studies have shown that trilineage proliferation of blood cells in bone marrow is monoclonal and arises in haematopoietic stem cell. In contrast, fibroblasts are not part of the neoplastic clone. Bone marrow fibrosis results from stimulation of fibroblastic proliferation and collagen synthesis by platelet derived growth factor and transforming growth factor-β, which are secreted by increased numbers of abnormal megakaryocytes.

PMF, a rare disease, manifests usually in the elderly, median age at diagnosis being 65 years. Sex incidence is equal. The disease has insidious onset with fatigue and weight loss. Splenomegaly (due to extramedullary haematopoiesis) is present in majority of patients and may be massive. Other manifestations include portal hypertension, bleeding varices, ascites, splenic pain due to infarction, and lymphadenopathy (due to extramedullary haematopoiesis). About one-third of patients are asymptomatic and detected incidentally.

Laboratory evaluation reveals —

- *Peripheral blood*
  - Anaemia
  - Marked anisopoikilocytosis with tear drop red cells
  - Leucoerythroblastic blood picture (presence of immature cells of erythroid and granulocytic series in peripheral blood Fig. 7.10)
  - Total leucocyte and platelet counts are raised in early stage; with disease progression, counts are reduced.
- *Bone marrow examination:* In fibrotic stage, bone marrow aspiration typically reveals a 'dry tap,' i.e. failure to obtain bone marrow with aspiration of only peripheral blood. Bone marrow trephine biopsy shows fibrosis, increase in the number of abnormal megakaryocytes that are often clustered together, osteosclerosis, and dilated marrow sinuses containing intrasinusoidal haematopoiesis. Reticulin and trichrome staining can assess degree of marrow fibrosis.

Differential diagnosis includes (1) other myeloproliferative diseases associated with fibrosis: CML, PV, and essential thrombocythaemia; (2) myelofibrosis secondary to metastasis in marrow, lymphoma, or disseminated tuberculosis;

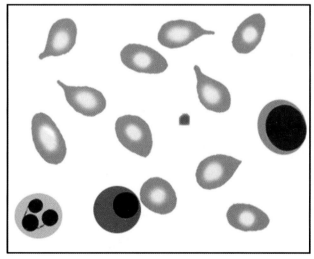

Figure 7.10: Blood smear in primary myelofibrosis showing many tear drop cells and leucoerythroblastic reaction

Table 7.7: Causes of bone marrow fibrosis

Haematologic disorders	Nonhaematologic disorders
1. Myeloproliferative neoplasms: chronic myelogenous leukaemia, primary myelofibrosis, essential thrombocythaemia, polycythaemia vera, systemic mastosytosis	1. Infections: tuberculosis, histoplasmosis, kala-azar, human immunodeficiency virus
2. Myelodysplastic syndromes	2. Metastatic carcinoma
3. Acute leukaemias	3. Autoimmune disorders
4. Lymphoma	4. Hyperparathyroidism
5. Multiple myeloma	5. Renal osteodystrophy
6. Hairy cell leukaemuia	6. Vitamin D deficiency
7. Gray platelet syndrome	7. Paget's disease of bone

(3) myelodysplastic syndrome with myelofibrosis; and (4) acute myelofibrosis. Causes of bone marrow fibrosis are listed in Table 7.7.

The median survival ranges from 3 to 5 years from diagnosis; however, it is highly variable. Common causes of death are infections, heart failure, haemorrhage, thrombosis, and transformation to AML (15% of patients).

Treatment is largely palliative. A trial of androgens and corticosteroids may alleviate anaemia, but regular transfusions are usually required. Chemotherapy (hydroxyurea) is used for control of elevated white cell and platelet counts and to reduce the size of spleen. Splenic irradiation can result in relief of splenic pain and reduction of spleen size. Splenectomy may be considered in the presence of unacceptable transfusion needs, enlarged and painful spleen, complications of portal hypertension, and life-threatening refractory thrombocytopaenia. However, splenectomy is associated with risk of considerable morbidity and mortality and should be undertaken with caution.

❏ ESSENTIAL THROMBOCYTHAEMIA

Syn: Primary thrombocythaemia

Essential thrombocythaemia (ET) is a clonal, myeloproliferative neoplasm characterised by marked proliferation of megakaryocytes in bone marrow causing thrombocytosis in peripheral blood. It usually occurs in the elderly (50–60 years of age). Patients manifest with bleeding and/or thrombotic (digital or cerebral ischaemia) manifestations. Splenomegaly is present at diagnosis in 50% of patients. Many patients are asymptomatic and are discovered incidentally on routine blood examination.

By definition, platelet count in ET is more than 4.5 lac/cmm; in the majority of patients it exceeds 1 million/cmm. Morphologic abnormalities of platelets such as giant forms, marked variation in size and shape, and megakaryocyte fragments are often seen in peripheral blood. Bone marrow shows markedly increased numbers of large or giant megakaryocytes, which are often arranged in clusters (Figs 7.11 and 7.12). Platelet function tests reveal defective aggregation with epinephrine.

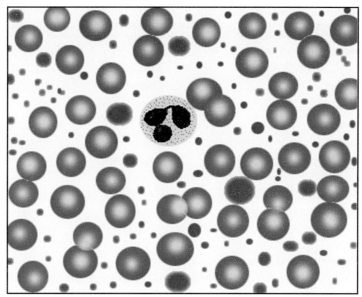

Figure 7.11: Blood smear in essential thrombocythaemia showing normal red blood cells, thrombocytosis, marked variation in size of platelets, and large and giant platelets

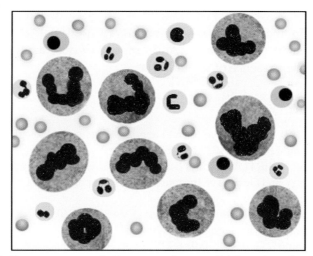

Figure 7.12: Bone marrow aspiration smear in essential thrombocythaemia showing increased number of diffusely scattered, mature, large, multilobated megakaryocytes

Differential diagnosis includes (i) other myeloproliferative disorders, and (ii) secondary (reactive) thrombocytosis which commonly occurs in infections, iron deficiency, chronic inflammatory disorders, malignant diseases, acute haemorrhage, and following splenectomy. Features that favour diagnosis of a clonal disorder against reactive thrombocytosis are:
• Haemorrhagic and/or thrombotic manifestations
• Splenomegaly

Table 7.8: Differences between essential thrombocythaemia and reactive thrombocytosis

Parameter	Essential thrombocythaemia	Reactive thrombocytosis
1. Underlying cause for thrombocytosis	Absent	Present
2. Thrombosis	Often	No
3. Haemorrhage	Often	No
4. Splenomegaly	May be present	Absent
5. *JAK2V617F* mutation	Present (50%)	Absent
6. C-reactive protein	-	Raised
7. Giant platelets and megakaryocyte fragments on blood smear	Often present	Absent
8. Defective platelet function	Present	Absent
9. Megakaryocytes	Abnormal	Normal

- Abnormal platelet function (reduced aggregation with epinephrine)
- Giant platelets on blood smear
- Abnormal megakaryocytes (e.g. giant forms) on bone marrow examination.

Features of essential thrombocythaemia and reactive thrombocytosis are compared in Table 7.8.

Median survival is 10 to 15 years after treatment. Causes of death include thrombosis, haemorrhage, and evolution to AML (<5% of patients). Patients with thrombotic or haemorrhagic episodes or with very high platelet counts are treated with cytotoxic (hydroxyurea) therapy. Addition of low dose aspirin (75 mg per day) may be helpful in the presence of thrombosis.

❑ BIBLIOGRAPHY

1. Goldman JM, Melo JV. Chronic myeloid leukaemia - Advances in biology and new approaches to treatment. N Engl J Med. 2003;349:1451-64.
2. Jaffe ES, Harris NL, Stein H, Vardiman JW (Eds): World Health Organisation Classification of Tumours. Pathology and Genetis of Tumours of Haematopoietic and Lymphoid Tissues. Lyon. IARC Press, 2001.
3. Sawyers CL. Chronic myeloid leukemia. N Engl J Med. 1999;340: 1330-40.
4. Schafer AI. Thrombocytosis. N Engl J Med. 2004;350: 1211-19.
5. Swerdlow SH, Campo E, Harris NL, Jaffe ES, Pileri SA, Stein H, Thiele J, Vardiman JW (Eds): WHO classification of tumours of haematopoietic and lymphoid tissues. 4th ed. Lyon. International Agency for Research on Cancer. 2008.
6. Tefferi A. Myelofibrosis with myeloid metaplasia. N Engl J Med. 2000;342: 1255-65.
7. Tefferi A. Polycuthemia vera: A comprehensive review and clinical recommendations. Mayo Clin Proc. 2003;78: 174-94.

CHAPTER

8

Chronic Lymphoid Leukaemias

These are a heterogeneous group of clonal, neoplastic disorders characterised by proliferation of mature B or T lymphoid cells (Table 8.1).

❑ CHRONIC LYMPHOCYTIC LEUKAEMIA

Chronic lymphocytic leukaemia (CLL) is a neoplastic disorder characterised by monoclonal proliferation of immunologically incompetent, slowly dividing, mature B-lymphocytes. CLL is the most common form of leukaemia in western countries, while it is the least common type in India.

Clinical Features

CLL occurs principally in persons over 50 years of age (median age at presentation: 65–70 years). It is twice as common in males as compared to females. First-degree

Table 8.1: Chronic lymphoid leukaemias

B cell type	T cell type
• Chronic lymphocytic leukaemia	• T-cell prolymphocytic leukaemia
• B-cell prolymphocytic leukaemia	• T-cell large granular lymphocytic leukaemia
• Waldenström macroglobulinaemia	• Adult T cell leukaemia/lymphoma
• Hairy cell leukaemia	• Sezary syndrome
• Plasma cell leukaemia	
• Leukaemic phase of non-Hodgkin's lymphoma	

relatives of the patient have significantly increased risk of developing CLL and other lymphoid malignancies. Patient may present with weakness, fatigue, and weight loss, repeated infections (due to hypogammaglobulinaemia) and symptoms related to anaemia or thrombocytopaenia. Generalised lymphadenopathy is the most common presenting feature; mild to moderate splenomegaly is present in two-thirds of cases. About 25% of patients are asymptomatic and are discovered incidentally on clinical or laboratory examination.

Laboratory Features

Peripheral Blood Examination

Anaemia develops with progressive marrow replacement by tumour cells and is normocytic and normochromic. Other causes of anaemia in CLL include hypersplenism and autoimmune haemolysis. Autoimmune haemolytic anaemia occurs in about 10% of patients and is characterised by mild hyperbilirubinaemia, increased reticulocytes and spherocytes, and positive Coombs' (antiglobulin) test.

Total leucocyte count is increased and is usually more than 50,000/cmm with >80% of cells being lymphocytes. Diagnosis of CLL should be considered if lymphocyte count is >5000/cmm in the absence of any other underlying cause.

In majority of cases, >90% of neoplastic cells are small, mature looking lymphocytes with high N/C ratio, scanty cytoplasm and dense, clumped chromatin. Nucleoli are not seen or are inconspicuous (Fig. 8.1). In about 15% of cases, in addition to small, mature-looking lymphocytes, >10% (but <55%) cells are prolymphocytes; this category is designated as CLL/PL. 'Smudge' or basket cells are a characteristic feature of CLL and are produced during spreading of blood film because of fragility of lymphocytes.

Platelet count may be normal or decreased. Thrombocytopaenia becomes severe with progressive replacement of bone marrow by leukaemic cells. Other causes of thrombocytopaenia are immune destruction of platelets and hypersplenism.

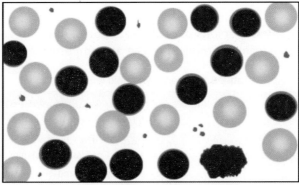

Figure 8.1: Blood smear in chronic lymphocytic leukaemia showing small, mature-looking lymphocytes with clumped chromatin. A smudge cell is seen at lower right

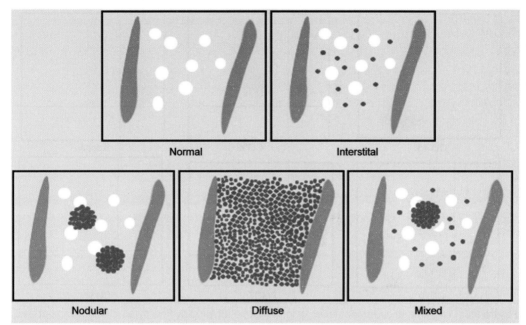

Figure 8.2: Patterns of bone marrow infiltration in CLL. Four patterns of infiltration can be seen in CLL: (1) Interstitial: Individual neoplastic cells are interspersed between haematopoietic cells and fat cells; (2) Nodular: Well-defined round or oval aggregates of neoplastic cells that are non-paratrabecular; (3) Diffuse: Extensive replacement of both haematopoietic and fat cells so that marrow architecture is effaced and appears 'packed'; (4) Mixed: Combination of nodular and interstitial pattern

Bone Marrow Examination

National Cancer Institute criteria for diagnosis of CLL require lymphocyte count above 5000/cmm and bone marrow lymphocytes more than 30%.

Assessment of pattern of infiltration of neoplastic cells in bone marrow has prognostic importance. Four patterns of infiltration can be recognised on bone marrow trephine biopsy—interstitial, nodular, diffuse, and a combination of these. Diffuse pattern is associated with aggressive disease and worse prognosis. Nodular pattern is associated with a favourable prognosis (Fig. 8.2).

Immunophenotyping

Immunophenotyping provides definitive diagnosis and should be done in all cases before beginning therapy. It is particularly helpful in situations where lymphocytosis is less than 5000/cmm or when lymphocyte morphology is atypical. CLL cells usually express membrane phenotype of early B cells. Characteristically CLL cells express CD19, CD20 (weak), CD5, CD23, weak surface membrane immunoglobulin, and absent reactivity with FMC7 and with CD2. A single light chain (either κ or λ) is expressed on the surface of cells supporting the clonal origin of lymphocytes (Fig. 8.3).

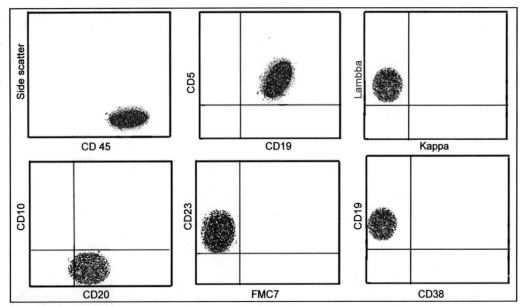

Figure 8.3: Diagrammatic representation of immunophenotyping by flow cytometry in a case of CLL. The cells express CD19, CD5, lambda light chain (dim), CD23, CD20 (dim), and are negative for CD10, FMC7, and CD38. Absence of CD38 expression is a good prognostic indicator

Cytogenetic Analysis

In CLL, conventional cytogenetic analysis is difficult due to the presence of only a few dividing neoplastic lymphocytes. Advent of fluorescent *in situ* hybridisation (FISH) (which can detect chromosomal abnormalities in non-dividing cells) has led to the identification of cytogenetic abnormalities in majority of patients with CLL. There is no single cytogenetic abnormality specific for CLL. The common abnormalities include 13q-, 11q-, trisomy 12, 17p-, and complex abnormalities. Some chromosomal abnormalities are associated with a poor outcome such as 11q- or 17p-.

Immunological Studies

Hypogammaglobulinaemia is observed in two-thirds of patients and becomes severe with progression of disease; it is associated with increased risk of bacterial infections. M band (monoclonal protein) is observed in about 5% of patients.

Diagnosis

Diagnosis of chronic lymphocytic leukaemia should be considered when an elderly patient presents with (i) absolute lymphocytosis in peripheral blood >5000/cmm; (ii) lymphocytes are small, mature-looking with high N/C ratio, round to oval nuclei and clumped chromatin; smudge cell is a characteristic feature; (iii) characteristic immunophenotyping: CD19+, CD20+ (dim), CD23+, CD5+, surface membrane immunoglobulin + (dim), monoclonal κ or λ light chain, FMC-, CD10-; and (iv) Bone marrow shows increased numbers (≥30%) of mature, small lymphocytes. Prolymphocytes are ≤55%.

Differential Diagnosis

Reactive Lymphocytosis

Reactive lymphocytosis occurs in infections by viruses (such as Epstein-Barr virus, cytomegalovirus, hepatitis, influenza), tuberculosis, toxoplasmosis, and rickettsia. Reactive lymphocytosis is transient and lymphocyte count is usually less than 5000/cmm. Morphology of reactive lymphocytes (large size, abundant cytoplasm, scalloping, dark blue edges) is also helpful. In doubtful cases surface marker analysis for monoclonality (κ or λ light chain restriction) can be done.

Other Chronic Lymphoid Leukaemias

CLL should be differentiated from prolymphocytic leukaemia, leukaemic phase of non-Hodgkin's lymphoma (especially mantle cell lymphoma and follicular lymphoma), and hairy cell leukaemia (Fig. 8.4 for comparative morphological features). Prolymphocytic leukaemia is characterised by massive splenomegaly, no lymphadenopathy, marked lymphocytosis, and predominance of prolymphocytes in peripheral blood (>55%). In leukaemic phase of follicular small-cleaved cell lymphoma, neoplastic small lymphocytes show deep nuclear clefts and immunophenotypic analysis shows CD5-, CD19+, CD20+, BCL-2+, and strong surface membrane immunoglobulin. FISH can identify t(14;18) in 70 to 95% of cases of follicular lymphomas. In mantle cell lymphoma involving peripheral blood, neoplastic cells are small cleaved lymphocytes with a characteristic immunophenotype: CD5+, CD19+, CD20+, CD23-, and strong surface membrane immunoglobulin. In about 75% of patients with mantle cell lymphoma, t(11;14) chromosomal abnormality is present. Hairy cell leukaemia is characterised by massive splenomegaly, pancytopaenia, lymphocytes with small, fine projections on cell surface, typical immunophenotype, and tartrate-resistant acid phosphatase activity (TRAP) (Table 8.2).

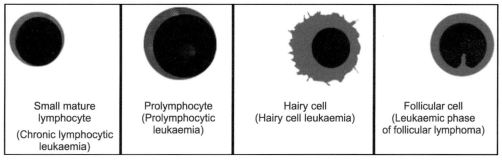

| Small mature lymphocyte (Chronic lymphocytic leukaemia) | Prolymphocyte (Prolymphocytic leukaemia) | Hairy cell (Hairy cell leukaemia) | Follicular cell (Leukaemic phase of follicular lymphoma) |

Figure 8.4: Comparative morphological features of chronic lymphoid leukaemias

Table 8.2: Differential diagnosis of chronic lymphoid leukaemias and
B-cell lymphomas that can involve peripheral blood

Parameter	CLL	MCL	SMZL/SLVL	HCL	FL	PLL
CD5	+	+	–	–	–	–
CD10	–	–/+	–	–	+	–/+
CD11c	–/+	–/+	+	+	–	+
CD19	+	+	+	+	+	+
CD20	+(dim)	+(bright)	+(bright)	+(bright)	+(bright)	+(bright)
CD23	+	–/+	–/+	–	–/+	–
CD79b	–	+	+	–/+	+	+
FMC7	–	+	+	+	+	+
SmIg	+(dim)	+(bright)	+(bright)	+(bright)	+(bright)	+(bright)

CLL: Chronic lymphocytic leukaemia; MCL: Mantle cell lymphoma; SMZL/SLVL: Splenic marginal zone
lymphoma/splenic lymphoma with villous lymphocytes; HCL: Hairy cell leukaemia; FL: Follicular lymphoma;
PLL: Prolymphocytic leukaemia

Monoclonal B-cell lymphocytosis: Monoclonal B-cell lymphocytosis is defined as low level (absolute lymphocyte count <5000/cmm) of asymptomatic proliferation of B lymphocytes and light chain restriction on immunophenotyping by flow cytometry. There is no lymphadenopathy, organomegaly, or cytopaenia and bone marrow lymphocytes are <30%. There is a small risk of progression to CLL. Recent investigations suggest that most cases of CLL are preceded by monoclonal B lymphocytosis.

Complications of CLL

1. **Infections:** Patients with CLL have increased risk of bacterial, viral, and fungal infections, due to disease itself (from hypogammaglobulinaemia) or following therapy (from neutropaenia and depletion of T lymphocytes).
2. **Autoimmune haemolytic anaemia and thrombocytopaenic purpura.**
3. **Second malignancies:** There is increased risk of second malignancies in CLL such as skin cancer and solid tumours.
4. **Aggressive transformation:** Progression to a more aggressive disorder can occur such as prolymphocytic leukaemia or Richter's syndrome. Richter's syndrome is development of a diffuse large cell lymphoma in a patient with pre-existing CLL. It occurs in approximately 3 to 5% of cases. It should be suspected when patient develops unexplained fever, weight loss, and localised lymphadenopathy, particularly abdominal, and elevation of lactate dehydrogenase. It is refractory to chemotherapy and median survival is about 4 months.

Prognosis

1. **Staging:** Prognosis depends primarily on the stage of the disease at diagnosis. There are two main staging systems for CLL: Rai (1975) and Binet (1981). These are shown in Table 8.3.

Table 8.3: Staging systems for CLL

Binet stages	Rai stages
A: < 3 lymphoid areas* enlarged	**0:** Lymphocytosis only
B: ≥ 3 lymphoid areas enlarged	**I:** Lymphadenopathy
C: Anaemia (Haemoglobin <10 g/dl) and/or thrombocytopaenia (Platelet count <1 lac/cmm)	**II:** Hepatomegaly and/or splenomegaly ± lymphadenopathy **III:** Haemoglobin <11 g/dl **IV:** Platelet count <1,00,000/cmm
* Lymphoid areas: lymph nodes (unilateral or bilateral cervical, axillary, and inguinal), liver and spleen	

Table 8.4: Prognostic factors in CLL

Low-risk	High-risk
• Early stage disease (Binet:A; Rai:0,I)	• Advanced stage disease (Binet:B, C; Rai: II, III, IV)
• Predominance of small mature lymphocytes	• >10% prolymphocytes
• Interstitial or nodular marrow infiltration	• Diffuse marrow infiltration
• Normal karyotype or 13q-	• 11q-, 12+, 17p-
• Antigen CD38-	• Antigen CD 38+
• Normal β_2 microglobulin	• Elevated β_2 microglobulin
• Mutated IgV_H gene	• Nonmutated IgV_H gene
• LDT>12 months	• LDT<12 months
• Female	• Male
• ZAP-70-	• ZAP-70+
• Thymidine kinase low or normal	• Thymidine kinase raised
LDT: Lymphocyte doubling time or time required for lymphocyte count to double in peripheral blood	

2. **Other prognostic factors:** There is a correlation between disease stage (as defined in Table 8.3) and median survival. However, the staging systems cannot accurately predict those patients in early stage who will have disease progression and those who will remain indolent. About 50% of patients in early stage will develop more advanced disease. Also, there is marked variation in disease progression amongst patients with similar stages. Assessment of risk of progression of disease can be done from various factors as shown in Table 8.4.

Treatment

Treatment is principally symptomatic and is not curative.

Early stage disease is relatively benign and patients are often asymptomatic. Median survival of these patients is >10 years and therefore no treatment is usually indicated. Early institution of therapy does not improve survival and increases the risk of second cancers and development of resistance to treatment.

Treatment is indicated when patient develops systemic symptoms related to disease (e.g. fever, weight loss, fatigue), evidence of disease progression (progressive worsening of anaemia or thrombocytopaenia, progressive enlargement of lymph nodes or spleen, lymphocyte doubling time <12 months), or presence of massively enlarged lymph nodes or spleen.

Various forms of therapy for suppression of disease include chemotherapy, corticosteroids, and radiotherapy. Chlorambucil is the commonly used drug in CLL. It is used either as high dose intermittent therapy every 4 to 6 weeks or as a continuous low dose treatment. Although both forms of therapy are equally effective, intermittent therapy is less toxic to bone marrow. Treatment, however, does not affect overall survival. Other chemotherapeutic drugs that are employed are— fludarabine, CHOP (cyclophosphamide, hydroxydaunomycin [daunorubicin], oncovin [vincristine], and prednisolone), pentostatin (2,3 deoxycoformycin), and cladribine (2 chlorodeoxyadenosine). Fludarabine is increasingly being used since it has been shown to produce a better and more durable response. Corticosteroids are helpful for treatment of autoimmune haemolytic anaemia and immune thrombocytopaenia. Local radiotherapy is given for treatment of splenic/lymph node enlargement causing compression problems. Splenectomy is indicated for hypersplenism, painful splenomegaly, and for immune haemolytic anaemia or thrombocytopaenia resistant to corticosteroids.

❏ PROLYMPHOCYTIC LEUKAEMIA

Prolymphocytic leukaemia (PLL) is an uncommon but a distinct form of chronic lymphoid leukaemia characterised by splenomegaly, marked lymphocytosis with predominance of prolymphocytes in the peripheral blood. PLL is of two types—B cell (75%), and T cell (25%). It is more aggressive than CLL.

Clinical Features

B-PLL occurs in elderly persons in the sixth or seventh decade of life. Mean age at presentation is about 10 years older than patients with typical CLL. The characteristic clinical feature is marked splenomegaly; there is minimal or no lymphadenopathy. (In typical CLL, lymph node enlargement is greater as compared to the size of the spleen). Anaemia and thrombocytopaenia are present in 50% of patients at diagnosis. In T-PLL, clinical features include hepatosplenomegaly, generalised lymphadenopathy, and skin involvement in the form of an erythematous, papular rash.

Laboratory Features

Total lymphocyte count is extremely high and is generally more than 1 lac/cmm. Prolymphocytes are the most numerous cells in peripheral blood and are more than 55%. Prolymphocyte is a large lymphoid cell (more than twice the size of a small lymphocyte) with low nuclear-cytoplasmic ratio, condensed nuclear chromatin, and a prominent vesicular nucleolus (Fig. 8.5).

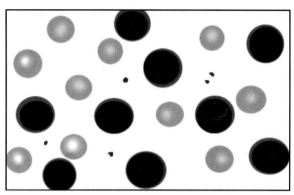

Figure 8.5: Blood smear in prolymphocytic leukaemia

Immunophenotypic analysis shows:
- B-PLL: CD19+, CD20+, CD22+, CD79a+, FMC7+, Surface membrane immunoglobulin **(SmIg)+ (strong)**, CD23-
- T-PLL: CD2+, CD3+, CD7+, and CD4+CD8- or CD4+CD8+ or CD4- CD8-
  M band (monoclonal protein) in serum is found in 30% of cases.

Cytogenetic analysis shows abnormality of 14q32 in most patients with B-PLL, and inv(14) in 80% of patients with T-PLL.

Differential Diagnosis

   i. **Chronic lymphocytic leukaemia with prolymphocytic transformation (CLL/PLL):** CLL/PLL differs from PLL in following:
     a. Age: PLL (70 years) occurs at more older age than CLL/PLL (60 years).
     b. Splenomegaly is more marked in PLL.
     c. Lymphadenopathy is moderate or marked in CLL/PLL, while it is minimal or absent in PLL.
     d. Cytogenetic abnormalities.
   ii. **CLL/PL:** Predominant cells are small, mature lymphocytes and prolymphocytes are >10% but less than 55%.
  iii. **Lymphosarcoma cell leukaemia:** This is the leukaemic phase of non-Hodgkin's lymphoma that occurs at relatively younger age. Total leucocyte count is moderately raised, and the neoplastic cells show characteristic indented or clefted nuclei.
  iv. **Acute lymphoblastic leukaemia:** In contrast to lymphoblasts in ALL, prolymphocytes have more condensed chromatin, a conspicuous and a prominent nucleolus, and lower nuclear-cytoplasmic ratio.

Course and Prognosis

The course is aggressive with poor response to treatment; median survival is less than 3 years in B-PLL and 6 to 7 months in T-PLL.

Treatment

Patients with PLL are frequently refractory to treatment and median survival is short. Chemotherapeutic agents used include CHOP (cyclophosphamide, doxorubicin, oncovin, and prednisone), fludarabine, and deoxycoformycin. Splenectomy can reduce tumour mass and cause partial improvement.

❑ HAIRY CELL LEUKAEMIA

Hairy cell leukaemia (HCL) is a rare chronic lymphoproliferative disorder of B cell origin characterised by occurrence in middle-aged persons, pancytopaenia, splenic enlargement, and hairy cells in bone marrow and other sites.

Clinical Features

The disease has male predominance. The usual symptoms are tiredness, abdominal distension, easy bruisability and repeated infections. These features result from cytopaenias and splenic enlargement. The characteristic physical sign is marked spleno-megaly. Mild hepatomegaly may be present. There is usually no lymphadenopathy. Some patients are asymptomatic and detected incidentally.

Laboratory Features

Peripheral Blood Examination

Cytopaenia affecting two or more cell lines is the main laboratory feature. Anaemia is mild to moderate and is normocytic and normochromic. Leucopaenia is frequently present. Neutropaenia and monocytopaenia are usual. Due to low TLC, hairy cells are difficult to demonstrate. In cases with TLC greater than normal, hairy cells are increased in proportion and easily identifiable. Hairy cells are large and are twice the size of a small lymphocyte. Their cytoplasm is clear to lightly basophilic and shows numerous fine, hair-like or broader projections on surface. Nuclear-cytoplasmic ratio is low. The nucleus is round, oval, or indented; chromatin is reticular and nucleoli are inconspicuous (Fig. 8.6). Hairy cells are best demonstrated by phase contrast or electron microscopy. Mild to moderate thrombocytopaenia is usual.

Bone Marrow Examination

Bone marrow is difficult to aspirate (dry tap) due to reticulin fibrosis. Bone marrow trephine biopsy is essential for definitive diagnosis. It shows diffuse or focal infiltration by mononuclear cells, which are characteristically loosely arranged; the individual nuclei are widely spaced from each other ('fried egg appearance'). This characteristic loosely structured appearance is attributed to artificial retraction of abundant cytoplasm in formalin-fixed tissues. (In other leukaemias and lymphomas, the nuclei of neoplastic cells are in close proximity).

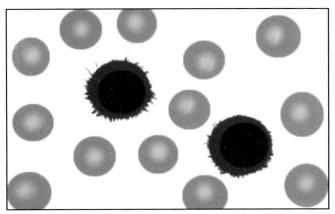

Figure 8.6: Blood smear in hairy cell leukaemia

The reticulin stain demonstrates increased bone marrow fibrosis with reticulin fibres often surrounding individual cells.

Cytochemistry

HCL cells show reactivity with tartrate-resistant acid phosphatase (TRAP) enzyme. Alternatively, antibody to TRAP can be used in flow cytometry.

Immunophenotypic Analysis

Cell surface immunologic marker analysis reveals B cell nature of hairy cells (CD19+, CD20+, and CD22+). Hairy cells express SmIg (strong), CD11c, CD25, CD103, and HC2.

Histology of Spleen

Histology of spleen shows infiltration of red pulp by hairy cells, broadening of splenic cords, and formation of pseudosinuses which are lined by hairy cells (instead of endothelial cells) and filled with red cells. White pulp is atrophic.

Diagnosis and Differential Diagnosis

Diagnosis of HCL can be made when a middle-aged patient presents with marked splenomegaly, pancytopaenia, hairy cells in peripheral blood which are TRAP-positive and showing activated B cell immunophenotype, and typical picture on bone marrow biopsy.

HCL should be differentiated from disorders presenting with splenomegaly and pancytopaenia, e.g. non-Hodgkin's lymphoma, agnogenic myeloid metaplasia with myelofibrosis, and Waldenström's macroglobulinaemia. Occasional patient of non-Hodgkin's lymphoma presents with splenomegaly with minimal lymphadenopathy and pancytopaenia due to bone marrow involvement. Cytology of neoplastic cells, pattern of bone marrow infiltration, close approximation of nuclei in lymphoma versus widely spaced nuclei in HCL, immunophenotyping, and histology of spleen help in arriving at the correct diagnosis. In agnogenic myeloid metaplasia with myelofibrosis, findings in peripheral blood (marked anisopoikilocytosis, leucoerythroblastosis, and tear drop cells) and in bone marrow (clusters of atypical megakaryocytes and marked myelofibrosis) allow correct diagnosis to be made. Diagnosis of Waldenström's macroglobulinaemia is based on typical clinical features, infiltration of lymphocytes, plasmacytoid lymphocytes, and plasma cells in bone marrow; and demonstration of IgM monoclonal protein in serum.

Cases of HCL presenting with leucocytosis should be differentiated from other lymphoproliferative disorders particularly chronic lymphocytic leukaemia with isolated splenomegaly, splenic lymphoma with villous lymphocytes, and leukaemic phase of non-Hodgkin's lymphoma.

Bone marrow involvement in systemic mastocytosis can resemble infiltration by hairy cells; clinical features and cytochemistry are helpful in making the correct diagnosis.

Complications of HCL

1. **Infections:** These are common in HCL due to reduction in granulocytes and monocytes. Common infections are those due to gram-negative bacteria, mycobacteria, and fungi.
2. **Anaemia and bleeding tendencies.**
3. **Skeletal infiltration**, particularly head of femur.
4. **Vasculitis** — This occurs in small number of cases.

Course and Prognosis

Prolonged survival is possible with current modes of therapy. Death usually results from complications related to pancytopaenia, particularly infections.

Treatment

In a small number of patients with HCL, manifestations of cytopaenia are not present and these patients do not need treatment. Such patients are regularly observed and treatment is instituted on development of complications.

Most of the patients have cytopaenia and are symptomatic at the time of diagnosis (anaemia, infections, or bleeding) and require therapy. Currently available modes of therapy for HCL are purine nucleoside analogues (pentostatin or cladribine), alpha interferon (IFN-α), and splenectomy. Either pentostatin or cladribine is highly effective in inducing high rate (80%) of complete remission for prolonged duration. Alpha interferon can be used in patients with severe cytopaenia till blood counts improve; this is then followed by nucleoside analogue therapy. Spleen is the major site of cellular proliferation and secondly hypersplenism further worsens pancytopaenia. Previously, splenectomy was the mainstay of treatment in HCL and caused improvement in blood counts in majority of patients. Splenectomy, however, is of no benefit in patients without enlargement of spleen. Splenectomy may be indicated in patients with splenic enlargement and moderate or little marrow involvement; this may be followed by a nucleoside analogue therapy when disease progression occurs.

❏ BIBLIOGRAPHY

1. Bennett JM, Catovsky D, Daniel MT, Flandrin G, Galton DAG, Gralnick HR, Sultan C. The French-American-British (FAB) Co-operative Group: Proposals for the classification of chronic (mature) B and T lymphoid leukaemias. J Clin Pathol. 1989;42: 567-584.

2. Binet JL, Auquier A, Dighiero G, Chastang C, Piguer H, Goasguen J, et al. A new prognostic classification of chronic lymphocytic leukemia derived from a multivariate survival analysis. Cancer. 1981;48: 198-206.

3. Bouroncle BA. Leukemic reticuloendotheliosis (Hairy cell leukemia). Blood. 1979;53: 412-436.

4. British Committee for Standards in Haematology: Guidelines on the diagnosis and management of chronic lymphocytic leukaemia. Br J Haematol. 2004;125: 294-17.

5. Catovsky D. Chronic lymphoid leukaemias. In Hoffbrand AV and Lewis SM (Eds.) : Postgraduate Haematology. 3rd ed. London. Heinemann Professional Publishing Ltd. 1989.

6. Flinn IW and Grever MR. Chronic lymphocytic leukemia. Cancer Treat Rev. 1996;22: 1-13.

7. Gale RP and Foon KA. Biology of chronic lymphocytic leukaemias. Semin Hematol. 1987;24: 230-39.

8. Galton DAG, Goldman JM, Wiltshaw E, Catovsky D, Henry K, Goldenberg J. Prolymphocytic leukaemia. Br J Haematol. 1974;27: 7-23.

9. International Workshop on Chronic Lymphocytic Leukemia. Chronic lymphocytic leukemia: Recommendations for diagnosis, staging and response criteria. Ann Intern Med. 1989;110: 236-238.

10. Kalil N, Cheson BD. Chronic lymphocytic leukemia. The Oncologist .1999;4: 352-69.

11. Melo JV, Catovsky D, and Galton DAG. The relationship between chronic lymphocytic leukaemia and prolymphocytic leukaemia. I. Clinical and laboratory features of 300 patients and characterization of an intermediate group. Br J Haematol. 1986;63: 377-87.

12. Morrison VA. Chronic leukemias. CA Cancer J Clin. 1994;44: 353-77.

13. Rai KR, Sawitsky A, Cronikite EP, Chanana AD, Levy RN, Pasternack BS. Clinical staging of chronic lymphocytic leukaemia. Blood. 1975;46: 219-34.

14. Rozman C and Montserrat E. Chronic lymphocytic leukemia. N Engl J Med 1995;333: 1052- 57.

15. Rozman C, Montserrat E, Rodriguez Fernandez JM, et al. Bone marrow histologic pattern.The best single prognostic parameter in chronic lymphocytic leukemia; a multivariate survival analysis of 329 cases. Blood. 1984;64: 642-48.

16. Shanafelt TD, Call TG. Current approach to diagnosis and management of chronic lymphocytic leukemia. Mayo Clin Proc. 2004;79: 388-98.

CHAPTER

9

Plasma Cell Dyscrasias

Plasma cell dyscrasias (also called as paraproteinaemias or monoclonal gammopathies) are a group of disorders characterised by neoplastic proliferation of plasma cells and increased production of a single homogeneous immunoglobulin (paraprotein, monoclonal protein, M protein). They are listed in Table 9.1.

❏ INVESTIGATIONS IN PLASMA CELL DYSCRASIAS

Peripheral Blood Examination

Rouleaux formation (Refer to Fig. 9.7) and markedly raised erythrocyte sedimentation rate (ESR) are typical features and result from hyperglobulinaemia.

Table 9.1: Plasma cell dyscrasias

Plasma cell neoplasms
- Plasma cell myeloma (multiple myeloma) and variants (smoldering myeloma, non-secretory myeloma, plasma cell leukaemia)
- Solitary plasmacytoma of bone
- Extramedullary plasmacytoma
- Primary amyloidosis
- Systemic light and heavy chain deposition diseases
- Osteosclerotic myeloma (POEMS syndrome)

Immunoglobulin-secreting neoplasms that are composed of both plasma cells and lymphocytes
- Waldenström macroglobulinaemia
- Heavy chain diseases

Bone Marrow Examination

Bone marrow involvement in plasma cell myeloma is often focal, and multiple aspirations from different sites may be needed. In myeloma, plasma cells are more than 10%. In Waldenström's macroglobulinaemia, bone marrow shows infiltration by lymphocytes, plasmacytoid lymphocytes, and plasma cells.

Immunological cell marker analysis (for demonstration of monoclonality) and cytogenetic studies can be performed on bone marrow plasma cells.

Investigation of Protein Abnormalities

The term M (monoclonal, malignant, or myeloma) protein refers to the presence of structurally and electrophoretically homogeneous protein in serum or urine, which is synthesised by a neoplastic clone of plasma cells.

The monoclonal protein may be complete immunoglobulin molecules of the same class, or immunoglobulin light chains of the same type, or heavy chains of the same class. In contrast to monoclonal proteins, polyclonal proteins are immunoglobulins of different types. Monoclonal proteins are produced by neoplastic plasma cells that arise from a single progenitor cell, while polyclonal proteins are produced in response to the antigenic stimulation by different plasma cell clones. Disorders associated with production of monoclonal immunoglobulins are listed in Table 9.2.

Demonstration of monoclonal protein in serum and/or urine is an important laboratory test in plasma cell dyscrasias. Techniques employed for identification and characterisations of M proteins are shown in Box 9.1.

Serum Protein Electrophoresis

This is the initial step in the identification of abnormal proteins (Box 9.2). In this technique, separation of different proteins is achieved on the basis of their charge.

Table 9.2: Disorders associated with synthesis of monoclonal immunoglobulins (M protein)

1. Plasma cell dyscrasias: plasma cell myeloma, solitary myeloma, extramedullary plasmacytoma, Waldenström's macroglobulinaemia, primary amyloidosis, heavy chain disease, monoclonal gammopathy of undetermined significance.
2. Lymphoproliferative disorders: non-Hodgkin's lymphoma, chronic lymphocytic leukaemia, Hodgkin's lymphoma.

Box 9.1 Investigations at diagnosis in plasma cell dyscrasias

- Blood: Complete blood count including haemoglobin, blood smear, erythrocyte sedimentation rate (ESR) or plasma viscosity
- Bone marrow: Plasma cell number and morphology, demonstration of clonality and immunophenotype
- Serum: Albumin, immunoglobulins, protein electrophoresis, immunofixation, serum free light chain assay, κ/λ ratio
- Urine: 24-hour protein, 24-hour protein electrophoresis, 24-hour immunofixation
- Skeletal radiological survey
- Skeletal MRI scan

Commonly employed supporting media are paper, agar, agarose, and cellulose acetate membrane. Serum to be tested is applied to the supporting medium that is then placed in the electrophoresis chamber containing alkaline buffer solution; electric current is applied till the desired separation is achieved. Abnormal protein is identified by visual inspection and by densitometry scanning (Fig. 9.2). Normal and abnormal patterns are shown in Figure 9.1.

Normally five zones of proteins can be distinguished from anode to cathode as shown below:

Anode (+) Albumin- α1 globulin-α2 globulin-β globulin-γ globulin Cathode(-)

Each zone is composed of different proteins as follows:
- Albumin
- α1 globulin—α1 antitrypsin, α1 acid glycoprotein, α1 lipoprotein, Gc-globulin
- α2 globulin—α2 macroglobulin, haptoglobin, ceruloplasmin, complement, haemopexin

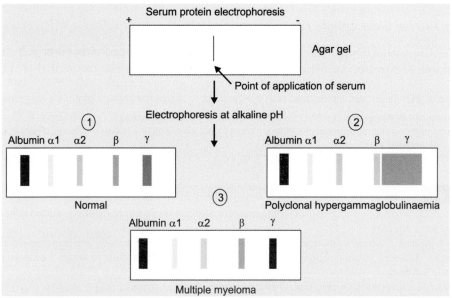

Figure 9.1: Diagrammatic representation of serum protein electrophoresis.
1: Normal pattern; 2: polyclonal hypergammaglobulinaemia; 3: M band in myeloma

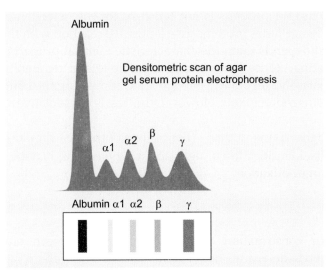

Figure 9.2: Diagrammatic representation of densitometric scanning of serum protein electrophoresis (normal)

- β globulin — β lipoprotein, transferrin
- γ globulin — Immunoglobulins.

Immunoglobulins migrate to the γ region and may extend to the β and α2 regions. A localised dense band with sharp margins in the γ to α2 region indicates M band. On densitometer tracing, a narrow-based, tall, sharply defined spike is seen. The position of the band may suggest the type of immunoglobulin, e.g. IgG is located in γ region while IgA migrates to the β region. A wide band with indistinct borders merging into the background on electrophoresis or a broad based peak in γ region on densitometric tracing is observed in polyclonal hypergammaglobulinaemia (e.g. in chronic infections or collagen vascular diseases) (Fig. 9.1).

In about 80% of patients with monoclonal gammopathies, M band will be detected. M band or spike in serum is not observed in nonsecretory myeloma, light chain disease, and primary amyloidosis. Urine sample must also be examined for the presence of M protein because if only light chains are being produced then they are not demonstrable in serum due to their rapid excretion in urine.

Urine Protein Electrophoresis

Both serum and urine protein electrophoresis should be performed in all suspected patients of plasma cell dyscrasias. In those plasma cell dyscrasias in which only light chains are synthesised, monoclonal protein may not be detected on serum protein electrophoresis. This is because, due to their low molecular weight, light chains are excreted in urine. Bence Jones protein in urine refers to either κ or λ light chains synthesised by a neoplastic clone of plasma cells.

Reagent strip test for proteins is not sensitive for the detection of light chains in urine. However, Bence Jones proteins give a positive reaction with the sulphosalicylic acid test. One test depends upon the characteristic thermal properties of Bence Jones proteins. On heating, Bence Jones proteins precipitate at temperature between 50° and 60° C and redissolve on boiling (90–100°C). On lowering the temperature to 60°C, Bence Jones proteins reprecipitate. However, this test is not sensitive and false negative reactions occur.

Monoclonal light chains in urine (Bence Jones proteins) should be demonstrated by electrophoresis. Identification of light chain type (κ or λ) is done by immunoelectrophoresis or immunofixation.

Immunoelectrophoresis

This is done for confirmation of monoclonal protein seen on serum protein electrophoresis and to determine heavy chain class and light chain type of monoclonal immunoglobulin (Box 9.3).

The procedure is as follows:
1. A well of appropriate size is cut with the template in agar gel, filled with the serum to be tested, which is then separated by electrophoresis.
2. Following this, a trough is cut parallel to electrophoretic migration and filled with polyvalent or mono-specific antiserum.
3. The separated serum proteins and the antiserum are allowed to diffuse into the gel for 24 hours.
4. Immunoprecipitin lines are formed (known as arcs) as antibodies meet their corresponding antigens.

Normal serum proteins are identified by the characteristic locations and shapes of the arcs. Pattern of the normal serum is compared with that of the test serum under similar conditions (two well and central trough pattern). Thickening and bowing of heavy chain or light chain arcs by monospecific antisera indicate presence of monoclonal protein.

Immunofixation

This technique is the gold standard for identification of nature of M protein and is particularly helpful for the identification of a small amount of M protein. In this technique, serum proteins are separated by electrophoresis in a gel and monospecific

---

Box 9.3   Immunoelectrophoresis

- This technique combines electrophoresis and immunodiffusion.
- Two uses in paraproteinaemias-
  1. Detection of M band—M band shows abnormalities such as thickening and bowing of arc, duplication, forking, and spoon shape.
  2. Identification of heavy and light chain type of M protein.

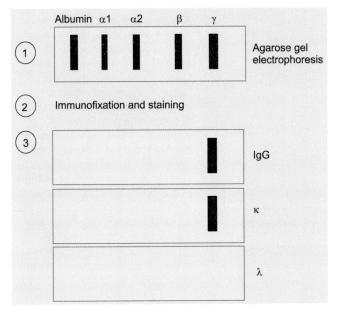

Figure 9.3: Principle of immunofixation.
(1) Serum proteins are separated by agarose gel electrophoresis.
(2) The M band in γ region is overlaid with monospecific antisera (IgG, IgA, IgM, and κ and γ light chains). Immunoprecipitation develops due to reaction between antigen and its corresponding antibody. Unbound material is removed by washing. Band is stained with a protein stain. (3) An example in which the M protein is identified as IgGκ. The M protein is IgGκ as there is development of immunoprecipitation with IgG and κ antisera. Anti-γ antibody shows no immunoprecipitation band

antiserum is applied directly over the surface of the gel. Immunoprecipitation band develops in the gel between corresponding protein antigen and the monospecific antiserum. The gel is washed to remove the unbound (unprecipitated) proteins and stained with a protein stain to demonstrate the immunoprecipitation band. The test is simple and requires shorter time than immunoelectrophoresis (Fig. 9.3).

Quantitation of Monoclonal Immunoglobulins

The quantitation of monoclonal and other immunoglobulins is necessary to assess the disease severity and follow response to treatment. The height of the peak on serum protein electrophoresis (on densitometer tracing) is directly proportional to the amount of M protein. However, exact quantitation can be done by single radial immunodiffusion. In this method, supporting gel has been impregnated with the specific antiserum. Test serum placed in the well diffuses into the antibody-incorporated gel and circular precipitates develop. The width of the circular precipitate is directly proportional to the concentration of immunoglobulin in the test serum (Fig. 9.4).

Radiological Studies

Complete skeletal survey should be obtained to detect bone lesions. This includes a series of radiographs of skull, spine, arms, ribs, pelvis, and legs. In some patients, magnetic resonance imaging or computerised axial tomography may be required. Magnetic resonance imaging is being increasingly used especially to assess spinal cord compression and extramedullary disease.

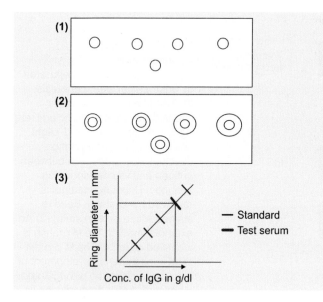

Figure 9.4: Principle of single radial immunodiffusion. (1) Agar gel into which antibody (e.g. anti-IgG) has been incorporated. Circular wells are cut in agar. Upper four wells are filled with increasing known concentrations of antigen, (e.g. IgG) i.e. standards, while the lower well is filled with the test (i.e. patient's) sample. Allow immunodiffusion by keeping the gel in a moist chamber at 4°C for 24 hours. (2) Formation of circular precipitates or rings due to radial diffusion of antigen into the antibody-incorporated gel. (3) Ring diameter is proportional to the concentration of the antigen (e.g. IgG)

❑ MULTIPLE MYELOMA

Multiple myeloma (MM) is a neoplasm of terminally differentiated B lymphocytes called plasma cells characterised by (i) formation of multifocal tumour masses composed of plasma cells at multiple (bone marrow-based) locations in the skeleton, (ii) suppression of normal immunoglobulin production (hypogammaglobulinaemia), and (iii) production of a monoclonal protein (paraprotein). This causes bone pain, osteolytic lesions, hypercalcaemia, and anaemia.

Pathogenesis

Myeloma cells originate from antigen-exposed post-germinal center B cells with somatic hypermutation, IgH gene rearrangement, and class switching. The progeny of this cell migrates to the bone marrow where maturation to terminally differentiated plasma cells occurs. An early event is chromosomal translocation involving 14q32 causing immortalisation of plasma cell clone. Further genetic changes like del13 lead to transformation to abnormal plasma cell clone (monoclonal gammopathy of undetermined significance or MGUS). It is now recognised that in almost all cases, multiple myeloma is preceded by asymptomatic MGUS. MGUS carries the same primary genetic abnormalities detected in multiple myeloma. Progression of MGUS to multiple myeloma is associated with acquisition of several genetic abnormalities (*RAS* mutations, p16 methylation, abnormalities of *MYC* oncogenes, secondary translocations, and *p53* mutation) and changes in marrow microenvironment. The bone marrow microenvironment undergoes marked changes with progression like increased angiogenesis and overproduction of cytokines and growth factors by stromal

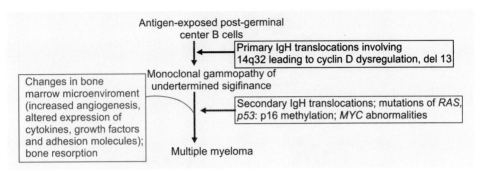

Figure 9.5: Pathogenesis of multiple myeloma

cells. The cytokines and growth factors later activate multiple signalling pathways that contribute to cell growth, survival, and drug resistance of myeloma cells (Fig. 9.5).

Bone lesions in myeloma result from imbalance between activity of osteoblasts and osteoclasts. Imbalance of two molecules, receptor activator of NFκB ligand or RANKL and osteoprotegerin leads to osteoclast activation and bone resorption. In addition, macrophage inflammatory protein-1α produced by myeloma cells contributes to overactivity of osteoclasts.

Aetiology

This is unknown. Risk factors include exposure to pesticides and herbicides (in farm workers), ionising radiation, prolonged use of hair colouring agents (cosmetologists), and chronic antigenic stimulation.

Clinical Features

MM occurs mainly in the older age (50–70 years) and has equal sex incidence. Manifestations are as follows:

Skeletal System

Bone pain in the back and ribs, which is aggravated by movement, is the most common symptom. Bone destruction is also responsible for spontaneous fractures in weight-bearing bones, osteolytic lesions, osteoporosis, spinal cord compression, and hypercalcaemia. Production of osteoclast-activating factor by myeloma cells is responsible for skeletal destruction (Fig. 9.6).

Renal Failure

This occurs in 50% of patients. Its causes are—formation of light-chain casts in renal tubules, hypercalcaemia (results from bone resorption), amyloid deposits, and pyelonephritis.

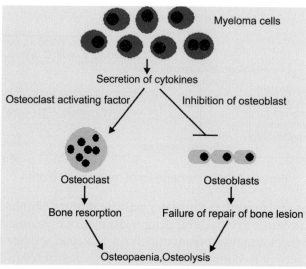

Figure 9.6: Pathogenesis of bone lesions in myeloma

Anaemia

Fatigue, weakness, and pallor result from anaemia. Anaemia can result from replacement of bone marrow by myeloma cells, suppression of haematopoiesis, renal failure, bleeding, infection or haemolysis.

Infections

Patients are susceptible to bacterial infections particularity of respiratory and urinary tracts. Hypogammaglobulinaemia due to suppression of normal B-lymphocytes by myeloma cells and neutropaenia secondary to marrow infiltration are responsible.

Haemorrhagic Tendencies

These can occur such as purpura or mucosal bleeding. They are due to thrombocytopaenia (bone marrow replacement), platelet dysfunction (due to coating of platelets by immunoglobulins which interfere with platelet aggregation), or antibodies against clotting factors.

Hyperviscosity syndrome

A triad of visual changes, bleeding, and neurologic impairment results from increase in blood viscosity by immunoglobulins.

Laboratory Features

Peripheral Blood Examination

Anaemia develops with progression of disease in all patients and is normocytic and normochromic.

A characteristic feature on peripheral blood smear is bluish background and red cell rouleaux formation (Fig. 9.7) due to hypergammaglobulinaemia.

Total leucocyte count may be normal or low. Differential count may show neutropaenia with relative lymphocytic predominance and few plasma cells. A

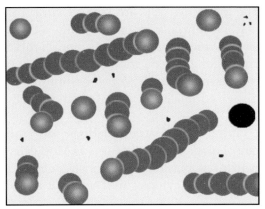

Figure 9.7: Peripheral blood smear in multiple myeloma showing rouleaux formation

leucoerythroblastic blood picture is observed in a minority of cases.

Platelet count is usually normal. Thrombocytopaenia, when present, is usually mild.

A markedly increased (or rapid) erythrocyte sedimentation rate is a typical feature. It is due to increased immunoglobulins.

Rouleaux formation may interfere with blood grouping.

Bone Marrow Examination

Bone marrow aspiration: This reveals plasmacytosis (>10%). Marrow involvement is often focal and percentage of plasma cells aspirated from different sites is variable.

The morphology of neoplastic cells varies from mature-looking plasma cells to immature cells resembling plasmablasts (Fig. 9.8). The mature cells have abundant, deeply basophilic cytoplasm with a perinuclear clear area or 'hof' representing Golgi zone, and an eccentrically placed nucleus with coarse chromatin and no nucleoli.

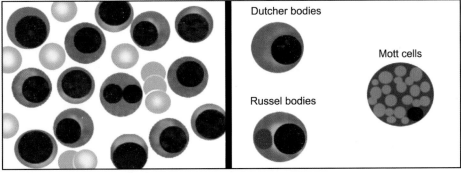

Figure 9.8: Bone marrow smear showing increased number of plasma cells in multiple myeloma. One binucleate plasma cell and one immature plasma cell with nucleolus are also seen. Panel on right shows some distinctive morphological features of plasma cells

The immature cells are larger than typical plasma cells with larger nucleus, which may be centrally or eccentrically located, finely dispersed nuclear chromatin, one or two prominent nucleoli, and light blue cytoplasm. Bi-or multinucleated cells and pleomorphism may be seen. The nuclear-cytoplasmic dissociation, i.e. relative cytoplasmic maturity (deep basophilia) in the presence of nuclear immaturity (finely dispersed nuclear chromatin) and pleomorphism are features of neoplastic plasma cells.

Intracellular accumulations of immunoglobulins may produce distinctive morphological features such as Mott cells or morula cells (numerous 'grape-like' pale bluish cytoplasmic inclusions), Dutcher bodies, and Russell bodies (round hyaline inclusions in cytoplasm). These features also occur in reactive plasmacytosis.

Bone marrow biopsy: Large clusters or sheets of plasma cells on marrow biopsy are highly suggestive of a neoplastic rather than a reactive disorder.

Immunoperoxidase or immunofluorescent techniques can be applied using antibodies to κ or λ chain to demonstrate monoclonality. Neoplastic plasma cells will show either κ or λ chain positivity, while reactive plasma cells are positive for both κ and λ light chains in a balanced proportion. Although these immunocytochemical techniques are not necessary for diagnosis of MM in most cases, they are helpful in establishing clonality in- (i) those cases in which clinical, radiologic, and immunologic features are suggestive of diagnosis of MM but plasma cells are mature-looking and relatively few in number; and (ii) non-secretory myeloma in which neoplastic plasma cells do not synthesise immunoglobulin.

Protein Alterations

Zone electrophoresis of serum proteins (see Fig. 9.1) shows a sharply defined M band in about 80% of patients. Usually it is located in the γ globulin region, but occasionally it migrates to β or α2 regions.

Immunoelectrophoresis or immunofixation using monospecific antisera reveals M protein to be IgG in 55 to 60%, light chains only in 20 to 25%, and IgA in 15 to 20% cases. Rarely myelomas are of IgD, IgE, IgM, and biclonal (synthesis of two M proteins) type. Non-secretory myeloma accounts for 1% myeloma cases. Approximately 70% cases show presence of both serum and urinary monoclonal protein. Conditions associated with the production of a monoclonal protein are shown in Table 9.2.

Normal immunoglobulins in serum are markedly decreased (hypogamma-globulinaemia).

Immunophenotyping

Neoplastic plasma cells express CD138 (bright), CD38 (bright), CD45 (dim), and either κ or λ immunoglobulin light chain. There is often abnormal acquisition of CD56 and CD117. In contrast to normal plasma cells, there is loss of CD19 expression.

Biochemical Abnormalities

Serum creatinine is raised in the presence of renal insufficiency. *Hypercalcaemia* is often present. *Serum alkaline phosphatase* is normal or slightly increased; this is helpful in differentiating MM from skeletal involvement due to hyperparathyroidism or metastatic carcinoma in which alkaline phosphatase is markedly raised. Measurement of *serum β2 microglobulin* at the time of diagnosis provides useful prognostic information. β2 microglobulin level more than 6 µg/ml is associated with high tumour mass and shorter survival as compared to patients with β2 microglobulin < 6 µg/ml. Serial estimation of β2 microglobulin is also helpful in assessing the growth rate of myeloma.

Cytogenetic Analysis

With fluorescent *in situ* hybridisation, chromosomal abnormalities are identified in majority of patients with myeloma. The most common abnormalities are translocations involving 14q and deletions of chromosome 13. A deletion of chromosome 13 is an adverse prognostic indicator (Table 9.4).

Radiological Features

A full skeletal X-ray survey is needed. Bone changes in MM include–diffuse osteoporosis, localised osteolytic lesions, and pathological fractures. The osteolytic lesions appear as multiple, rounded, punched out areas without sclerosis at the borders. Common sites for osteolytic lesions are vertebrae, ribs, skull, pelvis, and proximal areas of long bones. Rarely the localised lesions are osteosclerotic and associated with **p**olyneuropathy, **o**rganomegaly, **e**ndocrinopathy, **m**onoclonal protein, and **s**kin changes (POEMS syndrome). Diffuse osteoporosis may lead to compression fractures of thoracic or lumbar vertebrae.

Osteolytic lesions in MM are produced by activation of osteoclasts by certain factors secreted by myeloma cells. These osteoclast-activating factors (OAF) are tumour necrosis factor α and interleukin-1β.

Skeletal changes do not occur in about 20% of patients. About 3% of patients present with a solitary osteolytic lesion (plasmacytoma).

Diagnosis

Diagnosis of MM requires correlation of clinical, bone marrow, immunological, and radiological findings. This is because some of the findings in MM are also observed in other disorders (Fig. 9.9).

The parameters taken into consideration for diagnosis of multiple myeloma are shown in Box 9.5.

Criteria for diagnosis of multiple myeloma, smoldering myeloma, and monoclonal gammopathy of undetermined significance are shown in Box 9.4.

Plasmacytosis in bone marrow	Osteolytic lesions
Plasma cell dyscrasias Chronic infections Chronic inflammation Cirrhosis Carcinoma	Multiple myeloma Metastatic carcinoma Hyperparathyroidism
Monoclonal protein	Hypogamma-globulinaemia
Plasma cell dyscrasias Chronic lymphocytic leukaemia Non-Hodgkin's lymphoma	Plasma cell dyscrasias Leukaemias Lymphomas Autoimmune disease

Figure 9.9: Why multiple criteria are needed for diagnosis of myeloma? It can be seen that typical features of myeloma also occur in other acquired disorders and no single criterion is specific for myeloma

---

Box 9.4   Diagnostic criteria for multiple myeloma, smoldering myeloma, and monoclonal gammopathy of undetermined significance (International Myeloma Working Group 2003, adapted by WHO 2008 classification)

Multiple myeloma
- Presence of M protein in serum/urine
- Presence of clonal plasma cells in bone marrow or plasmacytoma on biopsy
- Presence of related organ or tissue impairment*

Smoldering myeloma (Asymptomatic myeloma)
- Serum M protein ≥3.0 g/dl and/or bone marrow clonal plasma cells ≥10%
- Absence of related organ or tissue impairment*

Monoclonal gammopathy of undetermined significance
- Serum M protein <3.0 g/dl
- Bone marrow clonal plasma cells <10% and low level of plasma cell infiltration on biopsy
- Absence of lytic bone lesions
- Absence of other B lymphoproliferative disorder
- Absence of related organ or tissue impairment*

*: Related organ or tissue impairment: hypercalcaemia, renal insufficiency, anaemia, bone lesions (CRAB)
Note: Patients with M protein and monoclonal plasma cells that are below the minimal criteria can still be diagnosed as multiple myeloma if evidence of tissue impairment (CRAB) is confirmed. This is because it has been observed that a small number of symptomatic patients have plasma cell <10% and M protein <3 g/dl.

Box 9.5   Typical features of multiple myeloma

- Symptomatic patient (especially bone pain, repeated infections, fatigue) >50 years of age
- Bone marrow plasma cells increased
- Osteolytic bone lesions on skeletal X-ray survey
- Presence of M component in serum and/or urine
- Hypogammaglobulinaemia (reduced levels of normal immunogolbulins)

Differential Diagnosis

Reactive Bone Marrow Plasmacytosis

This is seen in chronic granulomatous infections (e.g. tuberculosis), cirrhosis, chronic active hepatitis, carcinoma, and Hodgkin's disease. Following features are helpful in distinguishing reactive from neoplastic plasmacytosis: (a) Plasma cells arranged as solid sheets or clusters and showing nuclear cytoplasmic asynchrony favour neoplastic proliferation of plasma cells; (b) Serum protein electrophoresis shows a broad-based band of polyclonal hypergammaglobulinaemia in reactive plasmacytosis, and M band in γ to α2 region in MM; (c) Immunoperoxidase technique shows light chain restriction (predominantly κ or λ chain reactivity) in neoplastic plasma cells while both κ or λ light chain positivity in a balanced proportion in reactive plasma cells. κ/λ ratio is 2:1 in reactive plasmacytosis. (d) Reactive plasma cells are CD19+, CD56−, while myeloma cells are CD19− and CD56+.

Monoclonal Gammopathy of Undetermined Significance (MGUS)

Patients with MM must be distinguished from those with MGUS. MGUS is considered later (Refer to Table 9.6).

Waldenström's Macroglobulinaemia (WM)

In contrast to MM, in WM hyperviscosity syndrome, hepatosplenomegaly and lymphadenopathy are prominent, and osteolytic lesions and hypercalcaemia are rare. Bone marrow in WM shows diffuse infiltration by lymphocytes, plasmacytoid lymphocytes, and a few plasma cells; mast cells are also increased in number (Refer to Table 9.5).

Lymphoproliferative Disorders with Monoclonal Gammopathy

Some lymphoproliferative disorders are associated with production of monoclonal immunoglobulins, particularly small lymphocytic lymphoma, chronic lymphocytic leukaemia, and plasmacytoid lymphocyte type lymphoma. Correct diagnosis is usually possible by clinical examination, blood and bone marrow examination, and lymph node biopsy.

Metastatic Carcinoma

Carcinomas metastatic to bone can produce osteolytic lesions similar to multiple myeloma. Diagnosis is based on demonstration of malignant cells in bone marrow and identification of primary tumour.

Staging and Prognosis

There are two main staging systems of multiple myeloma: Durie and Salmon staging system and International staging system (Table 9.3). Importance of some factors affecting prognosis is as follows:

Serum β2 microglobulin

Estimation of serum β2 microglobulin, either alone or in combination with other parameters, is useful for predicting duration of survival and prognosis in MM.

In southwest Oncology Group study, median survival was found to be 3 years with pretreatment serum β2 microglobulin level ≤6 µg/ml, while median survival was less than 2 years for those with values >6 µg/ml. If combined with serum albumin or age, then patients could be stratified into three distinct groups–low-risk, intermediate risk, and high-risk with increasingly shorter median survival.

Plasma Cell Labelling Index

Proliferative activity of tumour cells measured as labelling index using [³H] thymidine has prognostic importance. A low plasma cell labelling index (<1%) is indicative of low percentage of plasma cells that are actively growing and longer median survival as compared to a high index.

Table 9.3: Staging systems in multiple myeloma

Durie and Salmon staging system	International staging system (ISS)
Stage I (All of following)	**Stage I**
• Haemoglobin >10.0 g/dl, normal serum calcium, normal immunoglobulin levels (non-M protein)	• Serum β2 microglobulin < 3.5 mg/L
• Low M protein: IgG < 50g/dl, IgA < 30g/dl, urine BJ protein <4 g/24 hours	• Serum albumin ≥ 3.5 g/dl
• Normal bone X-ray or single plasmacytoma of bone	**Stage II**
Stage II Values between stage I and stage III	Serum β2 microglobulin < 3.5 mg/L and serum albumin < 3.5 g/dl OR Serum β2-microglobulin 3.5–5.5 mg/L irrespective of serum albumin level
	Stage III
Stage III (≥ 1 of following)	Serum β2 microglobulin >5.5 mg/L
• Haemoglobin < 8.5 g/dl, serum calcium >12 mg/dl	
• Multiple lytic bone lesions	
• High M protein: IgG > 70 g/dl, IgA > 50 g/dl, urine light chains > 12 g/24 hours	
Subclassification: A: Serum creatinine < 2 mg/dl B: Serum creatinine ≥ 2 mg/dl	

Table 9.4: Prognostic significance of cytogenetic abnormalities in myeloma

Parameter	Unfavourable prognosis	Favourable prognosis
1. IgH translocations	t(4;14), t(14;16), t(14;20)	t(11;14), t(6;14)
2. Numerical abnormalities	del(13q), del(17p), hypodiploidy	Hyperdiploidy

Plasmablastic Morphology

Plasmablastic morphology and increased lactate dehydrogenase levels (indicative of increased tumour burden) have poor prognosis.

Cytogenetic abnormalities

The significance of cytogenetic abnormalities in myeloma is shown in Table 9.4.

Treatment

Although chemotherapy does not cure the disease, it relieves symptoms, controls the progression of disease, and prolongs survival. It is indicated in symptomatic patients and when evidence of disease progression develops. Melphalan with or without prednisone daily for 4 days every 4 to 6 weeks is the standard form of treatment. Chemotherapy causes reduction of tumour mass which results in fall in concentration of paraprotein in serum and urine, reduction in serum $\beta2$ microglobulin, and decrease in plasma cells in bone marrow which allows return of normal haemopoietic activity and normalisation of peripheral blood counts. This objective evidence of response to therapy develops gradually and occurs in 50 to 60% of patients. Patients should be regularly followed and when fall in paraprotein concentration becomes stabilised at lower level for at least 3 months (plateau phase), treatment is discontinued. The median remission time (plateau phase) is about 2 years and median survival 3 years with this treatment. Relapse eventually occurs after stopping treatment when chemotherapy (melphalan±prednisone) is reinstituted. Cumulative exposure to melphalan therapy is associated with risk of myelodysplasia and AML. Thalidomide has been shown to produce response in about 30% of relapsed or refractory patients.

Other forms of chemotherapy in MM include:

1. Cyclophosphamide with or without prednisone
2. Combination chemotherapy (vincristine, adriamycin, and dexamethasone or VAD)
3. Interferon alpha – This is given as a maintenance therapy following conventional chemotherapy and has been shown to prolong the remission achieved with chemotherapy.
4. High dose chemotherapy followed by autologous stem cell transplantation rescue: This option should be considered in newly diagnosed younger patients who will be able to tolerate the side effects. Although overall survival is improved, relapse eventually occurs in majority of patients (due to stem cell graft contaminated with tumour cells or incomplete eradication of minimal residual disease). Although

allogeneic stem cell transplantation is associated with long-term disease-free survival, treatment-related mortality is very high.

Supportive care consists of (1) treatment of anaemia: Current evidence indicates that recombinant human erythropoietin is effective in improving haemoglobin and reducing transfusion needs even in patients without renal impairment; (2) bone disease: bisphosphonates (pamidronate, clodronate) inhibit osteoclast activity and reduce skeletal pain, hypercalcaemia, and other skeletal morbidity and improve quality of life; they are recommended for all patients with myeloma needing treatment for their disease; local radiotherapy is given for localised bone pain and pathological fractures; (3) renal failure: is usually responsive to rehydration and chemotherapy (by reducing paraproteins and light chains); (4) hyperviscosity syndrome is treated with plasmapheresis followed by chemotherapy.

Causes of Death

With current chemotherapy, multiple myeloma is incurable with overall median survival of approximately 3 years. The common causes of death are infection secondary to hypogammaglobulinaemia and neutropaenia, haemorrhage, renal failure, myelodysplastic syndrome, and acute myeloid leukaemia. Myelodysplastic syndrome and acute myeloid leukaemia may occur as part of the natural history of myeloma or more commonly secondary to therapy with alkylating agents.

Other Forms of Plasma Cell Myeloma

Solitary Plasmacytoma of Bone

This is a rare condition in which neoplastic proliferation of plasma cells is limited to a single focus in the bone. Patient presents with bone pain or pathological fracture at the site of the lesion. In this condition there is only a single osteolytic bone lesion on skeletal radiological survey composed of plasma cells. Evidence of multiple myeloma (like myeloma cells in bone marrow, anaemia, renal disease and a monoclonal protein in serum and/or urine) is absent. Common sites are vertebrae, ribs, skull, ileum, femur, clavicle, and scapula. Regular follow-up with serum and urine protein electrophoresis for monoclonal protein is essential after radiotherapy. Most patients (55%) develop evidence of dissemination (multiple myeloma) within 10 years. A proportion of patients appear to be cured at 10 years, while some patients have recurrence or development of another plasmacytoma.

Extramedullary (Extraosseous) Plasmacytoma

This is a rare neoplasm of plasma cells, which arises in extramedullary or extraosseous site particularly upper respiratory tract such as oropharynx, paranasal sinuses, nasopharynx, and larynx. However, any site may be affected including gastrointestinal tract, breast, gonads, etc. Multiple myeloma should be excluded by relevant investigations. Risk of progression to multiple myeloma is low. Treatment consists of radiotherapy.

Smoldering Myeloma

These patients meet the minimal diagnostic criteria for multiple myeloma, but do not have myeloma-related symptoms and osteolytic bone lesions. The disease remains stable for many years; treatment is initiated when evidence of disease progression develops.

Nonsecretory Myeloma

This accounts for approximately 1% cases of multiple myeloma. Clinical, radiological, and haematological features are similar to those found in typical (secretory) myeloma except for the absence of monoclonal protein in serum and urine (since plasma cells synthesise but do not secrete immunoglobulins), and lower incidence of renal insufficiency. Immunofluorescence or immunoperoxidase studies will show monoclonal cytoplasmic immunoglobulin. Treatment is like MM. Monoclonal nature of plasma cell proliferation may be established by demonstration of light chain restriction.

Plasma Cell Leukaemia

Plasma cell leukaemia is a rare type of leukaemia defined as presence of >2000/cmm or >20% of plasma cells in peripheral blood. It may be primary (*de novo*) or secondary (which occurs during late stages of multiple myeloma).

Both primary and secondary types occur in adults between 50 and 60 years of age. Lymphadenopathy and hepatosplenomegaly occur more frequently in primary type than secondary type, while bone involvement is more common in secondary type.

Anaemia and thrombocytopaenia are frequent. Peripheral blood smear shows rouleaux formation, raised ESR, and plasma cells or plasmablasts. Many patients have M protein in serum and Bence Jones proteins in urine. Bone marrow shows infiltration by plasma cells. Immunological marker analysis typically shows monoclonal cytoplasmic immunoglobulin and expression of CD38 antigen on surface.

Primary leukaemia has aggressive clinical course, short survival (<6 months), and poor response to treatment. Treatment is similar to multiple myeloma.

❑ WALDENSTRÖM'S MACROGLOBULINAEMIA

Waldenström's macroglobulinaemia (WM) is a rare B-lymphoproliferative disorder characterised by (1) neoplastic proliferation of small lymphocytes, lymphoplasmacytoid cells, and plasma cells, and (2) production of monoclonal IgM immunoglobulins. Macroglobulins are IgM immunoglobulins, which have high molecular weight. Underlying lymphoplasmacytic lymphoma is present in majority of patients.

Clinical Features

WM is a disease of the old persons with highest occurrence between 60 and 70 years. It is more common in males. Fatigue, weakness, and weight loss are common symptoms. The physical presence of macroglobulins increases blood viscosity and may produce hyperviscosity syndrome. Manifestations of hyperviscosity syndrome include visual impairment, bleeding tendencies (purpura, epistaxis), and neurological changes (headache, ataxia, vertigo, altered mental state, coma). Retinal changes of hyperviscosity are distension and segmentation of retinal veins ("sausage link" pattern), haemorrhages, and exudates. Hyperviscosity syndrome usually develops when serum viscosity is more than four times normal. On physical examination, usual findings are lymphadenopathy and hepatosplenomegaly. Uncommon manifestations of WM are: (1) peripheral neuropathy, (2) cryoglobulinaemia (patient develops Raynaud's phenomenon, urticaria, purpura on exposure to cold), (3) cold haemagglutinin disease, and (4) amyloidosis.

Bone pain and lytic bone lesions are absent in contrast to multiple myeloma. Renal involvement is also rare.

Laboratory Features

Peripheral Blood Examination

Normocytic normochromic anaemia is present in majority of patients at diagnosis. Causes of anaemia include expansion of plasma volume, inhibition of haematopoiesis, and sometimes haemolysis. Rouleaux formation is prominent.

Leucopaenia may be present. Lymphocytes are frequently increased. Platelet count may be normal or low.

Erythrocyte sedimentation rate is usually markedly raised.

Bone Marrow Examination

This reveals intertrabecular infiltrate of small lymphocytes, plasmacytoid lymphocytes, and plasma cells in varying proportions. Mast cells are prominent. Periodic acid Schiff-positive inclusions in nucleus and cytoplasm of some of the cells may be seen.

Immunophenotyping

This shows surface and cytoplasmic IgM+, IgD-, CD19+, CD20+, CD22+, CD5-, CD10-, and CD23-.

Serum and Urine Protein Electrophoresis

Zone electrophoresis of serum shows a dense, well-localised band (and a narrow based spike on densitometer tracing) in γ region. Identification of monoclonal protein is made by immunoelectrophoresis or immunofixation using monospecific antisera. Monoclonal protein in WM shows reactivity against μ heavy chain and to one type of light chain either κ or λ. In symptomatic patients, concentration of paraprotein in serum is usually > 3 g/dl. Electrophoresis of concentrated urine will reveal monoclonal light chains in majority of patients.

Tests for Haemostasis

Coating of platelets by monoclonal IgM causes abnormalities in platelet function, e.g. prolongation of bleeding time, and defective platelet aggregation. Monoclonal proteins inhibit fibrin monomer polymerisation, which results in prolongation of thrombin time.

Lymph Node Biopsy

Shows histologic features of plasmacytoid type of lymphoma.

Differential Diagnosis

Multiple Myeloma

Some differences between MM and WM are outlined in Table 9.5.

Other Lymphoproliferative Disorders with IgM Monoclonal Gammopathy

Some cases of chronic lymphocytic leukaemia and non-Hodgkin's lymphoma may be associated with monoclonal macroglobulinaemia.

Table 9.5: Comparative features of multiple myeloma (MM) and Waldenström's macroglobulinaemia (WM)

Parameter	MM	WM
1. Organomegaly, hyperviscosity syndrome	Rare	Frequent
2. Skeletal disease	Frequent	Absent
3. Renal insufficiency	Frequent	Rare
4. Bone marrow findings	Increased plasma cells	Diffuse infiltration by lymphocytes, plasmacytoid lymphocytes, and plasma cells
5. Nature of monoclonal protein	Usually IgG, IgA, or light chains only	IgM
6. Drug of first choice	Melphalan+Prednisone	Chlorambucil
7. Median survival	3 years	5 years

Monoclonal Gammopathy of Undetermined Significance of IgM Type

These patients have increased monoclonal IgM in serum but do not have anaemia, organomegaly or manifestations of hyperviscosity. These patients need regular follow-up as WM may develop in an occasional patient.

Splenic Lymphoma with Villous Lymphocytes

Features favouring this disorder are marked enlargement of spleen without lymphadenopathy, moderately raised leucocyte count with villous lymphocytes, and IgM paraprotein concentration < 2 g/dl.

Prognosis

The disease is indolent with overall survival of 5 years. Adverse prognostic factors include advanced age (>60 years), cytopaenias in peripheral blood, neuropathies, and weight loss. Transformation to a high-grade diffuse large cell lymphoma occurs in a minority of patients.

Treatment

Patients should be treated when they develop clinical manifestations or evidence of disease progression. Chemotherapy (usually chlorambucil + prednisone) is given to control the proliferation of neoplastic cells. New therapeutic drugs are nucleoside analogues (cladribine and fludarabine) which have been tried in newly diagnosed and in cases resistant to chlorambucil + prednisone and appear to be effective. Plasmapheresis is helpful in alleviating manifestations of hyperviscosity.

❑ MONOCLONAL GAMMOPATHY OF UNDETERMINED SIGNIFICANCE

The presence of monoclonal protein in serum without clinical or laboratory manifestations attributable to underlying plasma cell disorder or lymphoproliferative disease is referred to as monoclonal gammopathy of undetermined significance (MGUS). Previously these disorders were called as benign monoclonal gammopathies. If such patients are followed regularly, majority remains stable over many years and consequently require no treatment. However, a small proportion will eventually develop some form of plasma cell dyscrasia such as multiple myeloma, Waldenström's macroglobulinaemia, or amyloidosis. Therefore, follow-up is necessary to determine the benign or malignant nature of these disorders. Thus, the designation monoclonal gammopathy of undetermined significance appears to be more appropriate for these disorders.

MGUS is reported to occur in 1% of individuals over 50 years of age. Features favouring MGUS are as follows:

Table 9.6: Comparison of multiple myeloma (MM) and MGUS

Parameter	MM	MGUS
1. Plasma cells in marrow	> 10%	< 10%
2. Anaemia, hypercalcaemia, lytic bone lesions, renal involvement	Frequent	Absent
3. Monoclonal protein	Variable	IgG < 3.0 g/dl
4. Normal immunoglobulins	Usually low	Usually normal
5. Plasma cell labelling index	> 1%	< 1%

1. Bone marrow plasma cells are within normal limits or are less than 10%. Morphologically plasma cells may be mature or immature.
2. Concentration of monoclonal protein in serum is <3.0 g/dl. Level of M protein remaining stable during long-term follow-up is the most reliable feature favouring MGUS. Bence Jones proteinuria is absent or if present its level is low. In most patients concentration of uninvolved immunoglobulins is normal, although it may be reduced in an occasional patient.
3. Anaemia, osteolytic lesions, hypercalcaemia, renal involvement, organomegaly, and extramedullary plasmacytoma are absent.
4. Plasma cell labelling index using [^{3}H] thymidine or immunofluorescence procedure is low indicating low proliferative activity.

Following features favour the diagnosis of plasma cell dyscrasia other than MGUS–bone marrow plasmacytosis greater than 10%, steadily rising M-component, significant Bence Jones proteinuria, anaemia, osteolytic lesions, hypercalcaemia, hepatosplenomegaly, or high plasma cell labelling index. Differences between MM and MGUS are listed in Table 9.6.

Most cases of MGUS are benign and remain stable over many years of follow-up. In a study by Kyle, when followed for more than 10 years, malignant plasma cell dyscrasia or a lymphoproliferative disorder developed in approximately 20% of patients with MGUS.

Patients with MGUS should not be treated unless progression to a neoplastic plasma cell disorder occurs.

❏ BIBLIOGRAPHY

1. Alexanian R and Dimopoulos MA. Management of multiple myeloma. Semin Hematol. 1975;32: 20-30.
2. Alexanian R. Localized and indolent myeloma. Blood. 1980;56: 521-25.
3. Barlogie B, Epstein J, Selvanayagam PI, Alexanian R. Plasma cell myeloma - new biological insights and advances in therapy. Blood. 1989;73:865-79.
4. Bataille R and Sany J. Solitary myeloma. Clinical and prognostic features of a review of 114 cases. Cancer. 1981;48:45-851.
5. British Committee for Standards in Haematology: Diagnosis and management of multiple myeloma. Br J Haematol. 2001;115:522-40.
6. Channing Rodgers RP. Clinical laboratory methods for detection of antigens and antibodies. In Stites DP, Terr AI, Parslow TG (Eds): Basic and Clinical Immunology. 8th ed. Connecticut. Appleton and Lange, 1994.

7. Dimopoulos MA and Alexanian R. Waldenstrom's macroglobulinaemia. Blood. 1994;83:1452-59.

8. Durie BGM and Salmon SE. A clinical staging system for multiple myeloma. Correlation of measured myeloma cell mass with presenting clinical features, response to treatment, and survival. Cancer. 1975;36:842-54.

9. Durie BGM, Salmon SE, and Moon IE. Pretreatment tumour mass, cell kinetics, and prognosis in multiple myeloma. Blood. 1980;55:364-72.

10. Durie BGM, Stock-Novack D, Salmon SE, Finley P, Beckord J, Crowley J, Coltman CA. Prognostic value of pre-treatment serum β2 microglobulin in myeloma: a Southwest Oncology Group study. Blood. 1990;75:823-30.

11. Gandara DR, Mackenzie MR. Differential diagnosis of monoclonal gammopathy. Med Clin North Am. 1988;72:55-1167.

12. Gertz MA, Fonseca R, Rajkumar SV. Waldenstrom's macroglobulinaemia. The Oncologist 2000;5:63-67.

13. Greipp P, San Miguel J, Durie B, et al. International Staging system for multiple myeloma. J Clin Oncol. 2005;23:3412.

14. Greipp PR and Kyle RA. Clinical, morphological, and cell kinetic differences among multiple myeloma, monoclonal gammopathy of undetermined significance, and smoldering multiple myeloma. Blood. 1983;62:166-71.

15. Greipp PR, Witzog TE, Gonchoroff NJ, Haberman TM, Katzman JA, O'Fallon WM, Kyle RA. Immunofluorescence labelling indices in myeloma and related monoclonal gammopathies. Mayo Clin Proc. 1987;62:969-77.

16. Joyner MV, Cassuto JP, Dujardin P, Schneider M, Ziegler G, Euller L, Masseyeff R. Nonexcretory multiple myeloma. Br J Haematol. 1979;43:559-66.

17. Klein B. Cytokine, cytokine receptors, transduction signals, and oncogenes in multiple myeloma. Semin Hematol. 1995;32:4-19.

18. Kohn J. The laboratory investigation of paraproteinemia. In Dyke SC (Ed): Recent Advances in Clinical Pathology. Series 6. Edinburgh and London. Churchill Livingstone. 1973.

19. Kosmo MA and Gale RP. Plasma cell leukemia. Semin Hematol. 1987;24:202-8.

20. Kyle RA and Greipp PR. Smoldering multiple myeloma. N Engl J Med. 1980;302:1347-49.

21. Kyle RA and Greipp PR. The laboratory investigation of monoclonal gammopathies. Mayo Clin Proc. 1978;53:719-39.

22. Kyle RA. 'Benign" monoclonal gammopathy. A misnomer? JAMA. 1984;251:1849-54.

23. Kyle RA. Monoclonal gammopathy of undetermined significance. Am J Med. 1978;64:814-26.

24. Kyle RA. Multiple myeloma. Review of 869 cases. Mayo Clin Proc. 1975;50:29-40

25. Kyle RA. Why better prognostic factors for multiple myeloma are needed? Blood. 1994;83: 1713-16.

26. Latrielle J, Barlogie B, Johnston D. Ploidy and proliferative characteristics in monoclonal gammopathies. Blood. 1982;59:43-51.

27. Lin P. Plasma cell myeloma. Haematol Oncol Clin N Am. 2009;23:709-27.

28. Shrikhande AV, Saoji AM, Chande CA, Thakar YS. Gel immunodiffusion and disc electrophoresis. A technical manual. Dept. of Microbiology, Govt. Medical College, Nagpur. 1994.

29. Swerdlow SH, Campo E, Harris NL, Jaffe ES, Pileri SA, Stein H, Thiele J, Vardiman JW (Eds): WHO classification of tumours of haematopoietic and lymphoid tissues. 4th ed. Lyon. International Agency for Research on Cancer. 2008.

30. The International Myeloma Working Group: Criteria for the classification of monoclonal gammopathies, multiple myeloma and related disorders: a report of the International Myeloma Working Group. Br J Haematol. 2003;121:749.

CHAPTER

10

Malignant Lymphomas

Lymphomas are a heterogeneous group of malignant neoplasms, which originate primarily in lymph nodes or other lymphoid tissues. They are divided into two major types—Hodgkin's lymphoma (HL) and non-Hodgkin's lymphoma (NHL). Clinical and biologic differences between these two are outlined in Table 10.1.

Cell of origin: NHL arises from B or T lymphocytes; cell of origin in majority of cases of Hodgkin's lymphoma is a mature B lymphocyte at the germinal centre stage of differentiation.

Clinical features: In NHL, involvement of multiple peripheral lymph nodes, extranodal disease, noncontiguous dissemination to distant organs, and bone marrow involvement are more common. In contrast, in HL, disease is usually limited to a single axial lymph node region (usually cervical), spread is in contiguous manner, and bone marrow involvement is rare. HL occurs predominantly in young adults, while NHL shows increasing incidence with age.

Table 10.1: Differences between Hodgkin's and non-Hodgkin's lymphoma

Parameter	Hodgkin's lymphoma	Non-Hodgkin's lymphoma
1. Incidence	Stable	Steadily increasing
2. Age	Usually in young adults	Incidence increases with age
3. Cell of origin	Usually B lymphocyte	B or T lymphocyte
4. Lymphadenopathy	Axial, especially cervical or mediastinal	Multiple, peripheral
5. Extranodal disease	Rare	More common
6. Defining morphological feature	Reed-Sternberg cell in a characteristic cellular milieu	—
7. Prognosis	Curable in majority of cases	Variable

Cytogenetic analysis: Clonal, non-random chromosomal abnormalities are frequent in NHL; specific and recurrent cytogenetic changes have not been demonstrated by conventional techniques in classical HL.

Morphology: The characteristic defining feature of HL is Reed-Sternberg cells against background of inflammatory cells; such morphology is not observed in NHL.

❏ HODGKIN'S LYMPHOMA

Thomas Hodgkin first described this disease in 1832. It is characterised histologically by presence of Reed-Sternberg (RS) cells in a background of reactive inflammatory cells such as lymphocytes, plasma cells, eosinophils, and fibroblasts. Hodgkin's lymphoma (HL) is usually localised to a single lymph node region in the initial stage; with progression it spreads to other lymph node regions by contiguity and disseminates to other organs.

Aetiopathogenesis

The RS cells and their mononuclear variants are the neoplastic or malignant cells in HL. Other cells in the background such as lymphocytes, plasma cells, and eosinophils are non-neoplastic. The characteristic cell of HL was described by Sternberg (1893) and Dorothy Reed (1902). A unique feature of HL is that the malignant cells form only a minor component of the tumour, majority being composed of reactive cells. The reactive cells (granulocytes, lymphocytes, plasma cells, and fibroblasts) probably represent the immune reaction of the host against the tumour cells.

Hodgkin's lymphoma comprises of two distinct disease entities (see classification): (1) nodular lymphocytic predominance HL, and (2) classical HL. Nature of RS cells in HL remained unknown for many years. Recent molecular studies have shown that RS cell is a B lymphocyte originating in germinal centre of lymph node in majority of cases, and hence the term 'Hodgkin's lymphoma' is more appropriate than the previous term 'Hodgkin's disease'.

Infection by Epstein-Barr virus (EBV) is thought to play a role in the causation of HL on the basis of identification of EBV DNA in lymph nodes and elevated antibody titres to EBV in some patients, and increased risk of HL in patients with infectious mononucleosis.

Various types of cytokines have been found to be elaborated by RS cells and lymphocytes in HL. Secretion of these cytokines may be responsible for certain histologic features such as fibrosis and eosinophilia. In addition B systemic symptoms may be related to secretion of certain cytokines.

Clinical Features

HL is a common form of malignancy in young adults (20–30 years). A second minor peak of increased incidence is noted after 50 years of age. Males are more commonly affected.

The usual mode of presentation is localised supradiaphragmatic lymph node enlargement, commonly in cervical region; the enlarged nodes are firm, painless, rubbery, freely mobile, and discrete. Mediastinal lymphadenopathy is frequent. Extranodal involvement is uncommon.

About one-third of patients have systemic symptoms related to disease. These are called B symptoms and include: fever, night sweats, and weight loss >10% in last 6 months. Presence of systemic symptoms is associated with unfavourable prognosis. Sometimes systemic symptoms are not associated with clinically evident lymphadenopathy and patient presents as a case of pyrexia of unknown origin (PUO); in these cases usually intra-abdominal disease is present. Some patients have alcohol-induced pain at the site of enlarged lymph nodes or pruritus. Splenomegaly and hepatomegaly occur in advanced stages.

Clinical features also depend on histologic type of HL.

Histopathology and Classification of Hodgkin's Lymphoma

Classical Reed-Sternberg Cell and its Variants

The identification of classical RS cells in the characteristic cytologic environment of normal inflammatory cells is essential for diagnosis of Hodgkin's lymphoma. The classical RS cell is a giant cell (20–30 μ) having two nuclei or two nuclear lobes, which may appear as mirror images. Each nuclear lobe or each nucleus contains a prominent inclusion-like eosinophilic nucleolus surrounded by a clear zone ("owl-eyed" nucleoli). The cytoplasm is usually abundant and faintly eosinophilic or amphophilic. The mononuclear form has the same morphological features as the classical RS cell except a single nucleus and is called as Hodgkin's cell.

Variants of RS cells include lacunar cell variant, lymphocytic and histiocytic (L and H or 'popcorn' cell) variant, and pleomorphic cell variant. These variants are important in the histological classification of HL. The lacunar cell variant is a large cell with abundant clear cytoplasm and a single multilobated nucleus with multiple small nucleoli. These cells appear to lie in clear spaces that are probably produced by artefactual retraction of cytoplasm during formalin-fixation. The lacunar cell variant is typically seen in nodular sclerosis HL. The L and H variant or 'popcorn' cell is particularly frequent in lymphocytic predominance type of HL and is characterised by a large, folded multilobed nucleus with multiple small nucleoli. The pleomorphic variant shows bizarre nuclear multilobation, marked variation in size and shape and is seen in lymphocyte depletion type of HL. Cells resembling RS cells are also found in other conditions (e.g. infectious mononucleosis, NHL, phenytoin-induced adenopathy, solid cancers) and therefore for diagnosis of HL, presence of RS cells in the typical background of normal inflammatory cells is essential.

Classification of Hodgkin's Lymphoma

World Health Organisation classification of HL is presented in Table 10.2.

Table 10.2: WHO classification

Hodgkin's lymphoma
1. *Nodular lymphocytic predominant Hodgkin's lymphoma*
2. *Classical Hodgkin's lymphoma*
   - Nodular sclerosis
   - Mixed cellularity
   - Lymphocyte-rich
   - Lymphocyte-depleted

Table 10.3: Salient features of different types of Hodgkin lymphoma

Type	% of HL	Median age, Sex	Clinical features	Microscopy	Course and prognosis
1. Nodular LPHL	5%	30–50 years; M>F	Localised peripheral lymph nodes; B symptoms rare	L & H variant; macronodules composed mostly of small B lymphocytes	Indolent; multiple late relapses; rarely fatal
2. Nodular sclerosis CHL	60–80% of CHL	Usually young adults; M=F	Mediastinal, supraclavicular; stage I or II	Lacunar variant; nodules composed of T lymphocytes, plasma cells, eosinophils, and histiocytes and surrounded by collagen bands	Related to stage
3. Mixed cellularity CHL	15–25% of CHL	Bimodal; M>F	Often high stage with B symptoms	Classic RS cells and Hodgkin cells against mixed cell background of T lymphocytes, plasma cells, eosinophils, histiocytes	Related to stage
4. Lymphocyte-rich CHL	5% of CHL	Older adults; M>F	Peripheral lymph node; low stage	Classic RS or Hodgkin cells; nodular or diffuse pattern with mostly small T lymphocytes	Related to stage
5. Lymphocyte-depleted CHL	< 1% of CHL	Older age; M>F	Advanced stage, B symptoms, often in HIV+ve	Bizarre pleomorphic RS cells; depletion of small lymphocytes; disorderly fibrosis	Related to stage

Note: Immunohistochemistry of RS cells and variants in all types of CHL is similar: CD30+, CD15+, CD45-, CD79a-, EMA-, CD20 weak or absent; immunohistochemistry of nodular LPHL: CD30-, CD15-, CD45+, CD79a+, EMA+, CD20+

Salient features of different types of Hodgkin's lymphoma are presented in Table 10.3. Differences between classical and nodular lymphocyte predominant Hodgkin's lymphoma are presented in Table 10.4.

Staging of Hodgkin's Lymphoma

The extent of disease is determined by staging which correlates with survival and prognosis. Staging determines the nature of treatment, and the outcome of therapy

Table 10.4: Comparison of classical and nodular lymphocyte predominance Hodgkin lymphoma (HL)

Parameter	Classical Hodgkin lymphoma (CHL)	Nodular lymphocyte predominance Hodgkin lymphoma (NLPHL)
1. Per cent of Hodgkin lymphoma	95%	5%
2. Age	Bimodal: Young adults and old age	Unimodal: Young adults
3. B symptoms	May be present	Rare
4. Association with Epstein-barr virus	Some cases	No
5. Behaviour	Aggressive; early stage can be cured with current therapy; late relapse very rare	Indolent; multiple late relapses common
6. Typical RS cells and mononuclear Hodgkin cells	+	–
7. L & H (popcorn) cells	–	+
8. Immunophenotype:		
• CD30	+	–
• CD15	+	–
• CD45, CD79a, EMA	–	+
• CD20	Weak or absent	Present
9. Pathology of relapse	CHL	NLPHL or diffuse large B-cell lymphoma

depends on accuracy of staging. The staging of Hodgkin's lymphoma is based on Ann Arbor staging system, which is as follows.

In **Stage I**, disease is limited to a single lymph node region (I); if the disease involves a single extralymphatic organ or site the stage is designated as IE.

In **Stage II**, two or more lymph node regions are involved but are limited to the same side of diaphragm (II); the stage is IIE if localised disease of extralymphatic organ or site is also present.

In **Stage III**, lymph node regions on both sides of diaphragm are involved (III); in addition, the disease may involve spleen (IIIS) or extralymphatic organ or site (IIIE) or both (IIISE).

Stage IV denotes disseminated or diffuse disease of one or more extralymphatic site. Involvement of liver or bone marrow indicates stage IV disease.

Each stage is again subdivided into A or B as follows:

A: No systemic symptoms

B: Presence of systemic symptoms: unexplained fever, night sweats, weight loss >10% in last 6 months.

Staging Procedures

Once the diagnosis of HL is confirmed histologically by biopsy, extent of disease is determined by staging procedures.

Previously used staging laparotomy for 'pathological staging' is no longer performed and clinical staging is usual.

History and physical examination: This includes presence or absence of B systemic symptoms, documentation of all sites of enlarged lymph nodes, presence or absence of splenomegaly or hepatomegaly.

Blood examination: Complete blood count, liver and kidney function tests, serum alkaline phosphatase level should be obtained.

Radiological examination: X-ray-chest is obtained to detect mediastinal and hilar lymph node enlargement, pleural effusion, or pulmonary involvement. CT scan precisely determines the extent of disease.

Chest and abdominopelvic CT scan are done to detect occult nodal or extranodal disease.

Bone marrow biopsy: This is indicated in selected situations such as presence of B systemic symptoms and stage III/IV disease. Bilateral iliac crest bone marrow biopsy is performed to increase the chance of detection of bone marrow involvement.

Liver biopsy: Liver biopsy needs to be performed in all patients with stage III disease.

Course and Prognosis

It should be noted that accuracy of staging decides the nature of treatment and prognosis in HL. Histological subtype of HL is not an independent prognostic factor.

With current methods of treatment, 5-year survival of patients with early disease (stages IA and IIA) is about 95% with many of them possible cured. In advanced disease (stages III and IV), 5-year survival is about 55%. Patients with HL have increased risk of radiotherapy- or chemotherapy-induced malignancies such as cancer of lung, sarcomas, cancer in head or neck region, acute myeloid leukaemia, and non-Hodgkin's lymphoma.

Treatment

Mode of therapy depends on stage of disease. Patients with early or localised HL are treated with curative intent. Patients with early stage disease (IA or IIA) with no risk factors are treated with combined chemotherapy and radiotherapy. Four courses of chemotherapy (ABVD: adriamycin, bleomycin, vinblastine, dacarbazine) followed by involved field radiation is the standard form of treatment in these patients. In advanced stage disease (III, IV, bulky I and II), combination chemotherapy (6–8 cycles of ABVD) is the usual form of treatment. For a small group of patients who are refractory to primary therapy or who relapse later, high dose chemotherapy and radiation followed by autologous stem cell rescue can be considered.

❏ NON-HODGKIN'S LYMPHOMA

The non-Hodgkin's lymphomas are a heterogeneous group of neoplastic disorders of lymphoid tissue, which includes distinct categories, defined by clinical, morphological, immunological, and genetic characteristics. The incidence of non-Hodgkin's lymphomas has been rising, while that of Hodgkin's lymphomas has remained stable. The reasons for rise may be related to increasing elderly population, human immunodeficiency virus infection, increasing use of immunosuppressive therapy, and availability of better diagnostic tools.

Predisposing Factors

The exact cause of non-Hodgkin's lymphoma (NHL) is unknown; however several disorders are associated with increased risk of development of NHL (Table 10.5).

Pathogenesis

During normal B cell development, (antigen-independent) rearrangement of immunoglobulin (Ig) genes occurs in progenitor B cells in bone marrow. This consists of somatic recombination of V (variable), D (diversity), and J (joining) segments of Ig heavy chain genes, and of V and J segments of Ig light chain genes. These 'naïve' B cells express both IgM and IgD on their surface and migrate to the germinal centres of lymphoid tissues. The variable region genes of these 'naïve' B cells are unmutated since they have not been exposed to an antigen. After exposure to an antigen in germinal centre, mutation of variable region genes occurs (so as to produce antibodies with increased affinity towards immunising antigen). B cell with mutated variable region gene may survive as a memory B cell or may undergo class switching to IgG, IgA, or IgE. The later cells evolve into immunoglobulin-producing plasma cells. Somatically mutated variable region genes are found in majority of B cell lymphomas (e.g. follicular lymphoma and Burkitt's lymphoma) indicating their origin from germinal centre or post-germinal centre B cells. Unmutated variable genes in neoplastic cells indicate derivation from naïve B cells (e.g. mantle cell lymphoma and some cases of chronic lymphocytic leukaemia/small lymphocytic lymphoma). In most cases of B cell lymphomas, nature of inciting antigen is unknown. *Helicobacter pylori* is implicated in gastric MALT lymphoma, and hepatitis C virus in some marginal zone lymphomas.

Table 10.5: Predisposing factors for NHL

Congenital disorders
- Ataxia telengiectasia
- Wiskott-Aldrich syndrome
- Severe combined immunodeficiency

Acquired disorders
- Organ transplant recipients
- Acquired immunodeficiency syndrome
- Autoimmune disorders
- Infections
    - *Helicobacter pylori* (for gastric MALT lymphoma)
    - Epstein-Barr virus (for endemic Burkitt's lymphoma)
    - Human T lymphotropic virus (for adult T cell leukaemia/lymphoma)

Chromosomal translocations involving immunoglobulin heavy chain genes have been described in several types of B cell lymphomas (Refer to Table 10.7). These translocations probably arise from errors of VDJ recombination, somatic hypermutation in germinal centres, or class switching. These translocations involve genes that regulate cell proliferation such as *MYC* or apoptosis such as *BCL2* and play a major role in the genesis of non-Hodgkin's lymphomas. In **Burkitt's lymphoma**, translocation between chromosomes 8 and 14 places *MYC* proto-oncogene close to transcriptionally active immunoglobulin locus. This leads to overexpression of MYC protein (Fig. 10.1). MYC is a transcription factor that controls growth-regulating genes.

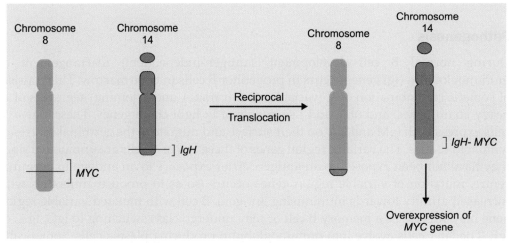

Figure 10.1: Molecular events in pathogenesis of Burkitt lymphoma

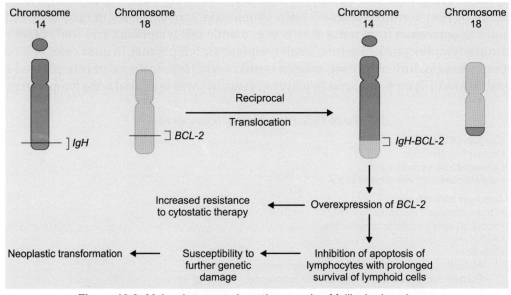

Figure 10.2: Molecular events in pathogenesis of follicular lymphoma

Constitutive expression of MYC enhances cell proliferation. In **follicular lymphoma**, reciprocal translocation between chromosomes 14 and 18 moves *BCL-2* from chromosome 18 into transcriptionally active *IgH* gene. BCL-2 is an anti-apoptotic protein. Overexpression of BCL-2 protein protects lymphocytes from cell death leading to their progressive accumulation (Fig. 10.2). In **mantle cell lymphoma**, gene for cyclin D on chromosome 11 is placed next to immunoglobulin heavy chain gene that is transcriptionally active. Cyclin D is a regulator of G1 phase of cell cycle and its overexpression leads to dysregulation of cell cycle.

Classification of Non-Hodgkin's Lymphomas

Various classification schemes employing different terminology and criteria have been proposed for NHL, e.g. Rappaport (1956), Lukes-Collins (1974), Kiel (1975), Working formulation of non-Hodgkin's lymphomas for clinical usage (1982), Revised European-American classification of Lymphoid Neoplasms (REAL) (1994), and World Health Organization (WHO) classification (2001 and 2008).

The WHO classification (Table 10.6) is based on REAL classification, which was proposed by International Lymphoma Study Group. In this classification, distinct disease categories have been defined based on clinical, morphological, immunophenotypic, and genetic features. Each disease category has distinctive natural history and prognosis that allows planning of specific treatment.

The two most common forms of NHL are follicular lymphoma and diffuse large B-cell lymphoma.

Currently, management is still based on biological behaviour of the neoplasm like low-grade (indolent) or high-grade (aggressive or highly aggressive) (Box 10.1). With the introduction of WHO classification and newer therapies, it is expected that treatment will be directed against specific disease entities in future.

Clinical Features of NHL

The usual presentation of NHL is in the form of peripheral lymphadenopathy. The salient features, which distinguish NHL from Hodgkin's lymphoma, are given earlier. Involvement of multiple peripheral lymph nodes with or without hepatosplenomegaly, extranodal disease (e.g. head, neck, gastrointestinal tract, skin, testis, CNS) and dissemination to bone marrow are more commonly observed in NHL than in HL. At presentation, many patients with NHL are in stage III or IV. Mediastinal mass (lymphoblastic lymphoma), jaw tumour (African Burkitt's lymphoma), skin plaques or nodules (mycosis fungoides) are other manifestations.

Patients with low-grade NHL (Box 10.1) have gradual progression of their disease and often have a long history. Patients may present with disseminated disease, disease limited to lymph nodes, or limited to extranodal location. Low-grade lymphomas have a tendency to recur, and transformation to a high-grade lymphoma can occur after some years.

Table 10.6: WHO classification of lymphoid neoplasms, 2008

I. Precursor lymphoid neoplasms
- B lymphoblastic leukaemia/lymphoma, NOS
- B lymphoblastic leukaemia/lymphoma with recurrent genetic abnormalities
- T lymphoblastic leukaemia/lymphoma

II. Mature B-cell neoplasms
- Chronic lymphocytic leukaemia/Small lymphocytic lymphoma
- B-cell prolymphocytic leukaemia
- Splenic marginal zone lymphoma
- Hairy cell leukaemia
- Splenic B-cell lymphoma/leukaemia, unclassifiable
- Lymphoplasmacytic lymphoma
- Heavy chain diseases
- Plasma cell neoplasms
- Extranodal marginal zone B-cell lymphoma (MALT lymphoma)
- Nodal marginal zone B-cell lymphoma
- Follicular lymphoma
- Primary cutaneous follicle center lymphoma
- Mantle cell lymphoma
- Diffuse large B-cell lymphoma, NOS
- Diffuse large B-cell lymphoma associated with chronic inflammation
- Lymphomatoid granulomatosis
- Primary mediastinal (thymic) large B-cell lymphoma
- Intravascular large B-cell lymphoma
- ALK positive large B-cell lymphoma
- Plasmablastic lymphoma
- Large B-cell lymphoma arising in HHV8-associated multicentric Castleman disease
- Primary effusion lymphoma
- Burkitt lymphoma
- B-cell lymphoma, unclassifiable with features intermediate between DLBCL and Burkitt lymphoma
- B-cell lymphoma, unclassifiable with features intermediate between DLBCL and classical Hodgkin lymphoma

III. Mature T- and NK-cell neoplasms
- T-cell prolymphocytic leukaemia
- T-cell large granular lymphocytic leukaemia
- Chronic lymphoproliferative disorder of NK cells
- Aggressive NK-cell leukaemia
- Epstein-Barr virus positive T-cell lymphoproliferative diseases of childhood
- Adult T-cell leukaemia/lymphoma
- Extranodal NK/T-cell lymphoma, nasal type
- Enteropathy-associated T-cell lymphoma
- Hepatosplenic T-cell lymphoma
- Subcutaneous panniculitis-like T-cell lymphoma
- Mycosis fungoides
- Sezary syndrome
- Primary cutaneous CD30 positive T-cell lymphoproliferative disorders
- Primary cutaneous peripheral T-cell lymphomas, rare types
- Peripheral T-cell lymphoma, unspecified
- Angioimmunoblastic T-cell lymphoma
- Anaplastic large cell lymphoma, ALK positive
- Anaplastic large cell lymphoma, ALK negative

IV. Hodgkin lymphoma

> **Box 10.1** Categories of lymphoma according to biological behaviour
>
> *Low-grade or indolent lymphomas*
> • Follicular lymphoma
> • Extranodal marginal zone B-cell lymphoma (MALT lymphoma)
> • Chronic lymphocytic leukaemia/small lymphocytic lymphoma
>
> *Aggressive lymphomas*
> • Diffuse large B-cell lymphoma
> • Mantle cell lymphoma
> • Peripheral T-cell lymphoma
>
> *Very aggressive lymphomas*
> • Burkitt lymphoma
> • Precursor T-cell lymphoblastic lymphoma

Extranodal lymphomas are lymphomas arising at sites other than lymphoid structures. Common sites are—gastrointestinal tract (especially stomach), lung, thyroid, salivary glands, and skin. Some of them originate from previous non-neoplastic disorder, e.g. *Helicobacter pylori* infection of stomach, autoimmune disorders, ulcerative colitis, etc. They are slowly growing tumours and remain localised for long duration. Surgery and radiotherapy are the usual forms of treatment and often control the disease.

Patients with high-grade or aggressive lymphoma have rapid progression of their disease that is often fatal if untreated. Systemic symptoms (fever, weight loss, night sweats) are commonly present at diagnosis.

Laboratory Investigations

Lymph Node Biopsy

If lymphadenopathy is generalised, lower cervical or axillary lymph nodes are selected. Biopsy of inguinal lymph nodes is usually avoided due to frequent presence of chronic nonspecific inflammation and fibrosis. The largest lymph node in the area should be excised. Distortion of lymph node should be avoided during removal. Sometimes radiologically guided biopsy may be required for deep-seated abdominal or thoracic lesions. Routinely, biopsied lymph node is fixed in 10% formol saline for paraffin embedding followed by haematoxylin and eosin staining.

Studies performed on biopsied lymph node are as follows:
• Morphological examination: For morphological classification; done on routinely processed tissue.
• Immunophenotyping: For subclassification into B- or T-cell and further types.
• Cytogenetic analysis: For detection of chromosomal abnormalities.
• Molecular studies: For gene rearrangement studies.
• Electron microscopy: For distinction between NHL and undifferentiated tumours.

Haematological Investigations

In all suspected cases of lymphoma, complete blood count and blood smear examination are initial investigations before biopsy. These are to rule out leukaemia (in leukaemia, lymph node biopsy is unnecessary for diagnosis) and to exclude lymphoma mimics (such as infectious mononucleosis). Bone marrow examination in NHL is mainly useful for determining the extent of disease or staging; involvement of bone marrow indicates stage IV disease.

Trephine bone marrow biopsy is preferred over marrow aspiration smears for assessment of marrow involvement. Bilateral posterior iliac crest trephine bone marrow biopsies have been advocated to increase the yield of positive bone marrow.

At presentation, marrow involvement in NHL occurs in about 50% cases. Involvement of bone marrow is common with certain types such as small lymphocytic, plasmacytoid lymphocytic, follicular small-cleaved cell, and lymphoblastic lymphomas.

Pattern of infiltration in bone marrow may be focal paratrabecular, focal nonparatrabecular (random), interstitial, or diffuse. Focal paratrabecular pattern consists of infiltration along the bony trabeculae. In focal nonparatrabecular pattern, lymphoma cells form nodules, which do not completely fill the intertrabecular space. In interstitial pattern, single or small groups of neoplastic cells infiltrate in between normal haematopoietic elements. Diffuse pattern consists of complete replacement of whole intertrabecular space by lymphoma cells.

Usually low-grade lymphomas (small lymphocytic and follicular small cleaved cell) show a focal (paratrabecular or nonparatrabecular) pattern of infiltration while high-grade (lymphoblastic and small noncleaved cell) lymphomas show a diffuse pattern.

Immunophenotyping

Identification of combination of cellular antigens (surface, cytoplasmic, or nuclear) present on a particular cell with the help of specific antibodies is called as immunophenotyping. It can be done on frozen or paraffin-embedded tissue sections or by flow cytometric analysis of cell suspensions. Applications of immunophenotyping in NHL are: (i) To differentiate neoplastic from non-neoplastic proliferation of lymphocytes, e.g. assessment of ratio of kappa to lambda light chains is helpful to demonstrate clonality in B cell neoplasms; light chain restriction is indicative of neoplastic proliferation; (ii) To differentiate lymphoma from undifferentiated neoplasms; (iii) To identify lineage (B or T cell) and the stage of differentiation of neoplastic cells.

Cytogenetic Analysis

With recent techniques, cytogenetic abnormalities can be identified in majority of patients with NHL. Common cytogenetic abnormalities are presented in Table 10.7. Some of the cytogenetic abnormalities are consistently observed in specific morphologic subtypes of NHL and play a role in the pathogenesis of lymphomas.

Table 10.7: Salient features of some NHLs

Type	Immunophenotype	Genetic abnormality	% of all NHLs
Mature B-cell type (Pan B markers+)			
1. Diffuse large B-cell lymphoma (DLBCL)	SIg±, CD5±, CD10±, Ki67<90%	t(14;18)(q32;q21) (*BCL2*) in 30%; 3q27 (*BCL6*) in 35%	30%
2. Follicular lymphoma	SIg+, CD5-, CD10+, CD23±, BCL2+	t(14;18)(q32;q21) (*BCL2*)	22%
3. Marginal zone (MALT) lymphoma	SIg+, CD5-, CD10-, CD23-	t(11;19)(q21;q21) in 50%	8%
4. Small lymphocytic lymphoma	SIg+ (weak), CD5+, CD10-, CD23+	Trisomy 3 in 60%; t(11;18) (q21;q21) in 25–50%	7%
5. Mantle cell lymphoma	SIg+, CD5+, CD10-, CD23-, cyclin D+	t(11;14)(q13;q32) (*CYCLIN D1*) in 70%	7%
6. Burkitt lymphoma	SIg+, CD5-, CD10+, Ki67>99% in contrast to DLBCL	t(8;14)(q24;q32) (*MYC*) in 80%	3%
Mature T-cell type (Pan T markers+)			
7. Peripheral T cell lymphoma	SIg-, CD5+, CD10-, CD4+, CD8-, TdT-	Many	8%

Gene Rearrangement Studies

Southern blot analysis using complementary DNA probes can be used to detect rearrangement of immunoglobulin or T cell receptor genes. Immunoglobulin gene rearrangement is indicative of B cell nature, while TCR gene rearrangement is indicative of T cell nature of the neoplasm. Uses of gene rearrangement studies are:

  i. To differentiate neoplastic from non-neoplastic proliferation of lymphocytes. TCR gene rearrangement is the only technique available for establishing clonal nature of T cell neoplasms;

  ii. To distinguish lymphoma from undifferentiated neoplasms;

  iii. To identify lineage (B or T) of lymphoid cells.

Gene rearrangement studies are especially useful in those cases in which surface antigen analysis by antibodies fails to establish the lineage or clonality of the disease.

Investigations for diagnosis of NHL are outlined in Box 10.2.

Box 10.2 Diagnosis of NHL

- Complete blood count including blood smear: This is done to rule out leukaemia (e.g. CLL) and reactive conditions clinically mimicking lymphoma. Bone marrow examination may be required in some cases.
- Excisional lymph node biopsy: This is subjected to morphological examination, immunophenotypic analysis (for validation of diagnosis, determination of lineage and degree of maturation of neoplastic cells, and assessment of prognosis), and cytogenetic and molecular studies (for assessing clonality, genetic abnormalities, and prognosis)
- Integration and correlation of clinical, haematological, morphological, immunological, cytogenetic, and molecular studies to reach final diagnosis.

Staging of NHL

Staging is necessary to plan treatment, assign prognosis, and for post-treatment evaluation. The Ann Arbor staging system for Hodgkin's lymphoma can also be used for non-Hodgkin's lymphoma. However, as mode of spread of NHL is non-contiguous and unpredictable and as progression to distant sites occurs early, this staging system is less useful for NHL. Most patients with NHL have stage III or IV disease at presentation, and localised stage I or II disease is rare. Thus, staging is not critical for majority of cases as chemotherapy is the mainstay of treatment and radiotherapy alone is rarely indicated. Staging investigations are given in Box 10.3.

An International Prognostic Index (IPI) is commonly used in aggressive NHL. This is based on age, stage (Ann Arbor), number of extranodal sites of disease, performance status, and serum lactate dehydrogenase level. Four risk groups are identified using a scoring system: low, low intermediate, high intermediate, and high with predicted 5-year survival of groups being 73%, 51%, 43%, and 26%, respectively. Such a system can help in treatment planning according to the risk group, e.g. in high-risk patients, intensive or experimental form of therapy can be tried, while in low-risk patients, intensive therapy is not warranted and established form of therapy is appropriate.

Treatment of NHL

Treatment of NHL is based on histological subtype, grade of lymphoma, stage of disease, and measurable prognostic factors.

Low-Grade NHL

Those patients who have localised disease (stage I or II) are treated with involved field radiotherapy. This leads to prolonged disease-free survival in 50% of patients.

Most patients with low-grade NHL have advanced (stage III or IV) disease at presentation. In many centres treatment is not initiated until evidence of disease progression develops (wait and watch policy). This is because low-grade NHLs are indolent neoplasms that are incurable and a period of deferral of treatment does not adversely affect the survival. Treatment options are single alkylating drug therapy

---

Box 10.3   Staging investigations in NHL

- History (B systemic symptoms), physical examination (sites of disease)
- Complete blood count, blood smear (for spillover, cytopaenias, haemolysis), bilateral bone marrow aspiration and biopsy (for infiltration)
- Chest X-ray (for mediastinal adenopathy, pleural effusion, lung involvement)
- Abdomino-pelvic CT scan (to assess lymphadenopathy and other organs)
- Biochemical tests: liver and kidney function tests, lactate dehydrogenase
- In selected cases, CT scan of chest (for precise delineation of disease if chest X-ray is abnormal), bone scan and skeletal X-rays (if bone pain, tenderness), magnetic resonance imaging (CNS involvement), CSF examination (in high-grade lymphomas).

(chloambucil or cyclophosphamide) or combination chemotherapy. With single alkylating agent therapy, relapse occurs in ≥70% of patients within 5 years. Treatment can be then repeated, although duration of response becomes shorter and the disease eventually becomes resistant to treatment. The survival of advanced stage NHL is 5 to 10 years.

There is increasing evidence that *Helicobacter pylori*-associated gastric MALT lymphoma can be successfully treated with antibiotics alone.

Aggressive NHL

Currently, cure can be achieved in many patients with combined chemotherapy and/ or radiotherapy. Intensive combination chemotherapy is instituted immediately after diagnosis and staging. About 50 to 60% achieve complete remission and a proportion of them are probably cured. The standard regimen is CHOP (cyclophosphamide, doxorubicin, vincristine, prednisolone). Patients who relapse can be considered for high dose chemotherapy followed by autologous bone marrow transplantation.

Intensive multi-agent chemotherapy is needed for very aggressive lymphoblastic lymphoma and Burkitt's lymphoma, which often spread to CNS and bone marrow.

❏ BIBLIOGRAPHY

1. Carbone PP, Kaplan HS, Musshoff K, Smithers DW, Tubiana M. Report of the Committee on Hodgkin's lymphoma Staging Classification. Cancer Res. 1971;31:1860-61.
2. Carde P. Hodgkin's lymphoma I. Identification and classification. Br Med J. 1992;305:99.
3. Jaffe ES, Harris NL, Stein H, Vardiman JW (Eds). World Health Organization Classification of Tumours. Pathology and Genetis of Tumours of Haematopoietic and Lymphoid Tissues. Lyon. IARC Press, 2001.
4. Kuppers R, Klein U, Hansmann ML, Rajewsky K. Cellular origin of human B-cell lymphomas. N Engl J Med. 1999;341:1520-29.
5. Mounter PJ, Lennard AL. Management of non-Hodgkin's lymphomas. Postgrad Med J. 1999;75: 2-6.
6. Skarin AT, Dorfman DM: Non-Hodgkin's lymphomas: Current classification and management. CA Cancer J Clin. 1997;47:351-72.
7. Swerdlow SH, Campo E, Harris NL, Jaffe ES, Pileri SA, Stein H, Thiele J, Vardiman JW (Eds). WHO classification of tumours of haematopoietic and lymphoid tissues. 4th ed. Lyon. International Agency for Research on Cancer. 2008.
8. Urba WJ, Longo DL: Hodgkin's lymphoma. N Engl J Med. 1992;326:678-87.

CHAPTER

11

Quantitative and Qualitative Disorders of Leucocytes

Disorders of leucocytes may be quantitative or qualitative. Quantitative disorders are related to the concentration of leucocytes (leucocyte counts) in peripheral blood. Qualitative disorders refer to the structural or functional abnormalities of white blood cells.

Leucocytosis is defined as an increase in the number of circulating leucocytes (total leucocyte count) above the upper level of normal. *Leucopaenia* refers to total leucocyte count below the lower limit of normal. An absolute rise or fall in the count can affect any white blood cell in peripheral blood, i.e. neutrophil, eosinophil, basophil, monocyte, or lymphocyte (Box 11.1). *Leucoerythroblastic reaction* refers to the presence of immature white blood cells as well as nucleated red cells in peripheral blood. *Leukaemoid reaction* refers to the presence of markedly increased leucocyte count (>50,000/cmm) and

Box 11.1 Quantitative disorders of leucocytes
Values in adults
• Leucocytosis: Total leucocyte count > 11,000/cmm
• Leucopaenia: Total leucocyte count < 4,000/cmm
• Neutrophilia: Absolute neutrophil count > 7,500/cmm
• Neutropaenia: Absolute neutrophil count < 2,000/cmm
• Lymphocytosis: Absolute lymphocyte count > 4,000/cmm
• Lymphocytopaenia: Absolute lymphocyte count < 1,500/cmm
• Eosinophilia: Absolute eosinophil count > 600/cmm
• Monocytosis: Absolute monocyte count > 1000/cmm
• Basophilia: Absolute basophil count > 100/cmm

immature white blood cells in peripheral blood resembling leukaemia but occurring in non-leukaemic conditions.

DISORDERS OF GRANULOCYTES

❑ NEUTROPHILIA

Neutrophilia or neutrophilic leucocytosis (Fig. 11.1) is an increase in the absolute neutrophil count above normal level (usually > 7,500/cmm). Causes of neutrophilia are listed in Table 11.1.

The most common cause of neutrophilic leucocytosis is bacterial infections particularly by Gram-positive cocci. Bacterial infections are frequently associated with following alterations in peripheral blood—(i) neutrophilic leucocytosis (Fig. 11.1) with shift to left (Figs 11.2 and 11.3): Although segmented neutrophils are mainly increased some band forms and occasional

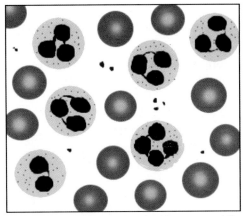

Figure 11.1: Blood smear showing neutrophilia

metamyelocyte may be found; (ii) toxic granules (Refer to Figs 11.4 and 11.6): These are dark blue or purple granules in the cytoplasm of segmented neutrophils, band forms, and metamyelocytes. They represent azurophil granules; toxic granules probably result from impaired cytoplasmic maturation while generating large number of neutrophils. (iii) Döhle inclusion bodies: These are small, pale blue inclusion bodies in the periphery of cytoplasm of neutrophils (Fig. 11.6). They represent rows of rough endoplasmic reticulum; (iv) Cytoplasmic vacuoles: They are indicative of phagocytosis.

Table 11.1: Causes of neutrophilia or neutrophilic leucocytosis

- Physiological: newborns, pregnancy, stress, exercise
- Bacterial infections, especially pyogenic
- Tissue destruction: surgical or other trauma, burns, myocardial infarction
- Inflammatory disorders: vasculitis, myositis, rheumatoid arthritis
- Acute haemorrhage
- Acute haemolysis
- Metabolic disorders: acidosis, uraemia, toxins, gout
- Drugs: corticosteroids, lithium, β-agonists, myeloid growth factors
- Solid tumours
- Haematological malignancies: myeloproliferative neoplasms, chronic myelomonocytic leukaemia, acute myeloid leukaemia
- Rare inherited disorders: Down syndrome (transient myeloproliferative disorder), hereditary neutrophilia, congenital leucocyte adhesion deficiency
- Other: cigarette smoking, asplenia

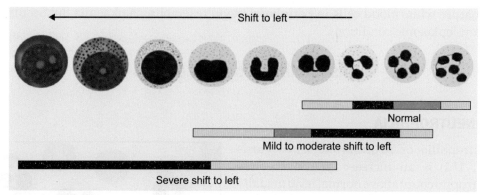

Figure 11.2: Shift to left in neutrophil series. Normally neutrophils with 3 lobes predominate, while some have 4 lobes and only a few have 2 or 5 lobes. In mild to moderate left shift, immature cells are limited to band forms and metamyelocytes. In severe left shift, immature cells like myeloblast, promyelocytes, and myelocytes are also seen

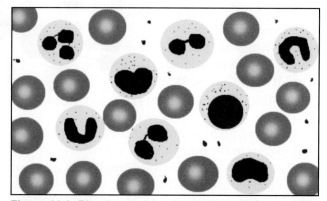

Figure 11.3: Blood smear showing shift to left in neutrophils

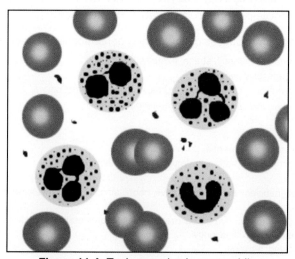

Figure 11.4: Toxic granules in neutrophils

❑ LEUCOERYTHROBLASTIC REACTION

Presence of immature cells of neutrophil series and nucleated red blood cells in peripheral blood (see Fig. 3.20) can be due to various causes (Table 11.2). Total leucocyte count may be normal or raised.

Bone marrow examination may be required to establish the underlying cause.

❑ LEUKAEMOID REACTION

Definition is given earlier. It is of two types—myeloid and lymphoid (Table 11.3).

In myeloid type, blood picture resembles either acute or chronic myeloid leukaemia.

Marked neutrophilic leucocytosis with presence of premature white cells of all stages (from myeloblasts to segmented neutrophils) may mimic chronic myeloid leukaemia (CML). Differentiation of CML from leukaemoid reaction is given in Table 7.3.

Lymphoid leukaemoid reaction is one in which peripheral blood picture resembles that of acute or chronic lymphoid leukaemia. Differentiation of reactive lymphocytosis from chronic lymphocytic leukaemia may sometimes be difficult and patient may have to be followed up to decide whether lymphocytosis is transient or persistent. (See also chapter on "Chronic lymphocytic leukaemia").

Table 11.2: Causes of leucoerythroblastic reaction

Infectious diseases
- Miliary tuberculosis

Cancers metastatic to bone marrow
- Carcinomas of lung, breast, prostate, gastrointestinal tract, thyroid, kidney

Haematological disorders
- Myelofibrosis
- Severe haemolysis, e.g. erythroblastosis foetalis
- Lymphoma
- Myeloma

Storage disorders
- Gaucher's disease
- Niemann-Pick disease

Table 11.3: Causes of leukaemoid reaction

Myeloid leukaemoid reaction
- Severe bacterial infection (e.g. pneumonia, endocarditis, septicaemia)
- Severe acute haemolysis
- Severe haemorrhage
- Cancers metastatic to bone marrow
- Other: eclampsia, burns, mercury poisoning

Lymphoid leukaemoid reaction
- Viral infections: infectious mononucleosis, infectious lymphocytosis
- Bacterial infections: tuberculosis, whooping cough

Differentiation of leukaemoid reaction from acute (myeloid or lymphoid) leukaemia is made by following features: (1) clinical presentation, (2) presence of underlying disease, (3) morphology on blood smear, (4) % of blasts in bone marrow, and (5) correction of leukaemoid blood picture after treatment of underlying disease.

Terms related to leucocytosis are shown in Box 11.2.

❏ NEUTROPAENIA

Neutropaenia refers to reduction in the number of neutrophils in the peripheral blood below the normal level (<2000/cmm).

Absolute neutrophil count more than 1000/cmm is usually considered as sufficient for phagocytic function of neutrophils. Neutropaenia has been divided into 3 grades as shown in Table 11.4.

Important causes of neutropaenia are given in Table 11.5.

Neutropaenia due to drugs may be dose-related or idiosyncratic. Idiosyncratic neutropaenia commonly occurs with following drugs-aminopyrine, phenylbutazone, chloramphenicol, sulphonamides, penicillin, anti-thyroid drugs, and phenothiazines.

Antigens on foetal granulocytes may enter maternal circulation and induce formation of anti-neutrophil antibodies. Transplacental passage of these antibodies from maternal to foetal circulation can cause neonatal isoimmune neutropaenia analogous to Rh haemolytic disease.

Pancytopaenia is a common laboratory manifestation of megaloblastic anaemia. Folic acid or vitamin B_{12} deficiency causes defective maturation of haematopoietic

Table 11.4: Grading of neutropaenia

Grade	Neutrophil count	Risk of infection
Mild	1500–1000/cmm	No increased risk
Moderate	1000–500/cmm	Mild risk
Severe	< 500/cmm	Significant risk

Box 11.2   Terms related to leucocytosis
• *Leucocytosis:* Total leucocyte count above the upper limit of normal for age
• *Shift to left:* Increased percentage of immature granulocytes in peripheral blood (usually up to bands and metamyelocytes)
• *Leukaemoid reaction (myeloid type):* Marked leucocytosis (total leukocyte count > 50,000/cmm) with presence of immature granulocytes in peripheral blood (up to promyelocytes or blasts)
• *Leucoerythroblastic reaction:* Presence of immature granulocytes and nucleated red cells in peripheral blood; total leucocyte count may or may not be high
• *Hyperleucocytosis:* Total leucocyte >100,000/cmm; it is seen almost exclusively in acute leukaemia (especially AML) and myeloproliferative neoplasms; it can result in life-threatening cerebral infarcts or pulmonary insufficiency due to sludging of blood flow in small vessels
• *Pseudoneutrophilia:* Leucocytosis following vigorous exercise and acute physical or emotional stress; it results from shift of cells (neutrophils, monocytes, and lymphocytes) from the marginal to the circulating pool.

Table 11.5: Causes of neutropaenia

1. *Infections:* overwhelming bacterial infections, septicaemia, miliary tuberculosis, human immunodeficiency virus infection, influenza, infectious mononucleosis
2. *Drugs:* antimicrobials (sulphonamides, chloramphenicol), analgesics (phenylbutazone, oxyphenbutazone), phenytoin, anti-thyroid drugs, cytotoxic drugs
3. *Immune neutropaenia:* Felty's syndrome, systemic lupus erythematosus, neonatal isoimmune neutropaenia, drug-induced
4. *Ineffective haematopoiesis:* megaloblastic anaemia
5. *Abnormal pooling:* hypersplenism
6. *Bone marrow replacement:* leukaemia, chronic myeloproliferative disorders, myelodysplastic syndrome, myeloma, lymphoma
7. *Bone marrow hypoplasia:* aplastic anaemia
8. *Other rare conditions:* Cyclic neutropaenia, Kostman syndrome, chronic familial neutropaenia, Fanconi anaemia, Schwachman-Diamond syndrome, dyskeratosis congenita, myelokathexis.

cells, which are destroyed prematurely in bone marrow (ineffective haematopoiesis). Although bone marrow is hypercellular, there is peripheral blood cytopaenia. Diagnosis is based on presence of macrocytosis and hypersegmented neutrophils in blood, megaloblastic maturation in marrow, and low levels of vitamin B_{12} or folate. In megaloblastic anaemia, neutropaenia is usually mild.

Haematologic malignancies, myelodysplasia, and aplastic anaemia require bone marrow examination for diagnosis.

Kostman syndrome is characterised by severe neutropaenia at birth along with maturation arrest at promyelocyte stage. Inheritance may be autosomal recessive (mutation in *HAX*1 gene) or autosomal dominant (mutation in *ELA2* gene). Mainstay of treatment is administration of G-CSF and antibiotics; haematopoietic stem cell transplantation may be curative for those who fail to respond to G-CSF. There is a risk of transformation to myelodysplasia or AML.

Repetitive and periodic neutropaenia and infections occur (usually every 3 weeks) in cyclic neutropaenia. Neutrophil count returns to normal between attacks. This is a rare hereditary disease that manifests in childhood with autosomal dominant mode of inheritance. Cyclic neutropaenia results from mutation in *ELA2* gene (gene for neutrophil elastase). There is a transient arrest at promyelocyte stage before each cycle. G-CSF is the effective form of treatment.

In chronic familial neutropaenia, neutrophil count is lower than 'normal' in some ethnic groups but is not associated with any risk of infections.

Clinical Features

Clinical manifestations are related to the underlying disorder and neutropaenia. Common sites of infection in neutropaenia are skin, urinary tract, respiratory tract, and oral cavity.

Agranulocytosis is a clinical syndrome characterised by rapidly developing severe neutropaenia in peripheral blood, along with fever, prostration, and painful necrotic ulcerations in oral and pharyngeal mucosa. It is of drug-induced origin.

❑ EOSINOPHILIA

Eosinophilia refers to increase in the absolute eosinophil count in the peripheral blood above 600/cmm (Fig. 11.5). Causes of eosinophilia are given in Table 11.6.

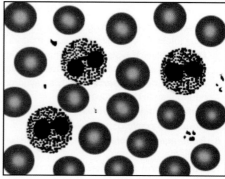

In allergic disorders, eosinophilia is transient and moderate. IgE causes release of granules from basophils and mast cells that contain chemotactic factors for eosinophils.

Eosinophilia is a regular feature of helminthic infections, particularly if the

Figure 11.5: Eosinophils in peripheral blood

parasite invades tissues. Parasites within the lumen of the intestine or encysted parasites do not evoke significant eosinophilic response.

Loeffler's syndrome consists of transient lung infiltrates on X-ray chest, eosinophilia, and cough. It is usually caused by migration of helminth larva through the lungs.

Tropical pulmonary eosinophilia occurs mainly in filaria-endemic regions (e.g. India, Southeast Asia) and is characterised by episodic cough with wheezing, lung infiltrates, and severe eosinophilia. High levels of antifilarial antibodies are present in the blood. Treatment is with diethylcarbamazine.

Hypereosinophilic syndrome is defined as persistent, high eosinophilia (> 1500/cmm for more than 6 months) without any identifiable cause and is present along with evidence of organ involvement and dysfunction. Organ damage results from tissue infiltration by eosinophils and from cytokines released from eosinophil granules. Organs commonly affected are heart, lungs, central nervous system, skin, and gastrointestinal tract. Treatment consists of corticosteroids, hydroxyurea, or α interferon. Cardiac failure is the usual cause of death.

Both hypereosinophilic syndrome and chronic eosinophilic leukaemia are associated with marked eosinophilia and organ involvement. Chronic eosinophilic leukaemia is characterised by increased blasts or presence of a clonal genetic abnormality. Hypereosinophilic syndrome, on the other hand, is a diagnosis of exclusion and is not associated with increased blasts or clonal abnormality.

Table 11.6: Causes of eosinophilia

1. Allergic diseases: asthma, urticaria, rhinitis, drug reactions
2. Parasites: filaria, trichinosis, toxocariasis, strongyloidiasis, echinococcosis
3. Dermatologic disorders: eczema, dermatitis herpetiformis, bullous pemphigoid
4. Carcinomas after radiotherapy
5. Pulmonary disorders: Loeffler's syndrome, tropical eosinophilia.
6. Haematologic malignancies: myeloproliferative disorders, Hodgkin's disease, eosinophilic leukaemia, peripheral T-cell lymphoma
7. Hypereosinophilic syndrome

❏ BASOPHILIA

Increased number of basophils in peripheral blood (>100/cmm) is observed in chronic myeloproliferative disorders especially chronic myeloid leukaemia, basophilic leukaemia, IgE-mediated allergic disorders, ulcerative colitis, and hypothyroidism.

❏ DISORDERS OF PHAGOCYTIC LEUCOCYTES CHARACTERISED BY MORPHOLOGIC CHANGES

These may be acquired or hereditary.

Acquired Morphologic Changes in Neutrophils

These include toxic granules, Döhle inclusion bodies, and cytoplasmic vacuoles that are seen in bacterial infections (Fig. 11.6). Hypersegmentation of nuclei (≥5 lobes in >5% neutrophils) is a characteristic feature of megaloblastic anaemia.

Inherited Morphologic Changes

Pelger-Huet Anomaly

In this autosomal dominant disorder, nuclear segmentation does not occur in granulocytes. Granulocyte nuclei may be rod-like, round, or at the most with two segments (spectacle-like or "pince-nez" nuclei) (Fig. 11.6). Survival and function of these granulocytes is normal. The abnormality results from mutation in laminin B receptor (LBR) gene located on chromosome 1q41-q43. Such granulocytes are also seen in some acquired disorders particularly myelodysplastic syndrome, acute myeloid

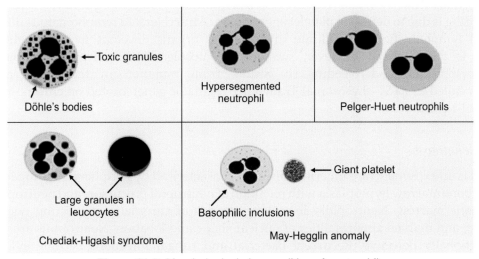

Figure 11.6: Morphological abnormalities of neutrophils

leukaemia, and myeloproliferative disorders and are then called as pseudo-Pelger-Huet cells.

Alder-Reilly Anomaly

This congenital abnormality of granulocytes is characterised by the presence of abnormally large, darkly staining granules resembling toxic granules in cytoplasm. The granules are also variably present in monocytes. This abnormality is commonly seen in mucopolysaccharidoses such as Hurler's and Hunter's syndrome.

May-Hegglin Anomaly

This uncommon condition with autosomal dominant inheritance is characterised by triad of thrombocytopaenia, giant platelets, and inclusion bodies in granulocytes. The inclusions resemble Döhle bodies. Most patients are asymptomatic, although bleeding manifestations have been reported in an occasional patient. Autosomal dominant giant platelet disorders include May-Hegglin anomaly, Fechtner syndrome, Sebastian syndrome, and Epstein syndrome. All these disorders have mutations in *MYH-9* gene located at chromosome 22q12.3-q13.2.

Chediak-Higashi Syndrome

This rare autosomal recessive disease is characterised by immune deficiency, poor resistance to bacterial infections (especially strepto- and staphylo-coccal), oculocutaneous albinism, bleeding tendency, multiple neurologic abnormalities, and giant peroxidase-positive lysosomal granules in granulocytes (Fig. 11.6). Similar lysosomal granules are also seen in other white blood cells and melanocytes. These abnormal inclusions result from the fusion of multiple cytoplasmic granules. Increased bleeding is due to defective platelet aggregation. An accelerated lymphomatous illness with lymphohistiocytic infiltrate in numerous organs develops in most patients and is characterised by fever, jaundice, hepatosplenomegaly, lymphadenopathy, pancytopaenia, and bleeding. It results from mutation in the *CHS1* gene (also called as *LYST*—Lysosomal Trafficking regulator gene) located on chromosome 1q42.1-1q42.2.

Myelokathexis

This is an extremely rare inherited disorder characterised by peripheral neutropaenia and bone marrow hyperplasia with retention of neutrophil precursors and neutrophils in bone marrow. Neutrophils show long strands of chromatin connecting nuclear lobes, and marked abnormalities of nuclear shape and lobation. Neutrophils are also functionally defective. Recurrent bacterial and fungal infections become evident during infancy. Molecular basis of this disorder is unknown.

WHIM syndrome is a rare autosomal dominant disorder characterised by warts, hypogammaglobulinaemia, infections, and myelokathexis. It is due to a mutation in *CXCR4* gene located on chromosome 2q21.

Functional Disorders of Phagocytic Leucocytes

Functional disorders of neutrophils can cause increased susceptibility to bacterial or fungal infections. Some disorders of neutrophil function are given in Table 11.7. Sites of defects in neutrophil function disorders are shown in Figure 11.7.

Congenital leucocyte adhesion deficiency: This is a heterogeneous group of rare autosomal recessive disorders characterised by marked leucocytosis (since leucocytes are unable to leave blood vessels), defective neutrophil adhesion to endothelium, absence of extravascular neutrophils, and recurrent life-threatening bacterial infections.

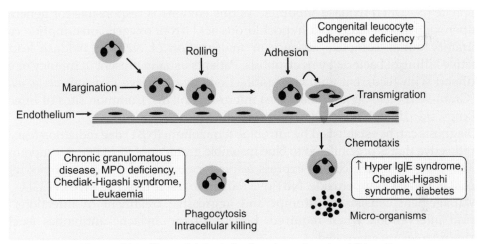

Figure 11.7: Sites of defects in disorders of neutrophil function

Table 11.7: Disorders characterised by neutrophil dysfunction

1. *Impaired adhesion:*
   - Congenital leucocyte adherence deficiency (Deficiency of CD11/CD18 surface glycoproteins)
   - Drugs: corticosteroids, alcohol
2. *Impaired motility:*
   - Hyperimmunoglobulin E syndrome
   - Chediak-Higashi syndrome
   - Diabetes mellitus, Hodgkin's disease, leprosy
3. *Impaired microbicidal killing:*
   - Chronic granulomatous disease
   - Myeloperoxidase deficiency
   - Chediak-Higashi syndrome
   - Leukaemias

Hyper IgE or Job's Syndrome

In this congenital disorder, defective neutrophil chemotaxis is present along with recurrent bacterial infections of skin and respiratory tract, recurrent cold, staphylococcal abscesses, dermatitis, eosinophilia, and markedly increased IgE.

Chronic Granulomatous Disease (CGD)

This is a group of hereditary disorders characterised by defective oxidative metabolism in phagocytic leucocytes with impaired generation of hydrogen peroxide and hydroxyl radical. There is marked chronic inflammatory reaction and granuloma formation at sites of infection.

In majority of patients, mode of inheritance is X-linked recessive while in some cases it is autosomal recessive. The disease results from mutation in one of the four genes (*CYBB, CYBA, NCF1, NCF2*) encoding phagocyte nicotinamide adenine dinucleotide phosphate (NADPH) oxidase subunits. As this enzyme is responsible for generation of superoxide anion, H_2O_2, and hypochlorous acid (from oxygen consumption called respiratory burst), complete absence or malfunction of NADPH oxidase leads to defective killing of bacteria by neutrophils. Patients usually present in infancy or early childhood with recurrent and severe infections by Gram+ve (*Staphylococcus aureus*) and Gram-ve (*E. coli, Serratia marcesens*) micro-organisms. Common sites of infection are lungs, skin, lymph nodes, gastrointestinal tract, and bones.

Diagnosis can be established by nitroblue tetrazolium (NBT) dye reduction test. NBT is a redox dye that is precipitated to blue insoluble granules of formazan by superoxide. In CGD, phagocytic cells cannot express respiratory burst and therefore do not reduce molecular oxygen to superoxide. NBT dye reduction test is thus negative in CGD.

Management consists of prompt and aggressive treatment of infections and surgical intervention when required. Long-term prophylactic antibiotics (such as co-trimoxazole) are advocated.

Myeloperoxidase (MPO) Deficiency

This is the most common hereditary neutrophil function defect. In MPO-deficient neutrophils, intracellular killing of micro-organisms is slow, but is ultimately achieved. There is susceptibility to candidal and bacterial (*Staph. aureus*) infections. Diagnosis is established by myeloperoxidase stain of blood smear that shows lack of peroxidase activity in neutrophils.

DISORDERS OF MONOCYTE MACROPHAGE SYSTEM

❏ MONOCYTOSIS

Monocytosis (Fig. 11.8) refers to an increase in the monocyte count above 1000/cmm. Causes of monocytosis are listed in Table 11.8.

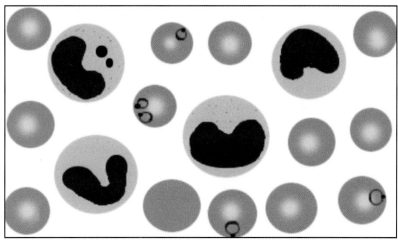

Figure 11.8: Blood smear showing monocytosis in a case of malaria. Ring forms of *Plasmodium falciparum* are seen in some red cells. One monocyte shows brown-black malarial pigment

Table 11.8: Causes of monocytosis

Infections: malaria, typhoid, tuberculosis, bacterial endocarditis, kala-azar

Haematological malignancies: acute myelomonocytic leukaemia (AML M4), acute monocytic leukaemia (AML M5), myeloproliferative neoplasms, chronic myelomonocytic leukaemia, myelodysplastic syndrome, Hodgkin's disease

Others: sarcoidosis, ulcerative colitis, regional enteritis, carcinomas

❏ STORAGE DISORDERS

Gaucher's Disease

Normally there is constant generation of glucocerebrosides from the breakdown of blood cell membranes. Glucocerebrosides are degraded enzymatically by lysosomal enzymes in macrophages. In Gaucher's disease, there is a hereditary deficiency of the enzyme glucocerebrosidase that is required for removing glucose from ceramide. This causes accumulation of glucocerebroside within the macrophages of the reticuloendothelial system. Such enlarged macrophages are also called as Gaucher's cells.

Gaucher's disease is an autosomal recessive disorder. A French physician Philippe Charles Ernest Gaucher first described this disease in 1882. Many different mutations in the glucocerebrosidase gene (located on chromosome 1q21) can cause Gaucher's disease. There are three clinically distinct types of Gaucher's disease–type I (chronic non-neuronopathic adult type), type II (acute infantile neuronopathic type), and type III (subacute neuronopathic juvenile type).

Clinical Features

Type I: This is the most frequent type. It occurs mainly in Ashkenazi Jews. Clinical manifestations appear usually during adulthood and neurological involvement is absent. Splenomegaly due to accumulation of Gaucher's cells is the usual finding. Manifestations of hypersplenism may be present. Marrow expansion may lead to bone pain or fractures. The Erlenmeyer flask deformity of distal femur is a typical feature on X-ray. Progression of the disease is slow.

Type II: This is the most severe form of Gaucher's disease occurring in infants and is characterised by prominent neurologic manifestations and hepatosplenomegaly. Bone involvement is uncommon. Death often occurs before 2 years of age.

Type III: In this type there is later onset of neurological involvement than in type II and more prolonged survival.

Diagnosis

Assay of glucocerebrosidase activity in leucocytes or cultured skin fibroblasts: The diagnosis is made by this test. This test can also be utilised for detection of heterozygotes and for prenatal diagnosis. However, as levels overlap in heterozygous and normal individuals, DNA analysis is preferred.

Demonstration of Gaucher's cells: Gaucher's cells (Fig. 11.9) are macrophages containing large amounts of accumulated glucocerebrosides. Morphologically these are large, round to oval cells with abundant, pale, fibrillary cytoplasm (likened to a crumpled tissue paper) and have one or more dark, eccentric nuclei.

These cells are PAS-positive. Gaucher's cells can be seen in bone marrow, spleen, lymph nodes, and liver.

Ideally, diagnosis of Gaucher's disease should be established by assay of enzyme activity rather than by demonstration of Gaucher's cells in bone marrow. This is because enzymatic assay is simple and convenient. Gaucher's cells may be few in number and thus may be missed in marrow, or presence of pseudo-Gaucher's cells may lead to a mistaken diagnosis of Gaucher's disease. Pseudo-Gaucher's cells can occur in various conditions such as chronic myeloid leukaemia, lymphoproliferative disorders, Hodgkin's lymphoma, acquired immunodeficiency syndrome, and mycobacterial infections.

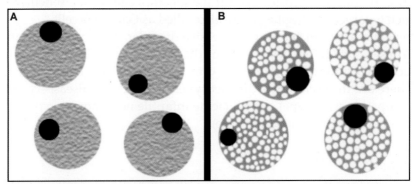

Figure 11.9: Comparative features of storage cells. Cytoplasm of Niemann-Pick cell (B) is vacuolated, while that of Gaucher's cell (A) is fibrillary (likened to crumpled tissue paper)

Treatment

Enzyme replacement therapy has become available and can arrest and reverse the symptoms of Gaucher's disease. It is given intravenously every 2 weeks on an outpatient basis. Splenectomy is indicated for bleeding secondary to severe thrombocytopaenia or when patient develops discomfort due to massive splenomegaly. Bone marrow transplantation has been attempted in a few patients. However due to increased morbidity and mortality associated with this procedure and good results of enzyme replacement therapy, bone marrow transplantation is not currently advocated. Transfer of normal glucocerebrosidase gene into autologous stem cells is being attempted and provides the prospect of cure in Gaucher's disease.

Niemann-Pick Disease

In this rare hereditary lipid storage disease, excessive deposition of sphingomyelin, cholesterol, and other lipids occurs in cells of the mononuclear phagocytic system. Parenchymal cells of organs are also frequently involved. Mode of inheritance is autosomal recessive.

Niemann-Pick disease is a heterogeneous disorder and different types have been described. The most common type is designated as type A (classical or infantile form) that accounts for three-fourth of the cases. It is common in Ashkenazi Jews. There is a severe deficiency of sphingomyelinase, which causes widespread accumulation of sphingomyelin and other lipids in various organs. Manifestations develop early during infancy and include failure to thrive, hepatosplenomegaly, generalised lymphadenopathy, and severe neurologic symptoms. A macular cherry red spot may be present. Death usually occurs before 3 to 4 years of age.

Other types of Niemann-Pick disease are rare.

Diagnosis

Demonstration of Niemann-Pick cells in bone marrow: Niemann-Pick cells are mononuclear phagocytic cells containing excessive accumulations of sphingomyelin and cholesterol within lysosomes. The cells are large with multiple small vacuoles of relatively uniform size in cytoplasm and a single, small eccentric nucleus (Fig. 11.9).

Assay of sphingomyelinase: Diagnosis requires assay of sphingomyelinase activity.

Treatment

Treatment is symptomatic.

Langerhans' Cell Histiocytosis

Langerhans' cell histiocytosis (LCH) is a group of disorders associated with neoplastic proliferation of Langerhans' cells. Previously these were called as histiocytosis X.

(Langerhans' cells are dendritic histiocytes normally residing in the epidermis. They function as antigen presenting cells).

Although LCH can occur at any age, it is most frequent in infants and children. Three major clinical syndromes are described:

- **Solitary eosinophilic granuloma:** A unifocal disease usually involving the bone (especially skull, femur, pelvic bones, ribs); more frequent in older children and adults.
- **Hand-Schuller-Christian disease:** A multifocal unisystem disease with involvement of multiple sites in one organ system, commonly bone; triad of lytic bone lesions, exophthalmos, and diabetes insipidus is characteristic. It usually occurs in young children.
- **Letterer-Siwe disease:** A multifocal multisystem progressive disease with involvement of multiple organs (skin, lymph nodes, spleen, liver, bones, and bone marrow). It occurs usually in infants.

The lesions in all the three syndromes are composed of Langerhans' cells in a milieu of reactive inflammatory cells (eosinophils, histiocytes, neutrophils, and small lymphocytes). Langerhans' cells are 10 to 15 μm in size with moderately abundant eosinophilic cytoplasm and grooved or lobulated nucleus. On immunophenotypic analysis, Langerhans' cells are positive for CD1a and S-100 protein. The ultrastructural hallmark of Langerhans' cells is Birbeck granules in cytoplasm.

Unifocal bone lesions can be effectively treated with surgical curettage. As spontaneous resolution occurs in some cases, stable and asymptomatic lesions can be followed without intervention. Disseminated disease and progressive or recurrent bone lesions are treated with chemotherapy and/or steroids. Widespread organ involvement is associated with poor outcome.

LYMPHOCYTOSIS

Lymphocytosis is defined as increase in the absolute lymphocyte count above upper limit of normal for age (>4000/cmm in adults). Causes of lymphocytosis are outlined in Table 11.9.

Table 11.9: Causes of lymphocytosis

1. Infections:
   Viral: infectious mononucleosis, acute infectious lymphocytosis, cytomegalovirus, infectious hepatitis, mumps, varicella
   Bacterial: tuberculosis, pertussis
   Protozoal: toxoplasmosis
2. Lymphoid malignancies: ALL, CLL, prolymphocytic leukaemia, leukaemic phase of NHL, large granular lymphocytic leukaemia
3. Monoclonal B-cell lymphocytosis
4. Persistent polyclonal B-cell lymphocytosis
5. Stress lymphocytosis: acute cardiovascular collapse, trauma, major surgery
6. Other: chronic infections, post-vaccination, autoimmune disorders

Acute infectious lymphocytosis: This is a contagious condition characterised by small mature-looking lymphocytosis occurring mainly in children; it may be related to coxsackie virus A, coxsackie virus B, echoviruses, and adenovirus type 12. Clinical manifestations are variable and leucocytosis varies from 20 to 50,000/cmm and lasts for 3 to 5 weeks.

Mononucleosis syndrome: Mononucleosis syndrome is characterised by presence of fever and reactive lymphocytes in blood (lymphocytes > 50% of blood leucocytes along with >10% atypical lymphocytes). The common causes are infection by Epstein-Barr virus and cytomegalovirus. Mononucleosis-like syndrome can also be caused by *Toxoplasma gondii*, HIV-1, and several other viruses.

Monoclonal B-cell lymphocytosis: This is a monoclonal proliferation (documented by light chain restriction) of B lymphocytes (B lymphocyte count < 5,000/cmm) seen in healthy elderly individuals that is asymptomatic, and there is absence of any evidence of a lymphoproliferative, infectious or autoimmune disorder. Monoclonal B cells may express CLL-like or non-CLL-like phenotype. Progression to CLL may occur, especially in individuals with CLL immunophenotype. Recent studies also indicate that nearly all cases of CLL are preceded by monoclonal B-cell lymphocytosis.

Persistent polyclonal B-cell lymphocytosis: This is a rare condition that is characterised by absolute lymphocytosis that is found to be polyclonal and B-cell in nature on immunophenotyping and is reported mainly in women who smoke and have a HLADR-7 phenotype. Small, atypical binucleated (having deep nuclear clefts) lymphocytes are characteristic. Most patients have a stable count and indolent course, but B-cell lymphomas have been reported to develop in rare patients. Patients should be followed up closely.

Stress lymphocytosis: This is a transient lymphocytosis in adults occurring immediately after acute events like trauma, surgery, acute myocardial infarction, etc. and is thus seen in emergency departments. It is usually mild and resolves shortly, and a re-evaluation after 2 to 4 weeks can allow distinction from a neoplastic process. It appears to be due to lymphocyte redistribution.

❏ INFECTIOUS MONONUCLEOSIS

Infectious mononucleosis (IM) is an acute infectious disease caused by Epstein-Barr virus (EBV) and characterised by fever, pharyngitis, lymphadenopathy, atypical lymphocytosis in peripheral blood, and heterophil and EBV-specific antibodies in serum.

Aetiopathogenesis

Epstein-Barr virus is a double-stranded DNA virus of the herpes virus family. Transmission occurs chiefly by transfer of saliva from infected persons into the oropharynx of susceptible individuals, usually by kissing. EBV infects B-lymphocytes of oropharyngeal tissue by binding to CD21 (which is the receptor for both C3d and EBV). EBV also spreads to other B-lymphoid sites in the body via circulation. Stimulation and proliferation of B-lymphocytes induces polyclonal hypergammaglobulinaemia and formation of IgM heterophil antibodies and autoantibodies.

EBV-infected B-lymphocytes express on their surface lymphocyte-determined membrane antigen (LYDMA). This is recognised by T cytotoxic/suppressor cells (CD 8+), which undergo activation and proliferation. The activated T cells represent most of the atypical or variant lymphocytes seen in peripheral blood. Multiplication of T cells also leads to enlargement of lymph nodes, spleen, and liver. Only small numbers of atypical lymphocytes are EBV-transformed B lymphocytes. EBV is characterised by its latency and EBV probably persists throughout life in the infected individual.

Clinical Features

IM is a disease of adolescents and young adults. Incubation period is 3 to 8 weeks. Patient usually presents with sore throat, fever, and generalised lymphadenopathy. Examination shows tonsillar enlargement, pharyngeal congestion, and transient palatal petechiae. Splenomegaly is present in 50% of patients. Less common manifestations of IM include–skin rash (resembling that occurring in typhoid fever), splenic rupture, Bell's palsy, Guillain-Barré syndrome, encephalitis, myocarditis, pericarditis, airway obstruction due to tonsillar hyperplasia, pneumonia, autoimmune haemolytic anaemia and thrombocytopaenia.

X-linked lymphoproliferative disorder (Duncan's syndrome) is a rare immunodeficiency disorder in which EBV infection in childhood produces fulminant infectious mononucleosis. There is a high-risk of later development of lymphoma and hypogammaglobulinaemia. The disorder is due to a mutation in *SH2D1A* (also called *SAP*) gene on chromosome Xq25 that encodes SH2 domain on a signal transducing protein called SLAM-associated protein (SAP).

Laboratory Features

Peripheral blood examination: Total leucocyte count is mild to moderately raised due to absolute lymphocytosis. On differential leucocyte count, lymphocytes constitute more than 50% of cells with many (>10%) of them being atypical. Atypical or variant lymphocytes are variable in size with more abundant amount of cytoplasm that may contain vacuoles or granules. Dark basophilia of peripheral cytoplasm at points of contact with other cells ('skirting')

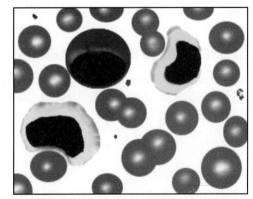

Figure 11.10: Atypical lymphocytes in blood in infectious mononucleosis

and scalloping of cytoplasmic border around erythrocytes are characteristic (Fig. 11.10). Nucleus may be oval or irregular with coarse, clumped chromatin pattern. Sometimes 1 or 2 nucleoli may be seen.

Mild to moderate neutropaenia and mild thrombocytopaenia can occur. In a few patients severe thrombocytopaenia with purpura occurs. Mild autoimmune haemolytic anaemia is observed in some cases.

Serological studies: Two types of serological tests are employed for diagnosis of IM-detection of heterophil antibodies and of EBV-specific antibodies.

(i) Detection of heterophil antibodies: An antibody, which is capable of reacting with an antigen that is completely unrelated to the antigen that had originally elicited its production, is called as a heterophil antibody. Heterophil antibodies are of the IgM class. Heterophil antibodies become detectable during the second week of illness and persist for about 2 months.

Paul-Bunnell test: Paul and Bunnell in 1932 described heterophil antibodies in the sera of patients with IM that agglutinated sheep erythrocytes. The test consists of mixing sheep erythrocytes with serial dilutions of patient's serum and finding the agglutination titre (i.e. the highest dilution at which agglutination is detected). In normal individuals agglutination titre is 1:56 or, less while in IM agglutination titres are increased (usually 1:224 or more). However, apart from IM high titres of heterophil antibodies are also found in leukaemias, lymphomas, and serum sickness. Therefore, high agglutination titres ($\geq$ 1:224) should be correlated with clinical and haematological findings to confirm the diagnosis of IM.

Paul-Bunnell-Davidsohn test (Differential absorption test): To distinguish heterophil antibodies in IM from those occurring in other disorders, Davidsohn in 1937 developed differential absorption test. It depends upon the finding that heterophil antibodies in IM and non-IM disorders have different antigen specificities, i.e. heterophil antibodies in IM are absorbed by beef red cells, but not completely by guinea pig kidney cells; while heterophil antibodies in other disorders are absorbed by guinea pig kidney cells, but not or only partially by beef red cells. Thus, blockage of sheep red cell agglutinating activity of patient's serum by prior absorption with beef red cells, but not by guinea pig kidney cells, indicates the presence of IM heterophil antibodies.

This test is usually employed when the agglutination titre with sheep erythrocytes is low, while clinical and haematological features are suggestive of IM.

Rapid slide tests: These are the simplest and the most widely used tests for the diagnosis of IM. Monospot test consists of mixing patients's serum with either beef red cell stromata or guinea pig kidney cell suspension on two halves of a glass slide. Horse erythrocytes are then added and presence or absence of agglutination is noted. (Substituting horse erythrocytes for sheep red cells enhances sensitivity of the test). Inhibition of agglutination by beef red cells but not by guinea pig kidney cells indicates the presence of IM heterophil antibodies.

(ii) Detection of EBV-specific antibodies: EBV-specific serologic studies detect antibodies directed against specific EBV antigens such as viral capsid antigen (VCA), early antigen (EA), and the Epstein-Barr nuclear antigen (EBNA). Presence of IgM anti-VCA antibodies, or anti-EA-D (in D or diffuse form of EA, the whole nucleus shows antigen positivity) antibodies, and absence of anti-EBNA antibodies are diagnostic of acute infectious mononucleosis.

Lymph node biopsy: Lymph node biopsy is not performed in infectious mononucleosis as diagnosis is established on the basis of typical clinical presentation, atypical lymphocytes in blood, and serologic studies. However, if presentation is atypical, a lymph node biopsy may be done to solve the diagnostic difficulty.

Lymph node biopsy shows hyperplasia of paracortical zones due to proliferation of T lymphocytes. Lymphocytes of varying sizes ranging from small lymphocytes to immunoblasts are present in these areas. Mitotic activity is increased. Immunoblasts may show binucleation thus mimicking Reed-Sternberg cells of Hodgkin's lymphoma. Follicles often show blurring of their margins due to paracortical hyperplasia. Sinuses are filled with lymphocytes of varying sizes including immunoblasts.

Other laboratory features:
  i. In addition to heterophil antibodies, a variety of autoantibodies may be found in IM, such as cold-reactive autoantibodies and antinuclear antibodies. These probably result from polyclonal B cell stimulation.
  ii. Liver function tests reveal mild elevations of liver enzymes and serum bilirubin, particularly during the second week of illness. Clinical jaundice, however, is rare.

Diagnosis and Differential Diagnosis

In majority of cases, diagnosis of IM is readily established on the basis of
* Typical clinical features (adolescent or young adult patient with sore throat, fever, lymphadenopathy, and splenomegaly);
* Lymphocytosis (> 50%) in peripheral blood with more than 10% atypical lymphocytes; and
* Positive heterophil antibody test in high titre with characteristic result on differential absorption test.

In approximately 10% cases of IM, heterophil antibody test is negative. In such cases, EBV- specific serologic tests should be done.

IM should be distinguished from CMV and toxoplasma-induced mononucleosis, human immunodeficiency virus seroconversion illness, streptococcal pharyngitis, other viral illnesses causing pharyngitis, and sometimes lymphoproliferative disorders.

Treatment

Treatment of IM is symptomatic and supportive.

IMMUNODEFICIENCY DISEASES

Immunodeficiency diseases are characterised by impairment of immune response against foreign antigens and susceptibility to infections. B and T lymphocytes, phagocytes, and complement are necessary for normal immune function and deficiency of any one of these can produce immunodeficiency.

When an immunodeficiency disorder is suspected, detailed clinical history and physical findings should be obtained. Clinical features highly suggestive of underlying immunological defect include: recurrent infections, infections by unusual organisms or by organisms of low virulence, opportunistic infections, or inadequate or slow response to treatment. Causative organisms may provide clue to the type of immunodeficiency, e.g. repeated infections with encapsulated bacteria indicate defective humoral (antibody-mediated) immunity or phagocytic defense, while viral, fungal, or parasitic infections suggest impaired T-cell-mediated immune response.

Procedures for evaluation of immune function are presented in Table 11.10.

Complete blood counts and examination of peripheral blood smear are helpful for detecting neutropaenia, lymphocytopaenia, and morphological abnormalities of neutrophils. In assessing B lymphocyte function, hypogammaglobulinaemia may be identified by serum protein electrophoresis. Quantitation of immunoglobulins can be done by single radial immunodiffusion, nephelometry, or by ELISA. IgG, IgA, and IgM are usually moderately to markedly reduced in X-linked hypogammaglobulinaemia and combined immunodeficiency. Isohaemagglutinin (anti-A, anti-B) titres should be greater than 1:4 after 1 year of age and is a useful test for assessment of IgM function. B lymphocyte function can also be assessed by measuring antibody levels before and after immunisation (e.g. with diphtheria or tetanus vaccines). CD19 and CD20 markers can be used for enumeration of B-lymphocytes by flow cytometry. A widely used test for evaluation of T cell function is delayed hypersensitivity skin test using purified protein derivative (PPD) or candida antigen. If reaction to this test is positive, then cell-mediated immunity is largely intact.

Table 11.10: Laboratory tests for evaluation of immune function

Parameter	Investigations
1. Basic blood studies	Total and absolute leucocyte counts, differential leucocyte count, morphology of neutrophils and platelets
2. B lymphocyte function	Serum protein electrophoresis and quantification of immunoglobulins (for hypogammaglobulinaemia), specific antibody titres following vaccination to diphtheria, tetanus, or pnumococci (for humoral response to antigens), quantitation of B cells by monoclonals (for deficiency of B cells)
3. T lymphocyte function	Delayed hypersensitivity skin test (for impaired cell-mediated response), absolute lymphocyte count, quantitation of T cells and T cell subsets
4. Neutrophil function	Absolute neutrophil count, Rebuck skin window test (for chemotaxis and motility), nitroblue tetrazolium dye reduction test (for phagocytic activity), cytochemical stain (myeloperoxidase)
5. Complement function	Total haemolytic complement (CH50)

❑ CLASSIFICATION OF IMMUNODEFICIENCY DISEASES

Immunodeficiency diseases are classified into two major types—primary and secondary. Primary immunodeficiency diseases are genetically determined disorders, which are subdivided according to the arm of the immune system that is defective (Table 11.11). Secondary immunodeficiency diseases are not intrinsic to the immune system and occur in a variety of acquired conditions such as acquired immune deficiency syndrome (AIDS), cytotoxic chemotherapy, radiotherapy, malnutrition, etc.

Only lymphocytic diseases are considered below. Figure 11.11 shows sites of involvement in primary immunodeficiency disorders.

Table 11.11: Selected primary immunodeficiency disorders

B cell immunodeficiency
• X-linked agammaglobulinaemia
• IgA deficiency
• Transient hypogammaglobulinaemia of infancy
• Common variable immunodeficiency

T cell immunodeficiency
• DiGeorge's syndrome
• Chronic mucocutaneous candidiasis

Both B cell and T cell immunodeficiency
• Severe combined immunodeficiency disease
• Wiskott-Aldrich syndrome
• Ataxia telangiectasia

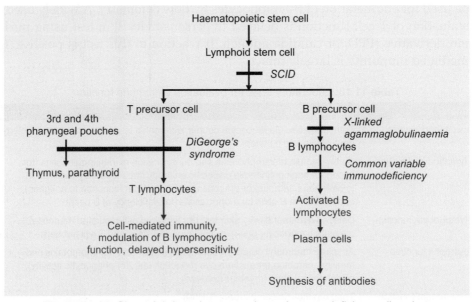

Figure 11.11: Sites of defects in some primary immunodeficiency disorders

Primary Immunodeficiency

X-linked Agammaglobulinaemia (Bruton's disease)

This inherited immune deficiency syndrome is caused by a mutation in *BTK* (Bruton tyrosine kinase) gene located on chromosme Xq21.3-q22. This gene encodes a nonreceptor tyrosine kinase that is essential for B-cell development. Infants with this disorder remain normal for first few months of life due to protection by transferred maternal IgG. Afterwards they start having repeated and severe bacterial infections. Although pre-B cells are identifiable in the bone marrow, they fail to differentiate into mature B cells. Lack of gammaglobulins can be detected by serum protein electrophoresis. Quantitation of immunoglobulins reveals virtual absence of IgA, IgM, IgD, and IgE (<200 mg/dl). B-lymphocytes are not detectable in the peripheral blood and plasma cells are absent in the lymphoid organs. There is inability to form antibodies after antigenic stimulation. Number and functions of T cells are adequate. Treatment consists of regular administration of intramuscular immunoglobulins. With recent availability of intravenous immunoglobulin, large doses can be given and adequate IgG levels can be achieved.

Selective Deficiency of IgA

Patients with isolated deficiency of IgA usually present with recurrent respiratory infections. IgA deficiency frequently occurs in autoimmune disorders (systemic lupus erythematosus, rheumatoid arthritis) and coeliac disease. IgA-deficient patients may form anti-IgA antibodies in high titre; when such patients receive blood transfusion containining IgA, anaphylactic reaction can occur.

There appears to be an impaired release of IgA or failure of differentiation of B-lymphocytes to IgA producing plasma cells.

Quantitation of immunoglobulins shows serum IgA to be less than 5 mg/dl and normal or increased levels of other immunoglobulins. Secretory IgA is also deficient.

Treatment is symptomatic. Therapeutic gammaglobulins or plasma contains small amounts of IgA. Patients requiring blood transfusion should be tested for anti-IgA antibodies and transfused washed red cells or blood from an IgA-deficient person.

Transient Hypogammaglobulinaemia of Infancy

Maternally derived immunoglobulins (IgG) in infants gradually decline over the first few months of life. Immunoglobulin levels subsequently rise due to their synthesis by the infant's immune system and normal adult levels are reached by the end of 1 year. In all infants there is a period of transient physiologic hypogammaglobulinaemia around 5 to 6 months of age. During this period maternally derived IgG is low while production of immunoglobulins is yet to start in the infant. In some cases, transient hypogammaglobulinaemia becomes unusually prolonged and severe due to unusual delay in beginning the synthesis of immunoglobulins; such infants may have increased susceptibility to infections. Regular follow-up is necessary to differentiate this disorder from other immunodeficiency diseases, particularly X-linked hypogammaglobulinaemia. Gammaglobulin therapy is indicated when severe infections develop. Routine immunisations are deferred till the infant's immune system is established.

Common Variable Immunodeficiency

Patients with this disease usually present with history of repeated pyogenic infections. Although it can occur at any age, onset of symptoms is commonly several years after birth (often 20–30 years of age). Males and females are equally affected. Association with autoimmune disorders such as systemic lupus erythematosus, rheumatoid arthritis, or pernicious anaemia is frequent. Other manifestations, which may be present, include chronic lung disease, chronic giardiasis, or malabsorption.

Common variable immunodeficiency may result from various mechanisms: intrinsically defective B cells, circulating autoantibodies against B cells, defective B cell function due to excessive suppressor T cell activity or reduced helper T cell activity.

DiGeorge's Syndrome (Thymic hypoplasia)

In this disease there is congenital aplasia or hypoplasia of thymus and parathyroid glands due to failure of development of 3rd and 4th pharyngeal pouches. These infants usually present with hypocalcaemic tetany (due to hypoparathyroidism). There may also be congenital cardiac defects and facial abnormalities such as low-set ears, short philtrum of upper lip, and hypertelorism. Later, defective cell-mediated immunity causes increased susceptibility to fungal, viral, bacterial, and protozoal infections. There is T cell lymphopaenia and lack of response to T cell mitogens such as phytohaemagglutinin. B cell immunity is variable. Thymic transplantation causes correction of defective cell-mediated immunity. In some cases spontaneous improvement occurs.

Severe Combined Immunodeficiency Disease (SCID)

SCID is characterised by marked deficiency of both B cell (humoral) and T cell (cell-mediated) immunity. There are two patterns of inheritance: X- linked and autosomal recessive. The basic defect may lie in the stem cell which fails to differentiate into mature B and T cells or there may be deficiency of cytokines necessary for maturation of lymphocytes. These patients usually develop symptoms of recurrent bacterial, viral, protozoal, or fungal infections during first few months of life. Candidiasis, chronic diarrhoea, and pneumonia are common. Administration of live virus vaccine may cause disseminated and fatal disease. Laboratory features include marked lymphopaenia, diminished T cells, lack of T lymphocyte response to phytohaemagglutinin, cutaneous anergy, low or absent B lymphocytes, hypogammaglobulinaemia, and lack of antibody formation after antigenic stimulation. Unless treated, death occurs before 1 year of age from severe infections. Bone marrow transplantation is the definitive form of treatment. Blood transfusions are contraindicated due to the risk of graft-versus-host disease.

Wiskott-Aldrich Syndrome

This is an inherited X-linked disorder characterised by severe eczema, recurrent pyogenic infections, and low platelets. It results from mutations in gene encoding *Wiskott-Aldrich syndrome protein (WASP)*, which is located at Xp11.22-11.23. Usual initial presentation is bleeding secondary to thrombocytopaenia in early infancy. Serum level of IgM is low, while IgA and IgE are increased. There is lack of antibody response to immunisation with polysaccharide antigen. There is progressive diminution of T cell immunity. Death usually occurs in childhood from haemorrhage, severe infection, or development of a lymphoproliferative disorder. Bone marrow transplantation from HLA- identical sibling donor offers the only prospect of cure.

Ataxia Telangiectasia

This is an autosomal recessive disorder characterised by triad of ataxia, oculocutaneous telangiectasia and increased susceptibility to infections. There is increased susceptibility to radiation-induced damage. DNA repair is defective and spontaneous chromosomal abnormalities are frequent. Alpha-fetoprotein levels are raised. Deficiency of IgA is common; some patients may have deficiency of IgE, IgG2, or IgG4. Defect in cell-mediated immunity is variable. Therapy consists of management of infections and of other complications.

Secondary Immunodeficiency

Immunodeficiency can occur in a variety of acquired disorders such as malnutrition, following radiotherapy or cytotoxic chemotherapy, administration of corticosteroids, haematological neoplasms such as chronic lymphocytic leukaemia, myeloma, and Hodgkin's disease, and viral infections such as AIDS.

Immunological Abnormalities in Acquired Immunodeficiency Syndrome (AIDS)

AIDS is caused by a retrovirus called as human immunodeficiency virus (HIV). Individuals at high-risk of HIV infection are male homosexuals or bisexuals, intravenous drug abusers sharing needles or syringes, haemophiliacs receiving F VIII concentrate, and heterosexual contacts of above high-risk individuals.

Immunodeficient persons are susceptible to (i) a variety of opportunistic infections especially *Pneumocystis carinii*, *Toxoplasma*, atypical mycobacteria, cytomegalovirus, Epstein-Barr virus, *Candida, Aspergillus,* and *Cryptococcus* and (ii) neoplasms such as Kaposi's sarcoma and non-Hodgkin's lymphomas.

Major alterations in immune system in AIDS are as follows:

T cells: HIV has tropism for CD4+ lymphocytes, which causes progressive loss of CD4+ cells and reversal of CD4/CD8 ratio. Depletion of CD4+ cells profoundly affects the immune system as CD4+ cells interact with other cells of the immune system and secrete a variety of lymphokines. T lymphocytes show decreased delayed hypersensitivity response to antigens, impaired proliferative response to phytohaemagglutinin, and decreased cytotoxic response.

B cells: Although polyclonal hypergammaglobulinaemia is present due to stimulation of B cells, effective antibody response to new antigens is lacking.

Monocytes and macrophages: Impairment of chemotaxis and phagocytosis is present.

Other: There is decreased synthesis of interleukin-2 and gamma interferon.

❏ BIBLIOGRAPHY

1. Beutler E, Saven A. Misuse of marrow examination in the diagnosis of Gaucher's disease. Blood. 1990;76:646-48.
2. Beutler E. Gaucher's disease. N Engl J Med. 1991;325:1354-60.
3. Cheeseman SH. Infectious mononucleosis. Semin Hematol. 1988;25:261-68.
4. Ebeli MH. Epstein-Barr virus infectious mononucleosis. Am Fam Physician. 2004;70:1279-87.
5. Gallin JI (Moderator). Recent advances in chronic granulomatous disease. Ann Intern Med. 1983;99:657-74.
6. McPherson RA, Pincus MR (Eds): Henry's clinical diagnosis and management by laboratory methods. 21st ed. Philadelphia. Elsevier Saunders. 2007.
7. Rosen FS, Cooper MD, Wedgwood RJ. The primary immunodeficiencies. N Engl J Med. 1984;311: 235-42 and 300-10.
8. Stites DP. Laboratory evaluation of immune competence. In Stites DP, Terr AI and Parslow TG (Eds): Basic and Clinical Immunology. 8th ed. Connecticut. Appleton and Lange, 1994.
9. Straus SE (Moderator). Epstein-Barr virus infections: Biology, pathogenesis, and management. Ann Intern Med. 1993;118:45-58.

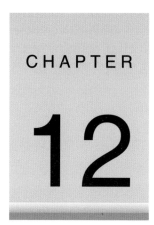

CHAPTER

12

Haematopoietic Stem Cell Transplantation

This is a therapeutic procedure in which normal haematopoietic stem cells from an appropriate donor are transferred to the patient having defective or diseased marrow to re-constitute normal haematopoiesis.

❑ TYPES OF HAEMATOPOIETIC STEM CELL TRANSPLANTATION (HSCT)

Depending on the 'relatedness' of the donor and the source of haematopoietic stem cells, three main types of HSCT are distinguished as shown in Box 12.1.

Allogeneic HSCT

In allogeneic HSCT, haematopoietic stem cells are obtained from a donor (a family member or a normal unrelated volunteer). Stem cells are best obtained from the HLA (human leucocyte antigen)-matched sibling, if available. As the genes for HLA

Box 12.1 Types of HSCT

- Allogeneic HSCT: Transplant from one individual to another of same species (peripheral blood or bone marrow).
  - Related: HLA-matched or mismatched
  - Unrelated: HLA-matched or mismatched
- Autologous: Transplant to the same individual (peripheral blood or bone marrow)
- Syngeneic: Transplant from one individual to another who are genetically identical, i.e. identical twins (peripheral blood or bone marrow).

are located on chromosome 6, and inheritance follows simple Mendelian pattern of inheritance, each sibling has 1:4 chance of finding complete HLA match. Only 30% of patients have HLA-matched sibling donor. Therefore registries of healthy volunteer donors have been set up in some western countries from which a matched-volunteer donor may be sought. It is necessary to fully or closely match HLA antigens of the recipient and the donor to reduce the risk of life-threatening complications (graft-versus-host disease or graft rejection).

Indications for Allogeneic HSCT

- Acute myeloid leukaemia in poor risk adults
- Acute lymphoblastic leukaemia in poor risk adults
- Chronic myeloid leukaemia
- Myelodysplasia
- Severe aplastic anaemia
- Severe primary immunodeficiency
- Haemoglobinopathies (thalassaemia major, sickle-cell disease)
- Inborn errors of metabolism

General Principles of Allogeneic HSCT

- *'Conditioning':* Patient is administered high dose chemotherapy (usually cyclophosphamide) alone or in combination with total body irradiation (TBI) to eradicate malignant cells, to ablate patient's marrow and create space for marrow graft, and to cause immunosuppression to prevent graft rejection. Conditioning regimen is usually administered over 1 week.
- *Transplantation:* One day after completion of 'conditioning,' stem cells are harvested from the selected donor (either peripheral blood or bone marrow), and infused intravenously into the recipient. As the patient is highly susceptible to infections due to 'conditioning,' reverse barrier nursing in a filtered air environment is necessary and prophylactic anti-infective agents are routinely administered.
- *Engraftment:* Stem cells from the donor start producing blood cells in the bone marrow 7 to 21 days following transplantation.
- *Prevention of Graft-versus-host disease (GVHD) and graft rejection:* Donor T lymphocytes recognise host tissues as foreign and cause graft-versus-host disease that is associated with high morbidity and mortality. To prevent GVHD and graft rejection, patient is routinely administered immunosuppressive therapy (methotrexate + cyclosporine) in allogeneic HSCT for 6 months.
- *Follow-up care:* Regular follow-up and care is necessary to assess and manage chronic GVHD, infections, and long-term side effects of conditioning regimen.

Graft versus leukaemia effect: Most of the curative effect of allogeneic HSCT in patients with leukaemia is due to graft versus leukaemia effect, which is mediated by donor lymphocytes. This is evident from reduced risk of relapse in patients with acute or chronic GVHD and increased risk of relapse with lymphocyte-depleted grafts.

Complications

Complications related to 'conditioning' regimen: These consist of early complications (<100 days post-transplantation) such as those associated with pancytopaenia, alopecia, oropharyngeal mucositis, diarrhoea, haemorrrhagic cystitis, cardiomyopathy, veno-occlusive disease of liver, convulsions, and interstitial pneumonitis. Late complications (>100 days) are cataracts (due to total body irradiation), sterility, early menopause, endocrine abnormalities, osteopaenia or osteoporosis, and increased risk of secondary malignancies (especially skin).

Graft rejection: Graft rejection by recipient's surviving immunocompetent T cells is more likely in the presence of HLA incompatibility and insufficient immunosuppression. It is more likely to occur in patients of aplastic anaemia. It is more common in patients who are sensitised to HLA antigens by previous blood transfusions. Transplatation of T cell-depleted graft is associated with significant reduction in its survival.

Graft-versus-host disease (GVHD): In GVHD, immunocompetent T lymphocytes in the transplanted graft recognise tissues of the host (who is immunodeficient) as foreign and react against them. It is of two types—acute and chronic. Risk of acute GVHD is more in unrelated HSCT and in HLA-mismatched HSCT.

Acute GVHD: Acute GVHD develops within 100 days of marrow transplantation. It principally affects skin, liver, and gastrointestinal tract and the severity is variable. Acute GVHD delays recovery of the immune system thus increasing susceptibility to infections. Diagnosis can be made by biopsy of the involved organ. GVHD can be prevented or its severity reduced by immunosuppressive therapy (usually methotrexate and cyclosporine). Another form of GVHD prophylaxis consists of depleting lymphocytes from the bone marrow graft; this procedure however increases the rate of graft rejection and also of relapse due to the loss of graft versus leukaemia effect. Treatment of acute GVHD is not satisfactory and involves corticosteroids, antithymocyte globulin, and monoclonal antibodies against lymphocytes.

Chronic GVHD: Chronic GVHD, developing after 100 days of transplantation, clinically resembles autoimmune disorder such as systemic lupus erythematosus, scleroderma, Sjögren's syndrome, or primary biliary cirrhosis. Treatment consists of immunosuppressive therapy

Infections: This is one of the major complications of HSCT. An association of certain infections with particular post-transplant period exists. During the early neutropaenic period, recipients are susceptible to bacterial, fungal, and herpes simplex infections. After engraftment, cytomegalovirus pneumonia is a frequent complication which may be life-threatening. Late infections by varicella zoster virus and encapsulated bacteria occur many months after transplantations.

Recurrence of malignancy: Recurrence of leukaemia, a major cause of graft failure, is less likely to occur when HSCT is done during first remission than in advanced stage of disease.

Autologous HSCT

In autologous HSCT, stem cells previously collected from the recipient are infused back, i.e. patient serves as his own source of stem cells.

- Stem cells are obtained from the patient during complete remission, processed to remove any contaminating malignant cells, and cryopreserved (frozen and stored in liquid nitrogen). Subsequent stem cell transplantation may be done within a few days or a few years of marrow harvest. In usual practice, conditioning regimen begins within a few days or weeks of marrow harvest
- Conditioning regimen is administered (high-dose chemotherapy)
- One day after completion of conditioning, stem cell product is rapidly thawed and infused intravenously.

As compared to allogeneic HSCT, immune restoration is quicker and there is no potential for GVHD. This permits the procedure to be performed in older patients. Length of hospital stay and transplant-related mortality are less as compared to allogeneic HSCT. The most common complication of autologous HSCT is relapse of underlying malignant disease; other late complications of conditioning regimen are similar to allogeneic HSCT but are less severe.

General principles of allogeneic and autologous HSCT are presented in Figure 12.1.

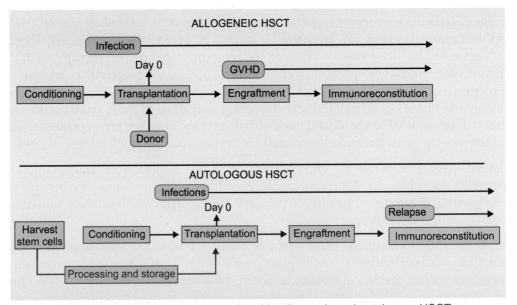

Figure 12.1: Sequence of events (blue) in allogeneic and autologous HSCT. Main complications of each type are shown in red

Indications for Autologous HSCT

- Relapsed aggressive non-Hodgkin's lymphoma
- Relapsed Hodgkin's lymphoma
- Multiple myeloma
- Solid tumours

Complications

Complications related to conditioning regimen are similar to allogeneic HSCT, although they are less frequent and less severe. The commonest late complication is relapse of the underlying malignant disease.

Allogeneic HSCT is an extremely stressful procedure associated with considerable morbidity and mortality and should be undertaken only in younger individuals (preferably less than 40 years). The major complications of allogeneic HSCT are graft -versus-host disease, graft rejection, and infections. In contrast to allogeneic HSCT, autologous transplantation can be carried out in elderly and there is no associated problem of graft-versus-host disease. However, autologous marrow for infusion may be contaminated with tumour cells with associated increased risk of post-transplantation relapse; also, autologous HSCT cannot be used for treatment of genetic disorders. An advantage of allogeneic HSCT is graft versus tumour (leukaemia) effect in which donor lymphocytes cause destruction of residual leukaemic cells by recognising them as non-self; this beneficial effect is lacking with autologous HSCT. Allogeneic and autologous HSCT are compared in Table 12.1.

Table 12.1: Comparison of allogeneic and autologous HSCT

Parameter	Allogeneic HSCT	Autologous HSCT
1. Source of stem cells	Family member or unrelated donor	Stem cells previously collected from the patient
2. Age of recipient	Young, < 55 years	Wide age range, can be done in older patients
3. Main indications	AML, ALL, MDS, CML, primary immunodeficiency, haemoglobinopathies	Relapsed NHL, relapsed Hodgkin's lymphoma, multiple myeloma, solid tumours
4. Risk of contamination of graft with malignant cells	Absent	Present
5. Risk of GVHD	Present	Absent
6. Graft versus tumour effect	Present	Absent
7. Main complication	GVHD	Relapse of malignancy
8. Overall procedure-related mortality	20–30% (if HLA-matched sibling donor), up to 45% (if unrelated donor)	5–10%
9. Treatment of inherited disease	Possible	Not possible
10. Restoration of immune function	Slower	Rapid

As identical twins are rarely encountered, syngeneic HSCT is not possible in majority of cases.

❑ SOURCES OF HAEMATOPOIETIC STEM CELLS

Haematopoietic stem cells for transplantation can be obtained from peripheral blood or from bone marrow of a donor. For allogeneic HSCT, donor should be healthy, HLA-compatible, and free from infections transmissible by the procedure.

Peripheral Blood Stem Cell Mobilisation and Harvesting

The current preferred method for harvesting haematopoietic stem cells or HSCs is from peripheral blood mononuclear cells. Although HSCs were known to circulate in peripheral blood, their very small number precluded their use for transplantation. Administration of recombinant haematopoietic growth factor (e.g. G-CSF ± chemotherapy) mobilises HSCs from bone marrow and enhances their subsequent yield from peripheral blood. The method of using HSCs isolated from peripheral blood for transplantation is known as peripheral blood stem cell transplantation (PBSCT). PBSCT is associated with more rapid engraftment as compared to bone marrow transplantation.

After administration of haematopoietic growth factor (+chemotherapy in autologous transplantation), donor is connected to an apheresis machine and mononuclear cells are collected. Timing of collection following administration of HGF is such that maximum yield of stem cells is obtained. The yield can be evaluated for adequacy by mononuclear cell count, CD34+ (a marker for haematopoietic stem cells) count, or assay for colony stimulating factor-granulocyte macrophage.

Bone Marrow Harvesting

Up to 1000 ml of marrow is aspirated from the donor from several sites in iliac crest under general anaesthesia. Aspirated marrow is collected in a harvest bag containing acid citrate dextrose solution. The yield is evaluated for adequacy by total white cell count of the harvest.

❑ RECENT ADVANCES IN HSCT

Umbilical Cord Blood Transplantation

Umbilical cord blood is an important and readily available source of haematopoietic stem cells. Due to the immaturity of immunocompetent cells in cord blood, risk of graft-versus-host disease is low. This allows for possibility of greater degree of HLA-mismatch between donor and recipient. However, number of stem cells in cord blood is limited and, therefore, most of the successful cord blood transplantations have been done in small children.

Non-myeloablative Allogeneic HSCT

In recent years, some investigators have reported encouraging results with a procedure that uses mild conditioning regimen (rather than usual intensive high-dose chemo-radiotherapy) in allogeneic HSCT for malignant disease. The aim of such mild conditioning is not to eliminate malignant cells and cause myeloablation, but to induce immunosuppression sufficient to promote engraftment and to cause slow generation of 'graft versus leukaemia' effect. It is thought that major therapeutic benefit of allogeneic HSCT results from this 'graft versus leukaemia' effect mediated by donor T lymphocytes (and not only from eradication of tumour cells by high-dose conditioning regimen). This procedure is relatively less toxic and can be performed in older patients. However, more studies are required before the role of this procedure in haematological cancers is established.

❑ BIBLIOGRAPHY

1. Appelbaum FR. Marrow transplantation for hematologic malignancies: A brief review of current status and future prospects. Semin Hematol. 1988;25:16-22.
2. Armitage JO. Bone marrow transplantation. N Engl J Med. 1994;330:827-38.
3. Klassen LW, Armitage JO, Warkentin PI. Bone marrow transplantation. In Koepke JA (Ed.): Practical Laboratory Hematology. New York. Churchill Livingstone. 1991.
4. Leger CS, Nevill TJ. Hematopoietic stem cell transplantation: a primer for primary care physician. CMAJ. 2004;170:1569-77.
5. Soutar RL, King DJ. Bone marrow transplantation. BMJ. 1995;310:31-36.

CHAPTER

13

Approach to the Diagnosis of Bleeding Disorders

Bleeding disorders result from defective haemostasis due to abnormality of vascular wall, platelets, or coagulation factors. They are one of the most commonly encountered problems in clinical haematology.

The evaluation of a patient suspected of having a bleeding disorder can be divided into two parts:
- Clinical evaluation–history, physical examination, family history
- Laboratory evaluation–screening tests, specific tests.

❑ CLINICAL EVALUATION

A carefully elicited history and physical examination are essential and provide clues regarding the nature of the disorder.

Clinically significant bleeding may be due to a local cause or a generalised defect in haemostasis. Features suggestive of a systemic haemostatic defect include–recurrent episodes of bleeding, bleeding from more than one site, spontaneous bleeding, and severe bleeding from trivial trauma.

In mild bleeding disorders it may be difficult to decide whether excessive bleeding is present. Such cases can be suspected by the amount of bleeding occurring following common surgical procedures such as tooth extraction, tonsillectomy, or circumcision.

Bleeding disorder may be hereditary or acquired. Hereditary nature of the disorder is suggested by presentation early in life (< 5 years) and history of similar complaints in close relatives of the patient with a definite inheritance pattern. There is also past history of bleeding episodes. Not all patients, however, present in childhood and mild defect may first become manifest during later years.

Family history is an essential part of the clinical evaluation as it enables to document the hereditary nature of the disorder, its pattern of inheritance and thus limits the number of diseases to be considered, and is also helpful in genetic counselling. There are three patterns of inheritance of a hereditary disorder–X-linked recessive, autosomal recessive, and autosomal dominant (Table 13.1). History of bleeding only in males and positive family history on maternal side spanning many generations is suggestive of X-**linked disorder** (e.g. haemophilia A or B). However, in 30% of cases of haemophilia, positive family history is lacking; therefore, negative family history does not rule out the possibility of haemophilia. In **autosomal recessive disease** (e.g. afibrinogenaemia, deficiency of F V or F X, von Willebrand disease), both males and females are affected (from current generation only) and history of consanguineous marriage is common. In **autosomal dominant disorders** (e.g. some forms of von Willebrand disease, hereditary haemorrhagic telangiectasia), bleeding manifests in both sexes, in one parent, and also in older generations.

Inheritance patterns of congenital bleeding disorders are presented in Box 13.1.

Table 13.1: Inherited haemorrhagic disorders

Deficiency	Mode of inheritance	Synonym	Incidence
Fibrinogen	AR	Afibrinogenaemia	Rare
Prothrombin	AR	-	Rare
F V	AR	Parahaemophilia	Rare
F VII	AR	-	1:500,000
F VIII	XR	Classical haemophilia, haemophilia A	1:10,000
F IX	XR	Haemophilia B, Christmas disease	1:60,000
F X	AR	-	Rare
F XI	AR	Haemophilia C	Rare
F XIII	AR	-	Rare
von Willebrand factor	AR or AD	von Willebrand disease	1:100

AR: Autosomal recessive; AD: Autosomal dominant; XR: X-linked recessive
Note: Deficiencies of Factor XII, high molecular weight kininogen, and prekallikrein are not associated with bleeding.

Box 13.1   Inheritance patterns of congenital bleeding disorders

- *X-linked recessive:* Haemophilia A, haemophilia B, Wiskott-Aldrich syndrome
- *Autosomal recessive:* Deficiencies of factors I, II, V, VII, X, XI, XIII; Bernard-Soulier syndrome, Glanzmann's thrombasthaenia, Gray platelet syndrome, von Willebrand disease (type 3), congenital amegakaryocytic thrombocytopaenia
- *Autosomal dominant:* Hereditary haemorrhagic telangiectasia, von Willebrand disease, May-Hegglin anomaly.

Generalised bleeding is a feature of many acquired conditions such as diseases of the liver, uraemia, haematological malignancies, carcinomas, sepsis, and administration of certain drugs (Table 13.2). In these cases the underlying disease dominates the clinical picture. Important features to look for on physical examination include fever, splenomegaly, hepatomegaly, lymphadenopathy, and icterus.

The most common inherited bleeding disorders are von Willebrand disease, haemophilia A, and haemophilia B.

Clinical history frequently indicates whether the disorder is due to abnormality of blood vessels/platelets (primary haemostasis) or coagulation factors (secondary haemostasis) (Table 13.3). Bleeding terminology is given in Box 13.2.

Table 13.2: Common drugs which can impair haemostasis and cause bleeding

Platelet phase
Aspirin, other nonsteroidal anti-inflammatory drugs, heparin, antibacterials, thiazides, chloroquine, quinine, cytotoxic drugs, ethyl alcohol

Coagulation phase
Oral anticoagulants, heparin

Table 13.3: Clinical differentiation between platelet/vascular and coagulation disorders

Parameter	Platelet/vascular disorder	Coagulation disorder
1. Commonly affected sex	Female	Male
2. Family history	Often negative (as most cases are acquired)	Often positive (as most cases are hereditary)
3. Petechiae, bleeding gums, epistaxis, menorrhagia	Common	Rare
4. Deep haematoma (muscle bleeding), haemarthrosis (joint bleeding)	Not seen	Common
5. Delayed bleeding (recurrence of bleeding from the same site hours or days following injury)	Not seen	Characteristic (12–24 hours after injury)
6. Previous h/o bleeding	Not present	Present since early childhood

Box 13.2 Bleeding terminology

- Petechiae: Tiny pinpoint areas of haemorrhage (≤ 2 mm in diameter) due to vascular or platelet disorder. They usually occur in clusters and do not blanch on pressure.
- Purpura: Areas of haemorrhage ≥ 3 mm but less than 1 cm in diameter. Appearance depends on age of lesion (red→purple→brown yellow). They do not blanch on pressure. They occur in vascular or platelet disorder. Palpable purpura is indicative of vasculitis. When occurring in mucosa, it is called as wet purpura.
- Ecchymosis (Bruise): An area of extravasated blood in skin greater than 1 cm in diameter. They result from trauma or haemostatic disorder.
- Telangiectasia: These are spots or areas resulting from localised dilated blood vessels. They blanch on pressure.
- Haematoma: A swelling resulting from a large area of haemorrhage in subcutaneous tissue or muscle. It does not blanch on pressure. It results from trauma or coagulation disorder.
- Haemarthrosis: Bleeding into a joint.

Table 13.4: Screening tests for haemostasis

Test	Assessment
Tests of primary haemostasis	
• Bleeding time	Platelet and vascular phases
• PFA-100 system	Platelet function
• Platelet count	Quantitation of platelets
• Blood smear	1. Quantitative and morphological abnormalities of platelets, 2. Detection of underlying haematological disorder
Tests of secondary haemostasis	
• Clotting time	Crude test of coagulation phase
• Prothrombin time	Extrinsic and common pathways
• Activated partial thromboplastin time	Intrinsic and common pathways

❏ LABORATORY EVALUATION

This can be divided into two parts—screening tests and specific tests. Screening tests are initial tests that are simple to perform, rapid and assess the integrity of primary or secondary haemostasis. These tests are non-specific and do not pinpoint the nature of the defect, but assess the function of one phase of the haemostatic system. Screening tests include: **tests of primary haemostasis** (Table 13.4) such as platelet count, peripheral smear examination, bleeding time, and PFA (Platelet function analyser)-100 test, and **tests of secondary haemostasis** (Table 13.4) such as prothrombin time and activated partial thromboplastin time. Directed by the results of the screening tests, appropriate specific tests are performed to define the precise nature of the defect. Specific tests include platelet function studies, specific coagulation factor assays, tests for fibrinolysis, etc.

❏ LABORATORY TESTS

Screening Tests for Primary Haemostasis

Bleeding Time (BT)

The bleeding time test is an *in vivo* measure of primary haemostasis (vascular and platelet components). It assesses the formation of primary haemostatic plug (following a skin puncture or incision), which is dependent on adequate functioning of platelets.

In this test, time required for bleeding to cease following a skin puncture/incision is measured. Stoppage of bleeding indicates formation of a primary haemostatic plug. Three methods—Duke's, Ivy's, and template—can measure bleeding time. Duke's method, which measures bleeding time following ear lobe puncture, is not recommended since, it cannot be standardised and can cause a large local haematoma. Both Ivy's and template are satisfactory methods. In Ivy's method, 2 to 3 standard punctures are made on the volar surface of the forearm with a lancet (cutting depth

2–2.5 mm) under standardised venous pressure (40 mm Hg). A stopwatch is started as soon as the punctures are made. Blood oozing from the puncture wounds is blotted with a filter paper at regular intervals. The time taken for each puncture wound to stop bleeding is noted. The average time is reported as the bleeding time. A disadvantage with this method is closure of puncture wound before stoppage of bleeding. Template method is similar to Ivy's, except that it uses a special surgical blade, which makes a larger cut (6–9 mm long and 1 mm deep).

Normal range for bleeding time is 2 to 7 minutes (Ivy's method).

Causes of prolongation of bleeding time:
- **Thrombocytopaenia:** Before carrying out a bleeding time test, a platelet count should be obtained. If platelet count is <100,000/cmm, bleeding time should not be carried out, as it will be prolonged.
- **Disorders of platelet function:** BT is markedly prolonged in hereditary disorders of platelet function like Glanzmann's thrombasthenia and Bernard-Soulier syndrome and mild to moderately prolonged in storage pool defect. Ingestion of aspirin (within last 7 days of the test) causes prolongation of BT. Uraemia, myeloproliferative disorders, leukaemias, myelodysplasia, and disseminated intravascular coagulation affect platelet function and prolong BT.
- **Inherited disorders of coagulation:** BT is prolonged in von Willebrand disease and afibrinogenaemia.
- **Vascular disorders.**

PFA (Platelet Function Analyser)-100

The conventional test for assessment of primary haemostasis has been measurement of bleeding time. However, this test is not sufficiently specific and sensitive, produces variable results, and does not correlate with significant bleeding. Recently, a new commercial automated device has been introduced, called as PFA-100 (Dade Behring) as a substitute for bleeding time. The instrument aspirates a small amount of citrated whole blood through a capillary and an aperture cut in a membrane. The membrane is coated with collagen and either epinephrine or adenosine diphosphate. Exposure of blood to these platelet agonists under high shear rates leads to binding of von Willebrand factor, platelet adhesion, activation, and aggregation. A stable platelet plug is formed which occludes the aperture. The time required for occlusion of aperture (called 'closure time') is prolonged as compared to normal in most cases of von Willebrand disease and some platelet function disorders. The test can also detect aspirin-induced platelet function defect.

It should be noted that bleeding time and PFA-100 tests are not necessary in thrombocytopaenia (since adequate number of platelets are required for assessment of platelet function).

If abnormal result is obtained with PFA-100, platelet aggregation studies should be performed for definitive diagnosis.

Platelet Count

Platelets can be counted manually under a microscope or by means of an automated haematology cell analyser.

In manual method, blood is mixed with 1% ammonium oxalate, number of platelets is counted in a counting chamber, and the result is reported as number of platelets per cubic mm. Under light microscope, platelets appear as small, roughly spherical, refractile particles. Differentiation of platelets from other particles is considerably aided by phase-contrast microscope. Normal range is 1,50,000 to 4,00,000/cmm.

Thrombocytopaenia is defined as platelet count below 1,50,000/cmm. Common causes of thrombocytopaenia are haematological malignancies, ingestion of certain drugs, disseminated intravascular coagulation, idiopathic thrombocytopaenic purpura, connective tissue diseases, megaloblastic anaemia, and aplastic anaemia. Thrombocytosis (platelet count >4,00,000/cmm) occurs in inflammation, following haemorrhage, and in myeloproliferative disorders.

Automated haematology analysers more precisely count platelets. However, these are expensive and have high running costs. Some electronic analysers can also measure platelet distribution width (PDW), mean platelet volume and reticulated platelets. **PDW** is a measure of degree of variation of platelet size present in a blood sample. High PDW is seen in myeloproliferative disorders due to the presence of marked variation in size of platelets (giant to small). In secondary or reactive thrombocytosis, PDW is normal. Thus PDW is of some value in differentiating essential thrombocythaemia from secondary or reactive thrombocytosis.

Mean platelet volume (MPV): It is increased when thrombocytopaenia is due to peripheral platelet destruction (since platelet production is stimulated with release of large platelets in circulation) and is normal or low when thrombocytopaenia is due to impaired platelet production. MPV is also increased in myeloproliferative disorders.

Young platelets with residual RNA are called as **reticulated platelets** (analogous to reticulocytes). They are considered as an index of platelet production. Increased values are observed in idiopathic thrombocytopaenic purpura and lower values in aplastic anaemia.

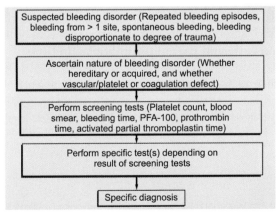

Figure 13.1: General approach for investigation of a bleeding disorder

Complete Blood Count and Blood Smear

A complete blood count and a blood smear can provide information in the form of:

- Presence of cytopaenia (anaemia, leucopaenia, thrombocytopaenia)
- Red cell abnormalities (especially fragmented red cells which may indicate disseminated intravascular coagulation)
- White cell abnormalities (like abnormal cells in leukaemias)
- Abnormalities of platelets–thrombocytopaenia (normally there is 1 platelet per 500–1000 red cells), giant platelets (seen in myeloproliferative disorders and Bernard-Soulier syndrome), and isolated discrete platelets without clumping in fingerprick smear (seen in uraemia, Glanzmann's thrombasthenia).

Direct platelet count should always be accompanied by examination of a stained blood film. It is helpful in assessing the correctness of direct count, adequacy of platelets and their morphological abnormalities; in addition underlying haematological disorders can be detected, if present.

Normally there are 8 to 20 platelets per oil immersion field or 15 to 30 platelets per high power field (400×). A rough estimate of platelet count can be obtained from blood smear which serves as a verification of platelet count obtained by automated analyser. Number of platelets are counted in 8 to 10 microscopic fields under oil immersion (1000×), average is taken, which is then multiplied by 20,000 to get the platelet count per cmm or per µl.

Some disorders are associated with giant platelets and bleeding tendency. These are listed in Table 13.5.

Screening Tests for Secondary Haemostasis

Previously, whole blood clotting time (Lee and White) was commonly done as a screening test for haemostatic abnormality. This is the time required for whole blood to clot in a glass test tube at 37°C. This is a crude test and is affected by a number of variables. It is usually prolonged when severe deficiency of a coagulation factor in intrinsic or common pathways is present (coagulation factor level <1%) and is often normal in mild/moderate deficiency. This test has now been replaced by activated partial thromboplastin time.

The most common screening tests for assessment of coagulation phase are prothrombin time and activated partial thromboplastin time.

Table 13.5: Causes of giant platelets in peripheral blood

Inherited disorders
MYH-9 syndromes*: May-Hegglin anomaly, Fechtner syndrome, Sebastain syndrome, Epstein syndrome
Other: Bernard-Soulier syndrome, Gray platelet syndrome, velocardiofacial syndrome, hereditary macrothrombocytopaenia with hearing loss, Mediterranean macrothrombocytopaenia, Montreal platelet syndrome

Acquired disorders
Myelodysplastic syndrome, myeloproliferative neoplasms, acute megakaryoblastic leukaemia, splenectomy, hyposplenism.

*All these disorders have mutations in *MYH-9* gene located at chromosome 22q12.3-q13.2.

Collection of Blood Sample for Coagulation Studies:

The pre-requisites for accurate results of coagulation studies are proper collection and subsequent handling of blood sample. Certain precautions should be followed for collection, handling, and storage of specimens for coagulation studies.

Venepuncture (usually from antecubital vein) should be smooth and non-traumatic to minimise tissue thromboplastin release. As far as possible blood for coagulation studies should not be collected from an indwelling catheter as it may be contaminated with tissue fluids, intravenous fluids, or heparin which will give rise to inaccurate results. Blood should be collected with a plastic or polypropylene syringe and a large bore needle (20 G1½ or 21 G1½). Glass syringe and glass test tubes/bottles should never be used for collection of blood for coagulation studies as glass activates contact factors and initiates coagulation through intrinsic pathway. Prolonged application of tourniquet should be avoided as stasis may cause increased fibrinolysis and activation of some coagulation factors. Blood container should be made of plastic in which liquid anticoagulant has been added earlier. The anticoagulant of choice for coagulation studies is aqueous trisodium citrate (3.2%); this is because it causes rapid chelation of calcium and factors V and VIII remain relatively more stable in it. Proportion of blood to anticoagulant should be 9:1. Blood from the syringe should be allowed to flow smoothly down the side of the container. Blood and anticoagulant should be gently but thoroughly mixed.

After collection, blood sample should be transported to the laboratory without delay and kept tightly stoppered to minimise pH changes. For assay of labile coagulation factors, maintenance at 4°C is advocated.

For most coagulation studies, platelet-poor plasma (PPP) is needed. Blood sample is centrifuged at 3000 to 4000 revolutions/min for 15 to 30 minutes to obtain PPP. Platelet-rich plasma (PRP) is required for platelet function studies; it is obtained either by slow centrifugation for 5 minutes or by allowing the anticoagulated blood to settle at room temperature.

Coagulation studies need to be carried out within 2 hours of collection and centrifugation of sample.

A control (standard) sample is prepared either locally or commercially and its value is determined earlier by a reference method. A control must be run along with the patient's sample to verify the accuracy of results and to assess the reproducibility of the test system.

Prothrombin Time

Tissue thromboplastin and calcium are added to platelet-poor plasma and clotting time of the mixture is noted. This test is a measure of extrinsic and common pathways. Commercial tissue thromboplastin is prepared from rabbit brain or rabbit lung. Tissue thromboplastin serves two functions. It activates extrinsic system and provides phospholipid surface for certain coagulation reactions. Calcium ions bind vitamin K-dependent factors (II, VII, IX, and X) to phospholipid. Normal range of PT is 11–16

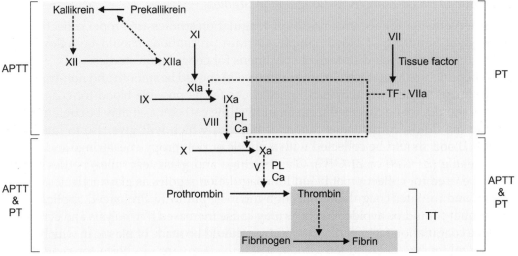

Figure 13.2: Coagulation factors measured by three screening tests: prothrombin time (PT), activated partial thromboplastin time (APTT), and thrombin time (TT)

seconds. Prothrombin time measures the activity of coagulation factors VII, X, V, II (prothrombin), and I (fibrinogen) (Fig. 13.2).

Causes of prolongation of PT:
1. *Vitamin K deficiency:* PT is a useful test for detection of vitamin K deficiency as it measures three vitamin K-dependent proteins out of four, i.e. II, VII and X.
2. *Oral anticoagulant therapy:* Oral anticoagulants interfere with the carboxylation of vitamin K-dependent factors. PT is the standard test for monitoring oral anticoagulant therapy.
3. *Disseminated intravascular coagulation*
4. *Inherited deficiency of a coagulation factor in extrinsic or common pathway,* i.e. VII, X, V, II, or I.

Activated Partial Thromboplastin Time (APTT)

In this test platelet-poor plasma is incubated with an activator. Then phospholipid and calcium are added and clotting time is noted. An activator serves to standardise the contact activation. Commonly used activators are kaolin, celite, ellagic acid, and silica. Phospholipid is also called as partial thromboplastin; it provides surface for certain coagulation reactions. APTT measures activity of coagulation factors in intrinsic and common pathways (Fig. 13.2). Normal range of APTT is 30 to 40 seconds.

Causes of prolongation of APTT:
1. *Inherited deficiency of F VIII or F IX:* APTT is the most widely used screening test for the detection of hereditary deficiency of F VIII and F IX. APTT is also prolonged in inherited deficiencies of other coagulation factors in intrinsic and common pathways.

2. *Circulating inhibitors:* Inhibitors may be of two types—specific and nonspecific. Specific inhibitors are directed against specific coagulation factors. The most common specific inhibitor is antibody against F VIII. Non-specific inhibitors are antibodies that are not directed against specific coagulation factors but block the interaction of clotting factors, e.g. lupus inhibitor.

3. *Disseminated intravascular coagulation*

4. *Heparin:* Heparin accelerates the action of antithrombin and thus inhibits thrombin and factors Xa, Xla, and IXa. Heparin therapy is monitored by regularly performing APTT.

5. *Liver disease:* Prolongation of APTT occurs in moderate to severe liver disease due to reduced synthesis of coagulation factors.

6. *Vitamin K deficiency:* Although vitamin K deficiency prolongs APTT, the test is not affected by F VII (a vitamin-K-dependent factor with the shortest half-life). Therefore, it is not as sensitive as PT to vitamin K deficiency.

   Shortening of APTT is observed in thrombosis and pregnancy.

   Approach to prolonged APTT is presented in Figure 13.3.

Thrombin Time

Thrombin reagent is added to platelet-poor plasma and the time required for clot formation is noted. Normal range is 8 to 12 seconds. Prolongation of thrombin time occurs in:

1. *Disorders of fibrinogen:* These include afibrinogenaemia (virtual absence of fibrinogen), hypofibrinogenaemia (fibrinogen level is detectable but less than 100 mg/dl), and dysfibrinogenaemia (qualitative defect of fibrinogen).

2. *Presence of heparin in plasma*

3. *Chronic liver disease*

4. *Fibrinogen/Fibrin degradation products.*

   In most patients suspected of having a bleeding disorder, it is possible to arrive at a presumptive diagnosis by performing a small battery of screening tests (Fig. 13.1 and Table 13.6). Depending upon the results of the screening tests, appropriate specific studies can be performed to arrive at the final diagnosis.

   In some bleeding disorders, haemostatic screening tests may be normal (Box 13.3).

❏ SPECIFIC TESTS

Specific Tests for Primary Haemostatic Disorders

Bleeding due to a defect in primary haemostasis results from following disorders:
- von Willebrand disease
- Thrombocytopaenia
- Vascular disorder
- Platelet function defect.

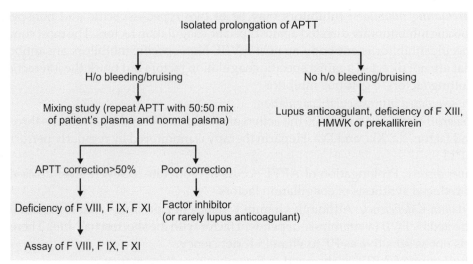

Figure 13.3: Approach to evaluation of isolated prolongation of APTT

Table 13.6: Interpretation of screening tests of haemostasis in a bleeding disorder

BT	PC	PT	APTT	Haemostatic defect	Common causes
I	N	N	N	Platelet function, vascular disorder	vWD, aspirin, uraemia, storage pool defect
I	D	N	N	Thrombocytopaenia	Secondary causes, drugs, ITP
N	N	I	N	Extrinsic pathway	Oral anticoagulants, vitamin K deficiency, deficiency of F VII
N	N	N	I	Intrinsic pathway	Heparin, haemophilia A or B, vWD, inhibitors
N	N	I	I	Common pathway	Heparin, liver disease, vitamin K deficiency, oral anticoagulants, deficiency of V, X, II, I
I	D	I	I	Multiple pathways	Disseminated intravascular coagulation, liver disease
N	N	N	N	-	Mild vWD, vascular disorder, platelet function defect, F XIII deficiency

N: Normal; I: Increased; D: Decreased; vWD: von Willebrand disease

---

Box 13.3 Bleeding disorders that may present with normal screening tests for haemostasis

- Coagulation disorders: mild haemophila A or B, mild von Willebrand disease, F XIII deficiency
- Platelet disorders: Glanzmann's thrombasthenia, platelet storage pool defect
- Vascular defects: Hereditary haemorrhagic telangiectasia, osteogenesis imperfecta, scurvy, Ehlers-Danlos syndrome
- Defects in fibrinolysis: α2-antiplasmin deficiency

Tests for specific Platelet Functions

Tests are available to define specific platelet functional abnormalities in adhesion, aggregation, release reaction, and platelet procoagulant activity.

Platelet adhesion studies: Whole blood is made to pass over a foreign surface and reduction occurring in the platelet count is estimated. In the glass bead column test, whole blood is passed through a column of non-siliconised glass beads. Proportion of platelets retained by the glass bead column is assessed from the platelet count done before and after the passage of blood through the column. Less than 25% retention of platelets is usually observed in von Willebrand's disease. Apart from adhesion, platelet retention is also caused by aggregation and thus the test is not specific. Due to the availability of more sensitive techniques, this test is rarely carried out.

Platelet aggregation studies: For platelet aggregation studies, a special instrument called as aggregometer is used. This instrument has a continuous stirring device to keep the platelets in platelet-rich plasma in an even suspension; when a platelet aggregating agent or agonist is added to platelet-rich plasma, change in light transmission occurs due to platelet aggregation which is recorded by a photometer.

When an aggregating agent is added to platelet-rich plasma, initially there is platelet shape change from discoid to spherical. This causes a small decrease in transmission of light. As aggregates of platelets form light transmission increases which is recorded on the strip chart.

Commonly employed aggregating agents are ADP, epinephrine, collagen, arachidonic acid, and ristocetin. ADP and epinephrine induce primary and secondary waves of aggregation (biphasic curve). Primary wave is due to the direct action of aggregating agent on platelets with formation of small aggregates. Secondary wave is associated with thromboxane A_2 synthesis and secretion from platelet granules. Collagen, arachidonic acid, and ristocetin induce a single wave of aggregation (monophasic curve).

Aggregation response is deficient or absent with ADP, epinephrine, collagen and arachidonic acid in Glanzmann's thrombasthenia. In this disorder there is congenital absence of platelet receptors GpIIb-IIIa necessary for fibrinogen binding during aggregation; platelet aggregation, however, is normal with ristocetin.

Defective aggregation with ristocetin but not with other agonists is a feature of von Willebrand disease and Bernard-Soulier syndrome. Addition of normal plasma (source of von Willebrand factor) corrects the abnormality in von Willebrand disease but not in Bernard-Soulier syndrome.

In release reaction defects, ADP and epinephrine induce primary wave of aggregation but no secondary wave is produced (Table 13.7).

Flow cytometric detection of glycoproteins on platelet surface: Analysis of membrane glycoproteins is necessary for diagnosis of Bernard-Soulier syndrome and Glanzmann's thrombasthenia.

Tests of platelet secretion or release reaction: Secondary wave of aggregation with ADP or epinephrine is an indirect evidence of release reaction. Various direct tests for assessing release reaction are available. Dense granule secretion may be assessed by quantitation of serotonin, and measuring ATP concentration by firefly bioluminescence technique. Measurements of platelet factor 4 and β thromboglobulin released from α

Table 13.7: Platelet aggregation studies in disorders of platelet function

Disorder	Aggregating agents			
	ADP/Epinephrine		Collagen	Ristocetin
	Primary wave	Secondary wave		
1. Bernard-Soulier syndrome (BSS)*	Normal	Normal	Normal	Deficient
2. von Willebrand disease (vWD)*	Normal	Normal	Normal	Deficient
3. Glanzmann's thrombasthenia	Deficient	Deficient	Deficient	Normal
4. Storage pool deficiency**	Normal	Deficient	Deficient	Normal
5. Aspirin-like defect**	Normal	Deficient	Deficient	Normal

*Cryoprecipitate corrects abnormality in vWD but not in BSS.
** Aggregation is defective with arachidonic acid in aspirin-like defect, but not in storage pool deficiency.

granules are sensitive indicators of platelet activation and have been applied in the study of hypercoagulable states.

Tests for detection of abnormalities in arachidonic acid metabolism: Arachidonic acid metabolism plays an important role in activation of platelets by generating thromboxane A_2 (Refer to Fig. 1.30). Defective platelet aggregation by arachidonic acid is indicative of abnormality in arachidonic acid metabolism. Techniques for quantitation of TxB_2, malondialdehyde, and other intermediate products in arachidonate pathway are available. Their use can lead to the identification of deficiencies of phospholipases, cyclooxygenase, and thromboxane synthetase.

Tests for platelet procoagulant activity: Platelet procagulant activity may be assessed by the prothrombin consumption test. This test assesses clotting activity or the amount of residual prothrombin remaining in serum after whole blood is allowed to clot completely. Prothrombin times of serum and of citrated plasma are performed and the result is expressed as their ratio. Presence of unconsumed prothrombin may be due to deficiency of coagulation factors or of platelet phospholipid.

Other platelet function tests: Clot retraction test: In this test citrated platelet-rich plasma is recalcified. The plasma clots, which subsequently undergoes retraction. Clot retraction is dependent upon adequate number and function of platelets. Poor clot retraction is observed in thrombocytopaenia and in Glanzmann's thrombasthenia.

Specific Tests for Coagulation Phase

Mixing Study Based on PT or APTT

If a coagulation factor deficiency is suspected and if there is isolated prolongation of either PT or APTT, mixing study should be performed to determine whether factor deficiency or an inhibitor is present. In this test, abnormal PT or APTT is repeated using 50:50 mixture of normal and patients's plasma and whether normalisation of previously prolonged test occurs should be noted. If deficiency of coagulation factor is present then the addition of normal plasma corrects prolonged clotting time. In the presence of inhibitors, result depends upon the type of inhibitor. Inhibitors may be of immediate-acting or delayed-acting types. If immediate-acting inhibitor is present APTT/PT performed using mixture of patient's plasma and normal plasma remains prolonged with no correction. If delayed-acting inhibitor is present, clotting time of the mixture immediately becomes normal; however, after incubation for 1 to 2 hours at 37°C, prolongation of clotting time is observed.

If mixing study indicates factor deficiency, it is necessary to identify the deficient factor. The deficient factor in patient's plasma can be identified by correction test using adsorbed normal plasma and aged normal human serum or by thromboplastin generation test.

Thromboplastin Generation Test (TGT)

This is a two-stage test.

Stage I (Generation of prothrombinase): Adsorbed plasma, serum, phospholipid, and calcium are incubated together. Adsorbed plasma supplies factors V and VIII; serum supplies factors IX and X, and both supply factors XI and XII. This leads to the generation of prothrombinase (F Xa-V-calcium-phospholipid complex).

StageII (Assessment of adequacy of prothrombinase generated): The coagulant activity of the prothrombinase formed is measured by its ability to clot substrate (normal) plasma. If the prothrombinase generated is deficient, then abnormal result (i.e. prolonged clotting time) is obtained. In such a case, substitution studies are carried out to localise the defect. The test is performed using patient's adsorbed plasma and normal serum, and patient's serum and normal adsorbed plasma to detect which substitution produces normal or abnormal result. A presumptive diagnosis of a particular factor deficiency can be made by also considering the results of PT and clinical history (Table 13.8).

Quantitative Estimation of Fibrinogen

A number of methods are available for estimation of plasma fibrinogen. Some of the methods are outlined below:

Table 13.8: Interpretation of thromboplastin generation test

History	Coagulation screen	TGT	Interpretation
Bleeding	PT-N, APTT-P	Plasma defect	F VIII deficiency
Bleeding	PT-P, APTT-P	Plasma defect	F V deficiency
Bleeding	PT-N, APTT-P	Serum defect	F IX deficiency
Bleeding	PT-P, APTT-P	Serum defect	F X deficiency
Bleeding	PT-N, APTT-P	Both plasma and serum defect	F XI deficiency
No bleeding	PT-N, APTT-P	Both plasma and serum defect	F XII deficiency

PT: Prothrombin time; APTT: Activated partial thromboplastin time; P: Prolonged; N: Normal

a. Coagulable protein method based on thrombin time: This is the most widely used reference method. This method makes use of the reaction between fibrinogen and thrombin in which there is formation of a fibrin clot. Clauss modified the thrombin time screening test so that it could be applied for estimation of fibrinogen. If thrombin in excess is added to the diluted plasma, then the clotting time is inversely proportional to the concentration of fibrinogen. The modifications of higher reagent concentration and lower plasma concentrations provide a linear relationship between clotting time and concentration of fibrinogen. The clotting time obtained is compared with clotting times of known fibrinogen standards in the same system to get the result.

b. Immunological methods: Immunologic procedures depend on reaction between plasma fibrinogen and anti-fibrinogen antibody. The methods include single radial immunodiffusion or radioimmunoassay. Immunologic methods, when applied together with functional (coagulable protein) method, are useful in diagnosing dysfibrinogenaemias. In the presence of dysfunctional fibrinogen molecules, low values are obtained with functional method (i.e. coagulable protein method), while normal results are obtained with immunologic method.

c. Other methods: Other methods of fibrinogen estimation are based on weighing of clot, and precipitation of fibrinogen by heat (56°C) or by chemicals (sodium sulphite). Normal level of fibrinogen in plasma is 200 to 400 mg/dl.

Low levels of fibrinogen are seen in a- or hypo-fibrinogenaemia, dysfibrinogenaemia, and disseminated intravascular coagulation. Transient hyperfibrinogenaemia occurs in inflammatory disorders, neoplasia, myocardial infarction, and trauma.

Coagulation Factor Assays

One-stage coagulation factor assays are commonly performed to diagnose factor deficiency and are based on APTT or PT. PT or APTT is performed using mixture of patient's plasma and factor-deficient plasma and the clotting time is noted. (Factor-deficient plasma contains all the coagulation factors, except the one to be assayed). Clotting time obtained is compared with a previously prepared reference graph, which has clotting time in seconds on one axis and percentage activity of coagulation factor on the other. Reference graph is prepared using various dilutions of standard (or normal) plasma mixed with factor-deficient plasma; 1:10 dilution of standard plasma represents 100% activity.

Normal level of all coagulation factors is 50 to 150% or 50 to 150 units/dl.

F XIII Qualitative Assay

F XIII is a transglutaminase that catalyses the formation of covalent bonds between fibrin monomers and imparts stability to the clot. In the absence of F XIII, fibrin clot is unstable and dissolves in 5M-urea solution or 1% monochloracetic acid.

In F XIII deficiency, all the screening tests of haemostasis are normal.

Paracoagulation Tests

Paracoagulation tests are employed for the detection of soluble (non-polymerised) fibrin monomers in plasma. These include protamine sulphate or ethanol gelation tests. In these tests, ethanol or protamine sulphate is added to platelet-poor plasma and formation of a gel is noted. Positive test is indicative of active or ongoing intravascular coagulation. Positive result is also obtained in lobar pneumonia, liver disease, and after major surgery.

Tests for Fibrinolysis

Detection of Fibrinogen/Fibrin Degradation Products by Latex Agglutination Test

FDPs are fragments produced by proteolytic digestion of fibrinogen or fibrin by plasmin (Refer to Figs 1.40 and 1.41).

Test for FDPs is performed on serum. Venous whole blood is mixed with thrombin and either soybean trypsin inhibitor or epsilon-amino-caproic acid. Thrombin removes all fibrinogen by converting it into a fibrin clot. Soybean trypsin inhibitor or epsilon-amino-caproic acid are inhibitors of fibrinolysis that prevent *in vitro* breakdown of fibrin.

A suspension of latex particles coated with anti-fibrinogen antibodies (FDPs share common antigenic determinants with fibrinogen) or with antibodies to specific FDPs is mixed with serum on a glass slide. If FDPs are present, then agglutination of latex particles occurs (Fig. 13.4). Apart from qualitative screening, a semiquantitative estimation of FDPs can also be done. These tests are simple, sensitive, and rapid but are expensive and false positive result with rheumatoid factor can occur.

Test for detection of FDPs are commonly employed for diagnosis of disseminated intravascular coagulation (DIC). Although FDPs are usually raised in most patients

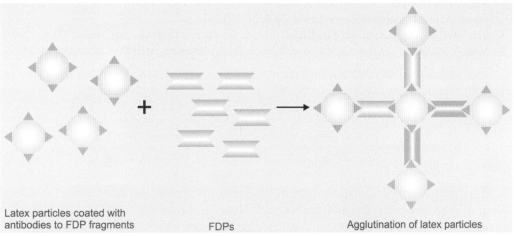

Latex particles coated with
antibodies to FDP fragments   FDPs   Agglutination of latex particles

Figure 13.4: Principle of latex agglutination test for fibrinogen/fibrin degradation products

with DIC, FDP test may sometimes be negative. This is because of removal of clottable FDP fragments X and Y along with fibrinogen by thrombin in blood collection tubes. In early DIC in which circulating plasmin levels are low, FDP fragments are mostly X and Y and their removal can produce a false negative test.

Apart from DIC, FDPs are also detected in pulmonary embolism, deep venous thrombosis, severe pneumonia, and recent myocardial infarction.

Detection of Cross-linked Fibrin D-dimers by Latex Agglutination Test

This test is similar to latex agglutination test for FDPs, except (1) latex particles are coated with monoclonal antibodies against D-dimers, and (2) test can also be done on plasma since there is no cross-reaction with fibrinogen. Positive test indicates that generation of both thrombin and plasmin has occurred, and distinguishes between fibrin and fibrinogen degradation products. D-dimer test is more specific for diagnosis of disseminated intravascular coagulation than FDP test.

❑ BIBLIOGRAPHY

1. Allen GA, Gladers B. Approach to the bleeding child. Ped Clin North Am. 2002;49:1239-56.
2. Day HJ, Rao AK. Evaluation of platelet function. Semin Hematol. 1986;23:89-101.
3. Greenberg CS, Devine DV, McCrae KM. Measurement of plasma fibrin antibody coupled to latex beads. Am J Clin Pathol. 1987;87: 94-100.
4. Marder VJ, Matchett MO, Sherry S. Detection of serum fibrinogen and fibrin degradation products. Comparison of six technics using purified products and application in clinical studies. Am J Med. 1971;51: 71-82.
5. Merskey C, Lalezari P, Johnson AJ. A rapid, simple, sensitive method for measuring fibrinolytic split products in human serum. Proc Soc Exp Biol Med. 1969;131: 871.
6. Mhawech P, Saleem A. Inherited giant platelet disorders. Classification and literature review. Am J Clin Pathol. 2000;113:176-190.
7. Moreno A, Menke D. Assessment of platelet numbers and morphology in the peripheral blood smear. Clinics in laboratory medicine. 2002; 22: 193-213.
8. Triplett DA. Coagulation and bleeding disorders: review and update. Clin Chem. 2000;46: 1260-9.
9. Vora A, Makris M. An approach to investigation of easy bruising. Arch Dis Child. 2001;84: 488-91.

CHAPTER

14

Bleeding Disorders Caused by Abnormalities of Blood Vessels
(The Vascular Purpuras)

Defective haemostasis occurs in a wide variety of vascular disorders (Table 14.1). In these diseases, clinical features are frequently distinctive, type of bleeding is superficial and laboratory tests of haemostasis yield normal results (Box 14.1).

Table 14.1: The vascular purpuras

Acquired	Inherited
1. Anaphylactoid purpura	1. Hereditary haemorrhagic telangiectasia
2. Infections	2. Hereditary connective tissue disorders
3. Scurvy	• Ehlers-Danlos syndrome
4. Senile purpura	• Osteogenesis imperfecta
5. Purpura simplex	• Marfan's syndrome
6. Mechanical purpura	• Pseudoxanthoma elasticum
7. Drugs, e.g. corticosteroids	
8. Cushing's syndrome	
9. Factitious purpura	

Box 14.1 Diagnosis of vascular purpuras
- Superficial, mild bleeding from skin and mucous membranes
- Bleeding from skin more in dependent portions of body
- Screening tests of haemostasis often normal
- Associated clinical features usually characteristic

❑ ANAPHYLACTOID PURPURA
(HENOCH-SCHÖNLEIN PURPURA, ALLERGIC PURPURA)

This is an immune complex disease in which purpura results from vasculitis (due to deposition of IgA-containing complexes). Manifestations of allergic purpura include:

- Predominant occurrence in children (2–8 years). Frequently there is a recent history of upper respiratory infection or of other inciting factor such as sensitivity to certain foods
- Rapid onset
- Skin: Palpable purpuric spots over extensor surfaces of extremities, associated with urticaria; sometimes haemorrhagic bullous and necrotic lesions occur
- Gastrointestinal tract: Abdominal pain (due possibly to mesenteric vasculitis), sometimes with bleeding
- Joints: Arthralgia
- Kidneys: Microscopic haematuria, proteinuria, acute glomerulonephritis, or nephrotic syndrome.

These features may occur in combination or one feature may predominate. The disease is self-limited but recurrent episodes are common. Chronic glomerulonephritis, and CNS bleeding are rare complications.

Diagnosis is based on typical clinical features and exclusion of haematological causes of purpura.

Glucocorticoids are sometimes administered for symptomatic relief.

❑ INFECTIONS

Infections can cause vascular damage by direct endothelial damage or by immune complex mechanism. Commonly responsible agents are meningococci, salmonella, measles virus, and rickettsial organisms. Severe infections can also cause bleeding by other mechanisms such as thrombocytopaenia or consumptive coagulopathy.

❑ SCURVY

Vitamin C deficiency is frequently associated with haemorrhagic manifestations such as perifollicular haemorrhages, petechiae, bleeding gums, subperiosteal haemorrhages, and deep-seated haematomas, The cause of bleeding is defective synthesis of collagen. Bleeding tendency is readily corrected by oral administration of ascorbic acid.

❑ SENILE PURPURA

Purpuric and ecchymotic lesions commonly develop in elderly persons over seventy years of age on forearms, hands, face, and neck. The lesions disappear after a few weeks leaving behind brown discolouration. There is atrophy of subendothelial collagen, subcutaneous fat and elastic tissue due to ageing which results in increased susceptibility of small blood vessels to trivial injury. No treatment is required.

❑ PURPURA SIMPLEX

Mild bruising may develop spontaneously on lower legs in young women of reproductive age, with aggravation during menstruation. It requires no treatment.

❑ MECHANICAL PURPURA

Violent and prolonged bouts of coughing may cause rupture of small blood vessels in face and neck area due to rise in local intravascular pressure. Prolonged upright posture in elderly may be associated with purpura in legs due to atrophy of perivascular connective tissue coupled with venous insufficiency (orthostatic purpura).

❑ HEREDITARY HAEMORRHAGIC TELANGIECTASIA (OSLER-WEBER-RENDU DISEASE)

This is a rare autosomal dominant disorder characterised by presence of multiple, small, telangiectatic lesions in skin, mucous membranes, and internal organs. Bleeding manifestations occur spontaneously or following minor trauma and are related to marked thinning of walls of dilated blood vessels. Onset of haemorrhages is usually in early adult life with recurrent epistaxis and gastrointestinal bleeding being common complaints. Bleeding tendencies increase with advancing age and commonly cause iron deficiency anaemia. Topical haemostatics, embolisation of pulmonary arteriovenous malformation, and administration of iron for correction of anaemia are the usual forms of therapy.

❑ BIBLIOGRAPHY

1. Kraft DM, McKee D, Scott C. Henoch-Schönlein Purpura: A review. Am Fam Physician. 1998; 58:405.
2. Lee GR, Bithell TC Foerster J, Athens JW, Lukens JN (Eds.): Wintrobe's Clinical Hematology. 9th ed. Philadelphia. Lea and Febiger. 1993.

Bleeding Disorders Caused by Abnormalities of Platelets

Disorders of platelets include (i) thrombocytopaenia (ii) thrombocytosis and (iii) platelet dysfunction.

❑ THROMBOCYTOPAENIA

Thrombocytopaenia refers to decrease in the number of platelets in peripheral blood below normal (<1.5 lacs/cmm). It may result from four main mechanisms (Table 15.1).
• Increased peripheral destruction of platelets
• Decreased production of platelets in bone marrow
• Dilutional thrombocytopaenia
• Sequestration in enlarged spleen.

The lower value of platelets is 1,50,000/cmm. Platelet count between 1,50,000 and 50,000/cmm is generally not associated with clinically significant bleeding. Platelet counts between 50,000 and 20,000/cmm usually cause bleeding with trauma or surgery or mild spontaneous bleeding. Platelet count below 20,000/cmm is associated with risk of spontaneous, severe haemorrhage.

Idiopathic Thrombocytopaenic Purpura (ITP)

In ITP, autoantibodies or immune complexes bind to platelets and cause their premature peripheral destruction. Megakaryocytes are normal or increased in bone marrow. ITP occurs in two forms—acute and chronic. Acute ITP is a short-lasting illness of sudden

Table 15.1: Causes of thrombocytopaenia

1. *Increased destruction of platelets*
   - *Immune*
     - Idiopathic thrombocytopaenic purpura (ITP)
     - Systemic lupus erythematosus
     - Drugs: heparin, gold salts, penicillin, quinidine, quinine
     - Infections: HIV, malaria, dengue, hepatitis C virus, *Helicobacter pylori,* other
     - Post transfusion purpura
     - Neonatal alloimmune purpura
   - *Nonimmune*
     - Disseminated intravascular coagulation
     - Thrombotic thrombocytopaenic purpura/Haemolytic uraemic syndrome
     - Giant haemangioma
2. *Decreased production of platelets*
   - *Hereditary*
     - Fanconi's anaemia
     - Wiskott-Aldrich syndrome
   - *Acquired*
     - Aplastic anaemia
     - Bone marrow infiltration (leukaemias, myelodysplasia, myelofibrosis, lymphoma, metastatic carcinoma)
     - Megaloblastic anaemia
     - Drugs (cytotoxic drugs, ethanol), Radiation
     - Viral infections
3. *Dilutional thrombocytopaenia*
   - Massive blood transfusion
4. *Increased sequestration*
   - Hypersplenism

onset which occurs in children following viral infection or vaccination. Chronic ITP is an indolent disorder of insidious onset with multiple remissions and relapses, occurs predominantly in adult women, and is not preceded by infection or associated with any underlying disease.

Pathogenesis

Acute ITP: In acute ITP, immune complexes of viral antigens and host anti-viral antibodies bind to Fc receptors on platelets that leads to immune destruction of platelets by macrophages in spleen. Alternatively, antiviral antibodies may cross-react with platelet antigens.

Chronic ITP: In chronic ITP, autoantibodies are predominantly IgG, and less commonly IgM. These antibodies are directed against specific platelet glycoproteins GpIIb/IIIa or GpIb/IX in majority of patients. GpIIb/IIIa are sites for fibrinogen binding during platelet aggregation. Thus, in addition to causing destruction of platelets, these autoantibodies also induce platelet dysfunction by blocking GpIIb/IIIa receptors. Antibody-coated platelets are recognised by Fc receptors on macrophages and destroyed mainly in spleen. Antibodies are also directed against megakaryocytes in ITP.

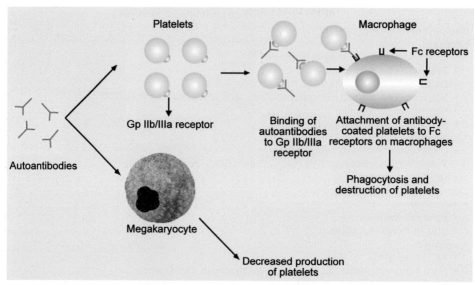

Figure 15.1: Pathogenesis of ITP

Antibody-coated platelets are rapidly destroyed in reticulo-endothelial organs particularly spleen (Fig. 15.1). Thrombocytopaenia results when peripheral destruction of platelets exceeds compensatory increase in thrombopoiesis in bone marrow. The cause of autoantibody formation is unknown.

Recent evidence indicates that thrombocytopaenia also results from suppression of platelet production due to megakaryocyte damage and dysfunction (mediated by autoantibodies).

Clinical Features

Incidence of ITP increases with age.

Clinical presentation varies from severe thrombocytopaenia and bleeding to asymptomatic mild thrombocytopaenia detected incidentally.

Acute ITP predominantly affects children between 2 and 6 years of age with sex ratio being 1:1. The disease often follows viral respiratory infection or vaccination after an interval of 2 to 3 weeks. There is increased incidence during winter and spring. The disease starts suddenly with cutaneous and mucous membrane bleeding in the form of purpuric spots and ecchymoses (especially on legs), bleeding from gums, nose, gastrointestinal tract and haematuria. Intracranial haemorrhage though rare can be fatal. Spleen tip may be palpable but significant splenomegaly is unusual. The disease is self-limited and spontaneous complete remissions usually occur within 2 to 6 weeks in more than 80% of patients. Recurrences are uncommon. In about 15 to 20% of children, thrombocytopaenia persists beyond 6 months.

Chronic ITP occurs in young adults. It is more common in females (3F:1M). There is an insidious onset of superficial bleeding from skin and mucous membrane;

Table 15.2: Differences between acute and chronic ITP

Parameter	Acute ITP	Chronic ITP
1. Age	Childhood	Young adults
2. Sex	No sex preference	More common in females
3. H/o preceding viral infection or vaccination	Common	No
4. Onset of bleeding	Sudden	Insidious
5. Degree of thrombocytopaenia	Severe	Moderate
6. Duration of disease	Self-limited (2–6 months)	Many years
7. Spontaneous remission	Usual	Rare

menorrhagia is particularly common in women. Chronic bleeding can cause iron deficiency anaemia. History of preceding viral infection or any underlying disease is lacking. Spleen is not palpable in chronic ITP and in the presence of splenomegaly alternative diagnosis should be considered. Some patients have asymptomatic thrombocytopaenia and are discovered incidentally during routine blood counts. Chronic ITP is an indolent disease with remissions and recurrences in bleeding occurring over many years.

Clinical features of acute and chronic ITP are contrasted in Table 15.2.

New terminology proposed by International Working Group (2009):
- The term immune thrombocytopaenia should be used in place of immune thrombocytopaenic purpura as bleeding is absent in majority of patients
- Primary ITP is defined as an autoimmune disorder with isolated thrombocytopaenia (platelet count <100,000/cmm) without any underlying cause.
- Secondary ITP refers to all other forms of immune thrombocytopaenia except primary ITP, e.g. drug-induced; associated with *Helicobacter pylori*, hepatitis C virus, or human immunodeficiency virus
- Phases of ITP:
  1. Newly diagnosed: First 3 months after diagnosis
  2. Persistent ITP: 3 to 12 months from diagnosis
  3. Chronic ITP: >12 months

Laboratory Features

Examination of peripheral blood: Blood loss may lead to anaemia. In children, lymphocytes and eosinophils are frequently increased. In acute ITP, platelets are markedly reduced (<20,000/cmm) while in chronic ITP platelet count is variable (usually moderately low, i.e. around 50,000/cmm). Morphologically, platelets are frequently large (megathrombocytes) (Fig. 15.2). In chronic ITP, bleeding manifestations are frequently mild as compared to the degree of thrombocytopaenia; this is due to the presence of large, giant platelets in circulation, which are functionally hyperactive. The number of large platelets is proportional to megakaryocyte number in marrow. Blood film is also necessary to rule out non-immune causes of thrombocytopaenia (e.g. aplastic anaemia,

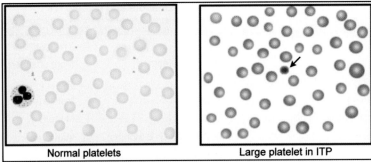

| Normal platelets | Large platelet in ITP |

Figure 15.2: Blood smear in ITP. Blood smear on left shows normal number and size of platelets. Blood smear on right shows reduced number of platelets with only a single large platelet (megathrombocyte) (arrow) in ITP

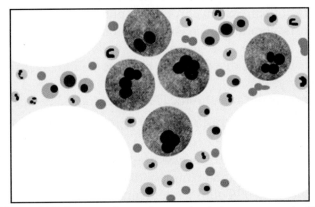

Figure 15.3: Increased megakaryocytes in bone marrow in ITP

leukaemia, myelodysplasia, megaloblastic anaemia, pseudothrombocytopaenia [see later], and inherited thrombocytopaenia).

Bone marrow examination: In bone marrow, megakaryocytes are normal or increased in number (Fig. 15.3) and frequently show morphological changes such as hypogranularity of cytoplasm, vacuolisation, lack of platelet budding, nuclear non-lobulation or hypolobulation and dense nuclear chromatin. These morphologic abnormalities are seen in any condition associated with accelerated platelet destruction and are not specific for ITP.

If clinical features, complete blood count, and blood smear are indicative of ITP, bone marrow examination is not necessary for diagnosis of ITP. However, it should be carried out if presentation is unusual (e.g. presence of splenomegaly or hepatosplenomegaly) and morphological abnormalities of leucocytes are present.

Coagulation profile: Prolonged bleeding time and deficient clot retraction are the usual abnormalities. Tests for blood coagulation are normal.

Platelet antibodies: Levels of platelet-associated immunoglobulins are raised in majority (more than 90%) of patients with ITP. This test, however, is neither sufficiently sensitive nor specific for ITP. Therefore, it is not necessary for diagnosis.

Differential Diagnosis (Table 15.3)

Diagnosis of ITP is one of exclusion since there are no specific clinical or laboratory features. In neonates and small children, maternal ITP, alloimmune neonatal thrombocytopaenia, and inherited thrombocytopaenia (Box 15.1) should be considered. Possibilities of drug-induced thrombocytopaenia and post transfusion isoimmune purpura are suggested by history. Isolated thrombocytopaenia may be the initial manifestation of systemic lupus erythematosus and antinuclear and anticardiolipin antibody tests should be carried out. If immune haemolytic anaemia is present along with thrombocytopaenia, diagnosis of Evans' syndrome should be considered. Autoimmune thrombocytopaenia can occur in lymphoproliferative disorders (lymphoma, chronic lymphocytic leukaemia) and in diseases of thyroid and these possibilities should be excluded by appropriate investigations. Human immunodeficiency virus (HIV) infection is emerging as a common cause of thrombocytopaenia and should be excluded in high-risk cases. Hereditary thrombocytopaenia (Bernard-Soulier syndrome, Wiskott-Aldrich syndrome, May-Hegglin anomaly) may mimick ITP and should be considered when recurrent thrombocytopaenia unresponsive to treatment is present since childhood and family history is positive. Fragmented red cells in peripheral blood or abnormal coagulation profile suggest disseminated intravascular coagulation or microangiopathic haemolytic anaemia. Distinctive clinical and laboratory features allow one to make the correct diagnosis in various other haematologic diseases in which thrombocytopaenia is a secondary feature (such as leukaemias, lymphomas, myeloma and aplastic anaemia).

Table 15.3: Differential diagnosis of ITP

Isolated thrombocytopaenia	Thrombocytopaenia associated with other haematological abnormalities
• Secondary immune thrombocytopaenia (HIV, HCV, *H. pylori*, autoimmune disorders) • Drug-induced thrombocytopaenia • Inherited thrombocytopaenia • Pseudothrombocytopaenia	• Megaloblastic anaemia • HELLP syndrome/Pre-eclampsia • Hypersplenism • Haematologic malignancies • Aplastic anaemia • Thrombotic thrombocytopaenic purpura/Haemolytic uraemic syndrome • Disseminated intravascular coagulation • Evans syndrome • Liver disease

Box 15.1 Causes of inherited thrombocytopaenia

• Small platelets: Wiskott-Aldrich syndrome
• Normal-sized platelets: Thrombocytopaenia absent radii syndrome, congenital amegakaryocytic thrombocytopaenia
• Giant platelets: MYH-9 syndrome (May-Hegglin anomaly, Fechtner syndrome, Epstein syndrome, Sebastian syndrome), Bernard-Soulier syndrome, Gray platelet syndrome, Montreal platelet syndrome

Diagnosis

Diagnosis of ITP is based on combination of following features:

- Mucocutaneous type of bleeding with abrupt onset (acute ITP) or insidious onset (chronic ITP)
- No other abnormality on physical examination with patient otherwise being normal
- Presence of isolated thrombocytopaenia with no other abnormality on complete blood count
- Bone marrow examination is normal (not required for diagnosis unless clinical presentation and course are unusual)
- Exclusion of other causes of thrombocytopaenia.

Treatment

Acute ITP: Acute ITP is a self-limited disorder with spontaneous remission occurring in majority of patients within 2 to 6 months. Therefore, the management of acute ITP is mainly supportive. In the absence of significant bleeding symptoms, simple observation without specific therapy to raise the platelet count is preferred. In children with severe bleeding symptoms, oral corticosteroids or intravenous immunoglobulins are given. Platelet transfusions along with high-dose intravenous steroids or intravenous immunoglobulin are indicated in life-threatening haemorrhage.

A few children go on to develop chronic ITP; even in these cases spontaneous remission is usual.

Chronic ITP: Patients with asymptomatic compensated thrombocytopaenia should be observed without any treatment. Symptomatic patients and platelet count <30,000/cmm are indications for treatment. The initial therapy in chronic ITP is corticosteroids. (Mode of action of corticosteroids is suppression of phagocytosis of antibody-coated platelets by macrophages and suppression of antibody production). In patients unresponsive to steroids, intravenous immunoglobulin can be tried (blocks Fc receptors of reticuloendothelial cells). Failure to respond to steroids, relapse, and very high doses of steroids to maintain remission are indications for splenectomy. With splenectomy, 75% of patients achieve remission. Intravenous immunoglobulin is usually administered before splenectomy to temporarily raise the platelet count.

See Box 15.2 for treatment of ITP and newer drugs available.

Approach for management of ITP is shown in Figure 15.4.

Box 15.2   Treatment of ITP
• First-line therapy: Corticosteroids, IV immunoglobulin, IV anti-D (only in RhD+ve individuals)
• Second-line therapy: Rituximab, TPO receptor agonists (romiplostim, eltrombopag), splenectomy
• Life-threatening bleeding: IV immunoglobulin, platelet transfusions

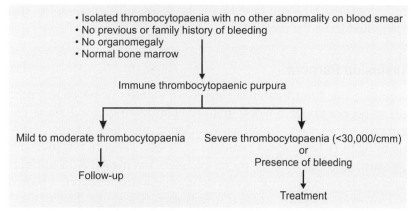

- Isolated thrombocytopaenia with no other abnormality on blood smear
- No previous or family history of bleeding
- No organomegaly
- Normal bone marrow

Immune thrombocytopaenic purpura

Mild to moderate thrombocytopaenia

Follow-up

Severe thrombocytopaenia (<30,000/cmm)
or
Presence of bleeding

Treatment

Figure 15.4: Approach for management of ITP

Alloimmune Neonatal Thrombocytopaenia

When the foetal platelets possessing paternally derived antigens lacking in the mother enter maternal circulation during gestation or delivery, formation of alloantibodies is stimulated. These maternal antibodies cross the placenta and cause destruction of foetal platelets. Firstborn babies are also frequently affected. The most common platelet antigen against which antibodies form is HPA-1a (PI^A1). The condition is self-limited and usually resolves by 3 weeks (maximum 3 months) after delivery. There is a risk of intracranial haemorrhage due to trauma during vaginal delivery. In severe cases purpura and haemorrhages are evident at birth or manifest within a few hours. Alloimmune neonatal thrombocytopaenia should be distinguished from other causes of neonatal thrombocytopaenia (Table 15.4).

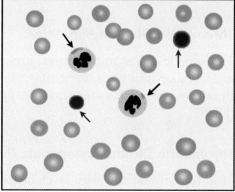

Figure 15.5: Blood smear in May-Hegglin anomaly showing giant platelets (red arrows) and Dohle-like inclusions within neutrophils (black arrow)

Table 15.4: Causes of neonatal thrombocytopaenia

Increased peripheral destruction of platelets
1. Immune destruction by maternal antibodies: autoimmune antibodies (maternal ITP or SLE), alloimmune neonatal thrombocytopaenia.
2. Non-immune mechanism: disseminated intravascular coagulation, intrauterine infections, giant haemangioma.

Decreased production of platelets
1. Thrombocytopaenia absent radii (TAR) syndrome
2. Wiskott-Aldrich Syndrome
3. May-Hegglin anomaly (Fig. 15.5)
4. Bernard- Soulier syndrome
5. Fanconi anaemia
6. Congenital malignancy.

Severe symptomatic thrombocytopaenia is usually treated by transfusion of platelets obtained from the mother.

Post-transfusion Purpura

In this very rare but life-threatening disorder, sudden onset of thrombocytopaenia and bleeding occurs about 1 week to 10 days following blood transfusion in some adult multiparous women. In all cases, donor platelets possess HPA-1a antigen while this antigen is lacking on patient's platelets. Patients are probably sensitised previously during pregnancy by foetal platelets having HPA-1a antigen. Following blood transfusion severe thrombocytopaenia due to destruction of patient's platelets develops. However, why the anti-HPA-1a antibodies cause destruction of patient's own platelets, which are HPA-1a-negative, is unknown. It has been suggested that HPA-1a antigen in donor binds with an alloantibody and these immune complexs are non-specifically adsorbed on patient's own platelets. Another explanation offered is HPA-1a antigen in donor plasma gets passively adsorbed on patient's platelets making them HPA-1a-positive and leading to their destruction by alloantibodies. The condition is treated by intravenous gamma globulin and plasmapheresis.

Thrombotic Microangiopathies

Thrombotic microangiopathies are characterised by microvascular thrombosis, microangiopathic haemolytic anaemia (MAHA), and thrombocytopaenia, and include thrombotic thrombocytopaenic purpura (TTP) and haemolytic uraemic syndrome (HUS).

Thrombotic Thrombocytopaenic Purpura

This uncommon disorder is characterised by formation of hyaline microthrombi in microcirculation of various organs due to aggregation of platelets. In idiopathic TTP, autoantibodies against ADAMTS13 (A disintegrin and metalloprotease with thrombospondin type 1 motif 13) lead to deficiency of ADAMTS13 and accumulation of ultra-large vWF multimers that bind large number of platelets. In familial TTP (Upshaw-Sohulman syndrome) ADAMTS13 deficiency results from mutations in *ADAMTS13* gene.

The disorder mainly affects young adults and is slightly more common in females. The pentad of manifestations includes: (i) Microangiopathic haemolytic anaemia: Haemolysis of red cells results from their passage across fibrin strands of microthrombi in circulation. Clinically patients have pallor and frequently icterus. Peripheral blood examination shows presence of fragmented and nucleated red cells and reticulocytosis (Fig. 15.6). Levels of lactate dehydrogenase and unconjugated bilirubin in serum are raised and indicate increased haemolysis; (ii) Bleeding manifestations secondary to severe thrombocytopaenia such as petechiae, ecchymoses, epistaxis,

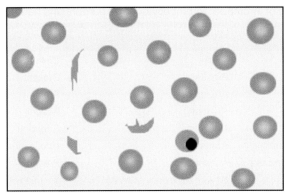

Figure 15.6: Blood smear in thrombotic thrombocytopaenic purpura showing schistocytes, thrombocytopaenia, and a late normoblast

and gastrointestinal/genitourinary bleeding. Coagulation studies (PT, APTT) are normal in most patients; (iii) Fluctuating neurologic dysfunction such as altered level of consciousness, seizures, visual field abnormalities, and hemiparesis, which may terminate in coma; (iv) Renal abnormalities: proteinuria, haematuria, azotaemia; (v) Fever. These five features may not be present in all patients. It is essential to make the correct diagnosis since platelet transfusions for correction of thrombocytopaenia can aggravate the predisposition to thrombosis. Most patients respond to transfusions of fresh frozen plasma or to plasmapheresis. In those patients who fail to respond, antiplatelet drugs, corticosteroids, or vincristine may be tried.

Haemolytic Uraemic Syndrome

Haemolytic uraemic syndrome is characterised by triad of acute renal failure, thrombocytopaenia, and microangiopathic haemolytic anaemia. HUS is classified into two types: typical and atypical. Typical HUS occurs predominantly in children <5 years of age and is associated with Shiga toxin-producing *Escherichia coli* O157:H7; it is characterised by a prodrome of diarrhoeal illness followed by MAHA, thrombocytopaenia, and renal failure. Atypical HUS has similar clinical features but is not preceded by diarrhoeal prodrome.

Differences between TTP an HUS are presented in Table 15.5. Microangiopathic haemolytic anaemia and thrombocytopaenia can also occur in pre-eclampsia, HELLP syndrome, autoimmune disorders, systemic infections, systemic malignancy, and malignant hypertension.

Massive Transfusion

Stored whole blood is deficient in viable platelets and in labile coagulation factors (F V and F VIII). Transfusion of massive amounts of such blood to individuals with severe blood loss can lead to thrombocytopaenia or coagulation factor deficiency by

Table 15.5: Comparison of thrombotic thrombocytopaenic purpura and haemolytic uraemic syndrome

Feature	Thrombotic thrombocytopaenic Purpura (TTP)	Haemolytic uraemic syndrome (HUS)
1. Age	Adults	Children < 5 years
2. MAHA	Present	Present
3. Thrombocytopaenia	Present	Present
4. Fever	Present	Absent
5. Severe renal failure	Uncommon	Common
6. Major neurologic abnormalities	Common	Uncommon
7. Prodrome of bloody diarrhaea	Absent	Present (in typical HUS)
8. Cause	Severe deficiency of ADAMTS13	Infection by *Escherichia coli* O157:H7 (in typical HUS)
9. Coagulation tests	Normal	Normal
10. Treatment	Plasma exchange	Supportive

MAHA: Microangiopathic haemolytic anaemia

dilutional effect. Bleeding due to massive transfusion can be prevented by transfusion of fresh frozen plasma and platelet concentrates along with stored blood.

Thrombocytopaenia due to Increased Platelet Sequestration or Pooling

Normally about 30% of total platelets in the body are sequestered in the spleen. In conditions associated with enlargement of spleen, splenic platelet pool expands and may reach up to 90% in some cases. Due to compensatory increase in platelet production in bone marrow, thrombocytopaenia is usually mild.

Pseudothrombocytopaenia

When platelet counts are determined by electronic cell counters on blood samples collected in EDTA, sometimes a falsely low result may be obtained. Examination of a parallel peripheral blood smear made from EDTA anticoagulated blood, however, reveals large clumps of platelets and platelets rosetting around neutrophils (Fig. 15.7). The platelet clumping results from presence of EDTA-dependent antiplatelet antibody in some patients. EDTA alters the conformation of GpIIb/IIIa complex and exposes neoantigen. The antibody reacts with this cryptic antigen and causes platelet clumping only *in vitro*. These antibodies do not have any clinical significance. Incorrect diagnosis of thrombocytopaenia can be avoided by simultaneous examination of peripheral blood film along with determination of direct platelet count.

Evaluation of a Thrombocytopaenic Patient

A thrombocytopaenic patient presents with purpuric spots, ecchymoses, or mucous membrane bleeding (epistaxis, gastrointestinal, genitourinary bleeding). The differ-

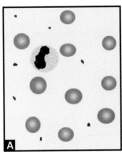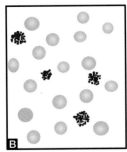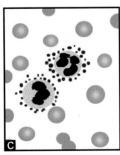

Figure 15.7: (A) Normal distribution of platelets on blood smear; (B) Blood smear showing aggregation of platelets; (C) Blood smear showing adherence of platelets to neutrophils (satellitism). Both (B) and (C) are examples of pseudothrombocytopaenia reported on automated haematology analyser in blood sample collected in EDTA anticoagulant

ential diagnosis is wide (Table 15.1: Causes of thrombocytopaenia). To ascertain the cause of thrombocytopaenia, complete clinical examination is essential including previous history of bleeding, family history, history of drug intake, presence of underlying disorder, and presence or absence of palpable spleen. Laboratory examination includes examination of peripheral blood smear, bone marrow examination and coagulation screen. A scheme for evaluation of a thrombocytopaenic patient is shown in Figure 15.8. Salient diagnostic features of platelet disorders are shown in Box 15.3.

❏ THROMBOCYTOSIS

This refers to increase in the platelet count above normal (> 4 lac/cmm). Causes of thrombocytosis are listed in Table 15.6.

Thrombocytosis due to myeloproliferative disorders is known as primary thrombocytosis. It can be usually distinguished from reactive (secondary) thrombocytosis by the presence in the former of leucocytosis and immature white cells and nucleated red cells in peripheral blood, defective platelet function (deficient

Table 15.6: Causes of thrombocytosis

- ***Reactive (Secondary):*** Haemorrhage, trauma, infections, iron deficiency, malignancy, splenectomy, chronic inflammatory disease
- ***Primary:*** Essential thrombocythaemia, polycythaemia vera, chronic myeloid leukaemia, idiopathic myelofibrosis

Box 15.3	Diagnosis of bleeding due to platelet disorders

- Superficial type of bleeding (mucocutaneous)
- Platelet count low (thrombocytopaenia) or normal (platelet function defect); bleeding time may be prolonged
- Coagulation screen (PT, APTT): Normal
- Specific laboratory evaluation is directed by results of screening tests for primary haemostasis, i.e. whether indicative of thrombocytopaenia (low platelet count) or platelet function defect (prolonged bleeding time with normal platelet count, abnormal PFA-100 test).

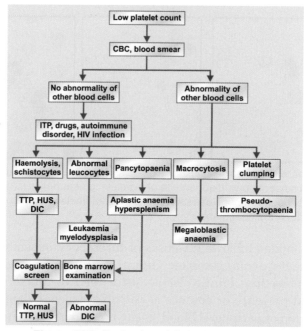

Figure 15.8: Evaluation of thrombocytopaenia

epinephrine-induced platelet aggregation) and splenomegaly. Also, in secondary thrombocytosis features of underlying causative disorder are evident.

Thrombocytosis in essential thrombocythaemia is associated with thromboembolic and bleeding manifestations. In reactive thrombocytosis, platelet count is modestly elevated and has no clinical significance. However, persistent thrombocytosis following splenectomy for chronic haemolytic anaemia may result in increased risk of thromboembolic complications if haemolysis is not completely corrected.

❑ DISORDERS OF PLATELET FUNCTION

Disorders of platelet function are classified into two broad categories: inherited and acquired (Table 15.7).

Inherited Disorders of Platelet Function

Bernard-Soulier Syndrome

This is a rare autosomal recessive congenital bleeding disorder. In this disease, adhesion of platelets to subendothelium is defective due to congenital absence of glycoprotein Ib receptor complex (which consists of GpIb, V and IX) on platelet surface. This receptor is essential for binding of platelets to subendothelium via von Willebrand factor (Fig. 15.10).

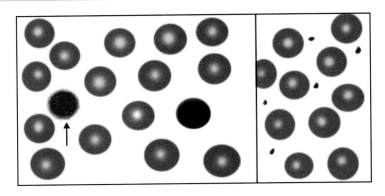

Figure 15.9: Blood smear showing a giant platelet (arrow). Panel on right shows normal platelets for comparison

Table 15.7: Disorders of platelet function

Inherited	Acquired
• Bernard-Soulier syndrome	• Haematopoietic stem cell disorders: myeloproliferative neoplasms, acute leukaemias, myelodysplastic syndrome, paroxysmal nocturnal haemoglobinuria
• Glanzmann's thrombasthenia	
• Storage pool deficiency	
• Dense granule	
• Alpha granule	• Paraproteinaemias
• Defective thromboxane synthesis	• Uraemia
	• Cardiopulmonary bypass
	• Drugs

It is caused by defects in *GP9* (located on 3q21.3), *GP1BB* (located on 22q11.21-q11.23), and *GP1BA* (located on 17pter-p12) genes.

The haemorrhagic manifestations usually begin in infancy or early childhood. They are of moderate to marked degree and consist of purpuric spots, easy or spontaneous bruising, and mucosal bleeding.

Characteristic laboratory abnormalities include giant platelets on peripheral blood smear (Fig. 15.9), mild to moderate thrombocytopaenia not proportional to the severity of bleeding, abnormal platelet function studies (in the form of prolonged bleeding time, impaired platelet aggregation with ristocetin not corrected by addition of normal plasma, normal platelet aggregation with other agonists), and absence of GpIb, V, and IX.

No satisfactory form of therapy is available. Severe haemorrhagic episodes are managed by platelet transfusions. Repeated platelet transfusions can induce alloimmunisation and formation of antibodies against glycoproteins that are absent.

Glanzmann's Thrombasthenia

In this very rare autosomal recessive bleeding disorder, platelet aggregation is deficient due to absence of GpIIb/IIIa recepter complex on platelets. The disorder results from mutations in genes *ITGB3* (located on 17q21.32) or *ITGA2B* (located on 17q21.32). Normally upon activation of platelets, GpIIb/IIIa receptors become exposed on platelet surface and serve as binding sites for fibrinogen. Fibrinogen molecules form bridges between adjacent platelets during aggregation.

In Glanzmann's thrombasthenia, the absence of fibrinogen binding due to lack of receptors is responsible for deficient aggregation (Fig. 15.10).

On peripheral blood smear, platelets appear small and discrete (i.e. they are not in clumps due to lack of aggregation), platelet count is normal, platelet function studies are abnormal (in the form of prolonged bleeding time, poor clot retraction, platelet aggregation is absent with ADP, epinephrine, collagen, and arachidonic acid and normal with ristocetin), and lack of GpIIb/IIIa complex.

No effective form of therapy is available. Severe haemorrhages are treated by platelet transfusions.

Storage Pool Deficiency

Deficiency of intracellular granules of platelets is referred to as storage pool deficiency. It may involve dense granules, alpha granules, or both.

Dense granule storage pool deficiency: This is the most common type of hereditary platelet function disorder. Patients usually present with mild mucocutaneous bleeding. Electron microscopy reveals absence of dense granules (Fig. 15.10). Intraplatelet levels of ADP, serotonin, and calcium are diminished. Platelet aggregation studies with ADP

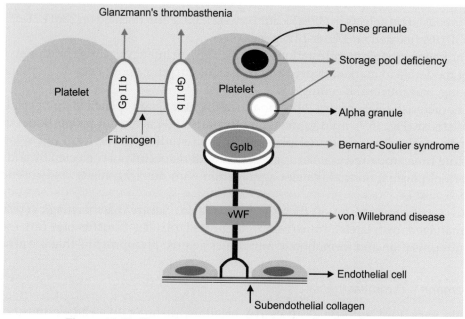

Figure 15.10: Sites of defects in some platelet function disorders

and epinephrine reveal primary wave of aggregation but secondary wave is absent. Aggregation with collagen is defective. Ristocetin-induced aggregation is normal.

Dense granule storage pool deficiency occurs most commonly as a sole abnormality. Less commonly it occurs in association with various congenital disorders such as Hermansky-Pudlak syndrome, Wiskott-Aldrich syndrome, etc. Hermansky-Pudlak syndrome is characterised by deficiency of dense granules, albinism, and presence of macrophages containing pigment (ceroid).

Bleeding episodes are managed with platelet concentrates.

Alpha granule storage pool deficiency (Gray platelet syndrome): In this condition, which has been described in only a few patients, alpha granules and their contents are diminished or absent (Fig. 15.10). These patients have a mild bleeding diathesis. Platelets are mildly decreased in number, are large in size, and appear pale-grey on stained blood smears. Defective platelet aggregation has also been described. Reticulin fibres are increased in bone marrow.

Defective Thromboxane Synthesis (Aspirin-like defect)

Thromboxane A_2 synthesised from arachidonic acid normally stimulates secretion from dense and alpha granules and is also a platelet agonist. Therefore, deficiencies of enzymes in arachidonic acid metabolism can impair release of granular contents from platelets (Refer to Fig. 1.30). Congenital deficiencies of cyclo-oxygenase and thromboxane synthetase are extremely rare in which platelet secretion is defective. Ingestion of aspirin inhibits cyclo-oxygenase and induces a similar defect. Patients have a mild bleeding disorder, prolonged bleeding time, normal primary wave but absent secondary wave with ADP and epinephrine, and deficient aggregation with collagen and arachidonic acid.

Basic laboratory studies for diagnosis of inherited disorders of platelet function have been presented earlier (Chapter 13).

Acquired Disorders of Platelet Function

Drugs

Aspirin inhibits the enzyme cyclo-oxygenase by causing its irreversible acetylation. This results in inability of the platelets to synthesise thromboxane A_2 and failure of platelet secretion. This forms the basis of use of aspirin as anti-platelet drug in practice. The inhibitory effect of aspirin on platelet function lasts for 7 to 10 days (life-span of affected platelets). Aspirin should be withheld for at least 10 days before performing platelet function studies. Platelet aggregation studies with ADP and epinephrine after aspirin ingestion reveal primary wave of aggregation but no secondary wave. Aspirin should be avoided in persons with bleeding disorders. In a patient taking aspirin, aspirin should be discontinued for at least 7 days before any surgical procedure. Other drugs affecting platelet function are other nonsteroidal analgesic anti-inflammatory drugs, penicillin, cephalosporins, local anaesthetics, dipyridamole, dextran, and heparin.

Myeloproliferative neoplasms

Bleeding manifestations occur in myeloproliferative neoplasms in the presence of normal or increased platelet count. A variety of platelet functional abnormalities have been described, the most common being defective aggregation response to epinephrine. Aggregation may also be defective with ADP and collagen.

Paraproteinaemias

Paraproteins in multiple myeloma and Waldenström's macroglobulinaemia coat the platelet surface and inhibit adhesion and aggregation. Paraproteins also interfere with interaction of coagulation factors.

Uraemia

The bleeding tendency associated with uraemia is usually in the form of petechiae, ecchymoses, and gastrointestinal haemorrhages, and may be severe. Platelet functional abnormalities are thought to play a major role. The usual laboratory abnormalities are prolongation of bleeding time and impaired platelet aggregation with ADP and epinephrine. The haemostatic abnormalities in uraemia are corrected by dialysis suggesting that a dialyzable substance causes them. The substances suspected include guanidinosuccinic acid, urea, and phenols. The usual form of treatment of bleeding diathesis in uraemia is haemodialysis. Cryoprecipitate and DDAVP (Desmopressin) may also be of benefit.

❑ BIBLIOGRAPHY

1. Bick AL. Platelet function defects associated with hemorrhage or thrombosis. Med Clin North Am. 1994;78:577-607.
2. British Committee for Standards in Haematology: Guidelines for the investigation and management of idiopathic thrombocytopaenic purpura in adults, children, and pregnancy. Br J Haematol. 2003;120:574-96.
3. Bromberg ME. Immune thrombocytopaenic purpura- The changing therapeutic landscape. N Engl J Med. 2006;355:1643-45
4. Cines D, Bussel J, Liebman H, et al. The ITP syndrome: pathogenic and clinical diversity. Blood. 2009;113:6511-21.
5. Cines DB, Blanchette VS. Immune thrombocytopaenic purpura. N Engl J Med. 2002;346:995-1008.
6. Cooper N, Bussel J. The pathogenesis of immune thrombocytopaenic purpura. Br J Haematol. 2006;133:364-74.
7. George JN, El-Harake MA, Raskob GE. Current concepts: Chronic idiopathic thrombocytopaenic purpura. N Engl J Med. 1994;331:1207-11.

8. George JN. How I treat patients with thrombotic thrombocytopaenic purpura: 2010. Blood. 2010;116:4060-9.

9. Hardisty AM and Caen JP. Disorders of platelet function. In Bloom AL and Thomas DP (Eds): Haemostasis and thrombosis. 2nd ed. Edinburgh. Churchill Livingstone. 1987.

10. Karpatkin S. Autoimmune thrombocytopaenic purpura. Blood. 1980;56:329-43.

11. Karpatkin S. Autoimmune thrombocytopaenic purpura. Semin Hematol. 1985;22:260-88.

12. Kiefel V, Santos S, Mueller-Eckhardt C. Serological, biochemical, and molecular aspects of platelet autoantigens. Semin Hematol. 1992;129:26-33.

13. Kunicki TJ, Newman PJ. The molecular immunology of human platelet proteins. Blood. 1992;80: 1386-404.

14. McCrae KR, Samuels P, Schreiber AD. Pregnancy-associated thrombocytopaenia: Pathogenesis and management. Blood. 1992;80:2697-714.

15. McMillan R. Chronic idiopathic thrombocytopaenic purpura. N Engl J Med. 1981;304:1135.

16. Rao AK, Holmsen H. Congenital disorders of platelet function. Semin Hematol. 1986;23:102-18.

17. Rodeghiero F, Stasi R, Gernsheimer T, et al. Standardization of terminology, definitions, and outcome criteria in immune thrombocytopaenic purpura of adults and children: Report from an International Working Group. Blood. 2009;113:2386-93.

18. Rutherford CJ, Frenkel EP. Thrombocytopaenia. Issues in diagnosis and therapy. Med Clin North Am. 1994;78:555-75.

19. Stasi R, Provan D. Management of immune thrombocytopaenic purpura in adults. Mayo Clin Proc. 2004;79:504-22.

20. Waters AH. Autoimmune thrombocytopaenia: Clinical aspects. Semin Hematol. 1992;29:18-25.

16 Disorders of Coagulation

INHERITED DISORDERS OF COAGULATION

❑ HAEMOPHILIA A

Haemophilia A (classical haemophilia) is the most common hereditary coagulation disorder. It occurs in approximately 1:10,000 individuals. It is caused by hereditary deficiency or dysfunction of Factor VIII. In India, about 1300 haemophilics are born every year and currently there are about 50,000 patients with severe disease.

Inheritance

The mode of inheritance of haemophilia A is X-linked recessive (Fig. 16.1). The abnormal gene (or the gene coding the synthesis of F VIII) is located on the X chromosome. The disease manifests only in males because they lack the complementary normal X chromosome. Females are carriers but do not manifest the disease as they have a normal allele on the complementary X chromosome. Typically positive family history is obtained in maternal grandfather, maternal uncles, and maternal male cousins. If a carrier female marries a normal male, then the male offspring has a 50% chance of being affected while the female offspring has a 50% chance of becoming a carrier. If a haemophilic male marries a normal female, all his sons will be normal while all his daughters will be carriers.

Positive family history is not obtained in about 30% of patients with haemophilia. These cases probably arise from spontaneous mutation. Therefore, negative family history does not rule out the possibility of haemophilia.

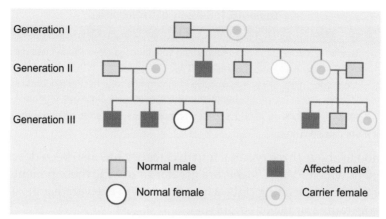

Figure 16.1: An example of X-linked pattern of inheritance in haemophilia A. Only males are affected. History of haemorrhagic diathesis is obtained in uncles and male cousins on maternal side. Carrier females transmit the disease

Majority of female carriers of haemophilia A do not suffer from haemorrhagic diathesis. This is because F VIII synthesised by complementary gene on the normal X chromosome is adequate to achieve haemostasis. However, haemophilia may develop in carrier females when there is lyonisation predominantly of normal X chromosomes during embryogenesis. Other mechanisms by which haemophilia can occur in females are homozygosity of haemophilic gene in the female offspring of carrier female and affected male, or hemizygosity of haemophilic gene due to chromosome anomalies such as Turner's (XO) syndrome. It should be noted, however, that a more common cause of F VIII deficiency in females is von Willebrand disease.

Pathogenesis of Bleeding in F VIII Deficiency

In vivo, extrinsic pathway controls bleeding after injury. Tissue factor-F VIIa complex activates F IX and F X and initiates a rapid but limited generation of thrombin on tissue injury. The initial formation of thrombin is subsequently amplified by a feed-back mechanism in which thrombin activates F XI and F VIII of intrinsic pathway. In F VIII deficiency, inadequate amounts of thrombin are generated. Secondly, increased amount of thrombin is required for activation of TAFI (thrombin-activated fibrinolysis inhibitor). Therefore, F VIII deficiency is associated with insufficient clot formation as well as rapid clot removal.

Clinical Features

Clinical severity of haemophilia A is variable and correlates with F VIII:C activity. Haemophilia A is classified into mild, moderate, and severe types based on the level of F VIII:C in patient's plasma (Table 16.1).

Table 16.1: Severity of haemophilia

F VIII:C level	Type	Frequency	Clinical features
<1%	Severe	70%	Frequent and spontaneous deep tissue haemorrhages and haemarthrosis
1–5%	Moderate	15%	Excessive haemorrhage after mild to moderate injury; occasional haemarthrosis; spontaneous bleeding infrequent
>5%	Mild	15%	Excessive haemorrhage only after major trauma or surgery

Normal level of F VIII:C is 50–150%.

In addition to above three types, a fourth category has also been described by some investigators in which FVIII:C levels are greater than 25%; these patients usually have moderately excessive bleeding only when exposed to a severe haemostatic challenge such as major trauma or major surgery.

In patients with mild disease, disorder may not be diagnosed until middle age (e.g. prolonged bleeding after major surgery).

Insufficiency of F VIII (haemophilia A) or F IX (haemophilia B) results in similar symptoms since the two coagulation factors are involved in the same step in the coagulation mechanism.

Petechiae are absent in haemophilia.

Factor VIII level and severity of bleeding are fairly similar in affected members of a particular haemophilic kindred.

In severe haemophilia, bleeding manifestations often start when the child begins to crawl or learns to walk. They include deep-seated haematomas and haemarthroses; mucous membrane bleeding from lips and tongue can occur after eruption of deciduous teeth.

Bleeding into weight-or stress-bearing joints (haemarthroses) is a characteristic feature of haemophilia A. Commonly affected joints are knees, ankles, hips, and elbows. Haemarthroses are a major cause of incapacitation in haemophilia. Onset of bleeding into the joint is preceded by tingling sensation, mild discomfort and slight restriction of movement. This is followed by pain, swelling, and stiffness of the affected joint. Blood induces inflammation of the synovium. Inflamed synovium, being hypervascular and friable, is vulnerable to re-bleeding following injury and a vicious cycle of repeated bleeding with progressive joint damage sets in. In the patient, often one specific joint is susceptible to repeated bleeding and damage and such a joint is called as target joint. Narrowing and irregularity of joint space due to destruction of cartilage, subchondral cysts, and osteoporosis develop and ultimately joint becomes disorganised and immobile. Cartilage and bone degeneration due to joint bleeding is known as haemophilic arthropathy.

Intramuscular haematomas are particularly common in muscles of calf, thigh, forearm, and buttocks. They can compress vital structures such as arteries (distal ischaemic injury) or peripheral nerves (sensory or motor neuropathy) and cause pressure necrosis of adjacent tissue.

Intracranial haemorrhage can occur following trivial trauma and is a common cause of death in haemophilia. Haematuria frequently occurs in severe haemophilia and may induce colicky pain (clot colick). Severe bleeding can occur postoperatively or after dental extractions in unrecognised haemophilics; such bleeding is typically of delayed onset.

Laboratory Features

Coagulation Profile

Tests for primary haemostasis (platelet count, bleeding time) and for extrinsic and common coagulation pathway (prothrombin time) are normal. The only abnormality in coagulation profile is prolongation of activated partial thromboplastin time (APTT), i.e. a measure of intrinsic and common pathways. The sensitivity of APTT to F VIII deficiency depends on the reagents used. Most APTT systems are prolonged in severe and moderate deficiencies of F VIII but results are variable in mild cases and may sometimes be normal. Results of APTT must be viewed in the light of the patient's complaints and F VIII:C assay should be performed in indicated cases even though APTT is normal.

Clotting time is a crude screening test for coagulation disorders and prolonged values are obtained mostly in severe cases (F VIII:C < 1%); it is often normal in mild/moderate cases. Therefore, clotting time has been replaced by APTT as a screening test for coagulation disorders.

Thromboplastin generation test (TGT) is a second-line test and reveals "plasma defect". The combination of normal PT, prolonged APTT, and plasma defect in TGT are highly suggestive of F VIII deficiency.

Factor VIII:C Assay

Clot-based assays are commonly employed particularly one stage assay based on APTT. Serial dilutions of normal reference plasma (normal pooled plasma) are made. To each dilution, F VIII-deficient substrate plasma is added and APTT of the mixture is determined. A reference graph is prepared showing relationship between APTT and F VIII: C per cent activity (1:10 dilution of reference plasma has 100% F VIII: C). APTT of mixture of diluted patient's plasma and substrate plasma is determined. From the APTT obtained F VIII:C content is derived from reference graph.

Normal F VIII:C level in plasma is 50 to 150%. It is affected by various factors such as venous stasis before collection of blood, prolonged storage of blood, severe exercise, pregnancy, inflammation, fever, liver diseases, hyperthyroidism, and haemolysis.

Apart from establishing the diagnosis of F VIII deficiency, F VIII:C assay is used to monitor F VIII replacement therapy.

Differential Diagnosis

Diagnosis of haemophilia A can be made when a male patient with appropriate family history presents with typical haemorrhagic manifestations, prolonged APTT with

Box 16.1 Diagnosis of haemophilia

- Haematomas, haemarthrosis, excessive post-traumatic bleeding, delayed bleeding
- Presentation in early childhood; family history often +ve (X-linked recessive)
- Bleeding time, platelet count - normal
- APTT - Prolonged
- Definitive diagnosis - Factor VIII assay.

Box 16.2 Causes of inherited deficiency of F VIII

- Haemophilia A
- von Willebrand disease (especially type 2N and type 3)
- Combined deficiency of F V and F VIII
- Some carriers of haemophilia A

normal prothrombin time and bleeding time, and a plasma defect in TGT. F VIII:C assay should be carried out for confirmation of diagnosis (Box 16.1).

Causes of F VIII: C deficiency include haemophilila A, von Willebrand disease, combined hereditary deficiency of Factors V and VIII, and acquired disorders such as F VIII inhibitors, and disseminated intravascular coagulation. Causes of inherited deficiency of F VIII are shown in Box 16.2.

von Willebrand disease occurs in both sexes and bleeding manifestations are mainly in the form of mucocutaneous haemorrhages such as petechiae and epistaxis, though haemarthrosis may occur. Laboratory investigations usually show prolonged bleeding time, prolonged APTT, and defective ristocetin induced platelet aggregation.

In **combined deficiency of Factors V and VIII**, both prothrombin time and APTT are prolonged.

Presence of **F VIII inhibitors** can be excluded by mixing experiment, i.e. APTT is repeated using mixture of patient's and normal plasma.

In **disseminated intravascular coagulation**, clinical features are usually dominated by the underlying disease and investigations reveal multiple coagulation abnormalities and thrombocytopaenia.

Clinically F VIII deficiency (haemophilia A) and **F IX deficiency (haemophilia B)** are indistinguishable. Distinction between them is critical as treatment of the two conditions is different. Thromboplastin generation test and specific factor assays allow one to make the correct diagnosis.

Differences between haemophilia A, haemophilia B, and von Willebrand disease are shown in Table 16.2.

Therapy of Haemophilia A

Therapeutic Agents

F VIII concentrate, cryoprecipitate, and desmopressin (DDAVP) are the three therapeutic options in haemophilia A.

Table 16.2: Comparison of haemophilia A, haemophilia B, and von Willebrand disease

Parameter	Haemophilia A	Haemophilia B	von Willebrand disease
1. Prevalence in general population	1:10,000	1:30,000	1:100
2. Pathogenesis	F VIII deficiency	F IX deficiency	Deficiency or qualitative abnormality of vWF
3. Inheritance	X-linked recessive	X-linked recessive	Autosomal dominant
4. Function of deficient factor	Cofactor; enhances conversion of F X to F Xa	Enzyme; conversion of F X to F Xa	Adhesion of platelets to subendothelium, carrier of factor VIII
5. Nature of bleeding	Deep tissues	Deep tissues	Superficial ± Deep
6. Abnormal screening tests	APTT	APTT	APTT, bleeding time
7. Diagnosis	F VIII assay	F IX assay	Ristocetin-induced platelet aggregation
8. Treatment	Cryoprecipitate, F VIII concentrate, desmopressin	F IX concentrate, prothrombin complex concentrate	Desmopressin, vWF concentrate

Factor VIII concentrate: They are of two types—plasma-derived and recombinant. Plasma-derived F VIII concentrate is derived by fractionation of pooled plasma obtained from multiple donors. It is available in the form of freeze-dried powder in vials labeled with the F V III content. It is reconstituted by the addition of a diluent and administered intravenously. F VIII concentrates are sterilised by heating or solvent detergent treatment by their manufacturers to inactivate viruses. As compared to cryoprecipitate, F VIII concentrate is stable when stored at 4°C and is relatively easy to administer. Its major drawback is high cost. Double inactivation procedures are nowadays employed to improve the safety. A purification process employing monoclonal antibodies against F VIII can now prepare highly purified F VIII concentrates.

Recombinant F VIII concentrates prepared by genetic engineering technology have recently been introduced and are found to be as effective as plasma-derived F VIII concentrates. They have the advantages of being free from infectious agents and a potential of large-scale production.

Cryoprecipitate: Preparation of cryoprecipitate: Plasma is separated from whole blood within 6 hours of collection of blood. Individual bags of freshly separated plasma are frozen at –70°C and then thawed at 4°C. A mixture of plasma and a flocculent precipitate is obtained which is then centrifuged. Most of the supernatant plasma is removed leaving behind sediment of cryoprecipitate and residual 10 to 15 ml of plasma. When stored at –25°C or lower, cryoprecipitate remains stable for 1 year. Before infusion required number of bags of cryoprecipitate are thawed at 37°C, and pooled together.

The cryoprecipitate has high content of F VIII:C, von Willebrand factor, fibrinogen, and fibronectin and also contains some amount of F XIII. On average, each bag of cryoprecipitate should have 80 units of F VIII:C.

As compared to F VIII concentrate, cryoprecipitate has low cost and is prepared from relatively few donors. However, cryoprecipitate is suitable mostly for hospitalised patients and cannot be used for treatment in home settings; in addition, viral attenuation of cryoprecipitate is difficult and F VIII content is variable from bag to bag. Haemolysis of recipient's red cells can occur due to the presence of anti-A or anti-B. Due to the availability of simpler and safer alternatives, cryoprecipitate is no longer used at major centres.

Desmopressin (DDAVP): This drug increases levels of F VIII and von Willebrand factor in plasma by stimulating their release from endothelial cells and platelets. Desmopressin is helpful in mild and moderate haemophilia but not in severe cases.

Management

Bleeding episodes in haemophilia A are treated by F VIII replacement therapy. The aim is attainment of a critical level of F VIII in the body sufficient to arrest the bleeding. Administration of one unit per kg body weight of F VIII raises plasma level by 2 units/dl. The approximate minimum desired F VIII levels required to control bleeding are- (i) Mild bleeding: 30% (0.3 units/ml), (ii) Serious or major bleeding: 50% (0.5 units/ml) and (iii) Major Surgery: 80–100% (0.8 units/ml). A formula for calculating units of F VIII to be infused to achieve the desired rise is as follows:

Units of F VIII to be administered = required rise in % units × weight in kg/2
Where,
Required rise in units/ml =
Required level of F VIII in patient's plasma in units/ml – Actual F VIII level before infusion;

To maintain the desired levels repeated doses are necessary as half-life of F VIII is about 8 to 12 hours. Severity of bleeding decides the duration of therapy.

Aside from treatment of bleeding episodes, another form of therapy in haemophilia A is prophylactic therapy. In this form of treatment, F VIII is regularly and periodically administered (every 2–3 days) to maintain the concentration of F VIII greater than 1% that prevents serious, and spontaneous haemorrhages, i.e. a severe disease is converted to a moderate disease. This form of therapy has been shown to significantly reduce the joint disease. However, prophylactic therapy is not commonly employed due to the high cost and limited supply of F VIII concentrates.

Antifibrinolytic agents such as epsilon-aminocaproic acid and tranexamic acid inhibit fibrinolysis and are used to prevent or treat oral haemorrhages (such as following dental extractions). (Saliva contains high concentration of fibrinolytic enzymes). Antiplatelet drugs (such as aspirin) and intramuscular injections should be avoided. Precautions should be observed to prevent injuries especially in children.

Complications of Replacement Therapy

Inhibitor antibodies against F VIII: Antibodies against F VIII develop in about 10 to 15% of patients with severe haemophilia who have received multiple transfusions. These antibodies may inactivate infused F VIII with patient becoming resistant to replacement therapy. There are two types of inhibitors–one type shows rise to a low titre while the other type shows anamnestic response to a high titre after administration of F VIII. Inhibitors are usually quantitated by Bethesda method. One Bethesda unit is the quantity of inhibitor that leaves 50% of residual F VIII when the mixture of patient's and normal pooled plasma is incubated at 37°C for 2 hours. Low titre inhibitors are usually treated by high doses of F VIII concentrates. Treatment of high titer inhibitors is difficult; products available to manage bleeding in these patients are prothrombin complex concentrates, porcine F VIII concentrates, and F VIIa. (Also see chapter on "Acquired inhibitors of coagulation").

Transmission of viral infections: Earlier generations of FVIII concentrates were associated with a significant risk of transmission of hepatitis B and C viruses (HBV and HCV) and human immunodeficiency virus (HIV). Before introduction of HIV screening tests for donor units and viral inactivation procedures for F VIII concentrates, about 60% of haemophilic patients got infected with HIV-1. Majority of these patients also were found to have developed antibodies to HCV. HBV and HCV infections carry the risk of chronic liver disease, cirrhosis, and hepatocellular carcinoma. Donor screening and viral inactivation procedures of F VIII concentrates (heat and solvent detergent treatment) have markedly reduced the risk of transmission of these agents. All newly diagnosed patients should receive HBV and HAV vaccines (if not immune).

Molecular Genetics of Haemophilia A

Genetic Defects in Haemophilia A

As in thalassemias, genetic defects in haemophilia A are diverse (Box 16.3). Recently **inversion in F VIII gene at intron 22** has been found to be responsible for 40 to 50% cases of severe haemophilia. The other common molecular lesions in haemophilia are deletions and point mutations. Majority of mild or moderate haemophilia are due to missense or frameshift mutations or deletions in F VIII gene. Majority of severe haemophilia are due to inversions (intron 22 or 1) in F VIII gene. Mechanism of inversion of intron 22 is shown in Figure 16.2. **Deletions** may involve some part or

Box 16.3	Genetic abnormalities in haemophilia A

- Inversions: Intron 22 inversion, Intron 1 inversion
- Point mutations: Missense mutation, nonsense mutation, frameshift mutation
- Deletion of part or whole of gene
- Insertion of repetitive sequences
- Splicing errors affecting production of mRNA

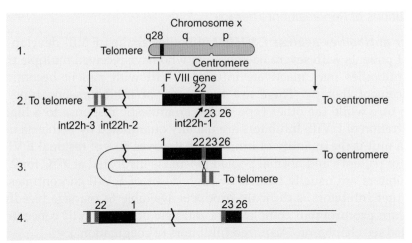

Figure 16.2: Mechanism of inversion of intron 22 leading to splitting of F VIII gene and severe haemophilia A. (1) Location of F VIII gene on Xq28 towards telomere. (2) Expanded region showing F VIII gene (black) and the homologous repeats (red) which are referred to as int22h-1, int22h-2, and int22h-3. (3) During meiosis in males, looping around of X chromosome occurs and homologous recombination can occur between two copies of int22h since the sequences are almost identical. (4) As a result of intrachromosomal recombination, 22 exons from 5' end of F VIII gene are moved to the telomeric end of X chromosome, while exons 23 to 26 from 3' end remain at the original position. This causes disruption of F VIII gene into two parts that cannot encode F VIII protein and severe haemophilia results

whole of the F VIII gene and are often associated with severe haemophilia. It has been suggested that haemophilic patients with large deletions, nonsense mutations, or intron 22 inversions are more likely to develop F VIII inhibitors than those with other molecular defects. Missense mutation (mutation which leads to the formation of a different amino acid) or small deletions have low risk of forming inhibitors. But these associations are not consistent. Some **point mutations** cause formation of a stop codon with premature termination of F VIII translation (nonsense mutation) and synthesis of a short non-functional protein; others lead to the formation of a complete but dysfunctional F VIII molecule due to single amino acid substitution. Recently, **insertion** of nonviral nucleotide sequences in F VIII gene has been described. Genetic defects have not been identified in a significant proportion of haemophilia A pedigrees. The molecular lesions in haemophilia A are constant in a given kindred.

Detection of Carriers

All the daughters of a haemophilic father are obligate carriers as they receive their father's defective X chromosome. Carrier state is also established in a female if she has a diseased son and a diseased relative or if she has more than one diseased son. In approximately 30% of cases, family history is negative as spontaneous mutation during gametogenesis is responsible for haemophilic state. Family history will also be negative if haemophilia has been silent in previous generations there being no male offsprings. Carrier testing may be done if carrier status of a female cannot be ascertained on the basis of family history alone. Documentation of carrier status of a woman provides the carrier and her spouse with options such as prenatal diagnosis or sterilisation.

There are two basic methods of carrier detection—phenotypic and genotypic.

Phenotypic Methods

Factor VIII: C assay: Normal level of F VIII:C in plasma is 50 to 150%. In female carriers F VIII:C levels are expected to be around half the normal, i.e. 50%. This is because during the process of lyonization half of the normal and half of the abnormal X chromosomes would be inactivated by random chance. However, as lyonisation is unpredictable, considerable overlap can occur between values obtained in normal and carrier females. Although the carrier state is suggested when F VIII:C level is 50% of normal or less, it cannot be ruled out even if F VIII:C levels are higher.

Determination of F VIII:C and vWF:Ag: Normally levels of vWF:Ag closely correlate with levels of F VIII:C. In carriers vWF:Ag levels are normal or slightly increased while F VIII:C levels are comparably less resulting in reduction of F VIII:C/vWF:Ag ratio. (F VIII: C/ vWF: Ag ratio less than 1 .0).

As F VIII:C levels may be normal in carriers (due to the process of random lyonisation) about 10 to 20% of carriers remain undetected by this method.

Genotypic Methods

A definitive method of establishing the carrier state is genotypic analysis. There are two methods—direct and indirect.

Direct methods: Identification of a specific defect in the F VIII gene may be accomplished by restriction enzyme analysis or by oligonucleotide probes. This analysis is suitable when the genetic abnormality in the affected kindred is known.

a. *Restriction endonuclease analysis:* When the point mutation in the F VIII gene alters (i.e. creates or abolishes) the cutting site of a particular restriction enzyme, then this method can be applied for detection of carriers. Steps of this analysis are - 1. DNA is isolated from leucocytes and separated into fragments by a restriction enzyme; 2. Fragments of DNA are separated by gel electrophoresis according to their size and then blotted on to the nitrocellulose membrane; 3. The fragments are hybridised with radioactive DNA probes followed by autoradiography. If cutting site of the restriction enzyme is altered due to a point mutation, then a fragment of a different size is produced.

Alternatively, polymerase chain reaction (PCR) can be used to amplify DNA followed by digestion of DNA by restriction enzyme. As DNA is amplified, digest can be analysed by direct inspection of the electrophoretically separated DNA fragments.

b. *Oligonucleotide probe analysis:* Desired normal and abnormal oligonudeotide probes are synthesised chemically and are radiolabelled. DNA isolated from leucocytes is digested by restriction enzyme and fragment to be analysed is separated by electrophoresis. Hybridisation is carried out with the labelled oligonucleotide probes followed by autoradiography. The normal and abnormal (mutant) probes hybridise with normal and mutant sequences respectively.

Indirect method: If the genetic defect in the affected family is unknown, then the indirect method, i.e. restriction fragment length polymorphism (RFLP) can be employed. Although the coding regions of the gene (exons) are highly conserved, DNA sequence variations can occur in the noncoding extragenic regions as well as in introns. These DNA sequence variations frequently alter the recognition site of a particular restriction enzyme resulting in formation of fragments of different sizes. The polymorphic restriction enzyme site, if linked closely to the abnormal gene and co-segregates in affected families, can be used as a genetic marker of the disease in the particular family. Key family members should be heterozygous for the polymorphism. Sources of error in RFLP analysis are recombination or crossing-over of genetic material during meiosis and non-paternity.

Three restriction enzymes, BcI, Bgl I, or Xba I are used for RFLP analysis. Although Southern blot analysis can be used, polymerase chain reaction technology is a rapid method that requires no radioactive gene probes. In the PCR-based method, the segment of DNA, which contains the restriction enzyme polymorphism, is amplified and then digested with the restriction enzyme. This is followed by agarose gel electrophoresis, ethidium bromide staining, and visualisation of fragments by ultraviolet fluorescence. If the cutting site of the restriction enzyme is altered, then a fragment of a different size is obtained. Presence or absence of a restriction site is used as a marker for tracking the haemophilia gene in pedigree analysis (Fig. 16.3).

Tests for detection of genetic abnormalities are shown in Box 16.4.

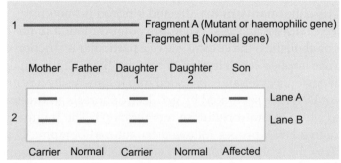

Figure 16.3: Analysis of haemophilia A pedigree. 1: Restriction enzyme digestion produces DNA fragments of different size in mutant and normal genes. 2: DNA is separated by electrophoresis and hybridised with labelled probe. Here, fragment A (larger) is linked with haemophilia A gene while fragment B (shorter) is linked with normal gene. Thus, status of family members can be ascertained

> **Box 16.4** Tests for detection of genetic abnormalities in haemophilia A
>
> Direct DNA testing
> - Southern blot analysis: Detection of intron 22 and intron 1 inversion
> - Amplification of regions of F VIII gene by polymerase chain reaction followed by agarose gel electrophoresis: Detection of insertions or deletions in F VIII gene
> - Single-stranded conformational polymorphism (SSCP) analysis: Detection of point mutations
>
> Indirect DNA testing
> - Linkage analysis for detection of restriction fragment length polymorphisms, if exact genetic defect has not been identified (for tracking defective gene in family members).

Prenatal Diagnosis

Prenatal diagnosis determines whether the foetus of female carrier is affected and thus offers the option of termination of pregnancy. Two methods of prenatal diagnosis are available—foetal blood sampling and genotypic analysis.

Foetal sex is determined by amniocentesis around 14 to 15 weeks of gestation. Foetal blood is obtained at 18 to 20 weeks by foetoscopy. Level of F VIII:CAg is determined by immunoradiometric assay which is capable of detecting minute amounts. F VIII:CAg is undetectable in haemophilia A. However, this assay is not suitable in kindreds with positive cross-reacting material in plasma.

For genotypic analysis, foetal DNA can be obtained either by amniocentesis (14–15 weeks) or by chorionic villus biopsy (9–12 weeks). Various methods of genetic analysis are outlined under "Detection of carriers".

Prenatal diagnosis by genetic analysis using chorion villus sampling is possible in the first trimester while foetal blood sampling can be applied only in the second trimester. Therefore genotypic analysis has the advantage of earlier (and thus safer) termination of pregnancy if required.

Preimplantation Diagnosis

Although prenatal diagnosis can avoid the birth of an affected child, it is traumatic for the parents due to the uncertainty involved during each pregnancy and the prospect of abortion of every affected foetus. Preimplantation diagnosis offers the genetic diagnosis in preimplantation embryos and thus eliminates the problem of termination of pregnancy. The advent of polymerase chain reaction and *in vitro* fertilisation techniques has made preimplantation diagnosis feasible. In this technique, a single cell is removed from the embryo (6–10 cell stage) following *in vitro* fertilisation and its DNA is amplified using polymerase chain reaction. Techniques for detection of mutation are applied on the amplified DNA. The unaffected embryo is implanted into the uterus. Preimplantation diagnosis has been applied to haemophilia A, β thalassaemia, sickle-cell anaemia, cystic fibrosis, Lesch-Nyhan syndrome, Tay-Sachs disease, and some other monogenic diseases.

Non-invasive Prenatal Diagnosis

It is known that foetal cells (such as erythroblasts and lymphocytes) are present in maternal circulation during pregnancy. These foetal cells though small in number, can be isolated from maternal blood by a method utilising antigenic differences between foetal and maternal cells. DNA is extracted from these foetal cells and analysed by a sensitive technique (polymerase chain reaction). If a mutation is detected, then it can be confirmed by doing chorionic villus biopsy in early pregnancy. The technique, at present, is in investigational stage.

❑ VON WILLEBRAND DISEASE

von Willebrand factor (vWF) is synthesised by endothelial cells and megakaryocytes. The vWF gene is located on chromosome 12. The basic mature vWF molecule is a monomer composed of 2050 amino acids. vWF monomers associate with each other through disulphide bonds to form multimers of varying sizes. The large multimers of vWF are more effective in haemostasis as they have greater binding sites for mediating adhesion of platelets to subendothelium.

Most of the vWF is synthesised by endothelial cells from where they are secreted constitutively or are stored in Weibel-Palade bodies for later secretion. In megakaryocytes vWF is stored in α granules and is secreted when platelets are activated. Soon after their secretion into the blood, vWF multimers are cleaved by the metalloprotease ADAMTS13 (A Disintegrin And Metalloprotease with Thrombospondin type 1 motif 13). ADAMTS13 cleaves a site within the A2 domain of vWF. In thromboctic thrombocytopaenic purpura, degradation of large vWF multimers does not occur due to deficiency of ADAMTS13. Structure of vWF is shown in Figure 16.4. In plasma, vWF and F VIII circulate as a non-covalently bound complex (Fig. 16.5).

Functions of vWF: There are two major functions of vWF in haemostasis–(i) vWF mediates adhesion of platelets to subendothelium by binding to platelet glycoprotein

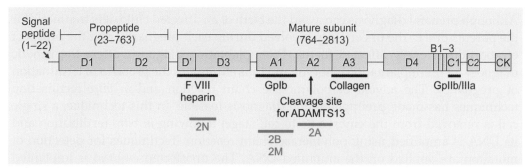

Figure 16.4: Structure of von Willebrand factor. The vWF precursor consists of a signal peptide (amino acids 1–22), propeptide (amino acids 23–763), and mature vWF subunit (amino acids 764–2813). Various domains, binding sites for F VIII, heparin, GpIb, collagen, and GpIIb/IIIa, and cleavage site for ADAMTS-13 are shown. Mutations causing type 2 VWD are mainly located within specific domains: type 2A within A2; types 2B and 2M within A1; and 2N within D' and D3 domains

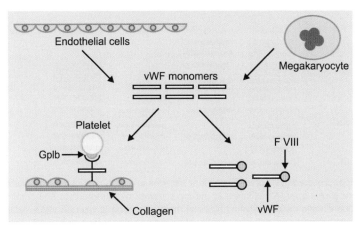

Figure 16.5: Synthesis and functions of von Willebrand factor. Endothelial cells and megakaryocytes synthesise vWF. Main functions of vWF are mediation of adhesion of platelets to subendothelial collagen and carriage of F VIII in circulation.

receptor Gp Ib (and also to Gp IIb/IIIa when platelets are activated) and subendothelium; and (ii) vWF forms a noncovalent complex with F VIII in circulation and serves to prevent the degradation and rapid removal of F VIII from circulation.

The multimeric vWF consists of different functional domains, which bind F VIII, Gp Ib, Gp IIb/IIIa, and collagen.

von Willebrand disease is a markedly heterogeneous congenital bleeding disorder characterised by deficiency or functional defect of vWF. von Willebrand disease is the most common congenital bleeding disorder with overall prevalence in the general population being 1%.

Terminology related to vWF and F VIII is given earlier in Chapter 1 "Overview of physiology of blood."

Classification

vWD is classified according to the criteria developed by The Working Party on von Willebrand Disease Classification (International Society on Thrombosis and Haemostasis, 1994 and 2006). (Table 16.3).

Type 1 vWD (classical vWD)

  i. There is a mild to moderate quantitative deficiency of all types of vWF multimers (i.e. small, intermediate and large); relative proportion of multimers is normal (Fig. 16.6).
 ii. This is the most common type of vWD accounting for 70% of all cases; bleeding manifestations are mild to moderate. Mode of inheritance is autosomal dominant.
iii. There is a corresponding reduction of vWF:Ag, vWF: RCo, and F VIII:C.

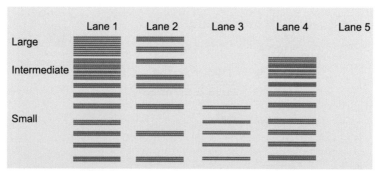

Figure 16.6: Electrophoretic analysis of vWF multimer patterns in different types of von Willebrand disease. lane 1: Normal multimers showing large multimers at the top followed by intermediate and small multimers; lane 2: type 1 vWD: Mild quantitative deficiency of all types of multimers; lane 3: type 2A vWD: deficiency of large and intermediate sized multimers along with abnormality of multimer pattern; lane 4: type 2B: selective loss of large vWF multimers; lane 5:type 3 vWD: complete deficiency of all types of vWF multimers

Table 16.3: Classification of von Willebrand disease

Parameter	Type 1	Type 2A	Type 2B	Type 2M	Type 2N	Type 3
1. Frequence of all vWDs	75–80%	~15%	~5%	Uncommon	Uncommon	Rare
2. Inheritance	AD	AD	AD	AD, AR	AR	AR
3. Bleeding	Mild	Mild to moderate	Mild to moderate	Mild to moderate	Mild to moderate	Severe
4. vWF:Ag	↓	↓ or N	↓ or N	↓ or N	↓ or N	Absent
5. vWF:RCo	↓	↓	↓	↓	↓ or N	Absent
6. F VIII	↓ or N	↓ or N	↓ or N	↓ or N	↓↓	↓↓↓
7. RIPA	N	↓	N	↓	N	Absent
8. LD-RIPA	Absent	Absent	↑↑↑	Absent	Absent	Absent
9. vWF multimer analysis	Mild ↓ of all multimers	Mild to moderate ↓ of intermediate and large multimers	Loss of large multimers + qualitative defect	Normal	Normal	Absence of all types of multimers

Abbreviations: ↓, ↓↓, ↓↓↓: Relative decrease; ↑↑↑: Markedly increased; N: Normal; AD: Autosomal dominant; AR: Autosomal recessive; vWF:Ag: vWF antigen; vWF:RCo: vWF ristocetin cofactor activity; RIPA: Ristocetin-induced platelet aggregation; LD-RIPA: Low dose ristocetin induced platelet aggregation

Type 2 vWD (variant vWD)

In type 2 vWD there is a qualitative abnormality of vWF with absence of large vWF multimers. Laboratory subclassification of type 2 vWD is based on multimeric analysis by electrophoresis (Fig. 16.6).

Type 2A:
  i. Deficiency of large and intermediate-size vWF multimers is due either to defective secretion into plasma or increased proteolysis of large vWF multimers after synthesis and secretion.

ii. Type II A comprises about 15% of all cases of vWD. Mode of inheritance is autosomal dominant and bleeding is mild to moderate.

iii. There is variable reduction in vWF:Ag, vWF:RCo, and F VIII:C

Type 2B:

i. Large vWF multimers have inappropriately increased affinity to bind to platelets; the abnormality resides in the GpIb-binding domain of vWF. This causes clearance from circulation of large vWF multimers along with platelets (to which they are bound) from circulation; this leads to reduction in their levels in plasma and mild thrombocytopaenia. Quantity of vWF multimers in platelets is normal.

ii. This is an uncommon type of vWD with autosomal dominant mode of inheritance and mild to moderate bleeding tendency.

iii. Laboratory abnormalities include variable reduction in vWF:Ag, vWF:RCo, and F VIII:C; increased responsiveness to small concentration of ristocetin in platelet aggregation studies, and mild thrombocytopaenia.

Type 2M:

i. There is reduced vWF-dependent platelet adhesion without selective deficiency of high molecular weight vWF multimers.

ii. Screening test results are similar in type 2M and type 2A vWD; distinction depends on multimer analysis.

Type 3

i. There is a severe quantitative deficiency of all forms of vWF multimers.

ii. This is a rare but severe bleeding disorder with autosomal recessive inheritance.

iii. vWF:Ag, vWF:RCo, and F VIII:C are markedly diminished.

Platelet-type vWD (Pseudo vWD):

i. There is an abnormal avidity of platelet membrane glycoprotein Gp Ib-IX complex to bind large vWF multimers leading to reduced levels of vWF multimers in plasma.

ii. This is a rare, mild to moderate bleeding disorder with autosomal dominant inheritance.

iii. Laboratory features are similar to type IIB vWD. Addition of cryoprecipitate (rich in vWF) to patient's platelet-rich plasma induces aggregation in platelet-type but not in type IIB vWD.

Type 2N:

i. There is a markedly reduced vWF binding affinity for F VIII due to a defect in the F VIII-binding domain of vWF.

ii. F VIII:C levels in plasma are reduced. The disease is called as autosomal haemophilia due to its resemblance to haemophilia A of mild to moderate type.

Clinical Features of vWD

vWD types 1, 2A, and 2B are inherited in an autosomal dominant manner. Bleeding manifestations in these patients are mild to moderate and superficial in type, i.e.

petechiae, ecchymoses, epistaxis, bleeding from gums and gastrointestinal tract, and menorrhagia. There is a marked heterogeneity in frequency, nature, and severity of bleeding. Often many patients are asymptomatic and come to attention because of abnormal bleeding time during a routine pre-operative coagulation screen or because of excessive post-traumatic bleeding.

Type 3 vWD is a severe autosomal recessive disorder with onset in early childhood. Bleeding manifestations are related to defective primary as well as secondary haemostasis such as mucocutaneous bleeding, deep haematomas, and haemarthroses.

Laboratory Features

The typical diagnostic features of von Willebrand disease are prolonged bleeding time, reduction (or qualitative abnormality) of vWF:Ag, and decrease in vWF:RCo, and F VIII:C levels.

However, there is a marked variability in the results of laboratory tests both among different individuals and in the same individual. The results of laboratory studies are influenced by many variables. Persons with blood group O have lower vWF values as compared to those with other blood groups. Higher vWF levels are obtained in older age, inflammatory states, pregnancy, physical exertion, and when oestrogen levels are raised. Mild and heterogeneous clinical nature of the disorder and non-availability of a specific and sensitive test for diagnosis further add to the difficulty. Frequently, repeated testing is required to unequivocally establish the diagnosis.

Bleeding time is prolonged in vWD, particularty in types 2 and 3. In type 1 vWD, a single bleeding time measurement may be normal and repeated testing is frequently necessary. Although platelet count is normal in most patients, it is slightly low in type 2B and platelet type vWD. Activated partial thromboplastin time (APTT) may be prolonged secondary to decreased F VIII:C levels in plasma (5–40%). In mild F VIII:C deficiency, APTT may be normal. Therefore, F VIII:C assay is required to definitively establish the deficiency.

vWF:Ag is commonly measured by Laurell rocket immunoelectrophoresis method. In this technique, antibody to vWF is incorporated into the agarose gel on a glass slide and patient's sample to be quantitated for vWF:Ag is placed in a well. After electrophoresis, immunoprecipitation develops in the form of rockets the length of which is proportional to the quantity of the antigen. The lower limit of normal for vWF:Ag is about 50%. In type 1 vWD, vWF:Ag is 20 to 50% while in type 2 it is markedly reduced or absent. Other quantitative techniques for vWF are radioimmunoassay and enzyme-linked immunosorbent assay.

The ristocetin-induced platelet aggregation (RIPA) is a commonly employed qualitative test for detection of von Willebrand disease. In this test ristocetin (1 mg/ml) is added to patient's platelet-rich plasma and aggregation response is observed. In vWD, RIPA is deficient, as it requires the presence of vWF-related ristocetin cofactor activity. In mild cases, however, this test may be normal; also it is not specific for vWD as positive test is also obtained in Bernard-Soulier syndrome and certain other

Table 16.4: Laboratory tests in von Willebrand disease

Initial tests

1. vWF:Ag (Laurell rocket immunoelectrophoresis, ELISA): Measures concentration of vWF protein in plasma

2. vWF:RCo (ELISA): Functional assay that measures binding of vWF (patient's plasma) to normal platelets in the presence of ristocetin

3. F VIII assay (one-stage assay based on APTT): Measures concentration of F VIII in plasma (In vWD, it assesses the ability of vWF to maintain F VIII in circulation)

Further tests

4. Low-dose ristocetin-induced platelet aggregation (platelet aggreagation with <0.6 mg/ml ristocetin): Measures aggregation response when patient's plasma is mixed with normal platelet-rich plasma and ristocetin

5. vWF multimer analysis (SDS electrophoresis): Assesses distribution of different vWF multimers

conditions. In type 2B and platelet-type vWD, enhanced responsiveness to small concentration of ristocetin (0.5mg/ml) is noted.

In the assay for ristocetin cofactor (RCoF) activity, ristocetin, formalinised normal platelets and patient's plasma are mixed and extent of aggregation is determined. Ristocetin facilitates binding of vWF to GpIb on platelets causing their agglutination. This test quantitates ability of the patient's vWF to bind to platelets (GpIb) and cause aggregation. Degree of agglutination is proportional to the amount of vWF. vWF:RCo is decreased in vWD.

In mild cases of vWD, bleeding time and APTT may be normal and assay for ristocetin cofactor activity inconclusive. Since many variables affect the laboratory results, repeated testing may be needed to establish the diagnosis.

vWF multimer analysis is done by sodium dodecyl sulphate-agarose gel electro-phoresis. Normally, small, intermediate, and large multimers are present. Type 1 vWD shows mild to moderate decrease in all types of multimers, type 2 has deficiency of large vWF multimers while in type 3, severe deficiency of all multimer types is observed. Subclassification of type 2 vWD is based on this technique (Fig. 16.6).

Laboratory tests in vWD are shown in Table 16.4.

Acquired von Willebrand disease: vWD can occur in various acquired disorders such as hypothyroidism, congenital heart disease, autoimmune diseases, lympho-proliferative disorders, monoclonal gammopathies, myeloproliferative disorders, and Wilms tumour. The underlying pathogenic mechanism may be autoantibodies directed against high molecular weight multimers of vWF, increased degradation of high molecular weight multimers by enzymes, or adsorption of vWF by tumour cells.

Treatment of vWD

For mild mucous membrane bleeding, antifibrinolytic agents tranexamic acid or ε-aminocaproic acid can be used. For significant bleeding, two treatment options in vWD are desmopressin and plasma-derived F VIII concentrate rich in high molecular weight multimers or cryoprecipitate. Desmopressin or 1-deamino-(8-D-arginine)-vasopressin (DDAVP), a synthetic vasopressin analogue, is the treatment of choice in type 1 vWD. It can be administered intravenously or as a nasal spray. Desmopressin raises vWF and F VIII:C levels by stimulating their release from storage sites. It is not much effective in vWD types 2A and 3. Desmopressin is contraindicated in type 2B as it aggravates thrombocytopaenia.

Plasma-derived F VIII concentrate rich in vWF or cryoprecipitate is the treatment of choice in those cases not responsive to desmopressin such as type 2 variant and type 3 vWD. The former preparation is preferred as it can be virus-inactivated.

In platelet-type vWD, platelet concentrates may be tried as both desmopressin and cryoprecipitate can induce thrombocytopaenia.

❑ HAEMOPHILIA B

Haemophilia B (also known as Christmas disease, after the first patient described) is a hereditary F IX deficiency state with X-linked recessive mode of inheritance. The incidence is about 1:60,000 populations.

Clinical features and inheritance pattern are similar to haemophilia A. It is essential to distinguish between haemophilia A and B in the laboratory because of different therapeutic products required.

Coagulation profile shows selective prolongation of activated partial thromboplastin time (APTT). In mild cases APTT may be normal and in such cases if clinical features are suggestive then specific F VIII and IX assay should be performed (F VIII assay should always be performed first). Thromboplastin generation test shows serum defect as against plasma defect in F VIII deficiency. F IX assay should be done in all cases; its principle is similar to that of F VIII assay. About 1 to 2% of patients with severe hamophilia B develop inhibitor antibodies against F IX.

The therapeutic products for haemophilia B are recombinant F IX (treatment of choice), fresh frozen plasma (for mild/moderate cases) and prothrombin complex concentrate (for severe cases). As half-life of infused F IX is about 24 hours, it is administered once per day. Prothrombin complex concentrate (PCC) contains all vitamin K dependent coagulation factors, i.e. F II, VII, IX and X. However, presence of minute amounts of activated coagulation factors in PCC may trigger the coagulation cascade leading to thromboembolic phenomena. Due to this potential risk, use of prothrombin complex concentrates is restricted to severe cases and is administered along with small amount of heparin.

Various genetic defects including gene deletions and point mutations are responsible for haemophilia B. Inhibitor antibodies against F IX develop more commonly in patients with gene deletions. Carrier detection in haemophilia B follows the same general principles as outlined for haemophilia A.

In contrast to haemophilia A, most cases of haemophilia B result from point mutations.

Haemophilia B Leiden: In this form of hemophila B, F IX levels in blood increase at the time of puberty followed by resolution of bleeding manifestations. It is seen in 3% of haemophilia B patients and results from specific F IX promoter mutations.

❑ INHERITED DISORDERS OF FIBRINOGEN

Hereditary disorders of fibrinogen are of two types—(i) deficiency: afibrinogenaemia or hypofibrinogenaemia; and (ii) dysfunction: dysfibrinogenaemias.

Hereditary Afibrinogenaemia

This rare autosomal recessive disorder is characterised by almost complete absence of fibrinogen in plasma. In the neonatal period there may be bleeding from the umbilical stump; afterwards common manifestations are excessive bleeding following trivial trauma, easy bruisability and bleeding from nose and gums. Intracranial haemorrhage is a frequent cause of death. Some patients present with haemarthrosis.

Coagulation profile reveals marked prolongation of all the screening tests of coagulation such as clotting time, prothrombin time, activated partial thromboplastin time, and thrombin time. Estimation of fibrinogen (outlined in "Approach to the diagnosis of bleeding disorders") reveals total absence or trace amounts (<5 mg/dl) of fibrinogen. Platelet function abnormalities are common and include prolongation of bleeding time and defective platelet aggregation with ADP, epinephrine, and collagen.

Fibrinogen level of 50 to 100 mg/dl is usually sufficient for control of bleeding. Treatment of bleeding episodes consists of administration of fibrinogen concentrate, fresh frozen plasma or cryoprecipitate.

Hypofibrinogenaemia

In this condition fibrinogen concentration in plasma is less than 100 mg/dl. Mode of inheritance is autosomal recessive or dominant. The condition may be asymptomatic or may manifest as a mild bleeding disorder. Thrombin time is usually prolonged and quantitative estimation of fibrinogen shows reduced levels. The condition should be differentiated from acquired causes of hypofibrinogenaemia such as disseminated intravascular coagulation, liver disease, and fibrinolytic therapy.

Bleeding, if present, may be managed by cryoprecipitate or fresh frozen plasma.

Dysfibrinogenaemias

Dysfibrinogenaemias are characterised by qualitative (or functional) abnormality of the fibrinogen molecule. Functional defects in dysfibrinogenaemias are diverse. Numerous dysfunctional fibrinogen molecules have been described which impair the formation of the fibrin clot by interfering in the formation of fibrin monomers (cleavage of fibrinopeptides by thrombin), spontaneous polymerisation of fibrin monomers, or cross-linking of fibrin monomers by F XIIIa.

Patients with dysfibrinogenaemia may be asymptomatic or may have mild bleeding tendency, a predisposition to thrombosis, or poor wound healing.

Prothrombin time, thrombin time, and reptilase time are frequently prolonged while activated partial thromboplastin time is variable. Typically estimation of fibrinogen by functional or clot-based assay shows reduced quantity of fibrinogen while immunologic method shows normal levels. Bleeding tendencies respond to cryoprecipitate.

ACQUIRED DISORDERS OF COAGULATION

Acquired disorders are more common than hereditary disorders of coagulation. They are usually secondary to some underlying disease and are frequently associated with multiple haemostatic defects. Some acquired coagulation disorders are presented in Table 16.5.

❑ VITAMIN K DEFICIENCY

Vitamin K is a fat-soluble vitamin that is absorbed in the proximal small intestine in the presence of bile salts. Green leafy vegetables are a good source of vitamin K. It is also synthesised by bacterial flora in the large intestine. It is stored in small amounts in the liver.

Vitamin K is required for gamma carboxylation of glutamic acid residues of four vitamin K-dependent factors II, VII, IX and X (Fig. 16.11). This post-translational modification is essential for binding of these coagulation factors to phospholipid in the presence of calcium. In the absence of vitamin K gamma carboxylation fails to occur and non-functional forms of vitamin K-dependent factors circulate in blood. These are called as acarboxy forms or PIVKAs (proteins induced by vitamin K absence or antagonism). Vitamin K is also necessary for gamma carboxylation of two natural anticoagulant proteins C and S.

Causes of vitamin K deficiency are haemorrhagic disease of newborn, poor dietary intake, impaired absorption due to obstructive jaundice or malabsorption syndromes, and drugs such as oral anticoagulants and broad-spectrum antibiotics.

Haemorrhagic Disease of the Newborn

In the normal newborn, levels of vitamin K-dependent clotting factors are depressed and show a further fall at 2 to 3 days of life. In premature infants levels are even lower. After a few days the levels gradually begin to rise. Vitamin K deficiency exaggerates the fall of these coagulation factors and causes bleeding.

Table 16.5: Acquired coagulation disorders

1. Disseminated intravascular coagulation	2. Liver disease
3. Vitamin K deficiency	4. Acquired inhibitors of coagulation
5. Heparin, oral anticoagulation, thrombolytic therapy	6. Renal disease
7. Paraproteinaemias	8. Cardiopulmonary bypass
9. Massive transfusion of stored blood	

Three forms of haemorrhagic disease of newborn are distinguished–early, classic, and late (Table 16.6). Early type is associated with maternal ingestion of oral anticoagulants or phenytoin and bleeding manifests at birth. Classic haemorrhagic disease of newborn typically occurs in exclusively breast-fed infants (breast milk is a poor source of vitamin K) and bleeding usually manifests at 2 to 3 days of life. Late type develops usually after 1 month and is associated with underlying disorder such as malabsorption or biliary atresia.

F VII falls quickly due to its short half-life leading to prolongation of prothrombin time. As factors IX and X subsequently decline, prolongation of activated partial thromboplastin time also occurs.

It is recommended that all neonates be administered prophylactic 0.5 to 1 mg of vitamin K at birth to prevent haemorrhagic disease of newborn. Treatment consists of parenteral vitamin K supplementation. If bleeding is severe and life-threatening, fresh frozen plasma may be administered.

❏ LIVER DISEASE (CIRRHOSIS OF LIVER)

The liver has a major role in haemostasis (Table 16.7). Because of this, chronic liver disease often produces complex coagulation abnormalities.

Causes of bleeding in liver disease (cirrhosis) include—(i) Oesophageal varices (secondary to portal hypertension) and peptic ulcer; (ii) Thrombocytopaenia (due to splenomegaly secondary to portal hypertension); (iii) Deficient synthesis of coagulation factors; (iv) Deficient utilisation of vitamin K; (v) Synthesis of dysfunctional fibrinogens (dysfibrinogenaemia) which leads to defective fibrin polymerisation; (vi) Defective platelet function due to raised FDPs; (vii) Disseminated intravascular

Table 16.6: Haemorrhagic disease of newborn

Parameter	Early	Classic	Late
1. Time of bleeding after birth	Within 24 hours	2–7 days	After 7 days to few months
2. Contributory factors	Maternal ingestion of anticonvulsants, oral anticoagulants, anti-TB drugs	Exclusive breast-feeding, low placental transfer of vitamin K, sterile gut	Malabsorption , chronic diarrhoea, prolonged breast-feeding with no supplementation, antibiotics
3. Nature of bleeding	Severe	Bruising, bleeding from GIT, umbilical stump or post-circumcision	Intracranial bleeding common

Table 16.7: Role of liver in haemostasis

1. Synthesis of proteins
   - Coagulation system—Factors I, II, V, VII, VIII, IX, X, XI, XII, XIII, prekallikrein, high molecular weight kininogen
   - Natural anticoagulants—Antithrombin III, protein C, protein S
   - Fibrinolytic system—Plasminogen, $\alpha 2$ antiplasmin
2. Utilisation of vitamin K for synthesis of vitamin K-dependent proteins (vitamin K is required for post-translational gammacarboxylation of Factors II, VII, IX, and X and proteins C and S).
3. Clearance of activated coagulation factors and plasminogen activators by reticuloendothelial cells of liver.

coagulation (DIC) due to inefficient clearance of activated coagulation factors and decreased synthesis of coagulation inhibitors-antithrombin III and protein C; and (viii) Increased fibrinogenolysis due to deficient clearance of plasminogen activators and α2-antiplasmin.

Laboratory abnormalities include prolongation of prothrombin time, activated partial thromboplastin time, and thrombin time (due to reduced synthesis of coagulation factors and production of dysfunctional fibrinogen). F VII, a vitamin K-dependent factor is the earliest to fall owing to its short half-life. Protein C, an anticoagulant also falls along with F VII. This is followed by decrease in the level of other coagulation factors. F VIII: C and von Willebrand factor levels are normal.

In advanced disease, fibrinolytic activity is increased leading to increase in the level of FDPs. Thrombocytopaenia due to splenomegaly, and platelet dysfunction due to inhibitory action of FDPs are also noted. Laboratory abnormalities in DIC in liver disease include reduction of F VIII:C, increased D-dimer, and raised thrombin-antithrombin complexes.

Therapy is given if bleeding especially from gastrointestinal tract is present and as a cover if surgery/biopsy is being considered. Various modes of therapy for haemostatic correction are–(i) Fresh frozen plasma - This provides all the coagulation factors. However, treatment of haemostatic defect needs large amounts of FFP, which can cause circulatory overload. (ii) Prothrombin complex concentrates - They supply vitamin K-dependent factors. They contain activated coagulation factors and thus may initiate DIC. (iii) Fibrinolytic inhibitors may be used if fibrinolysis is the major cause of bleeding and there is no DIC. Due to the risk of DIC, these agents have a limited role. (iv) Vitamin K is useful in liver disease with obstructive element.

❑ DISSEMINATED INTRAVASCULAR COAGULATION

Synonyms- Defibrination syndrome, Consumptive coagulopathy
Disseminated intravascular coagulation (DIC) is an acquired disorder occurring in a wide spectrum of underlying diseases and characterised by (i) Widespread systemic activation of coagulation with formation of microthrombi in small blood vessels and (ii) Bleeding diathesis secondary to depletion of coagulation factors and platelets (Fig. 16.7).

Aetiology

Important causes of DIC are listed in Table 16.8. Mechanisms initiating DIC in these conditions are as follows:
- **Sepsis and severe infections:** Membrane components of micro-organisms, such as lipopolysaccharides and endotoxins, or release of bacterial exotoxins cause release of inflammatory cytokines from mononuclear cells and endothelial cells.
- **Severe trauma:** Release of fat and phospholipids from damaged tissue, haemolysis, and endothelial damage cause systemic activation of coagulation. In patients with

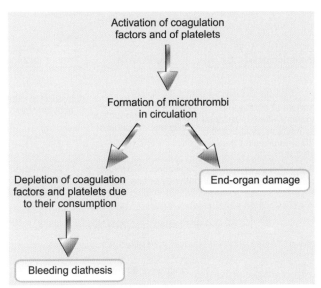

Figure 16.7: General mechanism of DIC

Table 16.8: Causes of DIC

1. Sepsis or severe infections
2. Trauma especially of brain or crush injury
3. Obstetric conditions: amniotic fluid embolism, abruptio placentae, septic abortion, eclampsia, intrauterine retention of dead foetus
4. Malignancy: disseminated solid cancers, acute promyelocytic leukaemia
5. Severe haemolytic transfusion reactions
6. Thermal injury- heat stroke, extensive burns
7. Snake bite, e.g. Russell's viper
8. Severe liver disease
9. Giant haemangioma (Kasabach-Merritt syndrome).

head trauma, DIC is especially common due to release of large amount of tissue factor from cerebral injury.

- **Obstetric conditions:** Leakage of thromboplastin-like material from placenta into the maternal circulation.
- **Malignancy:** Expression of tissue factor on malignant cells; release of procoagulant substances from promyelocytes in acute promyelocytic leukaemia.
- **Vascular disorders (Kasabach-Merritt syndrome):** Local activation of coagulation with consumption of coagulation factors and platelets.
- **Snakebite:** Proteolytic activation of coagulation factors. (Envenomation by Russell's viper and Echis carinatus induces DIC).

Pathogenesis

DIC is a systemic thrombo-haemorrhagic disorder characterised by (1) Intravascular activation of extrinsic pathway of coagulation with generation of thrombin and fibrin,

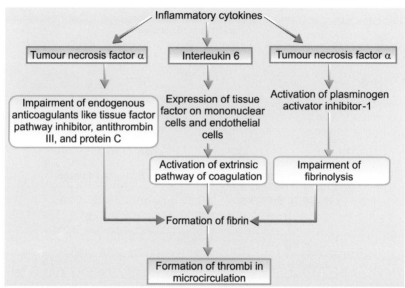

Figure 16.8: Pathogenesis of intravascular fibrin formation in DIC. Tissue factor is expressed on the surface of mononuclear cells and endothelial cells. This leads to initiation of extrinsic pathway of coagulation and generation of thrombin and fibrin. There is simultaneous inhibition of natural anticoagulants (antithrombin, protein C, and tissue factor pathway inhibitor) that further amplifies thrombin generation. At the same time fibrinolytic mechanism is suppressed by increased plasma levels of plasminogen activator inhibitor type 1 (PAI-1) that causes further propagation of fibrin formation. Inflammatory cytokines released from activated mononuclear cells and endothelial cells mediate these effects

(2) Reduction in levels of endogenous anticoagulants (antithrombin, protein C, and tissue factor pathway inhibitor), and (3) Suppression of fibrinolytic system which causes delayed and inadequate removal of fibrin. These three factors in combination lead to generalised deposition of fibrin (with formation of microthrombi) in circulation (Fig. 16.8). End-organ damage from generalised thrombotic occlusion of small blood vessels is responsible for most of the morbidity and mortality.

Depletion of coagulation factors and platelets results from their consumption in widespread microthrombi formation. This produces haemorrrhagic diathesis. There is secondary activation of fibrinolysis (though insufficient to remove all fibrin) that leads to generation of fibrinogen/fibrin degradation products. Plasminogen bound to platelet-fibrin thrombi is converted to plasmin by plasminogen activators. Plasmin cleaves fibrinogen as well as fibrin to generate fibrinogen/fibrin degradation products (FDPs). Fibrinogen degradation products are X, Y, D, and E fragments (Refer to Fig. 1.40). Fibrin degradation yields different fragments due to the presence of cross-linkages. A unique fibrin degradation product is D-dimer (Refer to Fig. 1.41). Circulating FDPs inhibit fibrin polymerisation and contribute to bleeding.

Mechanical damage to red cells by fibrin strands in circulation leads to microangiopathic haemolytic anaemia.

Clinical Features

Clinical features are largely determined by underlying disease that causes DIC. Two types of DIC are distinguished: acute and chronic.

- Acute or decompensated DIC: There is a rapid and extensive activation of coagulation leading to significant bleeding from consumption of coagulation factors and widespread microvascular thrombosis with consequent end-organ damage. Examples are DIC induced by sepsis and trauma.

- Chronic or compensated DIC: There is slow activation of coagulation in small amounts with slow consumption of coagulation factors; coagulation factor levels are normal or increased as they are replenished by enhanced synthesis. In chronic DIC, clinical features are minimal or absent and laboratory abnormalities are the only evidence of DIC. Examples of diseases initiating chronic DIC are intrauterine retention of dead foetus, liver disease, giant haemangioma, eclampsia, and malignancy.

In acute, fulminant DIC there is a sudden onset of spontaneous bleeding from multiple sites, such as skin (petechiae, ecchymoses), gastrointestinal tract, urinary system (haematuria), epistaxis and oozing from venepuncture sites. Intracranial haemorrhage can occur. Purpura fulminans (patchy areas of haemorrhagic skin necrosis) is a typical sign of fulminant DIC and results from thrombosis of small vessels of skin. Thrombotic occlusion may also affect vasculature of CNS, kidneys, heart, liver, lungs or adrenals.

Chronic DIC is a mild and protracted disease, which manifests usually with venous thrombosis; bleeding and microvascular thromboses are uncommon.

Laboratory Features

There is no single test that is diagnostic of DIC. Diagnosis is usually based on combination of clinical and laboratory features. Often multiple and frequent testing is required.

Acute DIC

In typical cases, all the coagulation screening tests (PT, APTT, and TT) are prolonged due to consumption of coagulation factors and inhibitory effect of FDPs (Box 16.5). It should be noted, however, that these tests might sometimes be normal. This is due

---

Box 16.5 Typical findings in acute DIC

- Presence of underlying disease known to be associated with DIC
- Low platelets or falling platelets on repeat testing
- Prolonged PT and APTT
- Low fibrinogen or falling levels on repeat testing
- Low plasma levels of coagulation inhibitors: ATIII or protein C
- Schistocytes (fragmented red cells) on blood smear
- FDP and D-dimer: Increased.

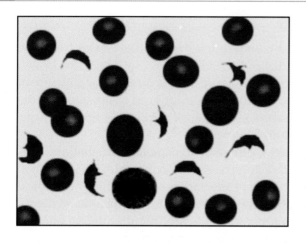

Figure 16.9: Blood smear in DIC. Schistocytes, polychromatic cells, a neutrophil with toxic granules, and thrombocytopaenia are present

to the presence of activated coagulation factors in circulation that cause rapid clot formation in the test system or the presence of X and Y FDP fragments which are coagulable by thrombin.

Quantitation of fibrinogen reveals hypofibrinogenaemia.

Peripheral blood examination shows fragmented red cells (schistocytes, helmet cells) on blood film and thrombocytopaenia (Fig. 16.9). Soluble fibrin monomers can be detected by 'paracoagulation tests'. In DIC, fibrin monomers combine with circulating FDPs to form soluble fibrin monomers. This inhibits fibrin monomer polymerisation. When ethanol or protamine sulphate is added to patient's plasma, fibrin monomers dissociate from FDPs and spontaneously polymerise to form a gel. This test is positive in early DIC but is not sufficiently sensitive. Positive test is also obtained in liver disease, lobar pneumonia and after major surgery.

Proteolytic action of plasmin on fibrinogen/fibrin generates FDPs. Latex agglutination test is commonly used for detection and quantitation of FDPs. This test has been outlined earlier. (See "Approach to the diagnosis of bleeding disorders"). FDPs are raised in most patients with DIC. However, FDP test may sometimes be negative.

Proteolysis of cross-linked fibrin by plasmin produces D-dimer fragments (Refer Fig. 1.41). Detection of D-dimers indicates both thrombin and plasmin generation. Latex particles coated with a monoclonal antibody against D-dimer are mixed with patient's serum and observed for agglutination. Amongst the currently available tests for DIC, D-dimer test is the most specific.

Chronic DIC

In chronic DIC, coagulation screening tests (PT, APTT, TT) are usually normal and platelet count is normal or slightly reduced. Test for FDPs and for fibrin monomers are abnormal (Box 16.6).

Box 16.6 Typical findings in chronic DIC
• Platelet count: Normal
• PT and APTT: Normal
• FDP and D-dimer: Increased

General Principles of Therapy

 i. Treatment of DIC depends on underlying cause and severity of clinical manifestations.
 ii. Management of the underlying disease process is the most effective measure in controlling DIC.
 iii. Transfusion of platelets or plasma components:
   • Platelets: In patients with DIC and bleeding and a platelet count <50,000/cmm
   • Fresh frozen plasma: In patients with DIC and bleeding and prolonged PT and APTT
   • Fibrinogen concentrate or cryoprecipitate: Severe hypofibrinogenaemia (<1 g/L) that persists despite FFP replacement.
 iv. Heparin: In DIC, where thrombosis predominates (arterial or venous thromboembolism, purpura fulminans with acral ischaemia).
 v. Recombinant human activated protein C: In severe sepsis with DIC; it should not be given to patients at high-risk of bleeding.

❑ ACQUIRED INHIBITORS OF COAGULATION (CIRCULATING ANTICOAGULANTS)

Acquired inhibitors of blood coagulation are substances that impair coagulation either by inactivating specific coagulation factors (specific inhibitors) or by interfering in coagulation reactions (nonspecific inhibitors).

Specific Inhibitors

These are antibodies that inhibit the activity of specific coagulation factors. They include inhibitors against F VIII, F IX, fibrinogen, von Willebrand factor, prothrombin, and factors V, XI, XIII, VII, XII and X. Inhibitors against F VIII are the most common followed by those against F IX.

F VIII Inhibitors

F VIII inhibitors develop in about 10 to 15% of patients with severe haemophilia A who have been exposed to multiple transfusions. They are uncommon in mild haemophilia. Their development causes refractoriness to F VIII replacement therapy. F VIII inhibitors are not restricted to haemophilic patients. They also occur in autoimmune disorders (rheumatoid arthritis, systemic lupus erythematosus), post partum females, malignancy, and during drug therapy especially penicillin. They also occur in elderly persons without any apparent cause. F VIII inhibitors in these patients cause bleeding but haemarthroses and deep haematomas are rare.

Coagulation profile reveals isolated prolongation of APTT. APTT performed using both patient's plasma and normal plasma (50:50) shows progressive (time-dependent) prolongation when incubated at 37°C for 2 hours.

The inhibitor antibodies against F VIII are commonly expressed in terms of Bethesda units. Patient's plasma (containing F VIII inhibitor) is mixed with normal pooled plasma (contains 100% F VIII activity), incubated at 37°C for 2 hours and residual F VIII activity in the mixture is assayed. The result is expressed as Bethesda units of inhibitor present per ml depending upon the reduction in the F VIII concentration in the incubation mixture.

Management of FVIII inhibitors is difficult. Various treatment options for F VIII inhibitors are: (i) High doses of F VIII concentrates along with plasmapheresis to remove inhibitor antibodies; (ii) Porcine F VIII concentrates which have low cross-reactivity against F VIII antibodies; (iii) Prothrombin complex concentrates and anti-inhibitor coagulant complex (Autoplex) which bypass F VIII; (iv) Immunosuppressive therapy and immunomodulation (IV immunoglobulin).

Non-Specific Inhibitors

They are not directed against specific coagulation factors. The prototype example is lupus anticoagulant.

Lupus anticoagulant (Lupus inhibitor): Lupus anticoagulants are acquired autoantibodies directed against phospholipid-protein complexes that can cause antiphospholipid syndrome. Antiphospholipid syndrome is an autoimmune disease characterised by venous or arterial thrombosis and/or recurrent foetal loss and presence of antiphospholipid antibodies in plasma. Types of antiphospholipid antibodies include anticardiolipin antibodies, anti-β2-glycoprotein I antibodies, and lupus anticoagulant. Anticardiolipin and anti-β2-glycoprotein I antibodies are detected by enzyme-linked immunosorbent assay, while lupus anticoagulant is identified by clot-based coagulation tests.

Antiphospholipid antibodies are encountered in systemic lupus erythematosus and other autoimmune diseases, neoplasia, lymphoproliferative disorders, viral infections particularly human immunodeficiency virus, in association with certain drugs, and in otherwise normal persons.

According to current guidelines, definite antiphospholipid syndrome is present if at least one clinical and one laboratory criteria are met:
1. Clinical criteria: vascular thrombosis, pregnancy morbidity
2. Laboratory criteria: anticardiolipin antibody, anti-β2-glycoprotein I antibody, lupus anticoagulant (laboratory test should be positive on ≥2 occasions at least 12 weeks apart).

Rarely, patients with antiphospholipid syndrome present with multiorgan failure of rapid onset that is associated with high mortality (catastrophic antiphospholipid syndrome). Acute thrombotic microangiopathy develops in multiple organs especially kidneys, lungs, central nervous system, heart, and skin.

Pathogenesis of thrombosis is unknown. Probably antiphospholipid antibodies activate endothelial cells, monocytes, and platelets causing increased synthesis of tissue

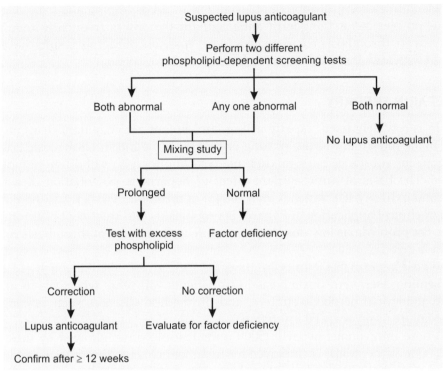

Figure 16.10: Strategy for laboratory identification of lupus anticoagulant

factor and thromboxane A2. Activation of complement cascade by antiphospholipid antibodies may trigger inflammatory reaction on the vessel wall or trophoblast surface. Interaction of antibodies with proteins like protein C, annexin 5, and plasmin may inhibit inactivation of procoagulant factors and impede fibrinolysis. A 'second hit' is possibly required for thrombosis or foetal loss to occur (like traumatic injury to vessesl, infections, oestrogens, etc).

The name 'lupus anticoagulant' is a misnomer since (i) most patients do not have systemic lupus erythematosus), and (ii) there is association with thrombosis rather than bleeding. The risk of foetal loss is high after 10th week of gestation.

Criteria for diagnosis of lupus anticoagulant are shown in Box 16.7 and Figure 16.10.

Box 16.7	Criteria for diagnosis of lupus anticoagulant (International Society on Thrombosis and Haemostasis)

- Prolongation of phospholipid-dependent screening test of coagulation*
- Failure of correction of prolonged screening test by mixing patient's plasma with normal platelet-poor plasma
- Correction of shortening of prolonged screening test by addition of excess phospholipids
- Exclusion of other coagulopathies like F VIII inhibitor or heparin

*At least two different screening tests (e.g. APTT, dilute Russell's viper venom time, kaolin clotting time, hexagonal phospholipids test) should be used before considering the sample as negative.

Note: For confirmation of diagnosis, re-testing of positive results is necessary after ≥12 weeks.

Incidental detection of lupus anticoagulant in an asymptomatic patient usually requires no treatment. Long-term anticoagulant therapy is frequently required in patients with thrombosis. In repeated foetal loss, encouraging results have been reported with low-dose subcutaneous heparin and/or aspirin.

❑ HEPARIN THERAPY

Heparin is a widely used, rapidly acting, and potent anticoagulant drug prepared from bovine intestinal mucosa or lung or from porcine intestinal mucosa. It is not a homogeneous substance but a mixture of glycosaminoglycans of different molecular weights. The basis of anticoagulant effect of heparin is potentiation of action of antithrombin III (AT III), which is an inhibitor of thrombin (F IIa), F Xa, and F IXa.

Major clinical application of heparin is prophylaxis and treatment of thromboembolism. For prophylaxis low-dose heparin while for treatment of thrombosis full dose heparin is given.

Low-dose heparin (5000 units 2–3 times per day) given subcutaneously is effective in preventing deep vein thrombosis in (i) patients >40 years who have to undergo elective abdominal or pelvic surgery, and (ii) medical diseases such as congestive cardiac failure or myocardial infarction.

Full dose intravenous heparin (5000 units loading dose followed by infusion of 1000–2000 units per hour) is employed for treatment of acute thrombosis and is given either as continuous infusion or intermittent injections.

Full dose intravenous heparin therapy for treatment of acute thrombosis is monitored usually by activated partial thromboplastin time (APTT) to maintain the dose within the therapeutic range. Therapeutic range is the level of anticoagulation that is sufficient to prevent thrombosis but does not cause spontaneous bleeding. Heparin level of 0.2 to 0.4 units/ml is considered as adequate anticoagulation. It is recommended to maintain the APTT of the patient between 1.5 and 2.5 times the control result to cover the therapeutic range.

Complications of heparin therapy include haemorrhage, thrombocytopaenia, thrombosis, and osteoporosis.

Heparin-induced thrombocytopaenia occurs in a small proportion of patients receiving standard heparin or low molecular weight heparin. It occurs in two forms— type I and type II.

Type I is a mild form of thrombocytopaenia (platelets >1 lac/cmm) which occurs early, i.e. during first few days of therapy and is often asymptomatic. It appears to be caused by aggregating effect of heparin on platelets.

Type II thrombocytopaenia is more severe (platelets <40,000/cmm), of delayed onset (usually develops after 4th day of treatment) and mediated by immune mechanism. Bleeding is rare despite marked thrombocytopaenia. Paradoxically many patients with type II thrombocytopaenia develop thrombosis (heparin-induced thrombocytopaenia with thrombosis or HITT). Thrombotic events include acute myocardial infarction, thrombotic stroke, peripheral arterial thromboses, and deep venous thrombosis.

The pathogenesis involves binding of IgG-heparin-platelet factor IV complex to Fc receptors on platelets that causes activation and aggregation of platelets as well as clearance of coated platelets by macrophages of reticuloendothelial system. Diagnosis is made by excluding other causes of thrombocytopaenia, by noting rise in platelet count after heparin withdrawal, and by demonstrating heparin-dependent platelet antibody by special tests. Platelet count gradually improves after cessation of heparin, but thrombocytopaenia develops on re-exposure. Treatment of thrombosis consists of immediate discontinuation of heparin and administration of inhibitors of thrombin like hirudin or danaparoid.

Low Molecular Weight Heparins (LMWH)

LMWH are prepared by enzymatic or chemical digestion of standard heparin. The anticoagulant action of LMWH is due to AT III-mediated inhibition predominantly of F Xa. The antithrombin action of LMWH is relatively weak. Duration of anticoagulation with LMWH is considerably longer than standard unfractionated heparin. LMWH is now the standard form of treatment in majority of patients since risk of heparin-induced thrombocytopaenia and thrombosis is low. Monitoring by APTT is not required. Because of longer duration of action, LMWH can be administered once daily. It is indicated for prevention and treatment of venous thrombosis and in acute coronary syndrome.

❑ ORAL ANTICOAGULANTS

Vitamin K is required for gamma carboxylation of coagulation factors II, VII, IX, and X. Oral anticoagulants interfere with the recycling of reduced vitamin K by inhibiting vitamin K epoxide reductase and also vitamin K reductase. This decreases availability of reduced form of vitamin K and thus inhibits gamma carboxylation (Fig. 16.11).

In the absence of vitamin K, functionally inactive forms of these coagulation factors circulate in plasma, which are unable to bind calcium. Such inactive forms are called as acarboxy forms or PIVKA (proteins induced by vitamin K absence or antagonism). These inactive coagulation factor precursors retain their antigenicity as detected by immunological assays but are unable to participate in the coagulation cascade.

Apart from factors II, VII, IX, and X, oral anticoagulants also inhibit two natural anticoagulant proteins C and S.

Time required for suppression of vitamin K-dependent coagulation factors depends on their half-lives. F VII, which has the shortest half-life (6 hour), disappears first followed by F IX (24 hour), F X (30 hour) and prothrombin (60 hour). Effective anticoagulation does not occur until all the pre-existing vitamin K-dependent coagulation factors are cleared from the circulation (3–4 days).

Oral anticoagulants are of two types—coumarins and the indanediones. Indanediones are rarely used due to the high risk of side effects. The most commonly used coumarin anticoagulant is warfarin sodium. A wide variety of drugs potentiate

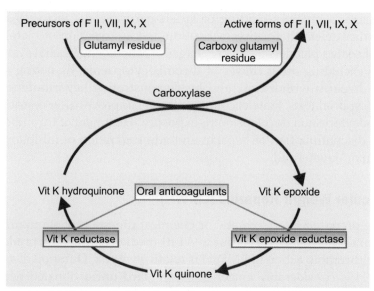

Figure 16.11: Vitamin K cycle. Oral anticoagulants inhibit vitamin
K epoxide reductase and vitamin K reductase

or inhibit the action of oral anticoagulants. This can increase the risk of bleeding or may reduce the anticoagulant effect. Dosage of oral anticoagulants may have to be adjusted when certain drugs are being given simultaneously.

Drugs may potentiate the action of oral anticoagulants by various mechanisms: (1) Impairment of platelet function (e.g. aspirin, non-steroidal anti-inflammatory drugs); (2) Impairment of warfarin metabolism (e.g. disulfiram); (3) Inhibition of recycling of vitamin K (cephalosporins); (4) Reduction of availability of vitamin K by interference with bacterial flora (broad-spectrum antibiotics); (5) Anticoagulant action (heparin); (6) Acceleration of clotting factor metabolism (thyroxine).

Drugs may inhibit the action of oral anticoagulants by: (1) Stimulating the hepatic microsomal enzymes and increasing the metabolism of warfarin (e.g. barbiturates, rifampicin, griseofulvin); (2) Reducing the absorption of warfarin from the gut (cholestyramine).

Indications for oral anticoagulants are (i) *Treatment of deep vein thrombosis (DVT):* DVT is a significant risk factor for pulmonary embolism. Initial treatment of DVT consists of immediate anticoagulation by intravenous heparin, which is given for 7 to 10 days. This is followed by warfarin which is started at least 2 to 3 days before discontinuing heparin; (ii) *Prevention of DVT in high-risk patients,* e.g. patients with previous history of venous thrombosis, patients undergoing hip surgery or surgery for cancer; (iii) *Cardiac conditions* such as myocardial infarction (for prevention of recurrence and stroke), valvular prostheses (to reduce the risk of thromboembolism), and atrial fibrillation (to decrease systemic embolisation), (iv) *Recurrent thromboembolic phenomena.*

Oral anticoagulant therapy is regularly monitored by prothrombin time (PT) that is a measure of three of the four vitamin K-dependent factors. The result is usually reported as ratio of PT of patient to PT of control. However, responsiveness of tissue thromboplastins (PT reagent), which are obtained from rabbit, bovine, or human sources, to decreased vitamin K-dependent factors is variable and the result of PT depends on type of thromboplastin used. Thus level of anticoagulation can vary widely even though identical PT results are obtained with different tissue thromboplastins. The therapeutic range with one thromboplastin reagent cannot be directly applied to another reagent. To achieve standardisation among laboratories, it is recommended to report the result of PT as International Normalized Ratio (INR) that is derived from the formula:

$$INR = \left(\frac{PT\ of\ patient}{PT\ of\ control} \right)^{ISI}$$

ISI (International Sensitivity Index) of a particular tissue thromboplastin is derived by comparing it with reference thromboplastin of known ISI.

The recommended therapeutic range depends on the indication for anticoagulation; for most cases, INR of 2.0 to 3.0 (commonly 2.5) is advised. Side effects of warfarin include: (1) Bleeding, (2) Skin necrosis due to microvascular thrombosis in subcutaneous tissue (protein C deficiency is thought to play a role), and (3) Teratogenic effect on the foetus if given during pregnancy.

❑ OTHER ACQUIRED COAGULATION DISORDERS

Renal Diseases

Excessive urinary loss of coagulation factor IX and antithrombin III may occur in nephrotic syndrome. Thrombotic tendencies in these patients are probably related to deficiency of antithrombin III.

Haemostatic abnormalities commonly develop in uraemia such as defective platelet function (which manifests as prolonged bleeding time and deficient platelet aggregation with ADP and epinephrine) and impairment of fibrin monomer polymerisation. These abnormalities are reversed by dialysis and are probably caused by a dialyzable substance. Bleeding diathesis usually responds to haemodialysis. Desmopressin and cryoprecipitate are other modes of therapy.

Paraproteinaemias

Paraproteinaemias are frequently associated with thrombocytopaenia, impairment of platelet function (due to coating of platelet surface by paraproteins causing blocking of platelet receptors), and defective fibrin monomer polymerisation. Treatment of primary disease with lowering of paraprotein level is followed by improvement.

Amyloidosis

Amyloid deposits in tissues avidly bind F X and can cause its secondary deficiency.

Cardiopulmonary Bypass

Haemostatic defects are frequent during and after cardiopulmonary bypass surgery and include platelet dysfunction, thrombocytopaenia, inadequate inactivation of heparin by protamine, and disseminated intravascular coagulation. Bleeding can be treated by platelet concentrates, desmopressin, and fresh frozen plasma or cryoprecipitate.

Massive Transfusion of Stored Blood

Massive transfusion refers to the transfusion equal to or greater than patient's blood volume within 24 hours. Stored blood is usually deficient in platelets and some coagulation factors (F V and VIII). Haemostatic defects in massively transfused patients are caused by dilution of platelets and coagulation factors. Disseminated intravascular coagulation secondary to shock and underlying disease is probably a more important cause of major bleeding in these patients than dilutional effect.

❑ BIBLIOGRAPHY

1. Aledort LM. Treatment of von Willebrand's disease. Mayo Clin Proc. 1991;66:841-46.
2. Antonarakis SE, Waber PG, Kittur SD, et al. Hemophilia A. Detection of molecular defects and of carriers by DNA analysis. N Engl J Med. 1985;313:842-48.
3. Baglin T. Disseminated intravascualr coagulation: Diagnosis and treatment. BMJ. 1996;312: 683-87.
4. Bakshi S, Arya LS. Diagnosis and treatment of disseminated intravascular coagulation. Indian Pediatrics. 2003;40:721-30.
5. Barrowcliffe TW. Low molecular weight heparin(s). Br J Haematol. 1995;90:1-7.
6. Bick RL, Baker WF. The antiphospholipid and thrombosis syndromes. Med Clin North Am. 1994;78:667-84.
7. Bick RL. Disseminated intravascular coagulation: Objective criteria for diagnosis and management. Med Clin North Am. 1994;78:511-43.
8. Bloom AL, Peake IR. Haemophilia. Diagnosis and management. In Poller L (Ed.): Recent Advances in Blood coagulation. No.5. Edinburgh. Churchill Livingstone. 1991.
9. Bowen DJ. Haemophilia A and Haemophilia B: Molecular insights. Mol Pathol. 2002;55: 127-44.
10. Chong BH. Heparin-induced thrombocytopaenia. Br J Haematol. 1995;l89:431-39.
11. Furie B, Limentani SA, Rosenfield CG. A practical guide to the evaluation and treatment of hemophilia. Blood. 1994;84:3-9.
12. Ginsburg D, Walter Bowie EJ. Molecular genetics of von Willebrand disease. Blood. 1992;79: 2507-19.
13. Graham JB, Green PP, McGraw RA, Davis LM. Application of molecular genetics to prenatal diagnosis and carrier detection in the hemophilias: some limitations. Blood. 1985;66:759-64.
14. Greaves M, Preston FE. Clinical and laboratory aspects of thrombophilia. In Poller L (Ed.): Recent Advances in Blood Coagulation. No.5 Edinburgh. Churchill Livingstone. 1991.
15. Hanly JG. Antiphospholipid syndrome: an overview. CMAJ. 2003;168:1675-82.
16. Hembleton J, Leung LL, Levi M. Coagulation: Consultative hemostasis. American Society of Hematology. Hematology. 2002;335-52.
17. Hirsh J, Dalen JE, Deykin D, Poller L. Heparin: Mechanism of action, pharmacokinetics, dosing considerations, monitoring, efficacy, and safety. Chest. 1992;102:337S-351S.

18. Hirsh J, Dalen JE, Deykin D, Poller L. Oral anticoagulants - Mechanism of action, clinical effectiveness, and optimal therapeutic range. Chest. 1992;102:312 S-326S.

19. Hirsh J. Oral anticoagulants. N Engl J Med. 1991;324:1865-75.

20. Hoyer LW, Carta CA, Golbus MS, Hobbins JC, Mahoney MJ. Prenatal diagnosis of classic hemophilia (Hemophilia A) by immunoradiometric assays. Blood. 1985;65:1312-17.

21. Hoyer LW. Hemophilia A. N Engl J Med. 1994;330:38-47.

22. Kanavakis E, Traeger-Synodinos J. Preimplantation diagnosis in clinical practice. J Med Genet. 2002;39:6-11.

23. Kashyap R, Choudhury VP. Hemophilia. Indian Pediatrics. 2000;37:45-53.

24. Kogan SC, Doherty M, Gitschier J. An improved method for prenatal diagnosis and carrier detection of genetic diseases by analysis of specifically amplified polymorphic sequences: application to haeophilia A. N Engl J Med. 1987;317:985-90.

25. Levi M, Cate HT. Disseminated intravascular coagulation. N Engl J Med. 1999;341:586-92.

26. Mammen EF. Coagulation defects in liver disease. Med Clin North Am. 1994;78:545-54.

27. Mannucci PM, Tuddenham EGD. The hemophilias - From royal genes to gene therapy. N Engl J Med. 2002; 344:1773-79.

28. McVey JH, Pattinson JK, Tuddenham EGD. Molecular biology in blood coagulation. In Poller L (Ed.): Recent Advances in Blood Coagulation No.5. Edinburgh. Churchill Livingstone. 1991.

29. Miyakis S, Lockshin MD, Atsumi T, Branch DW, Brey RL, Cervera R, Derksen RHWM, de Groot PG, Koike T, Meroni PL, Reber G, Shoenfeld Y, Tincani A, Vlachoyiannopoulos PG, Krilis SA. International consensus statement on an update of the classification criteria for definite antiphospholipid syndrome (APS). J Thromb Haemost. 2006;4:295–306.

30. Morrision AE and Ludlam CA.Acquired haemophilia and its management. Br J Haematol. 1995;89:231-36.

31. Newland AC, Evans TGJR. ABC of clinical haematology: Haematological disorders at the extremes of life. BMJ. 1997;314:1262.

32. Nilsson IM, Lethagen S. von Willebrand's disease. Indian J Pediatr. 1993;60:167-86.

33. Report of a WHO Scientific group: Control of hereditary diseases. WHO Technical Report series. 865. World Health Organization, Geneva. 1996.

34. Rick ME. Diagnosis and management of von Willebrands syndrome. Med Clin North Am. 1994;78:609-23.

35. Risberg B, Andreasson S, Eriksson E. Disseminated intravascular coagulation. Acta Anaesthesiol Scand. 1991;35 (suppl 95):60-71.

36. Ruggeri ZM, Zimmerman TS. von Willebrand factor and von Willebrand disease. Blood. 1987;70:895-904.

37. Sadler JE. A revised classification of von Willebrand disease. For the Subcommittee on von Willebrand Factor of the Scientific and Standardization Committee of the International Society on Thrombosis and Haemostasis. Thromb Haemost. 1994;71:520-5.

38. Sadler JE, Budde U, Eikenboom JC, et al. Update on the pathophysiology and classification of von Willebrand disease: areport of the Subcommittee on von Wilbrand factor. J Thromb Haemost. 2006;4:2103-14.

39. Smock KJ, Rodgers GM. Laboratory identification of lupus anticoagulants. Am J Hematol. 2009;84:440-2.

40. Toh CH, Dennis M. Disseminated intravascular coagulation: old disease, new hope. BMJ. 2003;327:974-7.

41. Triplett DA. Laboratory diagnosis of von Willebrand's disease. Mayo Clin Proc. 1991;66:832-40.

42. White GC II, Shoemaker CB. Factor VIII gene and hemophilia A. Blood. 1989;73:1-12.

CHAPTER

17

Blood Group Systems

International Society of Blood Transfusion (ISBT) Working Party recognises 30 blood group systems (Table 17.1). Red cell antigens that are produced by alleles (alternative forms of a specified gene) at a single gene locus or very closely linked loci constitute a blood group system.

Table 17.1: Blood group systems (International Society of Blood Transfusion or ISBT, 2008)

Traditional name	ISBT No	ISBT symbol	Traditional name	ISBT No	ISBT symbol
ABO	001	ABO	Landsteiner-Wiener	016	LW
MNS	002	MNS	Chido/Rodgers	017	CH/RG
P1Pk	003	P1	Hh	018	H
Rh	004	RHD, RHCE	Kx	019	XK
Lutheran	005	LU	Gerbich	020	GE
Kell	006	KEL	Cromer	021	CROM
Lewis	007	LE	Knobs	022	KN
Duffy	008	FY	Indian	023	IN
Kidd	009	JK	Ok	024	OK
Diego	010	DI	Raph	025	RAPH
Yt	011	YT	John Milton Hagen	026	JMH
Xg	012	XG	I	027	I
Scianna	013	SC	Globoside	028	GLOB
Dombrock	014	DO	GIL	029	GIL
Colton	015	CO	RHAG	030	RHAG

Blood group genes are inherited in a Mendelian manner and are mostly located on autosomes. Most of the blood group genes are expressed in a codominant manner (i.e. the two allelic forms are expressed equally if inherited in a heterozygous state). The particular alleles at a specified gene locus in an individual constitute the genotype. Phenotype is the outward expression of the genotype.

In blood transfusion practice, most important blood group systems are ABO and Rh. This is because, A, B, and Rh D antigens are the most immunogenic (i.e. capable of eliciting a strong antibody response on stimulation) and their alloantibodies can cause destruction of transfused red cells or induce haemolytic disease of newborn (HDN). ABO antigens are also important in organ transplantation.

Next to A and B, other antigens important in transfusion medicine due to their immunogenicity are D, K, C, Fy^a, c, E, k, e, Jk^a, S, and s.

❑ ABO SYSTEM

In ABO system, there are four main types of blood groups–A, B, AB, and O. Identification of these four blood groups is based on presence or absence of A and/or B antigens on red cells. According to Landsteiner's law, anti-A and/or anti-B antibodies are always present in plasma of individuals who lack corresponding antigen(s) on their red cells (Table 17.2). There are two major subgroups of A: A1 (80%) and A2 (20%). Thus ABO system comprises of six groups. Antigens and antibodies of these groups are–**A1**: anti-B; **A2**: anti-B, and in 1 to 8% cases anti-A1; **B**: anti-A; **A1B**: nil; **A2B**: anti-A1 in 22 to 35% cases; **O**: anti-A, anti-B. Usually, anti-A1 antibodies are weak and are of little clinical significance in routine practice.

Antigens of the ABO System

Antigens of the ABO system are: A (A1, A2), B, and H. In addition to red cells, they are also expressed on white cells, platelets, and various body tissues. They are also present in a soluble form in various body secretions (in secretors).

ABO antigens are carbohydrate structures on glycoproteins and glycolipids. ABO antigens are poorly expressed at birth, increase gradually in strength and become fully expressed around 1 year of age. In older age, they become slightly weak.

Table 17.2: ABO blood groups

Blood group	Approximate Indian frequency	Genotype	Antigen(s) on red cells	Antibody in plasma
A	27%	AA or AO	A	Anti-B
B	31%	BB or BO	B	Anti-A
AB	8%	AB	AB	Nil
O	34%	OO	Nil	Anti-A and anti-B

Note: *A* and *B* genes are dominant while *O* gene is recessive

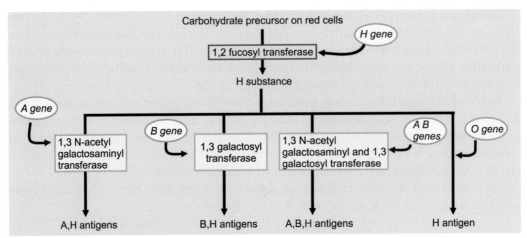

Figure 17.1: Formation of antigens of the ABO system

Formation of ABH antigens: The *H* gene (genotype *HH or Hh*) produces a transferase enzyme, which changes precursor substance (present on red cells) into H substance. The *A* and *B* genes produce specific transferase enzymes, which convert H substance into A and B antigens respectively. Some amount of H antigen remains unchanged on red cells. The *O* gene produces an inactive transferase so that H antigen persists unchanged on red cells (Fig. 17.1).

Some persons do not inherit the *H* gene (genotype *hh*) and thus cannot synthesise H substance. Such persons may inherit the *A* or *B* gene but cannot express it, as they are unable to produce the H substance. Such individuals are said to have Bombay phenotype or Bombay blood group (Oh). Their red cells type as group O; however, unlike group O individuals, Oh persons have no H antigen on their red cells and their plasma contains strong anti-H in addition to anti-A and anti-B. Therefore, Bombay group persons should be transfused only with Oh blood.

Secretors and non-secretors: Secretors are persons who secrete A, B, and H antigens into body fluids (such as plasma, gastric juice, saliva, sweat, tears, semen, milk, etc.). This ability is dependent on presence of a dominant secretor gene (*Se*). About 80% of individuals are secretors (genotype *Sese* or *SeSe*) and remaining are non-secretors (genotype *sese*). Both secretors and non-secretors express ABO antigens on red cells.

Antigens secreted by different ABO blood groups are:
- Group A: A, H
- Group B: B, H
- Group AB: A, B, H
- Group O: H

Antigens secreted in to body fluids are called as ABH substances. Testing for ABH substances in saliva may be helpful when red cell grouping yields uncertain results. Determining secretor status in saliva and semen can be helpful in forensic studies (e.g. semen sample collected from a rape victim revealing a soluble ABH antigen that does not match with the ABO blood group of the accused). *Inhibitor tests* are used to detect the presence of soluble blood group antigens in body secretions. If saliva contains a soluble antigen, and if corresponding antibody is added, the activity of the antibody is neutralised due to binding of antibody to antigen. When red cells carrying the appropriate antigens are subsequently added to the mixture, there will be inhibition of agglutination (i.e. the person is a secretor). If agglutination occurs, then the individual is a non-secretor.

Example:
    Blood group: B
    Step 1: Saliva + anti-B
    Step 2: Add B cells
    Result: No agglutination
    Interpretation: Secretor

Antibodies of the ABO System

The most important antibodies in transfusion practice are anti-A and anti-B. They are also called as naturally occurring antibodies because they arise without immune stimulation (i.e. transfusion or pregnancy) by relevant blood group antigens. They are not detectable in the blood of newborn infants due to their underdeveloped immune system and appear around 3 to 6 months of life. It is thought that they are produced in response to A- and B-like antigens of bacteria, which are present in the intestine and certain foods. If anti-A and/or anti-B are present at birth, they are of maternal origin (IgG). Anti-A and anti-B antibodies are usually of IgM class. They can efficiently fix the complement. Naturally occurring ABO antibodies can cause:
• Haemolytic transfusion reaction in case of ABO-mismatched blood transfusion,
• Acute graft rejection in case of ABO-incompatible solid organ transplantation, and
• Haemolysis of donor red cells following ABO-incompatible bone marrow transplantation.

Less commonly, some individuals have large amounts of ABO antibodies of immune nature. Usually, group O individuals following immune stimulation by transfusion, pregnancy, or injection of certain vaccines or toxoids (that contain bacterial A- and B-like antigens) produce them in large amounts. These antibodies are of IgG class, of high titre, and cannot be neutralised by soluble blood group antigens. If blood of such group O individuals (called dangerous universal group O donors) is transfused to group A or B individuals, serious haemolysis of recipient's red cells can occur. Therefore, group O donors should not be employed as universal donors. (Note: Red cells of group O donors are devoid of A and B antigens and cannot be agglutinated by anti-A and anti-B antibodies. Therefore, group O persons are traditionally considered as universal donors). In addition to causing haemolytic transfusion reaction, these IgG antibodies can cross the placenta and induce haemolytic disease of newborn.

❑ THE Rh SYSTEM

When Rhesus monkey red cells were injected into rabbits and guinea pigs, antibody, which was raised, was found to react with Rhesus monkey red cells as well as with 85% of human red cells. The antigen involved was called as Rh factor. Subsequently it was shown that the original antibody was different from anti-D antibody discovered later. The name of the antigen, however, has remained as Rhesus. According to the recent nomenclature by ISBT, the system has been named as Rh.

The Rh system is only next in importance to ABO system in transfusion practice. The importance of this system lies in the high immunogenicity of Rh D antigen, which readily induces formation of anti-D antibodies in Rh D-negative individuals. Anti-D antibodies can cause haemolytic transfusion reaction or, in pregnant women, Rh haemolytic disease of newborn.

Antigens of the Rh System

The important antigens of the Rh system are C, D, E, c, and e. D antigen is the most immunogenic. There are various nomenclature systems for Rh antigens. Fisher-Race or CDE nomenclature system is simpler and is outlined below.

According to Fisher and Race, three closely linked genes are inherited together on one chromosome (haplotype) from each parent. Allelic forms of these genes are C and c, D and d, and E and e with eight possible haplotypes–CDe, cde, cDE, cDe, cdE, Cde, CDE, and CdE. As an individual inherits one haplotype from each parent, 36 genotypes are possible such as Cde/cde, Cde/cDe, CDE/cde, etc. The presence of D in either homozygous (D/D) or heterozygous (D/d) state makes that individual **Rh positive**, while **Rh negative** persons are homozygous for d (d/d). It was thought that d gene was an amorph. Results of current genetic studies are consistent with Fisher-Race theory. It has been found that the *RH* locus is located on chromosome 1 and consists of two closely linked genes—*RHD* and *RHCE*. The alleles of *RHCE* are CE, Ce, ce, and cE (Fig. 17.2). In Rh negative persons, deletions, point mutations, or partial mutations of D gene have been found. Rh antigens are expressed only on red cells and not on any other tissues. They are also not secreted in body fluids. In contrast to ABO antigens, Rh antigens are fully expressed on red cells before birth and also on red cells of early foetuses.

Depending on the presence or absence of antigen D on red cells, a person is grouped either as Rh positive (when red cells express antigen D) or Rh negative (when D antigen is absent on red cells). Frequency of D antigen varies in different populations. **In India, approximately 95% of the people express D antigen on their red cells (Rh D-positive), while 5% are Rh D-negative.** Other forms of D antigen are weak D and partial D. Red cells having **weak D antigen** were formerly called as D^u cells which react weakly with anti-D reagent. There is a quantitative reduction in the number of D antigen sites on such red cells. D^u recipients do not make anti-D antibodies following stimulation by D antigen (e.g. following D+ve blood transfusion). D^u donors should

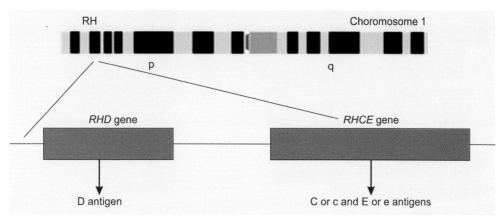

Figure 17.2: Genes of the Rh system. There are two genes of the Rh system: *RHD* gene that codes for D antigen and *RHCE* gene that codes for C or c and E or e antigens (giving rise to CE, Ce, cE, and ce antigen combinations). Presence of *RHD* gene confers Rh D positive phenotype while its absence Rh D negative phenotype

be considered as Rh positive and their blood should not be transfused to Rh-negative donors. In red cells having **partial D antigen,** parts of D antigen are missing. Variants of partial D antigen exist. Individuals with D^{VI} variant are able to produce anti-D antibody against the missing part of the antigen if exposed to D+ve antigen. Such recipients should be considered as Rh negative, while donors should be regarded as Rh positive. However, in practice, individuals with partial D antigen are typed as D negative and are identified only after they have produced anti-D antibodies.

Complete absence of all Rh antigens on red cells (Rh null cells) is associated with stomatocytosis (red cells have a slot-like area of central pallor, reminiscent of mouth) and compensated haemolysis.

Rh Antibodies

In general, most Rh antibodies are of immune type, i.e. they are the result of immunisation by blood transfusion or pregnancy. Most of these antibodies are of IgG class. Comparison of ABO and RhD groups is given in Table 17.3.

In practice, Rh antibodies can cause haemolytic transfusion reaction or haemolytic disease of newborn. Since Rh antibodies do not activate complement, haemolysis is extravascular and predominantly occurs in spleen. Due to high immunogenicity of D antigen, Rh-negative persons (especially women of child bearing age) should be transfused only with Rh-negative blood. During pregnancy, IgG anti-D can cross the placenta and induce haemolytic disease of newborn by causing immune haemolysis of foetal red cells. Rh haemolytic disease of newborn can be prevented by prophylactic administration of Rh immune globulin to all Rh-negative women during mid pregnancy and within 72 hours of delivery. Anti-D and anti-c can cause severe HDN. Anti-C, anti-E, and anti-e usually do not cause HDN or cause mild HDN.

Table 17.3: Comparison of ABO and RhD groups

Parameter	ABO group	RhD group
1. Location of gene	Chromosome 9	Chromosome 1
2. Antigens	A, B, AB	D
3. Distribution of antigens	Red cells, platelets, many tissues, body fluids	Red cells only
4. Development of antigens	Weak expression at birth	Fully developed at birth
5. Dosage effect*	No	Present
6. Nature of antibodies	Naturally occurring	Immune
7. Antibody class	IgM	IgG
8. Whether antibodies fix complement	Yes	No
9. Optimal reaction temperature of antibody	4°C	37°C
10. Optimal reaction medium	Saline	Antihuman globulin

* Dosage effect: A situation where antibody reacts more strongly with red cells having double the dose of antigen (due to homozygous state) than those having single dose (heterozygous state)

❏ BIBLIOGRAPHY

1. Contreras M, Lubenko A. Antigens in human blood. In Hoffbrand AV and Lewis SM (Eds.): Postgraduate Haematology. 3rd ed. London. Heinemann Professional Publishing Ltd. 1989.
2. Kelton JG, Heddle NM, Blajchman MA. Blood transfusion—A conceptual approach. New York. Churchill Livingstone. 1984.
3. Knowles SM. Blood cell antigens and antibodies: erythrocytes, platelets and granulocytes. In Lewis SM, Bain BJ, Bates I (Eds.): Dacie and Lewis Practical Haematology. 9th ed. London. Churchill Livingstone. 2001
4. World Health Organization: Safe blood and blood products. Module 3. Blood group serology. Geneva. World Health Organization. 2009.

Serologic and Microbiologic Techniques

❏ SEROLOGIC TECHNIQUES

ABO Grouping

In transfusion practice, test for ABO grouping is essential because of the consistent occurrence of haemolytic, naturally occurring antibodies in plasma of persons lacking the corresponding antigen on red cells (Box 18.1). There are **two methods for ABO grouping—cell grouping (forward grouping) and serum grouping (backward or reverse grouping).** Both cell and serum grouping should be done since each test acts as a check on the other thus reducing the risk of error in grouping. In cell grouping, red cells are tested for the presence of A and B antigens employing known specific anti-A and anti-B sera. In serum grouping, serum is tested for the presence of anti-A and anti-B antibodies by employing known group A and group B reagent red cells. Serum grouping should not be carried out in infants below 4 months since infants start producing anti-A and anti-B antibodies by 4 to 6 months of age. Elderly persons

Box 18.1	Blood grouping

- Routinely ABO and Rh grouping are done
- Importance of ABO grouping: Consistent presence of haemolytic, naturally occurring reciprocal antibodies in the plasma of all individuals lacking the corresponding antigen on red cells
- Importance of Rh grouping: Rh D antigen is highly immunogenic (next to A and B antigens) and induces formation of anti-D antibodies in persons lacking D antigen. Immune anti-D antibodies (IgG) can cause haemolytic transfusion reaction and haemolytic disease of newborn.

may also have depressed antibody levels. In both these cases, ABO grouping is reliably performed by cell grouping method.

There are five methods for blood grouping: slide, tube, microplate, column agglutination or gel technology, and solid phase adherence technology.

Slide Test (Forward grouping or cell grouping)

Principle: Red cells from the specimen are tested for A and/or B antigens by using known reagent antisera (anti-A and anti-B). Agglutination of red cells indicates presence of corresponding antigen on red cells.

Specimen: Specimen may be either capillary blood from finger prick, or venous blood collected in EDTA anticoagulant.

Reagents:
Antisera: Antisera are used to detect antigens on red cells. Previously, polyclonal anti-A, anti-B, and anti-AB sera obtained from humans were used for cell grouping. (Polyclonal antiserum contains many different antibodies directed against different epitopes of an antigen and are produced by different clones of plasma cells). These now have been replaced by anti-A and anti-B monoclonal antisera. (Monoclonal antiserum contains specific antibodies against a specific antigenic epitope and is produced by a single clone of plasma cells). Polyclonal antisera are obtained from human donors immunised with soluble antigens. Monoclonal antibodies are obtained by hybridoma technology. (Specific antibody producing mouse B-lymphocytes from immunised mice are artificially fused with mouse myeloma cells which are able to grow indefinitely in culture. The resulting hybrid cell, called hybridoma, is cloned and cultured to get large amounts of monoclonal antibodies). Monoclonal antisera are specific, avid, sensitive, and can detect weak antigens. Anti-A is colour coded blue and anti-B is colour coded yellow. A third antiserum called anti-A, B is also used in some blood banks (especially for grouping in newborns and to resolve ABO discrepancies); anti-A, B is colourless. Antisera also contain a preservative (0.1% sodium azide) to prevent growth of bacteria. They are stored at 2° to 8°C. Monoclonal antisera are free from infectious agents like HIV, HBV, or HCV, unlike sera obtained from humans. If monoclonal antisera are being used, third antiserum anti-AB is not required.

Method:
1. Divide a clean and dry glass slide into two sections with a glass marking pencil. Label the sections as anti-A and anti-B (Fig. 18.1).
2. Place one drop of anti-A and one drop of anti-B antiserum in the center of the corresponding section of the slide.
3. Add one drop of blood sample to be tested to each drop of antiserum.
4. Mix antiserum and blood by using a separate stick for each section.
5. By tilting the slide from side to side, observe for agglutination after exactly two minutes.

Table 18.1: Interpretation of cell grouping by slide test

Anti-A	Anti-B	Blood group
+	-	A
-	+	B
+	+	AB
-	-	O

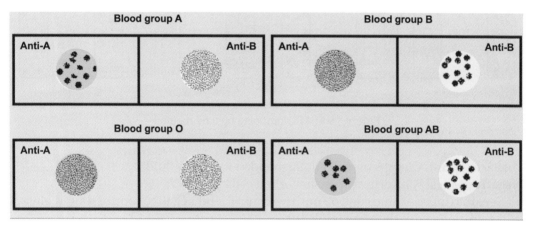

Figure 18.1: ABO blood grouping by slide method

6. Result:
   Positive (+): small clumps of red cells are seen floating in a clear liquid.
   Negative (-): Uniform suspension of red cells.
7. Interpretation: Interpret the result as shown in the Table 18.1.

Note: Slide test is rapid and simple. In practice, it is used: (1) As a preliminary grouping test before blood donation, (2) In blood donation camps, and (3) In case of an emergency. Results of slide test should always be confirmed by cell and serum grouping by tube method.

Weakly reactive antigens (like A1) may be missed by slide method. Slide test is also not suitable for serum grouping. Drying of the antiserum-blood mixture around the edges can be misinterpreted as agglutination. If the result is read before two minutes, weak antigens may be missed.

Tube Method

For **cell grouping**, known antiserum and patient's red cells are mixed in a test tube, incubated at room temperature for 5 minutes, and then centrifuged. In **serum or reverse grouping,** serum from the patient and reagent red cells of known group (available commercially or prepared in the laboratory) are used. Following centrifugation, a red cell button (sediment) will be seen at the bottom of the tube. Cell button is resuspended by gently tapping the base of the tube.

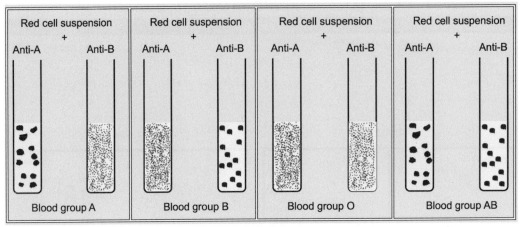

Figure 18.2: ABO grouping by tube method

Positive (+) test: Clumps of red cells suspended in a clear fluid
Negative (-) test: Uniform suspension of red cells (Fig. 18.2).

Separate tubes of auto control, positive control, and negative control should always be set up along with the test sample tube.

Auto control is necessary to rule out auto agglutination of patient's red cells, which occurs when autoantibodies are present in patient's serum. In auto control tube, patient's red cells are mixed with patient's own serum and the tube is centrifuged; if agglutination occurs, it is autoantibody-induced. Auto control test is particularly essential when ABO grouping is being done only by forward method and blood group is typed as AB.

In two **positive control** tubes, anti-A serum is mixed with group A red cells and anti-B is mixed with group B red cells, respectively. In two **negative control** tubes, anti-A serum is mixed with group B red cells and anti-B serum is mixed with group A red cells, respectively. These controls are necessary to confirm that reagents are working properly.

Test tube method of blood grouping is more reliable than slide method. This is because centrifugation brings antigen and antibodies closer together and allows detection of weaker antigen antibody reactions.

Microplate method: This technique is commonly used in many blood bank laboratories. A microwell plate consists of 96 small wells (U- or V- or flat-bottom) (Fig. 18.3). U-type is preferable since results are easier to read. Microplate method is more cost-effective since far less antisera is required as compared to the test tube method; also multiple samples can be tested at the same time because of 96 wells.

Column agglutination or gel technology: This method is easy, accurate, standardised, needs small sample volume, and reduces exposure to biohazardous samples. It does

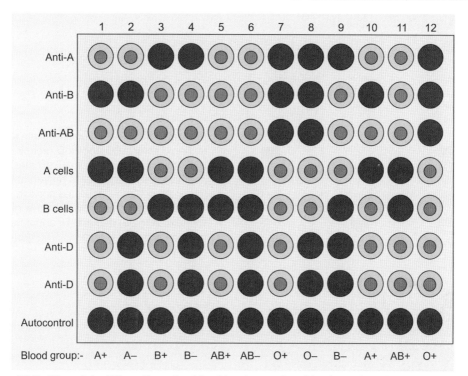

Figure 18.3: Microplate (96 well) method for blood grouping. Numbers 1 to 12 represent patient identification numbers. Reagents added to the patient sample are written on left, while interpretation (blood group of patient) is written at the bottom. Red compact button indicates agglutination, while uniform suspension indicates no agglutination

not require washing of red cells and microscopic examination. It is expensive and needs a special centrifuge.

Gel technology can be used for ABO and Rh grouping, compatibility testing, direct antiglobulin test, and antibody identification.

Method for cell grouping uses microtubes filled with dextran acrylamide gel (which functions both as a reaction medium and a size filter) and antisera. After addition of red cells to the top of the tube, haemagglutinates (if formed) are trapped at the top of the tube (positive test). Non-agglutinated cells pass through the gel and form a button at the bottom of the tube (negative test) (Fig. 18.4).

Solid phase adherence technology: This method of cell grouping uses a microplate in which wells (solid phase) are coated with reagent red cells or red cell stroma. Serum sample is added and antibodies, if present, are captured by the antigen on the coated red cells. Indicator red cells (coated with monoclonal IgG) are then added and the mixture is centrifuged. Indicator red cells attach to the antibody that was captured by coated red cells and agglutination is indicated by diffuse adherence of indicator red cells all along the microwell (positive test). If there is no haemagglutination, red cells form a button at the bottom of the microwell (negative test) (Fig. 18.5).

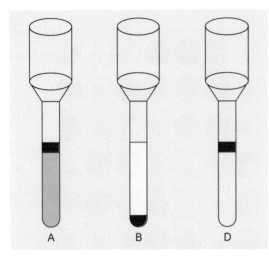

Figure 18.4: Gel or column agglutination technology for ABO and RhD grouping. If cells settle at the bottom it indicates a negative result, and if cells remain at the top of the column it indicates positive result. The above example shows positive reaction with anti-A (blue) and anti-D, and a negative reaction with anti-B (yellow). The group is A RhD+ve

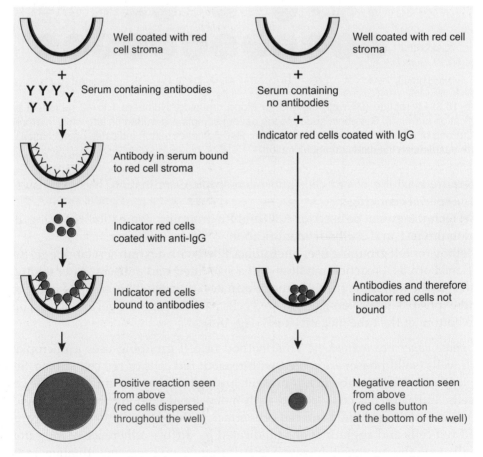

Figure 18.5: Principle of solid phase adherence test for blood grouping

False Reactions in ABO Grouping

Autoagglutination: Presence of IgM autoantibodies reactive at room temperature in patient's serum can lead to autoagglutination. If autocontrol is not used, blood group in such a case will be wrongly typed as AB. Therefore, for correct result, if autocontrol is also showing agglutination, cell grouping should be repeated after washing red cells with warm saline (to remove autoantibodies), and serum grouping should be repeated at 37°C.

Rouleaux formation: In rouleaux formation, red cells adhere to each other like a stack of coins. Rouleaux formation may be due to high levels of paraproteins in blood or intravenous administration of dextran. Rouleaux can be mistaken for agglutination during blood grouping test. Rouleaux formation is noted during serum grouping or if unwashed red cells are used for cell grouping. Rouleaux, but not agglutination, disappear on addition of normal saline.

False negative result due to inactivated antisera: Use of inactivated antisera or deterioration of reagent red cells will cause false negative result in ABO grouping. Antisera are inactivated if they are left at room temperature for long and are not kept stored at proper temperature.

Unexpected Results in Blood Grouping

Problems with cell grouping:
1. *Acquired B antigen:* Microbial enzyme D-acetylase can modify A antigen on red cells so that it resembles the terminal sugar (galactose) of B antigen. This is seen in Gram-negative septicaemia, carcinoma of colon/rectum, and intestinal obstruction.
2. *Chimerism:* A blood sample containing more than one population of red cells can result from (i) transfusion of ABO-compatible but not ABO-identical blood, (ii) bone marrow transplantation (when blood group of donor is different from that of recipient), and (iii) foeto-maternal haemorrhage.
3. *Polyagglutinable red cells:* Polyagglutination (agglutination of red cells by almost all normal adult human sera) results when certain antigens (like T or Tk) are exposed on red cells following action by some microorganisms. The cells return to normal following clearance of infection.
4. *Coating of red cells by Wharton's jelly of umbilical cord:* This can cause non-specific agglutination of red cells if blood sample is collected from umbilical cord of the newborn.
5. *Weakening or loss of red cell antigens:* This can occur in malignancies like leukaemia and some solid cancers giving rise to a false negative result.
6. *Excessive amounts of blood group substances:* Certain cancers are associated with excessive amounts of blood group substances in plasma; this can inhibit anti-A and anti-B sera causing a weak or negative result.
7. *ABO subgroups:* Anti-A1 is produced by a small proportion of patients with A2 and A2B group; this antibody agglutinates A1 and A1B red cells but not A2 and A2B cells.

Table 18.2: Causes of unexpected results in blood grouping

Unexpected positive	Unexpected negative
Cell grouping	
• Acquired B antigen (gastric or colonic cancer, intestinal obstruction)	• ABO subgroup
• Bone marrow transplantation	• Antigen suppression in leukaemia or cancer
• Out-of-group transfusion	• High levels of soluble blood group substances
• Foeto-maternal haemorrhage	
• Coating of red cells by Wharton's jelly of umbilical cord	• Improperly stored antisera
• Polyagglutinable red cells	
Serum grouping	
• Cold-reacting agglutinins	• Newborns and elderly
• Monoclonal immunoglobulins	• ABO subgroup
• Transfusion of plasma components	• Hypogammaglobulinaemia
	• Immunosuppresion

Problems with serum grouping:
1. *Lack of expected antibodies:* This occurs in immunosuppression, hypogammaglobu-linaemia, neonates, and elderly.
2. *Unexpected antibodies* are observed in cold-reacting auto- or allo-antibodies, paraproteinaemia, and following transfusion of plasma components.

Causes of unexpected results in ABO grouping are listed in Table 18.2.

Rh D Grouping

Out of the various antigens of the Rh system, D antigen is the most immunogenic and therefore, red cells are routinely tested for D. Individuals with D antigen on their red cells are called as Rh-positive, while those without D antigen are called as Rh-negative. If Rh-negative individuals are transfused with Rh-positive blood, 90% of them will produce anti-D antibodies. In such sensitised individuals, re-exposure to D antigen can cause haemolytic transfusion reaction or, in pregnant women, haemolytic disease of newborn. Rh grouping is especially important in young girls and in women of reproductive age group due to the risk of Rh haemolytic disease of newborn.

Rh D grouping is done only by forward or cell grouping method. Serum or reverse grouping is not carried out because of the absence of anti-D in majority of Rh-negative persons. Anti-D antibodies are not naturally occurring and develop only after exposure to Rh D positive red cells following transfusion or pregnancy.

Method of Rh D grouping is similar in principle to ABO grouping. Since serum or reverse grouping is not possible, each sample is tested in duplicate in blood banks. Autocontrol (patient's red cells + patient's serum) and positive and negative controls are included in every test run. With polyclonal antisera, if anti-D testing is negative, further testing for weak D should be performed. Positive reaction with either labels the unit as Rh D-positive. Blood units negative with both D and weak D are labelled as Rh-negative. Monoclonal IgM anti-D antiserum should be used for cell grouping, which allows Rh grouping to be carried out at the same time as ABO grouping at room temperature. With monoclonal antisera, most weak forms of D antigen are detected and further testing for weak forms of D antigen (D^u) is not required.

Compatibility Test (Cross match)

Compatibility testing refers to a set of procedures that are carried out before issuing blood for transfusion to the patient and consists of:

1. Checking of patient's blood request form and blood bank records for reason for transfusion, history of previous transfusions, result of previous blood grouping test, any clinically significant antibodies detected, and significant adverse effects to transfusion.

2. Performing ABO and Rh grouping of patient's blood sample and checking against previous results.

3. Antibody screening and identification

4. Confirmation of ABO and Rh blood group of donor unit

5. Cross matching: This is the final serologic compatibility test. This consists of testing patient' serum against donor red cells to detect any antibodies in patient reacting with donor red cells (major cross match) and testing patient's red cells against donor serum to detect any donor antibodies reacting with patient's red cells (minor cross match). Donor blood is considered to be compatible if there is no agglutination or haemolysis in major or minor cross match.

   Cross matching is performed to:
   • Confirm compatibility between ABO blood groups of the donor and the recipient, and
   • Detect any irregular antibodies present in recipient's serum reactive against donor red cells. (Those antibodies other than anti-A and anti-B are called as irregular or unexpected antibodies. They are capable of destroying transfused red cells carrying the relevant antigen [like D, C, c, E, e, K, k, Fya, Fyb]. They may be naturally occurring or immune).

   The name 'cross match' originated from the past practice of testing the recipient's serum against donor's red cells (major cross match) and donor's serum against recipient's red cells (minor cross match). However, minor cross match is considered as less important since antibodies in donor blood unit get diluted or neutralised in recipient's plasma. Also, if antibody screening and identification is being carried out, minor cross matching is not essential.

6. Labelling of blood product with identifying information of the recipient and compatibility test result.

   Tests for cross matching are listed in Box 18.2.

Box 18.2	Tests for cross matching

- Saline test at room temperature and 37°C: For detection of clinically significant IgM antibodies
- Indirect antiglobulin test (IAT) at 37°C, low ionic strength solution test at 37°C, or enzyme-treated red cell test at 37°C: For detection of clinically significant IgG antibodies

Note: (1) If agglutination or haemolysis is not observed in any of the above stages, donor unit is considered to be compatible with recipient's serum. Agglutination or haemolysis at any stage is indicative of incompatibility. (2) The commonly used major cross match test is a saline test at 37°C followed by conversion to IAT at 37°C.

The aim of compatibility testing is to prevent haemolytic transfusion reaction in the recipient. Before compatibility testing, ABO and Rh groups of the recipient are determined and group-compatible donor blood is selected. (In well-equipped blood banks, antibody screening of donor and recipient's blood is also carried out before cross matching to detect unexpected or irregular antibodies).

A single tube cross match consisting of three stages is recommended. Recipient's serum is tested against donor's red cells under three different conditions; agglutination or haemolysis in any one of the three stages indicates incompatibility. The three stages of compatibility test are as follows:

- Compatibility test at room temperature
- Compatibility test at 37° C
- Indirect antiglobulin test

1. **Compatibility test at room temperature (Immediate spin cross match):** The purpose of this test is to detect ABO incompatibility. Saline-suspended red cells of the donor and recipient's serum are mixed in a test tube, incubated briefly at room temperature, and centrifuged. Agglutination or haemolysis indicates incompatibility. If agglutination or haemolysis is absent, next step is performed.

2. **Compatibility test at 37°C:** The above test tube is incubated at 37° C for 20 minutes, centrifuged again, and examined for agglutination. If absent, perform the last stage.

3. **Indirect antiglobulin test:** The above mixture is incubated at 37° C for 30-60 minutes, washed in saline, and antiglobulin reagent is added. Following re-centrifugation, examine for agglutination or haemolysis. This test detects most of the clinically significant IgG antibodies. Principle of antiglobulin test has been described earlier in chapter on "Immune haemolytic anaemias".

If agglutination or haemolysis is not observed in any of the above stages, donor unit is considered to be compatible with recipient's serum. Agglutination or haemolysis at any stage is indicative of incompatibility.

False Reactions in Compatibility Testing

1. Autoagglutination: If autoantibodies are present in the recipient's serum, they can cause agglutination of recipient's own red cells as well as red cells of all donors. Autoantibodies are usually cold-reacting, and therefore, agglutination will be observed in saline stage at room temperature. To distinguish whether agglutination is due to auto- or alloantibodies, an auto control test is usually set up simultaneously.

If autoantibodies are present, agglutination will also be observed in autocontrol. If agglutination disappears by keeping the tube at 37°C for 10 minutes, presence of cold agglutinins is confirmed.

2. Rouleaux formation: Rouleaux may be mistaken for agglutination. Rouleaux has a characteristic 'stack of coins' appearance when seen under the microscope. Rouleaux (seen in multiple myeloma and after administration of dextran) disappear after addition of a drop of saline to the slide.

Limitations of Cross Match

Cross matching will not prevent sensitisation of recipient to new red cell antigens. This is because only those red cell antigens are detected for which corresponding antibodies are present in the recipient's serum. Also, all ABO and Rh grouping errors will not be detected.

Emergency Cross Match

If blood is required urgently, ABO and Rh grouping are carried out by rapid slide test and immediate spin cross match (saline test) is performed (to exclude ABO incompatibility). If the blood unit is compatible, then after issuing it, remaining stages of the cross match are completed. If any incompatibility is detected in these two tests, the concerned physician is immediately notified and transfusion is discontinued.

Antibody Screening and Identification

Screening for unexpected or irregular antibodies is carried out before transfusion in recipient's serum and in donor's blood (and during antenatal period in women). Sera of majority of recipients do not contain unexpected antibodies and are compatible with donor blood of same ABO and Rh type. Only about 1 to 3% of recipients demonstrate irregular antibodies for whom selection of blood lacking the corresponding red cell antigen is essential.

Antenatal patients should be screened for antibodies apart from anti-D, which can cause haemolytic disease of newborn (e.g. anti-c, anti-Kell, etc.). For antibody screening, serum of the recipient is tested against a set of three group O screening red cells of known antigenic type. Agglutination or haemolysis indicates presence of antibody reactive against red cell antigen.

❑ MICROBIOLOGIC TECHNIQUES

Microbiological agents that can be transmitted through transfusion are listed in Table 22.2. Donor blood should be screened for those pathogenic organisms that are frequent in a particular geographic region and which are transmissible by transfusion. In India, currently, it is mandatory to screen donor blood for following organisms:

- Hepatitis B virus
- Hepatitis C virus
- Human immunodeficiency virus types 1 and 2
- Syphilis
- Malaria

Hepatitis B Virus (HBV)

Blood samples from all donations are routinely tested for hepatitis B surface antigen (HbsAg). This antigen was previously called as 'Australia antigen' because it was first detected in the serum of an Australian aborigine. Screening of all blood donations for HbsAg has greatly reduced the risk of transmission of HBV through transfusion; the risk, however, is not completely eliminated. HbsAg-negative donor may transmit HBV when blood is collected in early incubation period or when very low levels of HbsAg, not detectable by presently employed methods, are present. This possibility, however, is very small.

An individual who has received HBV vaccine will have hepatitis B surface antibody but not HBSAg in blood.

Tests for screening donor blood for HbsAg are:
- Reverse passive haemagglutination assay (RPHA)
- Enzyme-linked immunosorbent assay (ELISA)
- Radioimmunoassay (RIA)

Commercial test kits for detection of HbsAg are available and the exact test procedure is provided with each kit. General principles of these tests are outlined below.

Reverse passive haemagglutination assay: In RPHA, red cells that are coated with anti-HBs antibody are mixed with donor's serum. If HbsAg is present in the serum, it will bind to the red cells and induce agglutination. Lack of agglutination indicates negative test. The test is called as 'reverse' agglutination because antibody, and not antigen, is coated on to the red cells. The test is called as 'passive' because the anti-HbsAg antibody coated onto the red cells is not an intrinsic component of the red cells and is coated onto the red cells artificially. The test is performed in U- or V-shaped wells of a microtitre plate.

Enzyme-linked immunosorbent assay: Serum sample to be tested is added to a well of the microtitre plate (which has been coated with anti-HbsAg antibody). A microtitre plate, wells of which have been pre-coated with anti-HBs, is called as solid phase support system. This is followed by a period of incubation (specified by the manufacturer) during which binding of antigen from serum (if present) and antibody (attached to the well) occurs. Washing of the solid phase removes the unbound antigen but not the antigen bound to the antibody on the surface of the well. This is followed by the addition of an enzyme-linked anti-HBs antibody (called as conjugate), which will combine with the bound antigen. After further incubation, a second wash is given to remove any unbound conjugate. A chromogenic substrate (for the enzyme) is then added and the mixture is incubated in the dark. If enzyme is present (bound to the antigen), then its action on the substrate will lead to the colour development. A stopping solution (an acid) is added to prevent any further reaction between the enzyme and the substrate. The result is read in a spectrophotometer at the specified wavelength. The cut-off value is obtained from the absorbance of negative and low positive controls (negative control + [low positive control × 0.2]). If the absorbance of test sample is greater than the cut-off value, the sample is considered as positive for HbsAg.

Radioimmunoassay: In principle, RIA is similar to ELISA. Serum samples to be tested are added to the wells of the microplate, which have been coated with anti-HBs antibody. If HbsAg is present in the test serum, it will bind to the coated antibody. This is followed by addition of radioactive iodine (I^{125})-linked anti-HBs antibody. A gamma counter measures the amount of bound radiolabelled anti-HBs. The mean for negative controls is also calculated. If the value of the test sample exceeds that of mean for negative controls, the sample is positive for HbsAg.

Hepatitis C Virus (HCV)

Amount of HCV antigen released in blood stream is small and cannot be detected readily. Therefore, screening of donor blood for HCV infection relies on detection of anti-HCV antibody in serum (which becomes detectable after 6 to 8 weeks of infection).

ELISA test for anti-HCV antibody is available from various commercial manufacturers. Sensitivity and specificity of these tests are variable. The earlier tests (first generation ELISAs) used recombinant proteins complementary to the NS4 region of the HCV genome. Second generation ELISAs incorporated recombinant or synthetic antigens from NS4 as well as NS3 regions of the genome, resulting in improvement in sensitivity and specificity over first generation tests. The third generation ELISAs, in addition to NS3 and NS4, also include antigens from NS5 region.

ELISA test for detection of antibody to HCV is expensive. It can detect about 95% of chronic infections and 50 to 70% of acute infections. False positive reactions are also known to occur. In clinical practice (but not in transfusion practice), a positive ELISA screening test for HCV needs to be confirmed by a recombinant immunoblot assay (RIBA) or by polymerase chain reaction.

Human Immunodeficiency Virus (HIV)

All blood units are routinely tested for antibodies against HIV-1 and HIV-2. Although many tests are available for detection of anti-HIV antibodies, ELISA test is usually employed for screening of blood donors.

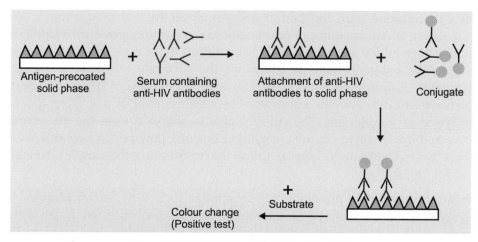

Figure 18.6: Principle of ELISA test for HIV

Enzyme-linked Immunosorbent Assay (ELISA)

In antiglobulin or indirect ELISA, serum to be tested is added to microwells of a microtitre plate, which have been coated with HIV antigens. If anti-HIV antibodies are present in the test serum, they will bind to antigens. After washing which removes unbound material, antihuman globulin antibody coupled to an enzyme is added which attaches to HIV antibodies. An appropriate enzyme substrate is added which gives a colour reaction. The intensity of colour developed is read in a spectrophotometer (Fig. 18.6).

Syphilis

Screening of donor blood for antibody to *Treponema pallidum* is usually carried out by Venereal Disease Research Laboratory (VDRL) test. In this non-specific test, donor serum (which has been heated to 56°C to inactivate the complement) is mixed with cardiolipin-lecithin-cholesterol antigen. If flocculation is observed, the test is reported as reactive.

Malaria Parasite

Sensitivity of blood smear for detection of malaria parasite is low. At least 100 parasites/µl of blood should be present for them to be detected on the blood smear.

❏ BIBLIOGRAPHY

1. Cheesbrough M. District Laboratory practice in Tropical Countries. Part 2. Cambridge. Cambridge University Press. 2000.
2. World Health Organization. Manual of Basic Techniques for a Health Laboratory. 2nd ed. Geneva. World Health Organization. 2003.

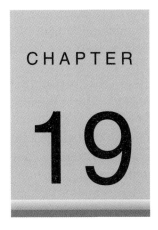

CHAPTER

19

Collection of Donor Blood, Processing and Storage

Collection of blood is a process whereby one unit (350 ml) of whole blood is collected from a suitable donor in an anticoagulant solution. Since all blood components and blood products are obtained from donor blood, safe transfusion practice begins with the proper selection of blood donors.

Risk of transmission of infectious diseases through transfusion depends on incidence and prevalence of infections in the blood donor population, effectiveness of donor selection process, and use of sensitive screening tests for infectious diseases.

A national comprehensive blood transfusion policy and a voluntary blood donation programme, should be implemented, which will serve as a foundation for safe blood supply. Blood donation should be entirely voluntary and non-remunerated.

❑ TYPES OF BLOOD DONORS

There are three main types of blood donors:
- Voluntary
- Professional
- Replacement

A **voluntary blood donor** donates blood out of his/her own free will and does not expect to receive any financial or other reward as an alternative to money. Voluntary donors donate blood on humanitarian grounds or out of sense of duty or responsibility towards community. Voluntary donors have lower incidence and prevalence of infections transmissible by transfusion as compared to paid or replacement donors. Since there is no monetary gain, they are not likely to hide any significant information or high-risk behaviour through which they might have been infected with transmissible micro-organisms. Voluntary donors often donate blood on regular basis, which helps in maintaining adequate blood supply. Voluntary blood donors are also more likely to come forward in response to an appeal for blood donation in an emergency.

Paid or professional donors donate blood for financial gain or other benefit that can be substituted for money. They donate blood solely for money and not because of any sense of duty or social commitment. Most of these blood sellers are alcoholics and drug abusers and sell their blood to earn money to engage in these vices. Paid donors have a very high incidence of infections transmissible by transfusion. They often donate blood at short intervals that puts them at risk of iron deficiency anaemia. Because of monetary benefit, they also conceal important medical information or their high-risk behaviour.

A **replacement blood donor** is a friend or a relative of the recipient whose donated blood unit is credited to the patient. Blood unit that has been donated replaces the blood unit used for the patient. The practice of replacement donation is carried out in many blood banks since blood supply through voluntary donation falls short of requirements. Replacement donation, however, is less suitable than voluntary donation. If relatives of the patient are unable to find a suitable blood donor known to them, they search for professional donors in order to meet the requirement. Also, because of pressure, replacement donor may hide significant medical information.

Directed donors are types of replacement donors who specifically request that their blood be given to a named patient; this is probably because of concerns regarding safety of blood from unknown donors. However, directed donation from mother to her child can induce transfusion-associated lung injury (due to formation in the mother of HLA antibodies to foetal antigens during pregnancy). Also, transfusion of blood from close relatives to prospective recipients of haematopoietic stem cell transplant carries the risk of HLA immunisation and graft rejection.

Practice of replacement donation is helpful where voluntary donation is inadequate. However, this practice is stressful for patient's relatives who have to find replacement donors at a time when they are already under stress due to patient's illness. Blood needs of the patient may not be met as the amount of blood donated may fall short of requirements.

❑ CRITERIA FOR SELECTION OF BLOOD DONORS

Careful selection of blood donors is an essential requirement for safe transfusion practice. It is necessary to ensure well-being of both the donor and the recipient.

Selection of blood donors should be carried out by a qualified physician or by a person working under his supervision.

Donor selection process consists of four parts:
- Predonation counselling
- Medical history
- Physical examination
- Haemoglobin estimation

The prospective donor should be assured that the personal information revealed shall be kept confidential.

Criteria for selection of blood donors are given below in short.

Predonation Counselling

This is an education programme in which information about health condition, high-risk behaviour, self-exclusion/self-deferral, and procedures involved in blood donation is given, donor's questions are answered, informed consent is obtained, and reassurance is given in case of anxiety.

Medical History

Age

The lower and higher age limits for blood donation are 18 and 60 years, respectively. These age limits are set because of -
- Age of consent and increased iron needs of the adolescents
- Risk of cardiovascular and cerebrovascular disease in old age following removal of large quantity of blood.

Donation Interval

The interval between two consecutive blood donations should be at least three months. This is to avoid iron depletion in the donor.

Volume of Donation

An individual weighing 45 kg or more can safely donate blood up to 350 ml. This limit intends to preclude the risk of vasovagal attack.

Pregnancy and Lactation

Pregnant women and lactating mothers (up to 1 year post-partum) should not donate blood.

Infectious Diseases

HIV-1 and HIV-2: Blood should not be collected from donors who give history suggestive of HIV infection (unexplained fever, weight loss, swollen lymph nodes, uncontrolled diarrhoea, or unusual skin lesions).

To eliminate the "window period" (early antibody-negative period in individuals infected with HIV) donations, individuals who have been exposed to the risk of HIV infection should be requested not to donate blood (such as homosexuals; intravenous drug abusers; or individuals having contact with commercial sex workers, with multiple sexual partners, or with known AIDS or HIV positive persons). Intention of this policy of "self-exclusion" of high-risk donors is elimination of donors in early (HIV antibody-negative) stage of HIV infection. Such individuals can be offered the choice of HIV antibody testing and counselling.

Hepatitis

An individual with history of jaundice within last 1 year or a positive test for HBsAg or anti-HCV antibodies should not be accepted for blood donation.

Malaria

In endemic areas, a donor may be accepted after 3 months of asymptomatic period following malarial attack and after full treatment.

Illness

Individuals with diabetes mellitus, hypertension, heart disease, renal disease, liver disease, lung disease, cancer, epilepsy, bleeding disorder, or allergic disease are not accepted.

Drugs

Many donors who are taking drugs are excluded because of their underlying disease. Other donors are excluded because of the nature of the drug they are taking, e.g. aspirin or other non-steroidal inflammatory drugs (which affect platelet function), and drugs with teratogenic action like finasteride, isotretinoin, acitretin, and etretinate, or cytotoxic drugs (like cyclophosphamide). Patients receiving human pituitary-derived growth hormone are permanently unfit due to the risk of Creutzfeldt-Jakob disease.

Dentistry

Due to the possibility of bacteraemia following tooth extraction or fillings, a 72-hour deferral period before donation is necessary.

Skin Piercing

Donors with history of tattooing, electrolysis, ear piercing, accidental needle stick in health care workers, or acupuncture during last 12 months should not be accepted.

Blood Transfusion

A person should not be accepted as blood donor for 6 months after receiving blood transfusion.

Immunisation

Donors who have received killed viral vaccines are acceptable as blood donors. Nature of vaccine received and respective deferral period are as follows.
- Attenuated live virus vaccine for measles, mumps, yellow fever, Sabin polio: 2 weeks
- German measles: 4 weeks
- Rabies: 1 year
- Passive immunisation with animal sera: 4 weeks
- Hepatitis B immune globulin: 1 year.

Physical Examination

This should consist of
- Weight: should be minimum 45 kg
- Blood pressure: Systolic blood pressure should be 100 to 180 mm of Hg and diastolic 50 to 100 mm of Hg
- Pulse: Pulse rate should be 50 to 100/min and regular
- Temperature: should be normal.
  Donor should be in good general health. Inspect donor's arms for possible evidence of intravenous drug abuse such as scars or infection at venepuncture site. Clinical examination of cardiovascular system, respiratory system, and abdomen should be normal.

Laboratory Test for Anaemia

Screening of donors for anaemia in blood bank is done by copper sulphate specific gravity method. This method is as follows.
  A drop of blood is allowed to fall in copper sulphate solution of specific gravity 1.053 from a height of 1 cm. Specific gravity of 1.053 is equivalent to haemoglobin concentration of 12.5 g/dl. The drop of blood gets covered with copper proteinate and remains discrete for 15 to 20 seconds. If the drop sinks within this time, its specific gravity is higher than that of copper sulphate solution (i.e. haemoglobin is >12.5 g/dl) and haemoglobin level is acceptable for donation. If it floats, haemoglobin level is unacceptable. However, specific gravity of whole blood is also affected by total

leucocyte count and concentration of plasma proteins. In the presence of leucocytosis (e.g. as in chronic myeloid leukaemia) or hypergammaglobulinaemia (e.g. multiple myeloma), haemoglobin value will be misleadingly high.

❑ COLLECTION OF DONOR BLOOD

In the blood bank, donor blood should be collected in a well-ventilated, hygienic, and air-conditioned room. Donor should be bled by a qualified physician or by an assistant who is well trained and is working under his supervision.

Equipments and Materials

1. Blood bag: Blood from a donor is collected in a sterile, disposable plastic bag (single, double, triple, or quadruple bag system) with capacity to hold 350 ml of blood. These bags contain a standard amount of anticoagulant preservative solution for specified amount of blood. Whole blood transfusion is still practiced in many blood banks, and therefore single bag is the most common type of blood bag used. Double, triple, and quadruple bag systems are used at places where facilities for separation of components are available.
2. Anticoagulant-preservative solution: The solution in the blood bag usually contains citrate phosphate dextrose adenine (CPDA)-1 (49 ml for 350 ml of blood). This solution prevents clotting of blood and also provides nutrients to maintain metabolism and viability of red cells. In CPDA-1, blood can be kept stored at 2 to 6°C for maximum of 35 days. Function of each component of this solution is as follows:
   • Citrate: Anticoagulation by binding of calcium in plasma
   • Phosphate: Acts as a buffer to minimise the effects of decreasing pH in blood
   • Dextrose: Maintenance of red cell membrane and metabolism
   • Adenine: Generation of ATP (energy source).
3. Sphygmomanometer, weighing balance, sealing clips or sealer, artery forceps.
4. 70% ethanol, sterile cotton gauze, adhesive tape
5. Emergency drugs and equipment
6. Blood tubes for collection of blood for testing (grouping, cross matching, screening for infectious diseases).

Technique

Blood bag should be labelled with the identification number of the donor before withdrawal of blood.

Blood is collected from a vein in the antecubital fossa. To make the veins prominent and palpable, a sphygmomanometer cuff is applied to the arm and inflated to 60 to 80 mm of Hg. The area selected for venepuncture is thoroughly cleansed with 70% ethanol and allowed to dry.

The blood collection bag is placed on a weighing balance that has been kept about 30 cm below the level of the arm. A loose knot is tied in the tubing near the venepuncture needle.

Venepuncture is performed, and the needle is secured in place with an adhesive tape after ensuring free flow of blood.

The pressure is reduced to 40 to 60 mm of Hg. The donor is asked to squeeze a rubber ball or a similar object slowly for the duration of donation. The blood and the anticoagulant are mixed at short intervals in the blood bag. The amount of blood collected should be monitored on the weighing balance. When the blood bag weighs 400 to 450 g, the required amount of blood has been collected.

The pressure cuff is completely deflated and the tubing is clamped with forceps about 10 cm away from the needle. The knot made earlier (close to the needle) is tightened or a sealing clip is applied.

The tubing is cut between the clamp and the knot/sealing clip. The clamp is removed from the tubing and blood samples (for grouping, cross matching, infectious disease screening) are collected in appropriate tubes. The tubing is then reclamped.

Needle is removed from the vein and pressure is applied over the puncture site with sterile cotton gauze. The needle is disposed of in a special "sharps" container.

Blood remaining in the tubing is non-anticoagulated and is forced back ('stripped') into the blood bag. Bag is inverted gently several times to mix the blood and the anticoagulant. Anticoagulated blood is then allowed to run back into the tubing.

Time required for blood collection should be between 7 to 10 minutes.

Blood sample tubes should be labelled with the donor identification number.

After cessation of bleeding, the venepuncture site is covered with sterile gauze and an adhesive tape. After a few minutes, the donor is allowed to sit up and taken to the refreshment area, where liquids are given. The donor is thanked for donation and is issued a donation card. Donor is given information about need to drink fluids, activities permissible, and care of venepuncture site.

Blood bag is stored in the refrigerator at 2 to 6°C.

At no time during the donation period, donor should be left unattended.

Donor Reactions

Occurrence of donor reactions is rare. One relatively common problem is a fainting attack or loss of consciousness due to sudden deprivation of blood supply to the brain *(syncope or vasovagal attack)*. It is due to the action of the autonomic nervous system and is induced by anxiety, sight of blood, or pain. Its features are sweating, slowing of pulse rate, pallor, coldness of skin, sudden hypotension, and sometimes fainting or vomiting. In such a case, donation should be discontinued. Legs should be elevated above the level of the head to augment the venous return and increase blood flow to the brain. Oral fluids are given if the donor is conscious. If there is prolonged hypotension, intravenous fluids may have to be administered. A severe vasovagal reaction is a contraindication for future donations.

Table 19.1: Tests done on donor blood

- Grouping
  - ABO grouping—cell and serum grouping
  - RhD grouping
- Screening and identification of unexpected antibodies
- Screening tests for infectious organisms
  - Hepatitis B surface antigen
  - Anti-HCV antibodies
  - HIV-1 and HIV-2 antibodies
  - VDRL test
  - Blood smear for malaria parasite

If the donor is highly apprehensive, he may hyperventilate which may cause excessive loss of carbon dioxide and respiratory alkalosis. This may result in tonic-clonic muscle contractions. **Hyperventilation** can be corrected by breathing in a paper bag.

Other reactions include formation of a bruise, haematoma, infection at venepuncture site, thrombophlebitis, and puncture of an artery.

It is necessary to mention occurrence of any adverse reaction on the card issued to the donor.

❏ PROCESSING OF DONOR BLOOD

This refers to various tests and procedures carried out on the donor blood after collection but prior to cross matching. Tests done on donor blood are listed in Table 19.1.

❏ STORAGE OF DONOR BLOOD UNIT

Whole blood is stored at a temperature between 2° to 6°C in a refrigerator specifically designed for blood storage. These temperature limits are set because:
- At temperatures below 2°C, freezing and lysis of red cells will occur; transfusion of such haemolysed blood will lead to disseminated intravascular coagulation and acute renal failure in the recipient
- Proliferation of any contaminating bacteria, which may have gained entry during venepuncture, is kept at a minimum level (up to 6° C)
- Glycolysis in red blood cells is kept at a minimum level in this temperature range so that dextrose in anticoagulant preservative solution is not utilised rapidly.

Changes which Occur in Stored Blood

Certain changes occur in blood with increasing duration of storage. These are:
- **Loss of viability of red cells:** Viability refers to the ability of red blood cells to survive following transfusion in recipient's circulation. It gradually decreases

with increasing length of storage. A proportion of red cells are removed from the circulation within the first 24 hours post-transfusion. Storage conditions should be such that, after transfusion, at least 75% of transfused red cells should survive at 24 hours in the recipient's circulation. Shelf-life of the stored whole blood is based on this criterion. For whole blood stored in CPDA-1 and maintained at 2° to 6°C, shelf-life is 35 days.

- **Loss of ATP:** Loss of ATP (energy source) occurs with increasing duration of storage leading to spherocytic shape change, membrane lipid loss, and increasing rigidity. Such cells have reduced survival. Adenine in CPDA-1 solution provides ATP and improves viability of red cells.
- **Depletion of 2,3-diphosphoglycerate (2,3-DPG):** Appropriate levels of 2,3-DPG in red cells are essential for a low oxygen affinity of haemoglobin and ready release of oxygen to the tissues. Progressive reduction of 2,3-DPG with storage increases oxygen affinity and reduces release of oxygen at tissue level. Restoration of 2,3-DPG in red cells occurs within 24 hours of transfusion; therefore, depleted 2,3-DPG levels are likely to be of significance mainly in patients with severe anaemia.
- **Loss of granulocyte function** occurs within 24 hours and **loss of platelet function** occurs within 48 hours of blood collection.
- **Decrease in pH of blood**
- **Increase in plasma potassium level**
- **Decrease in Factor VIII level** to 10 to 20% of normal occurs within 48 hours of blood collection
- **Formation of microaggregates:** In stored blood, tiny aggregates of cell debris, aged platelets, leucocytes, fibrin strands, and cold insoluble globulin form.

❏ BIBLIOGRAPHY

1. Cheesbrough M. District Laboratory Practice in Tropical Countries. Part 2. Cambridge. Cambridge University Press. 2000.
2. Saran RK, Makroo RN. Transfusion Medicine Technical Manual. Directorate General of Health Services. 1991.

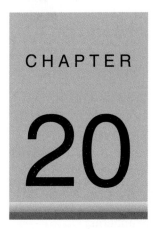

CHAPTER

20

Whole Blood, Blood Components and Blood Derivatives

In the past whole blood was the only preparation that could be administered to replace red cells, platelets, coagulation factors, etc. in a patient. In addition to what patient required, this caused unnecessary administration of unwanted cell or plasma constituents. Large volume of whole blood needed to achieve satisfactory replacement of a particular component also posed an important limitation. A significant advance in transfusion medicine was made when techniques became available for separation of blood components in a closed system and patient could be administered specific replacement therapy. One unit of donor blood can be utilised for preparation of different components and thus can benefit more than one patient. Nowadays, whole blood can be separated into various blood components and further derivatives can be obtained from plasma by fractionation (Table 20.1 and Fig. 20.1). This permits administration of specific replacement therapy as per the patient's requirements, and avoids transfusion of unwanted constituents of blood. One unit of donor blood can benefit more than one patient after its separation into plasma, red cell, and platelet components.

Separation of blood components from one another by centrifugation is possible due to differences in their specific gravities. Preparation of blood components has been greatly facilitated by the introduction of double and triple bags having closed integral tubing. After their separation, various components can be transferred from one bag to another in a closed circuit thus maintaining the sterility (Fig. 20.2). Venepuncture should be clean with little trauma to tissues. Blood and anticoagulant should be mixed

Table 20.1: Blood products

Whole blood
One unit of donor blood collected in a suitable anticoagulant-preservative solution and which contains blood cells and plasma.

Blood components
A constituent separated from whole blood, by differential centrifugation of one donor unit or by apheresis.

Blood derivatives
A product obtained from multiple donor units of plasma by fractionation.

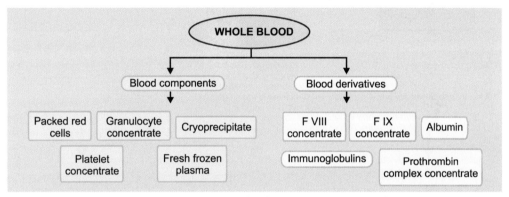

Figure 20.1: Blood components and derivatives that can be made from whole blood

constantly, and blood collection should be completed within 8 to 10 minutes. Blood should be processed for component separation within 6 hours of collection.

❏ WHOLE BLOOD

Whole blood still remains a commonly employed blood product at some places because of the lack of facility for component separation.

Whole blood is one unit of donor blood collected in a suitable anticoagulant-preservative solution. Its total volume is about 400 ml (350 ml of blood + 49 ml of anticoagulant). It consists of cellular elements and plasma. Whole blood is stored in a properly maintained blood bank refrigerator at 2° to 6°C and shelf-life of such blood (collected in CPDA anticoagulant) is 35 days (Box 20.1).

Before ordering whole blood transfusion, following should be noted:
• Transfusion of one unit raises haemoglobin by 1 g/dl or haematocrit by 3%.
• Whole blood stored at 2° to 6°C does not contain functionally effective platelets after 48 hours of collection and also labile coagulation factors (i.e. F V and F VIII). Therefore stored whole blood should not be used to replace platelets, granulocytes, or coagulation factors.
• Whole blood transfusion is associated with the risk of volume overload in patients with chronic severe anaemia and compromised cardiovascular function.

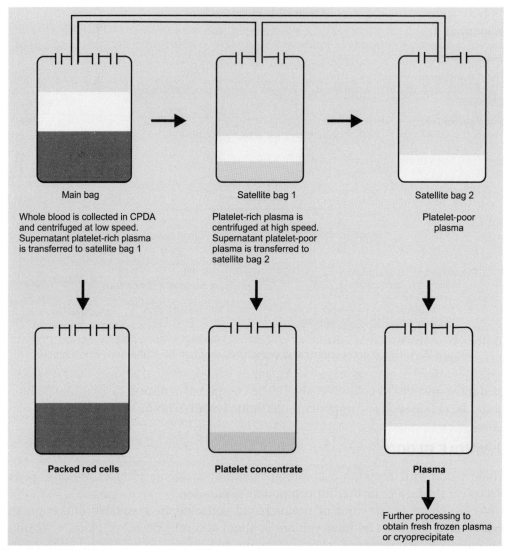

Figure 20.2: Principle of preparation of blood components from a single unit of whole blood. Packed red cells, platelet concentrate, and plasma thus obtained can be utilised for three different patients

Box 20.1	Whole blood

- One unit of blood collected in a suitable anticoagulant solution
- Haematocrit 35–45% and haemoglobin 12.0 g/dl
- Contains no functionally effective platelets and no labile coagulation factors
- Storage temperature: 2–6°C in appropriate blood bank refrigerator
- Shelf-life: 35 days (in CPDA-1)
- Indication: Acute massive blood loss, exchange transfusion, non-availability of packed red cells
- Risk of volume overload in patients with chronic anaemia and compromised cardiovascular function.

Transfusion of whole blood to the recipient should commence within 30 minutes of removing the blood bag from the refrigerator and should be completed within maximum of 4 hours of starting transfusion.

Many times, the clinician requests 'fresh' blood (i.e. one which is less than 24 hours old). After collection, blood can be issued only after all the necessary tests are completed (which may take 24 hours). Such 'fresh' blood can be utilised for infants, thalassaemics (who need red cells with maximal survival), and bleeding disorders (since platelets and labile coagulation factors become functionally ineffective after 48 hours of storage). However, if available, packed red cells, plasma components, or platelet concentrates are more effective and preferred forms of therapy for such patients.

In this era of blood component therapy, the only indication for whole blood transfusion is acute massive blood loss, i.e. correction of both hypovolaemia and red cell mass. (In these patients also, packed red cells along with a crystalloid solution are preferable). For all other indications, specific component therapy is administered.

❏ BLOOD COMPONENTS

Blood components can be separated from one another by centrifugation due to differences in their specific gravities. Separation of blood components is carried in double or triple bags with closed integral tubing. After collection from donor, blood should be processed for component separation within 6 hours. Blood components are listed in Table 20.2. Storage temperatures and duration of storage of some blood products are shown in Box 20.2.

Red Cell Components

Packed Red Cells

Packed red cells are prepared by removing most of the plasma from one unit of whole blood. Whole blood is either allowed to sediment overnight in a refrigerator at 2° to 6°C or is spun in a refrigerated centrifuge. Supernatant plasma is then separated from red cells in a closed system by transferring it to the attached empty satellite bag. Red cells and a small amount of plasma are left behind in the primary blood bag.

Table 20.2: Blood components

Red cells
- Packed red cells
- Red cells in additive solution
- Leucocyte-poor red cells
- Washed red cells
- Frozen red cells
- Irradiated red cells

Platelets
- Platelet concentrate

Granulocytes
- Granulocyte concentrate

Plasma
- Fresh frozen plasma
- Cryoprecipitate

Box 20.2	Temperature and duration of storage of blood products

- Whole blood, packed red cells: 2–6°C for 35 days
- Platelet concentrates: 20–24°C for 3 days with continuous agitation
- Fresh frozen plasma: Below –25°C for 1 year
- Cryoprecipitate: Below –25°C for 1 year

Main indication for packed red cells is replacement of red cells in anaemia (chronic anaemia, severe anaemia with congestive cardiac failure, anaemia in elderly).

Transfusion of packed red cells lowers the risk of volume overload. In contrast to whole blood, for a given volume, double the amount of red cells can be infused, i.e. total volume of whole blood is 400 ml (150 ml red cells + 250 ml plasma) while that of packed red cells is 250 ml (150 ml red cells + 100 ml plasma). Haematocrit of whole blood is about 40% while that of packed red cells is 55 to 75%. Normal saline can be added using Y-pattern infusion set to increase the speed of transfusion by reducing the viscosity. Packed red cells have a high viscosity and therefore the rate of infusion is slow.

Transfusion of one unit of red cells increases haemoglobin by 1 g% (or increases PCV by 3%). This rise becomes detectable 24 hours after transfusion (Box 20.3).

Red Cells in Additive Solution (Red cell suspension)

Commonly used additive solution is SAGM (which contains saline, adenine, glucose, and mannitol). After collection of whole blood in the primary collection bag (containing CPDA-1), maximum amount of plasma is removed (after centrifugation) and transferred to one satellite bag. The additive solution from the second satellite bag is transferred into the primary collection bag (containing packed red cells) in a closed circuit.

Advantages of this method are :
- Maximum amount of plasma can be removed for preparation of plasma components
- Red cells with improved viability are obtained (shelf-life increases from 35 days to 42 days)
- Flow of infusion is improved due to reduction in viscosity.

Indications for red cells in SAGM are similar to those for packed red cells. Red cells in SAGM are contraindicated for exchange transfusion in neonates.

Leucocyte-poor red Cells

These are the red cells from which most of the white cells have been removed. By definition, leucocyte-depleted red cells should contain less than 5×10^6 white cells per bag. They are obtained by passing blood through a special leucocyte-depletion filter at the time of transfusion; they can also be prepared in the blood bank.

Box 20.3 Packed red cells (Red cell concentrate)

- Red cells from which most of plasma has been removed
- Haematocrit 55–75% or haemoglobin 20 g/dl
- Raises haemoglobin by 1 g% or haematocrit by 3%
- Storage temperature: 2°–6°C and shelf-life 35 days (in CPDA)
- Indication: Replacement of red cells in anaemia and in acute/massive blood loss (along with crystalloid or colloid)
- Volume: 250 ml

Leucocyte-poor red cells are indicated:
- To avoid sensitisation to HLA antigens (e.g. in patients with severe aplastic anaemia who are likely to receive allogeneic bone marrow transplant)
- To avoid febrile transfusion reactions in persons who require repeated transfusions or who have earlier been sensitised to white cell antigens
- To reduce the risk of transmission of cytomegalovirus (CMV) in certain patients (if CMV-seronegative blood is not available)
  Leucocyte-depleted red cells cannot prevent graft-versus-host disease.

Washed Red Cells

Packed red cells can be washed with normal saline to remove plasma proteins, white cells, and platelets. Use of such red cells is restricted for IgA-deficient individuals who have developed anti-IgA antibodies.

Frozen Red Cells

Red cells can be stored frozen for up to 10 years. To prevent haemolysis of red cells during freezing and thawing, a cryoprotective agent such as glycerol is added. Donor red cells with rare blood groups can be stored frozen for recipients who have developed antibodies against frequently-occurring red cell antigens. Similarly, red cells can be stored frozen for future autologous transfusion, if blood group is rare. Before transfusion, red cells are thawed and glycerol removed gradually by using progressively less hypertonic solutions. Such red cells are virtually free from leucocytes, platelets, and plasma and thus their use is associated with low-risk of nonhaemolytic transfusion reactions.

Irradiated Red Cells

Transfusion of gamma-irradiated red cells is indicated for prevention of graft-versus-host disease in susceptible individuals like:
- Immunodeficient individuals, and
- Patients receiving blood from first-degree relatives.

Lymphocytes from donor blood react against the tissues of the recipient. Gamma irradiation (25 Gy) inhibits replication of donor lymphocytes.

Platelets

There are two methods for obtaining platelets (Box 20.4) for transfusion:
- Differential centrifugation of a unit of whole blood (platelet concentrate).
- Plateletpheresis (Box 20.5 for principle of pheresis).

> **Box 20.4** Platelets
>
> - Obtained either from single donor units of whole blood by centrifugation or by plateletpheresis
> - Platelets prepared from whole blood donation are supplied either as a single unit or as a pooled unit (i.e. platelets obtained from 4–6 donor whole blood units are 'pooled' together in one bag). Platelets obtained from plateletpheresis are supplied as one pack of single donor platelets.
> - Storage: 20–24°C with constant agitation up to 72 hours.
> - Common indications are thrombocytopaenia due to decreased platelet production and hereditary platelet function defect.

> **Box 20.5** Pheresis
>
> - Donor pheresis is a procedure in which a suitable donor is connected to an automated cell separator machine through which whole blood is withdrawn, the desired blood component is retained, and the remainder of the blood is returned back to the donor. Depending on the component that is separated and removed, the procedure is called as plateletpheresis, leucapheresis, or plasmapheresis.
> - Therapeutic pheresis consists of removing the undesirable blood component and returning the remaining blood portion to the patient's circulation. The undesirable component is discarded. Examples are therapeutic plasmapheresis in hyperviscosity syndrome in plasma cell dyscrasias, and leucapheresis in hyperleucocytosis in AML or CML.

Platelet Concentrate (Random Donor Platelets)

Platelet concentrate is prepared by differential centrifugation of one unit of whole blood within 6 hours of donation and before refrigeration. One unit of whole blood is centrifuged at low speed to obtain platelet-rich plasma (PRP). PRP is then transferred to the attached satellite bag and spun at high speed to get platelet aggregates (at the bottom) and platelet-poor plasma or PPP (at the top). Most of the PPP is returned back to the primary collection bag or to another satellite bag, leaving behind 50 to 60 ml of PPP with the platelets.

Platelets are stored at 20° to 24°C with continuous agitation (in a storage device called platelet agitator). Maximum period of storage is 3 to 5 days.

One unit of platelet concentrate contains $>45 \times 10^9$ platelets. Transfusion of one unit will raise the platelet count in the recipient by about 5000/μl.

The usual adult dose is 4 to 6 units of platelet concentrate (or 1 unit/10 kg of body weight). These units (which are from different donors) are pooled into one bag before transfusion. This dose will raise the platelet count by 20,000 to 40,000/μl.

Plateletpheresis (Single donor platelets)

In plateletpheresis, a donor is connected to a blood cell separator machine in which whole blood is collected in an anticoagulant solution, platelets are separated and retained, and remaining components are returned back to the donor. With this method, a large number of platelets can be obtained from a single donor (equivalent to 6 units). This method is especially suitable if HLA-matched platelets are required (i.e. if patient has developed refractoriness to platelet transfusion due to the formation of alloantibodies against HLA antigens).

Platelets are administered for prevention and treatment of bleeding due to thrombocytopaenia or platelet dysfunction. The usual indications are:
- Thrombocytopaenia due to decreased platelet production, e.g. aplastic anaemia, haematologic malignancies, following chemotherapy or radiotherapy, etc.
- Hereditary disorders of platelet function
- Massive blood transfusion.

Most of the adverse reactions associated with platelet transfusions are due to the presence of contaminating leucocytes or plasma (e.g. febrile non-haemolytic transfusion reactions, allergic reactions, etc.).

Platelet concentrates are contraindicated in thrombotic thrombocytopaenic purpura and in haemolytic uraemic syndrome.

Transfusion of multiple platelet concentrates from random donors can induce alloimmunisation to HLA antigens. This causes resistance to further platelet transfusions and predicted post-transfusion rise in platelet count fails to occur due to rapid clearance of infused platelets by anti-HLA antibodies. Such patients should receive HLA-compatible platelets obtained from a single donor by plateletpheresis.

Bacterial proliferation can occur in platelet concentrates since they are stored at room temperature; consequently septicaemia can occur in the recipient.

As platelet concentrates also contain a small amount of red cells, it is preferable to transfuse platelet concentrates of same or compatible ABO group and same Rh group; this precaution is especially important if recipient is a woman of childbearing age.

Granulocyte Concentrate

Granulocyte concentrates are rarely used because:
- Most infections can be effectively controlled by appropriate antibiotic therapy
- A granulocyte concentrate prepared from a single donor unit has insufficient granulocytes and is also heavily contaminated with red cells.
- Transfusion of granulocyte concentrate is associated with significant risks (like non-haemolytic transfusion reactions, lung infiltrates, transmission of cell-associated viruses like cytomegalovirus, etc.).

Granulocytes for transfusion can be obtained either from a single donor unit by differential centrifugation or by leucapheresis. Leucapheresis is preferred because of better granulocyte yield, which can further be enhanced by administration of corticosteroids to the donor.

Administration of granulocyte concentrates can be considered in a patient with severe neutropaenia with documented bacterial or fungal infection, which is not responding to appropriate antibiotic therapy.

Plasma Components

Plasma can be obtained either by centrifugation of a unit of whole blood or by plasmapheresis. Various components can be prepared from plasma, the important ones being fresh frozen plasma and cryoprecipitate.

Fresh Frozen Plasma (FFP)

For preparation of FFP, plasma is separated from whole blood by centrifugation, transferred into the attached satellite bag, and rapidly frozen at –25°C or at lower temperature. This process is carried out within 6 hours of collection because after this time, labile coagulation factors (F V and F VIII) are lost. Volume of FFP is 200 to 250 ml. FFP contains all the coagulation factors (Box 20.6).

FFP can be stored for 1 year if temperature is maintained below –25°C. When required for transfusion, FFP is thawed between 30°C and 37°C and then stored in the refrigerator at 2 to 6°C. Since labile coagulation factors rapidly deteriorate, FFP should be transfused within 2 hours of thawing.

Indications for FFP are:
- Deficiency of multiple coagulation factors as in liver disease, massive transfusion, disseminated intravascular coagulation, and thrombotic thrombocytopaenic purpura
- Reversal of warfarin overdose
- Inherited deficiency of a coagulation factor for which no specific concentrate is available.

FFP should not be used for volume expansion alone, for which synthetic crystalloids or colloids are safer alternatives.

FFP should be administered in a dose of 15 ml/kg of body weight over 1 to 2 hours. ABO-compatible FFP is preferred to avoid the risk of haemolysis of recipient's red cells by antibodies in donor plasma.

Cryoprecipitate

Cryoprecipitate is prepared by slowly thawing 1 unit of FFP at 4° to 6°C. Plasma and a white precipitate are obtained. After centrifugation, most of the supernatant plasma is removed leaving behind sediment of cryoprecipitate suspended in 10 to 20 ml of plasma. The unit is then refrozen (–25°C or colder) for storage and can be kept for 1 year at this temperature. When required for transfusion, cryoprecipitate is thawed at 30° to 37°C and then kept in the refrigerator at 2° to 6°C till transfusion (for maximum of 6 hours).

Cryoprecipitate contains F VIII (about 80 units), von Willebrand factor, fibrinogen, F XIII, and fibronectin. If specific factor concentrates are not available, cryoprecipitate can be used for treatment of F VIII deficiency, von Willebrand disease, F XIII deficiency, and hypofibrinogenaemia.

Box 20.6 Fresh frozen plasma
• Plasma separated from whole blood within 6 hours of collection and then rapidly frozen to –25°C or lower
• Contains all the coagulation factors
• Storage: At –25°C or lower up to 1 year
• Volume: 200–300 ml
• Indications: Multiple coagulation factor deficiencies (liver disease, warfarin overdose), disseminated intravascular coagulation, and massive blood transfusion.

❑ BLOOD DERIVATIVES

Blood derivatives are manufactured by fractionation of large pools (obtained from many thousand donations) of human plasma. Some form of viral inactivation treatment is incorporated during manufacturing process to reduce the risk of viral transmission. Important plasma derivatives are listed in Table 20.3.

Table 20.3: Blood derivatives

1. Human albumin solutions
2. F VIII concentrate
3. F IX concentrate
4. Prothrombin complex concentrate
5. Immunoglobulins

Human Albumin Solutions

Albumin is prepared by cold ethanol fractionation of pooled plasma and is available as 5% and 20% solutions. Albumin solutions are heat-treated (at 60° C for 10 hours) to inactivate any contaminating viruses.

Physiological functions of albumin are maintenance of normal colloid osmotic pressure of plasma and to act as a carrier protein for certain substances in circulation.

Albumin is used as a replacement fluid in therapeutic plasma exchange, and for treatment of diuretic-resistant oedema of hypoproteinaemia.

F VIII Concentrate

F VIII concentrate, prepared by fractionation from large pools of donated plasma, is supplied as a freeze-dried powder in vials. During manufacturing process, it is treated with heat or chemicals to destroy lipid-enveloped viruses like HIV, HBV, HCV, and HTLV. It is stored in the refrigerator at 2° to 6° C. Before administration, it is reconstituted as per manufacturer's directions and given intravenously.

F VIII concentrate is indicated for treatment of:
• Haemophilia A
• Severe von Willebrand disease.

Apart from plasma-derived F VIII concentrate, F VIII prepared by recombinant DNA technology is now commercially available. It is free from infectious viruses and thus safer than plasma-derived F VIII.

F IX Concentrate

Both plasma-derived and recombinant F IX concentrates are available for treatment of haemophilia B.

Prothrombin Complex Concentrate (PCC)

PCC contains factors II, IX, and X, and sometimes also F VII. PCC contains trace amounts of activated coagulation factors and can induce thrombotic complications in patients with liver disease and in patients prone to thrombosis.

Indications for PCC are:
- Inherited deficiency of F IX, II or F X.
- Haemophilia A with inhibitor antibodies against F VIII and who are nonresponsive to F VIII concentrate.

Immunoglobulins

Immunoglobulins are prepared by cold ethanol fractionation of pooled plasma and are used for passive immunisation against infections. They are of two main types—(i) non-specific ("normal") immunoglobulins, and (ii) specific immunoglobulins.

Non-specific or "Normal" Immunoglobulins

These are prepared from the pooled plasma of non-selected donors and are composed of antibodies against infectious agents that are prevalent in the donor population. Some preparations are only for intramuscular administration, while others can be given intravenously.

Indications for non-specific immunoglobulins are:
- Passive prophylaxis against hepatitis A
- Congenital or acquired hypogammaglobulinaemia
- Autoimmune thrombocytopaenic purpura to temporarily raise platelet count.

Specific Immunoglobulins

They are prepared from donors who have specific high titre IgG antibodies (e.g. from patients convalescing from infectious diseases or who are already immunised).

Specific immunoglobulins include:
- Specific immunoglobulins for passive prophylaxis against hepatitis B, varicella zoster, cytomegalovirus, or tetanus.
- Anti-RhD immunoglobulin, which is used for prevention of immunisation against RhD antigen in Rh D-negative mothers during pregnancy. It is obtained from Rh-negative persons immunised to Rh D antigen.

❏ BIBLIOGRAPHY

1. Nanu A. Blood components: Preparation and quality control. Indian J Hematol Blood Transf. 1991: 9: 159-70.
2. World Health Organization. Blood Transfusion Safety: The Clinical Use of Blood. Geneva. World Health Organization. 2002.

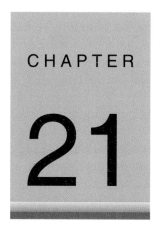

CHAPTER

21

Transfusion of Blood to the Recipient

Once it is decided that blood transfusion is required for a particular patient, a properly filled blood requisition form accompanied with labelled blood samples from the prospective recipient should be sent to the blood bank. It is the responsibility of the attending clinician to properly fill the request form. It should provide following information:

1. Name of the patient
2. Hospital registration number
3. Age/Sex
4. Ward number
5. Clinical diagnosis
6. Indication for transfusion, number of blood units required
7. Nature of product required, whether whole blood, packed red cells, platelets, fresh frozen plasma, cryoprecipitate, etc.
8. Date and time when required
9. Blood group of the patient, if known
10. Previous history of transfusion, transfusion reactions

Before withdrawing blood sample, the prospective recipient should be positively identified. Blood is collected in a plain tube (for serum grouping and compatibility testing) and also in a tube containing EDTA anticoagulant (for cell grouping). Sample tubes should be carefully labelled at the bedside. It should be kept in mind that **the most common cause of a haemolytic transfusion reaction is clerical error,** i.e. collecting blood from the wrong patient and incorrect labelling of sample tubes.

❏ SELECTION OF DONOR BLOOD FOR WHOLE BLOOD OR PACKED RED CELL TRANSFUSION

The first choice is the donor blood of the same ABO group as that of the recipient. If blood supply is inadequate, blood of the same ABO group may occasionally be not available; in such a case, if blood transfusion is likely to be potentially life saving and urgent, blood of an alternate but compatible group may be transfused (Table 21.1). Possible benefits and risks should be carefully assessed before considering such a transfusion.

To reduce the risk of haemolysis in a case of non-identical but compatible ABO transfusion, packed red cells instead of whole blood should be transfused (i.e. most of the plasma which contains anti-A and/or anti-B should be removed). This is especially important with group O donor blood, which can contain immune anti-A and anti-B antibodies that will cause serious haemolysis in a non-group O recipient.

For AB group recipients, if red cells of group AB are not available, group A donor blood is preferred over other alternatives since anti-B in group A is weaker than anti-A in group B.

Transfusion of Rh-positive blood to Rh-negative persons carries the risk of evoking the formation of anti-D antibodies (after about 3 months). Subsequent transfusion of Rh-positive blood to such sensitised individuals will cause haemolytic transfusion reaction. In the Rh system, **individuals with Rh-negative blood group should be transfused only with Rh-negative blood,** especially Rh-negative females of childbearing age and young girls (to prevent Rh immunisation and future haemolytic disease of newborn). In an emergency, Rh-positive blood may be transfused to non-immunised Rh-negative men and older women, if Rh-negative blood is not available and if blood transfusion will be potentially lifesaving. However, if such individuals are likely to need regular transfusions in future also, they should preferably be not exposed to Rh-positive blood.

Although persons with Rh-positive group can receive either Rh-positive or Rh-negative blood, they should be transfused with Rh-positive blood (owing to the rarity of Rh-negative blood which should be reserved only for Rh-negative recipients).

Currently, enzymatic removal of A and/or B antigens from red cells of A, B, and AB groups is being tried experimentally to convert all A, B, and AB donor units to group O unit. Since group O is an universal donor group, success in this strategy will

Table 21.1: Selection of donor blood group for transfusion of whole blood or packed red cells

Recipient blood group	Donor blood group	
	First choice	Alternative
A	A	O
B	B	O
AB	AB	A, B, O (in this order)
O	O	Nil

Table 21.2: Selection of donor blood group for transfusion of plasma

Donor blood (plasma) group	Recipient blood group
AB plasma (contains neither anti-A nor anti-B antibodies)	AB, A, B, O
A plasma (contains anti-B)	A, O
B plasma (contains anti-A)	B, O
O plasma (contains both anti-A and anti-B)	O only

hopefully make finding ABO-compatible blood less of a problem and will also reduce the risk of ABO mismatched transfusion reactions.

❑ SELECTION OF DONOR PLASMA

For transfusion of plasma and plasma components, selection of blood group of donor is given in Table 21.2.

❑ ANTIBODY SCREENING AND IDENTIFICATION

In well-equipped blood banks, screening for unexpected or irregular antibodies against red cell antigens is carried out before transfusion in both recipient's and donor's sera. For recipients demonstrating irregular antibodies, selection of donor blood lacking the corresponding antigen is selected.

❑ COMPATIBILITY TEST

The final check of compatibility between recipient and donor blood is cross-matching or compatibility test. There are two types of compatibility test: major and minor. The aim of cross matching is detection of ABO incompatibility and presence of clinically significant unexpected antibodies. If cross match is compatible, a compatibility label should be attached to the blood bag showing patient's (recipient's) name, hospital registration number, ward number, blood group, donation identification number, date of expiry of unit, and date of compatibility test.

❑ ISSUE OF DONOR BLOOD UNIT

Before issuing the blood unit for the recipient, information on the blood bag, request form, and compatibility label should be checked by the blood bank for any discrepancy.
Blood bag should be inspected for (Fig. 21.1):
- Evidence of haemolysis (pink discolouration of plasma, or red colouration of plasma just above the red cell layer)
- Large clots in plasma
- Black or purple discolouration of red cells indicative of bacterial contamination
- Leakage.

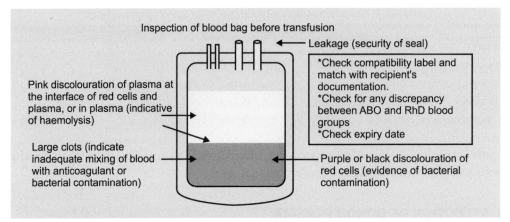

Figure 21.1: Checking of blood bag is essential on its arrival in ward or operating room and before beginning transfusion

The physician at the bedside should also carry out similar inspection before beginning transfusion. If any abnormality is detected, blood should not be transfused and blood bank is notified.

Blood bag should be procured from the blood bank only at the time of transfusion (i.e. when the intravenous line is in place in the recipient). Transfusion should commence within 30 minutes of removing the blood bag from the refrigerator of the blood bank. Blood unit should not be transfused if the blood bag is out of refrigerator for more than 30 minutes, since it increases the risk of proliferation of contaminating bacteria.

Do not transfuse blood unit if it shows evidence of haemolysis, clots, discolouration of red cells, or leakage.

❑ TRANSFUSION OF BLOOD UNIT

Before beginning transfusion, it is necessary to check the label on the blood bag, compatibility label, blood bag itself (for evidence of haemolysis, clots, discolouration of red cells, or leakage), and identity of the recipient. Check ABO and Rh D groups of both the recipient and donor written on the blood bag and the date of expiry of the blood unit.

It is necessary to correctly identify the recipient during sample collection and before beginning transfusion.

Blood should be transfused through a sterile, disposable administration set incorporating a standard filter (170 μm pore size). This filter retains small clots or cellular aggregates but permits passage of single cells and microaggregates. The usual needle size is 18- or 19-gauge. Microaggregate or leucocyte depletion filters are available which are used to prevent or decrease the febrile transfusion reactions in multiply transfused patients.

It is not necessary to warm blood before transfusion when rate of infusion is slow. However, rapid infusion of large volume of cold blood can induce ventricular arrhythmias or cardiac arrest. Blood warmer is used to warm blood in such cases. Blood should be warmed only by blood warmer and not by any other means such as hot water bowl since high temperature will induce haemolysis and release of potassium from red cells, which may prove fatal for the recipient.

No drugs of any kind should be added to the blood. Ringer's lactate (which contains calcium) or 5% dextrose cause formation of clots and haemolysis respectively. If fluids are to be added, the only acceptable one is normal saline. Normal saline is used for starting transfusion and also can be added to packed red cells to reduce viscosity. Addition of a drug may induce haemolysis; also if a reaction occurs it may be difficult to decide whether it is drug-induced or is related to blood transfusion.

The patient should be monitored closely during transfusion (by regularly noting general appearance, pulse, respiratory rate, temperature, and blood pressure). The patient should be closely observed especially during first 15 minutes, as most life-threatening haemolytic transfusion reactions are likely to occur during this period. Following this, patient is observed every hour, at the end of transfusion, and 4 hours after the end of transfusion.

Transfusion should be initiated within 30 minutes of removing blood unit from the storage refrigerator in the blood bank. Transfusion of whole blood or packed red cells should be completed within maximum of 4 hours of starting transfusion. If ambient temperature is high, infusion should be completed within a shorter period. This is because of the risk of bacterial proliferation in the blood unit, which increases with time at room temperature. (Bacteria may have gained entry into the blood unit during blood collection, storage, or transfusion).

After transfusion is over, details of transfusion such as time of starting and completion, nature of blood product transfused, donation identification number, and any adverse reactions should be recorded in the case records of the recipient.

❏ BIBLIOGRAPHY

1. Boral LI, Weiss ED, Henry JB. Transfusion Medicine. In Henry JB (Ed.): Clinical Diagnosis and Management by Laboratory Methods. 20th ed. Philadelphia. WB Saunders Compay. 2001.
2. World Health Organization. Blood Transfusion Safety: The Clinical Use of Blood. Geneva. World Health Organization. 2002.

CHAPTER 22

Adverse Effects of Transfusion

Blood transfusion is a life saving but a potentially hazardous procedure. It should be considered only if there are no alternative means (like intravenous fluids, specific treatment of anaemia) of treating the condition. Before contemplating transfusion, risks and benefits should be assessed. This is because even with best possible blood banking standards, transmission of infections or other complications can occur.

Benefits of blood transfusion include improvement of oxygen-carrying capacity and replacement of coagulation factors, platelets, immunoglobulins and other proteins. Potential risks of transfusion are transmission of infections like hepatitis and AIDS, transfusion reactions, and immunisation to antigens. Fluids such as saline or dextrose should be used when only volume replacement is required. Adverse effects of transfusion are listed in Table 22.1.

At many places, blood transfusion consists of giving a single unit of blood (which in most cases is unnecessary) and whole blood (for

Table 22.1: Adverse effects of transfusion

Immediate
Immunological
• Febrile nonhaemolytic transfusion reactions
• Haemolytic transfusion reactions
• Allergic reactions
• Anaphylactic reactions
• Transfusion-associated lung injury
Non-immunological
• Circulatory overload
• Bacterial contamination of donor blood unit
Delayed
Immunological
• Haemolytic transfusion reactions
• Post transfusion purpura
• Graft-versus-host disease
Non-immunological
• Transmission of infectious organisms
• Iron overload
Complications associated with massive transfusion

which there are very few indications and which exposes the recipient to unwanted components). Risks of such practice should be realised before undertaking single unit transfusion.

❑ IMMEDIATE COMPLICATIONS

Febrile Non-haemolytic Transfusion Reaction (FNHTR)

This manifests with fever, and sometimes with chills, flushing, headache, anxiety, itching, and tachycardia. The reaction begins 30 to 60 minutes following start of transfusion. FNHTR is common in recipients of multiple transfusions and in women who have had multiple pregnancies (due to previous sensitisation).

FNHTR is caused by:

* Release of cytokines from leucocytes during storage of blood, and
* Reaction of alloantibodies in the recipient with transfused white cells leading to release of pyrogens.

Diagnosis of FNHTR is based on eliminating other causes of fever such as haemolytic transfusion reaction, bacterial contamination of donor blood unit, transfusion associated lung injury, or underlying disease in the patient.

Management consists of:
* Stopping transfusion
* Workup for haemolytic transfusion reaction (see below) and for bacterial contamination of blood unit
* Administration of oral or rectal antipyretics (paracetamol) and i.m. /i.v. antihistaminic.

In regularly transfused patients, prevention of FNTHR involves slow speed of transfusion (up to 4 hours for 1 unit of whole blood) and administration of antipyretics before starting transfusion. If these measures are unsuccessful, leucocyte-depleted blood should be given (i.e. prior removal of buffy coat or transfusion through leucocyte depletion filters).

Haemolytic Transfusion Reaction (HTR)

Acute intravascular haemolysis is caused by transfusion of incompatible red cells. Binding of antibodies in patient's circulation to donor red cells leads to activation of full complement cascade and haemolysis (Fig. 22.1).

Acute HTR most often results from ABO incompatibility and is mediated by IgM (or sometimes IgG) anti-A or anti-B antibodies. ABO incompatibility almost always results in HTR because of consistent occurrence of potent and lytic IgM antibodies in plasma of patients lacking corresponding antigen on their red cells.

Mismatched ABO blood transfusion usually results from clerical error. This error may be:

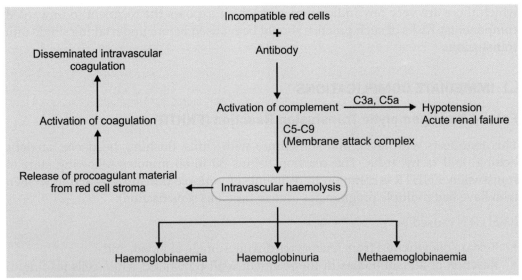

Figure 22.1: Pathogenesis of intravascular acute HTR following ABO incompatibility

- Incorrect identification of recipient during sample collection or during transfusion.
- Incorrect labelling of sample tubes or incorrect filling of request form.

Signs and symptoms of acute HTR usually appear within minutes of starting transfusion since only a small amount of blood (5–10 ml) can trigger the reaction.

Patient complains of pain or heat at the infusion site, substernal pain, restlessness, and loin or back pain. There is development of fever, rigors, breathlessness, tachycardia, hypotension, and bleeding manifestations. In severe cases, renal failure may follow. The reaction may be fatal and patient may die from shock, acute renal failure, or disseminated intravascular coagulation.

In unconscious or anaesthetised patients, the only indicators of HTR may be hypotension and excess bleeding.

Acute HTR is an emergency. Treatment consists of:
- Immediate discontinuation of transfusion
- Maintenance of intravenous access with normal saline
- Management of hypotension, renal failure, and disseminated intravascular coagulation.

Investigation of a Haemolytic Transfusion Reaction

If acute HTR is suspected, blood transfusion should be immediately stopped. This is because severity of reaction partly depends on the amount of incompatible red cells transfused. The transfusion set should be removed, but the intravenous line should be maintained with normal saline. The concerned physician is immediately notified.

As the clerical error is the most common cause of HTR, the label on the blood bag and the affixed compatibility label should be checked against the identity of the recipient. If there is a discrepancy, blood bank should be immediately notified since another patient may be involved in the possible mix up.

Diagnosis of acute HTR depends on demonstration of intravascular haemolysis in the recipient and of ABO incompatibility between the donor and the recipient.

Following samples should be collected from the recipient:

1. Venous blood in a plain tube and in a tube containing EDTA anticoagulant, and
2. First urine passed following transfusion.

Diagnosis of intravascular haemolysis is based on the presence of following findings in the post transfusion sample from the recipient:

- Pink colouration of plasma (after centrifugation of EDTA blood sample)
- Spherocytes and fragmented red cells on a stained blood smear
- Haemoglobinuria
- Reduced haptoglobin in blood
- Increased indirect serum bilirubin in blood.

Demonstration of blood group incompatibility between the donor and the recipient depends on following investigations:

- Repeat ABO blood grouping and Rh typing on recipient's pre- and post-transfusion blood samples and on donor blood unit
- Repeat cross matching of donor blood against recipient's pre-transfusion and post-transfusion samples
- Direct antiglobulin test (DAT) on recipient's pre- and post-transfusion samples. Positive DAT with post-transfusion sample and negative DAT with pre-transfusion sample indicate occurrence of antigen-antibody reaction.

In addition, **investigations for identification of complications** associated with HTR can be carried out as follows:

- Tests for disseminated intravascular coagulation: Coagulation screen, platelet count, fibrin degradation products
- Tests for renal failure: serum creatinine, blood urea.

It is to be noted that haemolysis of donor red cells can also result from following causes:

1. Bacterial contamination of donor unit: Infected blood shows black or purple discolouration of red cells and evidence of haemolysis. Blood from the donor unit should be sent for Gram's stain and bacterial culture.
2. Thermal damage: Keeping the blood bag in the freezer compartment of the ward refrigerator or keeping the blood unit in the hot water bowl for warming result in haemolysis.
3. Addition of drugs to the donor unit.

If no cause of haemolysis is found, possibility of a haemolytic anaemia like paroxysmal nocturnal haemoglobinuria or glucose-6-phosphate dehydrogenase deficiency should be considered.

Allergic Reactions

Mild urticaria, rash, and pruritus may develop within minutes of initiating transfusion. This results from reaction between some plasma proteins and corresponding IgE antibodies in recipient's plasma (with local release of histamine). Rate of transfusion should be slowed and an antihistamine given.

Anaphylactic Reaction

Anaphylactic reaction is rare and characterised mainly by hypotension, shock, and breathlessness. There is no fever. The reaction develops within minutes of starting transfusion. A very severe anaphylaxis occurs in individuals with IgA deficiency; in these patients, anti-IgA antibodies react with IgA of donor plasma leading to activation of complement and generation of anaphylatoxins (C3a and C5a). Transfusion should be immediately stopped and patient is given adrenaline and hydrocortisone.

Transfusion Associated Lung Injury (TRALI)

TRALI manifests within 1 to 4 hours of starting transfusion and is characterised by fever, chills, respiratory distress, and dry cough. X ray shows diffuse pulmonary infiltrates.

Potent leucoagglutinins in donor blood incompatible with granulocytes of the recipient react with leucocytes in recipient's circulation leading to the formation of leucocyte aggregates. After lodging in pulmonary microcirculation, they cause increase in vascular permeability.

Donors are generally multiparous women who develop leucoagglutinins at the time of pregnancy.

Treatment is supportive.

Circulatory Overload

Circulatory overload can develop if the rate of transfusion is too rapid (before compensatory fluid redistribution can occur), or is excessive, or if there is impairment of renal or cardiac function. It results in cardiac failure and pulmonary oedema.

It is especially likely to occur in patients with chronic severe anaemia and in patients with compromised cardiovascular function.

Treatment consists of propping up the patient in a sitting position, and administration of oxygen and intravenous diuretics.

Bacterial Contamination of Donor Unit

Transfusion of blood that is contaminated with bacteria can cause septicaemic shock. Bacterial contamination is more common with platelet concentrates (1–2% cases) than with whole blood or packed red cells (0.4%). This is because platelet concentrates are stored at a higher temperature (20–24°C) that favours proliferation of contaminating bacteria

Causes of bacterial contamination of a blood unit are:
- Incomplete sterilisation of skin during venepuncture for blood collection
- Asymptomatic bacteraemia in the donor at the time of blood collection (especially occurs with *Yersinia enterocolitica*)
- Tiny breaks in plastic bag leading to the entry of bacteria during storage.
- Thawing of cryoprecipitate or fresh frozen plasma in a water bath.

The usual contaminating organism in blood stored at 2 to 6°C is *Pseudomonas*. *Staphylococcus* is the common contaminant in platelet concentrates.

Clinical features resemble those of an acute haemolytic transfusion reaction. After starting transfusion, patient rapidly develops high-grade fever with rigors, hypotension, and shock. Treatment consists of high doses of intravenous antibiotics and supportive measures.

Diagnosis depends on Gram staining and culture of blood from blood bag.

❑ DELAYED COMPLICATIONS

Delayed Haemolytic Transfusion Reaction

Delayed HTR occurs in individuals who have been sensitised earlier to certain red cell antigens by previous transfusion or pregnancy. The concentration of antibody, however, is so low that it cannot be detected by tests before transfusion. On re-exposure to the same red cell antigen, there is a secondary immune response that causes destruction (predominantly extravascular) of transfused red cells bearing the particular antigen.

Clinically, patient develops fever, anaemia, and jaundice about 5 to 10 days after transfusion. Severe reaction is rare. Direct antiglobulin test is positive.

The usual antigens implicated are Rh and Kidd.

Post-transfusion Purpura

Severe thrombocytopaenia can rarely develop in some adult multiparous women about 5 to 10 days following blood transfusion. There is previous sensitisation of the recipient to a platelet antigen (HPA-1a or Pl^{A1}) during pregnancy; following re-exposure to the same antigen through transfusion, the antibodies paradoxically cause destruction of patient's own platelets (which are negative for HPA-1a or Pl^{A1}).

The condition is potentially fatal. Treatment consists of plasma exchange and intravenous immunoglobulins.

Transfusion Associated Graft-versus-Host Disease (GvHD)

GvHD can develop following:
- Blood transfusion in immunodeficient individuals (e.g. recipients of bone marrow transplant, premature infants, etc.), or

- Blood transfusion from a first-degree relative in immunocompetent individuals. GvHD results from engraftment in the recipient of donor lymphocytes that react against host tissues.

About 10 to 12 days following transfusion, patient develops fever, skin rash, vomiting, diarrhoea, hepatitis, and pancytopaenia (bone marrow suppression). The condition is usually fatal.

Irradiation of blood (25 Gy) before transfusion is recommended to prevent proliferation of donor lymphocytes and avoid GvHD.

Transmission of Infectious Organisms

The organisms likely to be transmitted by transfusion are usually those, which are prevalent in a particular geographic area or population. Organisms transmissible by transfusion are listed in Table 22.2.

In India, pre-transfusion testing of donor blood for following agents is currently mandatory (i.e. prior consent of prospective donor is not necessary) for

Table 22.2: Micro-organisms transmissible by transfusion

Viruses
- Hepatitis viruses
  - Hepatitis A virus
  - Hepatitis B virus
  - Hepatitis C virus
- Human immunodeficiency virus (HIV)
  - HIV-1
  - HIV-2
- Cytomegalovirus (of significance in immunocompromised recipients)
- Epstein-Barr virus (rare)
- Human T cell leukaemia virus (HTLV) (endemic in Japan and the Carribbean)
  - HTLV-I
  - HTLV-II
- Human parvovirus B 19 (of significance in patients with chronic haemolysis)

Prions
- Creutzfeldt-Jakob disease (CJD) and variant CJD (not proven)

Bacteria
- *Treponema pallidum* (syphilis)
- Bacterial contamination of donor unit (*Pseudomonas*, Staphylococci)
- Brucellosis (rare)

Parasites
- Malaria parasites
- *Trypanosoma cruzi* (prevalent in Latin America)
- *Toxoplasma gondii* (of significance only in immunocompromised recipients receiving granulocyte transfusion)
- *Babesia microti* (prevalent in North America)
- *Leishmania donovani* (rare)

- Hepatitis B virus
- Hepatitis C virus
- HIV-1 and HIV-2
- *Treponema pallidum* (Syphilis)
- Malaria parasite
  Infection by hepatitis B and C viruses and HIV-1 and HIV-2 is characterised by:
- Persistence of organisms in circulation for prolonged duration without necessarily causing clinical manifestations
- Long incubation period
- Ability to cause chronic carrier state
- Viability of organisms in blood stored at 4 to 6°C.
  Following two principal measures can prevent transmission of infection through transfusion:
- Blood should be collected only from voluntary, non-remunerated donors. All high risk (intravenous drug abusers, homosexuals, prostitutes, and sexual partners of such persons) and professional donors should be excluded. Standard criteria for selection of blood donors should be followed.
- All blood donations should be tested for infectious agents by screening tests.

Reliance solely on laboratory screening tests to exclude infections transmissible by transfusion is inadequate to ensure safe blood supply.

Hepatitis B Virus (HBV)

HBV is a partially double-stranded DNA virus of 42 nm diameter. It can cause:
- Acute hepatitis
- Chronic hepatitis
- Asymptomatic carrier state
- Cirrhosis
- Hepatocellular carcinoma.
  According to WHO, more than 10% of potential blood donors in developing countries are HBV carriers. HBV is highly infectious (50–100 times more so than human immunodeficiency virus). It is transmitted through all blood components and most of the blood derivatives.

Infected hepatocytes release large amounts of hepatitis B surface antigen (HbsAg) into the blood stream. Presence of HbsAg indicates active infection.

Screening of all blood donations for HbsAg has greatly reduced the risk of transmission of HBV through transfusion; the risk, however, is not completely eliminated. HbsAg-negative donor may transmit HBV when blood is collected in early incubation period or when very low levels of HbsAg, not detectable by presently employed methods, are present.

An individual who has received HBV vaccine will have hepatitis B surface antibody but not HbsAg in blood.

Hepatitis C Virus (HCV)

HCV is a single-stranded RNA virus of flaviviridae family, which was first identified in 1989. Prior to its discovery, it was known as non-A, non-B (NANB) hepatitis virus. Incubation period following infection is about 8 weeks. Most cases of HCV infection are asymptomatic. Following infection, chronic hepatitis develops in majority of cases. Cirrhosis (10–20% cases) and hepatocellular carcinoma (1–5% cases) are late sequelae in patients with chronic infection.

According to estimates of WHO (1999), prevalence rate of HCV in Southeast Asia is 2.15%.

Amount of HCV antigen released in blood stream is small and cannot be detected readily. Therefore, screening of donor blood for HCV infection relies on detection of anti-HCV antibody in serum (which becomes detectable after 6–8 weeks of infection).

Human Immunodeficiency Virus

Human immunodeficiency virus or HIV is RNA retrovirus, which causes slowly progressive immunodeficiency in infected persons. HIV infects CD4+ T lymphocytes, which play a central role in immune system. Infection leads to destruction of CD4+ lymphocytes with slowly progressive impairment of the immune system. The infected individual becomes susceptible to a range of opportunistic infections and malignancies. The most advanced stage of HIV disease is acquired immune deficiency syndrome or AIDS. HIV also infects nerve cells and causes neurological damage. HIV infection is lifelong and the infected individual remains infectious for life.

There is a wide variation in the prevalence of HIV infection between and within countries. Majority (95%) of cases of HIV infection occurring in the world are in the developing countries, the most affected region being sub-Saharan Africa. Southeast Asia is the second most affected region in the world, with majority of cases occurring in India, Myanmar, and Thailand.

According to the estimates of India's National AIDS Control Organisation (NACO), adult prevalence of HIV infection is 0.7% with approximately 4 million HIV infections, 90% of which are in the age group of 15 to 45 years.

In industrialised nations, HIV infection occurs chiefly in homosexual men and intravenous drug abusers.

In developing countries, HIV is transmitted mainly by following routes:
- Heterosexual intercourse (80% cases)
- Parenteral (i.e. transfusion of infected blood or blood products; use of blood-contaminated needles, syringes, or other skin-piercing instruments)
- Mother to child (during delivery or breastfeeding)

There are two types of HIV—HIV-1 and HIV-2.
- *HIV-1:* This is the most common type found worldwide. It is divided into two groups—M and O. There are eight subtypes of M (A to H). In India, subtype C is prevalent.
- *HIV-2:* This is found mainly in West Africa, India, and Sri Lanka.

Following HIV infection, viraemia becomes detectable after a few days and lasts for several weeks. During this period, the infected person may remain asymptomatic or develop a glandular fever-like illness. Anti-HIV antibodies appear 6 to 12 weeks after infection (called as seroconversion). **Window period** is the period between the onset of HIV infection and appearance of detectable antibodies in serum; it is the infectious but seronegative period (i.e. the test for anti-HIV antibodies is yet to become positive). Transfusion of donor blood collected during the window period will transmit HIV to the recipient. Collection of blood from the donor during the window period of HIV infection is, however, a rare event.

Following are main measures for the prevention of transmission of HIV through blood transfusion (Box 22.1):

- Recruitment only of voluntary, non-paid donors and exclusion of all professional or high-risk donors
- Self-exclusion of high-risk donors
- Screening test of donor blood for anti-HIV antibodies
- Avoidance of unnecessary blood transfusions.

Treponema Pallidum

Transmission of *Treponema (T.) pallidum* through blood transfusion causes syphilis. However, only fresh blood or platelet concentrates can transmit these organisms since storage of donor blood unit at 2 to 6°C for 48 to 72 hours inactivates *T. pallidum*. Transfusion-transmission of syphilis is, therefore, rare. The main value of testing donor blood for *T. pallidum* is to identify and exclude donors with high-risk behaviour and thus who are at risk of having sexually transmitted infections.

Plasmodium Species

Malaria parasite can be transmitted through all blood components. In endemic areas, testing of all blood units for malaria parasite is not feasible; it is also not practical to reject all potential donors who have had malaria in the past. Therefore, it is essential to maintain a high degree of suspicion if a transfusion-recipient develops symptoms suggestive of malaria and appropriate treatment should be given.

Box 22.1 Measures to prevent transmission by transfusion of hepatitis and HIV infections

- Transfuse only when essential. Avoid single unit transfusions
- Exclusion of all high-risk donors such as homosexuals, bisexuals, intravenous drug abusers, prostitutes, and sexual partners of these persons
- Reliance solely on voluntary donations. Exclude all professional donors
- Screening of all blood donations for HbsAg, anti-HCV, and anti-HIV before transfusion
- Use autologous transfusions wherever possible
- Viral inactivation of blood components and derivatives
- Patients requiring regular transfusion therapy (e.g. haemophilics and thalassaemics) should be given HBV vaccine.

Iron Overload

Each unit of blood contains about 200 mg of iron, while the daily physiologic loss of iron is only 1 mg. There is no physiologic mechanism for removal of excess iron. Therefore, patients receiving regular long-term blood transfusion therapy (such as thalassaemics) inevitably develop iron overload. Deposition of excess iron in heart, liver, and endocrine glands can cause respective organ failure. Iron chelating therapy with desferrioxamine should be instituted early in these patients to minimise iron accumulation.

❑ COMPLICATIONS ASSOCIATED WITH MASSIVE BLOOD TRANSFUSION

Massive blood transfusion refers to the replacement of patient's blood loss with transfusion of stored blood equivalent to total blood volume within 24 hours. The need for massive transfusion is usually an emergency that arises following an accident or an obstetric problem. Rapid loss of large amount of blood needs urgent correction to restore blood volume and to maintain tissue perfusion, oxygenation, and haemostasis.

Morbidity and mortality in these patients is usually due to the underlying condition coupled with major haemorrhage. In addition, massive blood transfusion is also associated with certain complications. Storage of blood at 2 to 6°C for 48 hours is associated with loss of platelet function and loss of labile coagulation factors (F V and F VIII). Therefore, rapid infusion of large volumes of stored blood will lead to dilution of platelets and coagulation factors. Prolongation of prothrombin time, activated partial thromboplastin time, thrombocytopaenia, or bleeding manifestations are indications for platelet transfusions or fresh frozen plasma.

Hyperkalaemia (due to release of potassium from stored red cells), hypocalcaemia (due to binding of calcium by citrate anticoagulant), and hypothermia (due to rapid infusion of large quantity of cold blood) can induce cardiac arrhythmias.

Microaggregates composed of platelets and leucocytes form gradually in stored blood. Following massive transfusion, these microaggregates can migrate to the lungs and induce adult respiratory distress syndrome. Microaggregates can be removed during transfusion through special filters.

❑ BIBLIOGRAPHY

1. Contreras M (Ed.). ABC of Transfusion. 3rd ed. London. BMJ Books. 1998.
2. Regan F, Taylor C. Recent developments. Blood Transfusion Medicine. BMJ. 2002;325:143-47.
3. World Health Organization. Blood Transfusion Safety: The Clinical Use of Blood. Geneva. World Health Organisation. 2002.

CHAPTER

23

Autologous Transfusion

In autologous transfusion, patient's blood is collected and is re-infused back subsequently when required. Although having a limited scope, autologous transfusion has certain advantages as shown in Box 23.1.

There are three methods of autologous transfusion:
- Predeposit (preoperative blood donation)
- Acute normovolaemic haemodilution
- Blood salvage.

❏ PREDEPOSIT AUTOLOGOUS BLOOD TRANSFUSION

This technique is applicable to those patients who are posted for elective surgery, are otherwise fit, and are likely to need blood since significant operative blood losses are expected. Patient's blood is collected in a blood bag before elective surgery, stored in the blood bank, and is re-infused back after surgery to replace the operative blood losses. Blood collection from the patient starts 5 weeks before surgery. One unit of

Box 23.1	Advantages of autologous transfusion

- Avoids transmission of infectious organisms
- Avoids immunologic complications associated with homologous transfusion (such as haemolysis, alloimmunisation, graft-versus-host disease, TRALI, allergic reactions)
- Reduces need for blood from homologous donors
- Avoids problem of finding compatible blood for a patient with a rare blood group or multiple red cell antibodies.

blood is collected every 7 days. Patient should be living near the transfusion centre. Maximum of total 4 units can be collected, with the number depending on the nature of surgery. The last donation is collected at least 4 days before operation to allow restoration of plasma volume. Patient is put on oral iron supplements to maintain haemoglobin level. Before each donation, haemoglobin level should be >11.0 g/dl. Blood bag(s) should be properly labelled and stored in the blood bank refrigerator. Pre-transfusion testing is carried out as for other homologous blood units.

If patient's blood group is rare or multiple antibodies against common red cell antigens are present, compatible blood may be difficult to find. In such cases, patient's red cells can be stored frozen for many years for any future requirement.

This technique is contraindicated in patients with cancer, significant cardiovascular disease, anaemia, trauma, uncontrolled hypertension, epilepsy, and pregnancy. Patients with bacteraemia should be excluded because proliferation of bacteria during storage can induce septicaemic shock following transfusion. Patients having infections transmissible by transfusion should also not be considered since clerical or administrative error may cause blood to be transfused inadvertently to the wrong recipient.

Wastage of donated blood unit(s) can occur in the event of cancellation of surgery or if the amount of blood donated exceeds the required amount. Unused blood is often not suitable for other donors because strict criteria for selection of donors are not followed.

Predeposit auto-transfusion cannot prevent the risk of circulatory overload, clerical error leading to haemolytic transfusion reaction, and bacterial contamination (during collection).

Close co-ordination between patient, surgeon, and blood bank is required. Implementation of this technique requires considerable planning and organisation.

❑ ACUTE NORMOVOLAEMIC HAEMODILUTION

Immediately before beginning surgery, patient's whole blood (1 or 2 units) is collected in blood bag(s) containing suitable anticoagulant. To maintain the blood volume, equivalent amount of crystalloid (at least 3 ml for every 1 ml of blood collected) or colloid (1 ml for every 1 ml collected) solution is infused. During surgery, the artificially created acute normovolaemic haemodilution will reduce the red cell loss for the given amount of bleeding. The collected blood units are returned back to the patient after surgical bleeding is controlled. Blood collected from the patient is labelled and kept near the patient. It remains at room temperature for only a short period so that there is minimal loss of coagulation factors and platelets. Testing and cross matching are not carried out. Keeping the blood bag near the patient minimises the risk of administrative error (i.e. transfusing blood to the wrong patient). This procedure can be carried out if significant blood loss is anticipated during surgery, i.e. greater than 1000 ml or 20% of blood volume. It should not be carried out in patients who will be unable to tolerate reduction in oxygen supply due to haemodilution (e.g. those having cardiopulmonary disease). Careful monitoring of the patient during surgery is essential.

❑ BLOOD SALVAGE

Blood salvage consists of collection of blood that is shed during surgery (intraoperative blood salvage) or following surgery (postoperative blood salvage) and subsequent re-infusion of the recovered blood to the same patient.

Blood salvage can be carried out in elective as well as emergency surgery when expected blood loss is extensive, e.g. cardiac surgery, total knee replacement, trauma surgery, ruptured ectopic pregnancy, or ruptured spleen. This procedure should not be carried out if salvaged blood is contaminated with bowel contents, urine, bacteria, amniotic fluid, or malignant cells. Re-infusion of blood that was collected more than 6 hours back can be harmful due to red cell lysis, hyperkalaemia, and bacterial contamination.

In intraoperative blood salvage, blood lost during surgery is aspirated from the operative field, anticoagulated, filtered to remove clots and debris, centrifuged, washed, and suspended in sterile saline before re-infusion. A red cell product free of contaminants is thus obtained. The technique requires an expensive automated blood salvage device and for each patient costly disposable materials.

In postoperative blood salvage, blood is recovered from wound drains and re-infused back directly through a filter.

❑ BIBLIOGRAPHY

1. Vanderlinde ES, Heal JM, Blumberg N. Autologous transfusion. BMJ. 2002;324:772-75.
2. World Health Organization. Blood Transfusion Safety: The Clinical Use of Blood. Geneva. World Health Organization. 2002.

CHAPTER 24

Alternatives to Blood Transfusion

Although blood transfusion can be lifesaving, it is associated with a risk of serious complications and of transmission of infections (see 'Adverse effects of transfusion'). Therefore, blood transfusion should be considered only if there are no alternative means of therapy and there is a likelihood of significant morbidity or mortality without transfusion. Blood transfusion can be avoided or its use minimised through following measures:

- **Avoidance of single unit transfusions**. One unit of blood raises haemoglobin only by 1 g/dl and rarely provides clinical benefit in chronic anaemia
- **Avoidance of unnecessary administration of blood** (e.g. before surgery to raise haemoglobin level, to effect early discharge from hospital, etc.)
- **Early diagnosis and specific treatment of anaemia**
- **Use of safer alternatives,** like synthetic crystalloids or colloids if only volume replacement is required
- **Meticulous surgical and anaesthetic techniques** to minimise operative blood losses
- **Consideration of autologous transfusion** in healthy patients undergoing elective surgery
- **Use of drugs to reduce bleeding during surgery** like aprotinin, tranexamic acid, fibrin glues, and sealants
- **Exploration of alternatives to blood transfusion:** (a) Haematopoietic growth factors, (b) Recombinant blood coagulation factors, or (c) Red cell substitutes.

❏ HAEMATOPOIETIC GROWTH FACTORS (HGFS)

These are polypeptides that regulate proliferation, differentiation, and maturation of haematopoietic progenitor cells. Erythropoietin, granulocyte macrophage-colony stimulating factor (GM-CSF), and granulocyte-colony stimulating factor (G-CSF) are the HGFs that are currently available commercially. They are produced by recombinant DNA technology.

Erythropoietin

This is produced in kidneys (90%) and in liver (10%). It stimulates erythroid precursors to proliferate, differentiate, and mature. Recombinant erythropoietin is the treatment of choice in anaemia of chronic renal failure and significantly reduces the need for red cell transfusions in end-stage renal disease. It is also helpful in anaemia of cancer and in anaemia in HIV-positive patients receiving zidovudine. Desirable response is obtained after several weeks of therapy with erythropoietin. Therefore, it is not helpful in acutely developing anaemias.

Granulocyte Macrophage-colony Stimulating Factor (GM-CSF)

GM-CSF stimulates proliferation, differentiation, and maturation of precursor cells of neutrophil and monocyte/macrophage cell lines. Recombinant GM-CSF accelerates myeloid recovery following bone marrow transplantation, and shortens duration of neutropaenia after chemotherapy-induced myelosuppression.

Granulocyte-colony Stimulating Factor (G-CSF)

G-CSF stimulates myeloid progenitor cells to form mature neutrophils. Recombinant G-CSF is used to shorten the period of neutropaenia following myelosuppressive chemotherapy.

❏ RED CELL SUBSTITUTES

Red cell substitutes are being developed which will transport oxygen from the lungs to the tissues similar to red cells. To be effective, red cell substitutes should bind oxygen in the lungs, readily release oxygen at the tissue level, should be non-toxic and non-immunogenic, sterilisable, and should remain functional in circulation for long duration. Currently, haemoglobin solutions and perfluorocarbons are undergoing clinical trials, but their major problem is short half-lives in circulation.

Red cell substitutes include:
* Haemoglobin solutions
* Perfluorocarbons.

Haemoglobin Solutions

Haemoglobin solutions are obtained from various sources:
- Human red cells (outdated blood units)
- Bovine red cells
  Haemoglobin solutions prepared from human and bovine sources carry the risk of transmission of infections.
- Transgenic animals: Haemoglobin gene is introduced into the embryo of animals like mice or pigs at an early stage of development. This leads to the synthesis of human haemoglobin in the transgenic animal.
- Recombinant DNA technique.

Disadvantages of Haemoglobin Solutions

- *Short survival in circulation*: Free haemoglobin molecules rapidly disintegrate into smaller fragments in circulation, which are then cleared by the kidneys. To increase the survival of haemoglobin in circulation, following modifications have been tried – 1. Intramolecular cross-linking of a haemoglobin molecule; 2. Intermolecular cross-linking of many haemoglobin molecules to form large polymers of haemoglobin; 3. Attaching haemoglobin to a polymer; and 4. Enclosure of haemoglobin molecule in a lipid membrane (encapsulated haemoglobin).
- *Kidney damage*: Haemoglobin solutions contaminated with red cell stroma or fragmented molecules of haemoglobin can induce disseminated intravascular coagulation and renal damage.
- *Vasoconstriction* with marked rise in blood pressure and reduction in cardiac output.
- *Increased oxygen affinity:* Once outside the red cell, haemoglobin loses its ability to bind 2,3-DPG with consequent increase in oxygen affinity. To decrease the oxygen affinity of free haemoglobin molecule, haemoglobin is treated with pyridoxal-5-phosphate.

Perfluorocarbons (PFCs)

These are organic molecules in which hydrogen atoms have been replaced by fluorine. They can dissolve large amount of oxygen molecules. Oxygen dissociation curve of PFCs is linear (not sigmoid like that of haemoglobin). They are emulsified before infusion since they are not miscible with water and blood.

They circulate in blood for only a short duration and are considered as a temporary red cell substitute. One indication is maintaining oxygenation of distal myocardium during balloon angioplasty.

❏ BIBLIOGRAPHY

1. Boral LI, Weiss ED, Henry JB. Transfusion Medicine. In Henry JB (Ed.): Clinical Diagnosis and Management by Laboratory Methods. 20th ed. Philadelphia. WB Saunders Compay. 2001
2. Lowe KC. Red cell substitutes. In Contreras M (Ed.): ABC of Transfusion. 3rd ed. London. BMJ Books. 1998.

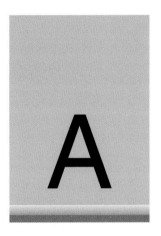

Reference Ranges

Reference ranges differ in different populations and also vary from laboratory to laboratory. Values obtained in an individual patient are best compared with the reference range established locally and interpreted in the context of clinical features and other investigations. Following reference values should be considered only as a rough guideline.

Haemoglobin:
- Adult males: 13.0–17.0 g/dl
- Adult females (nonpregnant): 12.0–15.0 g/dl
- Adult females (pregnant): 11.0–14.0 g/dl
- Children 6–12 years: 11.5–15.5 g/dl
- Children 6 months–6 years: 11.0–14.0 g/dl
- Infants 2–6 months: 9.5–14.0 g/dl
- Newborns: 13.6–19.6 g/dl

Packed cell volume:
- Adult males: 40–50%
- Adult females (nonpregnant): 38–45%
- Adult females (pregnant): 36–42%
- Children 6–12 years: 37–46%
- Children 6 months–6 years: 36–42%
- Infants 2–6 months: 32–42%
- Newborns: 44–60%

Red cell count:
- Adult males: 4.5–5.5 million/cmm
- Adult females: 3.8–4.8 million/cmm

Red cell indices:
- Mean cell volume (MCV): 80–100 fl
- Mean corpuscular haemoglobin (MCH): 27.0–32.0 pg
- Mean corpuscular haemoglobin concentration (MCHC): 32.0–36.0 g/dl

Reticulocyte count:
- Reticulocyte percentage: 0.5–2.5%
- Absolute reticulocyte count: 50,000–1,00,000/cmm

Relative proportions of haemoglobins:
- HbA: 95–97%
- HbA2: 1.5–3.5%
- HbF: <1%

Erythrocyte sedimentation rate (Westergren) (Upper limits):
- Adult males: 10 mm
- Adult females: 15 mm
- Children: 10 mm
- Elderly: Males—14 mm; females—20 mm

Osmotic fragility of red cells:
- Starts at 0.5% of sodium chloride or lower
- Complete at 0.3% of sodium chloride

Total leucocyte count (Adults): 4000–11000/cmm

Differential leucocyte count (Adults):
- Neutrophils: 40–75%
- Lymphocytes: 20–40%
- Monocytes: 2–10%
- Eosinophils: 1–6%
- Basophils: <1%

Neutrophil alkaline phosphatase (NAP) score: 40–100

Platelet count: 1,50,000–4,00,000/cmm

Iron studies:
- Serum iron: 50–150 µg/dl
- Total iron binding capacity (TIBC): 300–400 µg/dl
- Percent transferrin saturation: 20–55%
- Free erythrocyte protoporphyrin (FEP): < 80 µg/dl
- Serum transferrin receptor: 2.8–8.5 mg/L
- Serum ferritin: 15–300 µg/L

Vitamin B$_{12}$ and folate studies:
- Serum vitamin B$_{12}$: 150–700 ng/L
- Serum folate: 3–20 µg/L
- Red cell folate: 150–700 µg/L

Coagulation studies:
- Bleeding time (BT):
  - Ivy method: 2–7 minutes
  - Template method: 2.5–9.5 minutes
- Prothrombin time (PT): 11–16 seconds
- Activated partial thromboplastin time (APTT): 30–40 seconds
- Thrombin time (TT): ±3 seconds of control
- Plasma fibrinogen: 200–400 mg/dl
- Fibrinogen/fibrin degradation products (FDPs): <10 µg/ml
- D-dimer: <200 mg/L
- Factors II, V, VII, VIII, IX, X, XI, XII (per cent activity): 50–150%
- vWF:Ag: 50–150%

Differential count in bone marrow in adults:
- Myeloblasts: 0–3%
- Promyelocytes: 2–5%
- Neutrophil myelocytes: 8–15%
- Metamyelocytes: 9–24%
- Neutrophils (including band forms): 14–26%
- Erythroblasts: 15–36%
- Lymphocytes: 5–20%
- Plasma cells: 0–3%
- Myeloid:Erythroid (M:E) ratio: 2:1 to 4:1

Iron staining of bone marrow smears:
- Sideroblasts 30 to 50% of all erythroblasts
- No ringed sideroblasts

Biochemical studies:
- Serum bilirubin:
  - Total: <1.0 mg/dl
  - Direct: 0–0.2 mg/dl
- Total serum proteins: 6.0–8.0 g/dl
- Serum albumin: 3.5–5.0 g/dl
- Serum immunoglobulins:
  - IgG: 700–1500 mg/dl
  - IgA: 100–500 mg/dl
  - IgM: 50–250 mg/dl
- Serum creatinine: 0.5–1.2 mg/dl
- Serum lactate dehydrogenase: 200–450 IU/L
- Serum uric acid: 3.0–8.0 mg/dl
- Serum calcium (total): 9.0–11.0 mg/dl
- Serum β2 microglobuilin: 1.2–2.4 mg/L
- Serum haptoglobin: 0.8–2.7 g/L

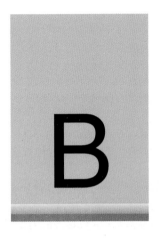

B   Selected CD Antigens

The CD (cluster of differentiation) antigen system is a nomenclature system for differentiation antigens on the surface of white blood cells and certain other cells. Each CD antigen is ascribed a number (CD1, CD2, etc.). A variety of monoclonal antibodies bearing different names are available commercially for identification of these antigens. Functions of some of these molecules are cell adhesion, signalling, cell protection, etc; while those of other molecules are unknown.

Applications of CD antigen analysis in haematology are summarised below:

- **Human immunodeficiency virus infection:** Enumeration of CD4+ and CD8+ cells (CD4/CD8 ratio)
- **Leukaemias and lymphomas:**
  - Classification and diagnosis of specific subtypes of leukaemias
  - Identification of prognostic groups
  - Assessment of clonality to distinguish a reactive from a neoplastic disorder
  - Monitoring of minimal residual disease (by identification of unique leukaemia phenotype on a cell amongst numerous normal cells)
  - To monitor effectiveness of monoclonal antibody therapy directed against antigens present on leukaemic cells (e.g. rituximab directed against CD20 antigen)
- **Haematopoietic stem cell transplantation:** Enumeration of CD34+ cells for evaluation of yield of stem cells in the harvest.
- **Paroxysmal nocturnal haemoglobinuria:** To detect deficiency of PIG transmembrane protein anchors CD59 or CD55.
- **Immunodeficiency disorders:** Enumeration of B and T lymphocytes

Methods for immunophenotyping: (1) Immunofluorescence, (2) Flow cytometry, and (3) Immunohistochemistry.

CD designation	Main reactivity	Comments
CD1a	Cortical thymocytes, Langerhans cells	Expressed on Langerhans cells in histiocytosis X
CD2	T lymphocytes	Pan T marker
CD3	T lymphocytes	Pan T marker; associated with T cell receptor
CD4	Helper inducer T lymphocytes	MHC class II receptor, HIV receptor
CD5	T lymphocytes, some B lymphocytes	Pan T marker; expressed by B-CLL cells
CD7	Pluripotent haematopoietic stem cells, T lymphocytes	Pan T marker; expressed by T-ALL and pluripotent stem cell leukaemias
CD8	Cytotoxic suppressor T lymphocytes	MHC class I antigen receptor
CD10	Precursor B lymphocytes	Expressed by pre B-ALL (CALLA) cells and follicular lymphoma cells
CD11c	Monocytes, granulocytes, activated T lymphocytes	Strongly expressed in hairy cell leukaemia
CD13	Myelomonocytic cells	Expressed in AML
CD14	Myelomonocytic cells	Expressed in AML
CD19	B lymphocytes	Pan B marker; Expressed on Precursor B ALL
CD20	B lymphocytes	Pan B marker
CD21	B lymphocytes and B precursors	Receptor for Epstein-Barr virus and C3d
CD22	B lymphocytes and B precursors	Pan B marker; Expressed in some B-ALL; Strongly expressed in hairy cell leukaemia
CD23	B lymphocyte subsets	Expressed on B-CLL cells
CD25	Activated B and T lymphocytes	Strongly expressed in hairy cell leukaemia
CD33	Myeloid precursors, monocytes	Expressed on AML blasts
CD34	Haematopoietic stem cells	
CD35	Granulocytes, monocytes	C3b receptor
CD36	Megakaryocytes, platelets, monocytes, macrophages	GpIIIb receptor
CD38	Plasma cells, Activated T and B cells	–
CD41	Megakaryocytes, platelets	GpIIb receptor
CD42b	Megakaryocytes, platelets	GpIb receptor

Contd...

Contd...

CD designation	Main reactivity	Comments
CD45	Leucocyte common antigen (LCA)	Present on almost all lymphoid cells
CD55	Multilineage	Decay accelerating factor; Absent on PNH cells
CD56	NK cells	Marker for NK cell neoplasms
CD59	Multilineage	Membrane inhibitor of reactive lysis (MIRL); Absent on PNH cells
CD61	Megakaryocytes, platelets	GpIIIa
CD64	Monocytes, macrophages	IgG receptor
CD71	Proliferating cells	Transferrin receptor
CD77	Activated B cells	Expressed in Burkitt lymphoma
CD79	B cells	Surface immunoglobulin receptor
CD103	–	Expressed in hairy cell leukaemia
CD117	Haematopoietic progenitor cells	C-kit; stem cell factor

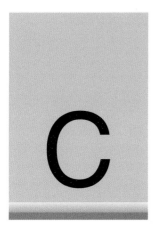

C

Critical Values in Haematology

Critical values (also called as action values or callback values) refer to the laboratory results that need to be notified urgently to the concerned clinician since they may be indicative of a critical or sometimes life-threatening condition of the patient and thus need for urgent clinical intervention. Haematological critical values are listed below.

Critical values in haematology	
Laboratory test result	**Interpretation/Risk**
1. Activated partial thromboplastin time ≥ 75 sec	Bleeding
2. D-dimer: Positive	Disseminated intravascular coagulation
3. Plasma fibrinogen < 100 mg/dl	Bleeding
4. Fibrin monomer: Positive	Disseminated intravascular coagulation
5. Haemoglobin < 7.0 g/dl	Myocardial ischaemia
6. Haemoglobin > 20 g/dl	Hyperviscosity syndrome
7. Total leucocyte count < 2000/cmm	Infection especially if absolute neutrophil count < 500/cmm
8. Total leucocyte count > 50,000/cmm	Leukaemoid reaction, leukaemia
9. Prothrombin time > 30 sec or > 3 times control	Bleeding
10. Platelet count < 20,000/cmm	Bleeding
11. Platelet count > 1 million/cmm	Thrombosis
12. Blood smear showing blast cells	Leukaemoid reaction, leukaemia
13. Blood smear showing sickle cells	Crises
14. Blood smear showing *Plasmodium falciparum* ring forms	Cerebral malaria
15. New diagnosis of aplastic anaemia	
16. New diagnosis of haematological malignancy	

Suggested Reading

❏ SECTION 1: PHYSIOLOGY OF BLOOD

1. Colman RW, Hirsh J, Marder VJ, Salzman EW (Eds). Hemostasis and thrombosis: Basic principles and clinical practice. Philadelphia: JB Lippincott Co. 1982.
2. Greer JP, Foerster J, Rodgers GM, Paraskevas F, Glader B, Arber DA, Means Jr RT (Eds): Wintrobe's clinical hematology. 12th ed. Philadelphia. Lippincott Williams & Wilkins. 2009.
3. Howard MR, Hamilton PJ. An Illustrated Colour Text. Haematology. 2nd ed. Edinburgh: Churchill Livingstone. 2002.
4. McPherson RA, Pincus MR (Eds): Henry's clinical diagnosis and management by laboratory methods. 21st ed. Philadelphia. Elsevier Saunders. 2007.
5. Stites DP, Terr AL, Parslow TG (Eds): Basic and Clinical Immunology. 8th ed. Connecticut: Appleton and Lange. 1994.
6. Swerdlow SH, Campo E, Harris NL, Jaffe ES, Pileri SA, Stein H, Thiele J, Vardiman JW (Eds): WHO classification of tumours of haematopoietic and lymphoid tissues. 4th ed. Lyon. International Agency for Research on Cancer. 2008.
7. Williams WJ, Beutler E, Erslev AJ, Lichtman MA (Eds). Hematology. 4th ed. New York: McGraw Hill Publishing Co. 1991.

❏ SECTION 2: DISORDERS OF RED BLOOD CELLS (ANAEMIAS)

1. Cheesbrough M. District Laboratory Practice in Tropical Countries. Part 2. Cambridge University Press. 2000.
2. Evatt BL, Gibbs WN, Lewis SM, McArthur JR, Fundamental diagnostic hematology. Anemia. 2nd ed. U.S. Department of Health and Human Services, Georgia, and World Health Organization, Switzerland, 1992.
3. Greer JP, Foerster J, RodgeRs GM, ParasKevas F, Glader B, Arber DA, Means Jr RT (Eds): Wintrobe's clinical hematology. 12th ed. Philadelphia. Lippincott Williams & Wilkins. 2009.
4. Hoffman R, Benz EJ, Shattil SJ, Furie B, Silberstein LE, McGlave P, Heslop H

5. Howard MR, Hamilton PJ. An illustrated colour text. Haematolgy. 2nd ed. Edinburgh: Churchill Livingstone. 2002.
6. Lewis SM, Bain BJ, Bates I (Eds). Dacie and Lewis Practical Haematology. 9th ed. London: Churchill Livingstone. 2001.
7. Provan D, Singer CRJ, Baglin T, Lilleyman J. Oxford Handbook of Clinical Haematology. 2nd ed. Oxford University Press. 2004.
8. Williams WJ, Beutler E, Erslev AJ, Lichtman MA (Eds). Hematology. 4th ed. New York: McGraw Hill Publishing Co. 1991.

❑ SECTION 3: DISORDERS OF WHITE BLOOD CELLS

1. Greer JP, Foerster J, Rodgers GM, Paraskevas F, Glader B, Arber DA, Means Jr RT (Eds): Wintrobe's clinical hematology. 12th ed. Philadelphia. Lippincott Williams & Wilkins. 2009.
2. Howard MR, Hamilton PJ. An Illustrated Colour Text. Haematolgy. 2nd ed. Edinburgh: Churchill Livingstone. 2002.
3. Lewis SM, Bain BJ, Bates I (Eds). Dacie and Lewis Practical Haematology. 9th ed. London: Churchill Livingstone. 2001.
4. Provan D, Singer CRJ, Baglin T, Lilleyman J: Oxford Handbook of Clinical Haematology. 2nd ed. Oxford University Press. 2004.
5. Swerdlow SH, Campo E, Harris NL, Jaffe ES, Pileri SA, Stein H, Thiele J, Vardiman JW (Eds): WHO classification of tumours of haematopoietic and lymphoid tissues. 4th ed. Lyon. International Agency for Research on Cancer. 2008.
6. Williams WJ, Beutler E, Erslev AJ, Lichtman MA (Eds). Hematology. 4th ed. New York: McGraw Hill Publishing Co. 1991.

❑ SECTION 4: DISORDERS OF HAEMOSTASIS

1. Colman RW, Hirsh J, Marder VJ, Salzman EW (Eds). Hemostasis and Thrombosis: Basic Principles and Clinical Practice. Philadelphia: JB Lippincott Co. 1982.
2. Greer JP, Foerster J, RodgeRs GM, ParasKevas F, Glader B, Arber DA, Means Jr RT (Eds): Wintrobe's clinical hematology. 12th ed. Philadelphia. Lippincott Williams & Wilkins. 2009.
3. Howard MR, Hamilton PJ. An illustrated colour text. Haematolgy. Second ed. Edinburgh: Churchill Livingstone. 2002.
4. Lewis SM, Bain BJ, Bates I (Eds). Dacie and Lewis Practical Haematology. 9th ed. London: Churchill Livingstone. 2001.
5. Provan D, Singer CRJ, Baglin T, Lilleyman J. Oxford Handbook of Clinical Haematology. Second ed. Oxford University Press. 2004.
6. Thomson JM (Ed). Blood Coagulation and Haemostasis. A Practical Guide. 3rd ed. Edinburgh: Churchill Livingstone. 1985.
7. Williams WJ, Beutler E, Erslev AJ, Lichtman MA (Eds). Hematology. 4th ed. New York: McGraw Hill Publishing Co. 1991.

6. Thomson JM (Ed). Blood Coagulation and Haemostasis. A Practical Guide. 3rd ed. Edinburgh: Churchill Livingstone. 1985.

7. Williams WJ, Beutler E, Erslev AJ, Lichtman MA (Eds). Hematology. 4th ed. New York: McGraw Hill Publishing Co. 1991.

❑ SECTION 5: BLOOD TRANSFUSION

1. Borker A, Warrier RP. Current practices in transfusion medicine. Indian Pediatrics. 2001;38: 227-30.

2. Brecher ME (Ed): Technical manual. American Association of Blood Banks. 15th ed. American Association of Blood Banks. Bethesda Maryland. 2005.

3. Cheesbrough M. District laboratory practice in tropical countries. Part 2. Cambridge University Press. 2000.

4. Contreras M (Ed). ABC of transfusion. 3rd ed. London: BMJ Books. 1998.

5. Mollison PL, Engelfriet CP, Contreras M. Blood transfusion in clinical medicine. 9th ed. London: Blackwell Scientific Publications. 1993.

6. Ness PM. Transfusion medicine: An overview and update. Clin Chem 2000;46: 1270-76.

7. Regan F, Taylor C. Recent developments. Blood transfusion medicine. BMJ 2003;325: 143-47.

8. Saran RK, Makroo RN. Transfusion medicine technical manual. Directorate General of Health Services. 1991.

9. World Health Organization. Blood Transfusion Safety: The clinical use of blood. Geneva. World Health Organization. 2002.

10. World Health Organization: Safe blood and blood products. Module 1. Safe blood donation. Geneva. World Health Organization. 2009.

11. World Health Organization: Safe blood and blood products. Module 2. Screening for HIV and other infectious agents. Geneva. World Health Organization. 2009.

12. World Health Organization: Safe blood and blood products. Module 3. Blood group serology. Geneva. World Health Organization. 2009.

Index

Page numbers followed by *f* refer to figure and *t* refer to table